# The Role of Fats in Human Nutrition

# The Role of Fats in Human Nutrition

*Edited by*

A. J. VERGROESEN

*Unilever Research, Vlaardingen/Duiven, Vlaardingen, The Netherlands*

1975

ACADEMIC PRESS

LONDON
NEW YORK
SAN FRANCISCO

A Subsidiary of Harcourt Brace Jovanovich, Publishers

ACADEMIC PRESS INC. (LONDON) LTD.
24/28 Oval Road,
London NW1

*United States Edition published by*
ACADEMIC PRESS INC.
111 Fifth Avenue
New York, New York 10003



Library of Congress Catalog Card Number 7418505
ISBN: 0-12-718050-8



Text set in 11/12 pt. Monotype Baskerville, printed by letterpress, and bound in Great Britain at The Pitman Press, Bath

# Contributors

G. S. BOYD *Department of Biochemistry, Edinburgh University Medical School, Edinburgh, Scotland*

J. J. GOTTENBOS *Unilever Research, Vlaardingen, The Netherlands*

D. M. HEGSTED *Department of Nutrition, Harvard School of Public Health, Boston, Massachusetts, U.S.A.*

S. HEYDEN *Department of Community Health Sciences, Duke University Medical Center, Durham, North Carolina, U.S.A.*

G. HORNSTRA *Unilever Research, Vlaardingen, The Netherlands*

A. J. HOUTSMULLER *Erasmus University, Rotterdam, The Netherlands*

U. M. T. HOUTSMULLER *Unilever Research, Vlaardingen, The Netherlands*

F. C. JAGER *Unilever Research, Vlaardingen. The Netherlands*

R. B. McGANDY *Department of Nutrition, Harvard School of Public Health, Boston, Massachusetts, U.S.A.*

K. SICKINGER *Krankenhaus Waldshut, Waldshut, Germany*

A. J. VERGROESEN *Unilever Research, Vlaardingen, The Netherlands*

R. O. VLES *Unilever Research, Vlaardingen, The Netherlands*

# Preface

This book reviews the present knowledge of the physiological and pathological effects of dietary lipids on the development and treatment of such common diseases as atherosclerosis, diabetes mellitus, obesity, fat malabsorption and arterial thrombosis. It also discusses the consequences of possible vitamin E deficiency, the normal regulation of cholesterol absorption and the pathophysiological effects of long-chain monoenoic fatty acids with more than 20 C-atoms in human nutrition. Where possible, the practical implications of these effects for human nutrition are given, but without detailed dietary prescriptions, as these have to be adapted to the different food habits and living conditions of various population groups.

The varied academic background of the authors includes biochemistry, veterinary medicine, biology, epidemiology and various specialities of human medicine: their selection was based on their active involvement in both research and clinical treatment. Although each has tried to give a fair presentation of the results and conclusions of many other investigators studying the role of fats in nutrition, it has been impossible to cover all fields of lipid metabolism; those areas of research where the practical consequences for human nutrition cannot yet be evaluated are not discussed extensively.

This volume has been written mainly for readers interested in the optimal fat composition of human diet; a reasonable background knowledge of physiology and biochemistry is presupposed. Each chapter can be read independently of the others. Some subjects have been discussed by more than one author and may thus have received different emphasis or interpretation because of a different approach to the problem. The subject index will facilitate a comparison of the various views.

A. J. VERGROESEN *June 1975*

# Contents

## 7 Specific Biological Effects of Polyunsaturated Fatty Acids
U. M. T. HOUTSMULLER



## 8 Cholesterol Absorption
G. S. BOYD



## 9 Linoleic Acid Intake and Vitamin E Requirement
F. C. JAGER

## 10 Nutritional Aspects of Rapeseed Oil

R. O. VLES

# 1 The Role of Fats in Human Nutrition: An Introduction

A. J. VERGROESEN and J. J. GOTTENBOS

*Unilever Research, Vlaardingen, The Netherlands*



It is many years since dietary fat was considered to be merely a useful and concentrated source of energy and a carrier of the fat soluble vitamins A, D, E and K. The vital importance of the essential fatty acids (EFA) to both man and animals, and the various effects of dietary fats on the metabolism of cholesterol and atherosclerosis and its complications are now generally recognized. This new insight has promoted many research activities in other, related fields, leading to a better understanding of fat metabolism. In this book, which sets out to show the very different approaches to the study of the role of fats, the more recent developments in fat nutrition are discussed. This chapter introduces the various subjects dealt with more specifically in subsequent chapters, and attempts to bridge the gaps between contributions. It also gives the results of some recent investigations in areas which could not be fully covered by other contributors, and has two Appendixes covering, firstly, diet and coronary heart disease (a joint statement by several American scientific societies) and secondly, the recommendations of the Netherlands Nutrition Council on the amount and nature of fats in the diet.

## I. LIPID–CARBOHYDRATE INTERACTION

We are now gradually realizing that fat as a source of energy cannot simply be replaced by carbohydrates without affecting, for example, liver metabolism to a great extent. A. J. Houtsmuller in Chapter 5 discusses why such a dietary change, which is frequently advocated to reduce saturated fat intake as a useful measure in the prevention of atherosclerosis, can be much less innocuous than is generally accepted. In the light of our present knowledge it is probable that in an appreciable percentage of the world population a high carbohydrate intake, especially in combination with an overconsumption of calories, may lead to a gradual induction of diabetes mellitus. Although it is known that most diabetics do not die from diabetes *per se*, but from the cardiovascular complications of a severe and generalized form of atherosclerosis which they normally develop, this knowledge has not yet led to intensive research into the relationship between these two disease entities. However, sufficient information is already available for a critical revaluation of whether the above-mentioned "simple" dietary modification really is advisable.

In diabetic adults and in juvenile diabetics, during periods of inadequate control, abnormal serum lipid compositions are commonly observed (Chance *et al.*, 1969a); it is now recognized that this hyperlipidaemia is associated with atheromatous lesions which tend to appear at an early age and which progress rapidly. Thus prevention of hyperlipidaemia is an important consideration in diabetes, particularly in children. The investigation by A. J. Houtsmuller (see Chapter 5) on the influence of various diets on diurnal levels of plasma glucose, plasma insulin and plasma lipids in obese and insulin-independent diabetic patients merits special attention. The disappointing results of Lloyd (1966) and of Chance *et al.* (1969b) obtained during long-term treatment of diabetic children given corn oil diets can be fully explained by the poor dietary adherence when the children reached adolescence. Nowadays, modern food industry in some countries can provide fully acceptable alternative products with the proper fatty acid composition, making it unnecessary to confine consumption to those pure oils which have a limited acceptability for reasons of palatability and local cooking habits.

## II. ESSENTIAL FATTY ACIDS

Our present preoccupation with the prevention and treatment of atherosclerosis, obesity and diabetes mellitus—diseases which have reached epidemic proportions in the more prosperous part of the world population—should not completely distract our attention from the serious nutritional problems in most of the developing countries. Normally the solution to these problems is sought in an increase in total caloric intake and especially in protein intake, without sufficient attention being given to an adequate fat intake. The elaborate research done since the discovery of the essential fatty acids (EFA) by Burr and Burr (1929) has demonstrated beyond any doubt that many, if not all, animal species will develop EFA-deficiency symptoms when raised on fat-free diets. For recent reviews see Holman (1971) and Söderhjelm *et al.* (1971). Paulsrud *et al.* (1972) recently showed that infants, given for various reasons intravenous fat-free alimentation, develop perceptible depletion of EFA reserves after only 5–10 days. One child, maintained for 4–5 months on such a regimen, reached in the serum phospholipids a ratio of the 20:3 (*n*-9) to 20:4 (*n*-6) fatty acids of 18 (instead of less than 1). Severe dermal lesions developed and, what is probably even more important, there was an increased susceptibility to infections. The implications of these findings in the large-scale treatment of children with kwashiorkor or with marasmus are evident and may explain why the present therapeutic approach, in which for instance, skim-milk powder is used to supplement locally available carbohydrate sources is far from optimal as both are extremely low in EFA content. In the more prosperous countries the syndrome of EFA deficiency is a rare phenomenon, except in cases of chronic fat malabsorption or diets of abnormal composition and even these exceptions can readily be corrected by the addition of a little linoleic acid to the diet, if necessary by parenteral nutrition. However, Kingsbury *et al.* (1969, 1974) have observed in an unexpectedly high percentage of patients with peripheral vascular disease a definite increase in the 20:3 (*n*-9) to 20:4 (*n*-6) fatty acid ratio of their plasma cholesteryl ester, one of the classical signs of EFA deficiency, although these patients apparently consumed a normal English diet. This interesting observation leads one to question why this condition develops. The possibility that some people have a greater need of EFA, whether genetically based or secondarily acquired as a result of abnormalities in their carbohydrate metabolism, which most of them clearly demonstrate, merits further investigation. Besides, it cannot be excluded that some dietary lipid components can increase the EFA requirement. Due to the lack of sufficient experimental data nothing more definitive can be said for the time being.

In addition, the question which fatty acids are the most efficient in combatting EFA deficiency has not yet been fully answered. U. M. T. Houtsmuller discusses some aspects of the differentiation in the biological activity of polyunsaturated fatty acids in Chapter 7, using the following symptoms of EFA deficiency as the main criteria: decreased body weight, increased skin permeability to water, increased spontaneous swelling of liver mitochondria *in vitro* and the altered fatty acid pattern of liver mitochondria. Depending on the various criteria, different amounts of linoleic acid are required to cure or prevent a specific symptom. To complicate the situation it appears that many, but not all, polyunsaturated fatty acids can replace linoleic acid for the correction of growth rate and swelling of liver mitochondria, but only a few fatty acids can restore the increased skin permeability to normal. The uncertainties remaining after the elaborate studies by Thomasson (1962) of the relation between the chemical structure of polyunsaturated fatty acids and their EFA activity can now be better understood.

Our understanding of the subject as a whole, however, does not yet enable us to draw up a full list of EFA-deficiency symptoms. Especially intriguing is the proposition put forward by Sinclair (1956) that atherosclerosis might perhaps be a special form of EFA deficiency. In our opinion this may be an acceptable proposition, but much larger amounts of EFA would be needed to cure this disease than are normally used for prevention of other more classical manifestations.

## III. ATHEROSCLEROSIS AND BLOOD LIPID LEVELS

The epidemiology of atherosclerosis is reviewed by Heyden in Chapter 2. Although not usually diagnosed before the age of 40, the onset of this disease occurs in infancy and childhood. Therefore, in recent papers (Kannel and Dawber, 1972; Fredrickson, 1972; De Haas, 1973) the necessity is underlined for a reorientation in the prevention of cardiovascular diseases by giving priority to children instead of adults. Both from epidemiological evidence and from direct nutritional experiments on animals and man, it is generally concluded that blood lipid concentrations—especially that of cholesterol—are closely related to the development of atherosclerotic vascular lesions and, moreover, that the type of dietary fat can influence the degree of atherosclerosis and the frequency of its complications. The results of the epidemiological investigations and the nutritional experiments on man are discussed in the contribution of McGandy and Hegsted (Chapter 4). Long-term (up to 10 years) experiments with rabbits invariably proved the correlation between blood cholesterol levels and degree of atherosclerosis and showed that the type of fat does indeed influence the atherosclerotic process and the frequency of its complications. Dietary fats rich in saturated fatty acids and poor in linoleic acid induce a higher degree of atherosclerosis than fats rich in linoleic acid and poor in saturated fatty acids (Gottenbos and Thomasson, 1961; Vles *et al.*, 1964; Vles *et al.*, to be published). The histological picture in the rabbit bears a striking resemblance to that in man. Actually, the similarity with human atherosclerosis becomes greater, the longer the duration of the animal experiments. Similar experiments with rabbits and other animal species (monkeys, pigs, chickens and pigeons) have been carried out by other investigators. They are reviewed and discussed by Constantinides (1965), Roberts and Strauss (1965), Wissler and Vesselinovitch (1968), Malmros (1969), Kritchevsky (1969), Eggen *et al.* (1969), Portman (1970) and many others. In many experiments it was found that the degree of atherosclerosis was correlated with a sustained elevation of serum cholesterol and appeared to be dependent on the type of dietary fat; and as Wissler and Vesselinovitch concluded:

> "No species appears to be immune to the development of atheromatous change if it is subjected to a sustained elevation of its blood lipids, especially the cholesterol-rich, low density lipoproteins, for several months."

However, it has still not definitely been proved that the level of the blood lipids is the primary factor in atherogenesis, as the atherosclerotic syndrome is the result of the interaction of a number of factors acting on the arterial endothelium and the intima. These factors are partly derived from the blood and partly caused by changes in the arterial wall (Adams, 1970; Haust, 1970). With respect to the blood factors a distinction can be made between normal blood constituents, e.g. lipoproteins and thrombocytes, and abnormal substances also transported by the blood, e.g. carbon monoxide and nicotine. The influence of blood cholesterol concentration on the development of atherosclerosis is related to the varying permeability of the arterial wall to lipoproteins, of which mainly the $\beta$-fraction is responsible for the cholesterol transport. The secondary and also the primary hyperlipoproteinaemias (with the exception of the rare essential hyperchylomicronaemia type I according to Fredrickson's classification) are held responsible for the occurrence of the atherosclerotic lesions, especially at those places where the arterial wall is damaged in some way [chemically by e.g. carbon monoxide (Astrup, 1972), or mechanically as in hypertension, local platelet thrombi], possibly in combination with local vessel-wall factors such as an abnormal mucopolysaccharide structure of the intimal layer. Genetic factors strongly determine the degree of either hypercholesterolaemia or hypertriglyceridaemia, and their mixed forms, which an individual will develop on a given diet: type II and type IV, Glueck *et al.* (1973) and Fredrickson and Levy (1972).

A continuous debate is still going on in respect to the levels which should be considered pathological. This discussion is confused by several factors.

1. The lack of standardization of laboratory techniques for the measurement of, say, plasma cholesterol, may easily result in variations of 25% or more, even in one and the same laboratory.
2. The lack of standardization of the diet consumed in the period preceding the analysis. Triglyceride levels are strongly influenced, even within 24–48 hours, by hypo- or hypercaloric diets, alcohol consumption, degree of control of chemical or manifest diabetes mellitus. Cholesterol levels can vary in an individual by about 20%, depending on the fatty acid composition and the cholesterol concentration of the diet in the preceding 10–14 days' period (see Chapter 4).
3. So-called "seasonal" variations which can sometimes induce 8–10% fluctuations in plasma cholesterol concentration and which are largely unexplainable.
4. Age. The newborn has a low cholesterol concentration of less than 80 mg/100 ml plasma (2·1 mmol/l). This level will rise rapidly in a few weeks to about 100 mg/100 ml plasma (2·6 mmol/l). Mexican school children between 5–9 and 10–14 years still have a mean blood cholesterol level of 100 mg/100 ml, but school children in Wisconsin (USA) in the same age groups have by then reached 186 mg/100 ml (Golubjatnikov *et al.*, 1972). It is important to note here that the majority of the world population of all age groups maintain a blood cholesterol level of less than 150 mg/100 ml, while only those population groups which are characterized by plenty, or even an excess, of food, lack of physical exercise, low incidence of acute or chronic infectious diseases, abnormal smoking and drinking habits, etc., demonstrate the "normal" age-dependent rise of plasma cholesterol levels to a mean adult level of about 230–240 mg/100 ml. It can confidently be said that most, if not all, of the adults living under prosperous conditions have too high a

blood lipid concentration, this being supported by the fact that on autopsy a moderate-to-severe degree of atherosclerosis is nearly always found, also in individuals dying from causes other than cardiovascular diseases. However, independent of age, in all larger-scale population studies about 30% of the subjects have a genetically determined higher plasma cholesterol level. An interesting study has been published by Weis and Wilcox (1972), who followed a group of 86 children from infancy to early adulthood and found that about 35% of this group constantly had significantly increased cholesterol levels. Apparently, blood lipid patterns are already established early in life by social and nutritional habits; preventive measures should therefore be taken as early as possible. Another subgroup of the population—those with familial-type II hyperlipoproteinaemia (Fredrickson's classification)—can also be recognized to have this condition independent of age and, in fact, it has been diagnosed in about 1% of 1800 consecutive unselected live births in a general hospital (Glueck and Tsang, 1972). Early recognition of this condition is important, as the disease may be fatal even in childhood if left untreated, whereas blood cholesterol levels can be normalized—probably, with a consequent increase in life expectancy—to a large extent by dietary measures (Kwiterovich *et al.*, 1970).

Summarizing the above-mentioned data, it seems that independent of age three subgroups based on blood-cholesterol levels, can be recognized in the general population:

a. a majority of about 70% who, given unfavourable living conditions, will demonstrate a moderate, age-dependent rise in plasma cholesterol levels up to a maximum of 240 mg/100 ml (6·2 mmol/l) as adults, constituting only a moderate risk factor for the development of cardiovascular disease. In the absence of other risk factors, e.g. hypertension and smoking, the symptoms will not manifest themselves before 60 years of age;
b. an important minority (probably heterozygous for the gene(s) responsible for the abnormality in their cholesterol metabolism) of about 30%, who—if left untreated—as adults will have plasma cholesterol levels of more than 240 mg/100 ml (6·2 mmol/l), which forms a serious risk factor leading to a very high incidence of coronary heart disease, manifesting itself prematurely at middle age;
c. an epidemiologically unimportant, but easily recognizable

group of less than 1 %, apparently homozygous for this gene, who will develop extremely high cholesterol levels if left untreated. Their abnormal cholesterol metabolism is difficult to control, but most of them will also respond favourably to dietary modification. To what extent this will affect their high death rate due to severe atherosclerosis at ages as young as 10 years is still unknown, but a beneficial effect may be expected.

Although hypertriglyceridaemia [triglyceride levels in fasting blood of over 150 mg/100 ml plasma (1·7 mmol/l)] is very common in the adult population of the prosperous countries of the world, this abnormality is seldom recognized in children and adolescents. This is not only because for technical and economic reasons, triglyceride levels are, not normally measured in population surveys, but also because in those studies where these levels have been measured a much lower incidence was found in children than in adults. The underlying abnormality apparently manifests itself much more slowly than the abnormal cholesterol metabolism forming the basis for hypercholesterolaemia. For further information the reader is referred to the chapters by Boyd (Chapter 8) and A. J. Houtsmuller (Chapter 5).

5. Diseases. For reasons largely unknown there are many acute or chronic diseases which can quite seriously influence blood lipid levels and if not recognized can lead to wrong conclusions. Viral diseases, especially those accompanied by diarrhoea, can lower plasma cholesterol levels by up to 50 % for an undefined period (probably for weeks). The early stages of maturity-onset diabetes are accompanied by hypertriglyceridaemia, which might even be considered an early symptom of this disease. Neoplastic diseases can reduce blood cholesterol levels, so obscuring a preceding period of hypercholesterolaemia. The same holds for ischaemic heart disease which is normally characterized by strong fluctuations in plasma cholesterol level in the period preceding the myocardial infarct and which is followed by a period of many weeks during which plasma cholesterol levels are abnormally low for the particular patient.

The efficacy of diets to lower blood lipids is discussed by McGandy and Hegsted in Chapter 4. For many dietary changes a satisfactory prediction of the serum cholesterol level in man can be made by the use of one of the equations developed by Hegsted *et al.* (1965), or by Keys *et al.* (1965).

However, it should be realized that these equations are of limited value and are applicable only to the dietary compositions which were actually studied. The generally accepted interpretation of the formula, namely, that a reduction in saturated fatty acids is twice as effective as the same increase in polyunsaturated fatty acids, seems simple and therefore attractive. The actual situation is, however, much more complex. In the first place, the various saturated fatty acids have different quantitative effects on blood cholesterol levels—lauric (12:0), myristic (14:0) and palmitic acid (16:0) probably being the most effective—and the saturated fatty acids with less than 12 carbon atoms being comparable to oleic acid (Vergroesen, 1972; Keys *et al.*, 1965; Hegsted *et al.*, 1965; Hegsted *et al.*, 1968).

Furthermore, in these equations no attention is paid to the *trans*-isomers of the natural *cis*-oleic acid (18 : 1, *n*-9 *cis*) which may be present in partially hydrogenated oils such as soyabean, cottonseed and olive oil in a relatively high percentage (theoretically up to 60% of total fatty acids).*

The influence of elaidic acid (18 : 1, *n*-9 *trans*) on blood lipid concentration is a complicated one as can be seen from the results of two experiments performed with the collaboration of Trappist nuns and monks who were given a liquid-formula diet (LFD) as the main source of food. A preliminary report on these experiments has been published (Vergroesen 1972).

The composition of diets A and B and the number of volunteers in each dietary group are given in Table 1A and 1B. From the results given in Fig. 1A it may be concluded that, under these conditions, elaidic acid in the presence—but not in the absence—of dietary cholesterol (one egg yolk per day = about 250 mg cholesterol) has a serum-cholesterol-increasing effect in comparison with oleic acid and even in comparison with palmitic acid. The course of experiment 1A was not flawless—for unknown reasons the initial serum cholesterol levels fluctuated more than normally, causing rather large variations in these concentrations at the start of the actual experiment. These results explain the apparent discrepancies in the results of Anderson *et al.* (1961), who described significant rises in blood lipid concentrations caused by

* Partial hydrogenation of vegetable oils with a high percentage of unsaturated fatty acids is a common procedure for changing product properties. As special analysis to differentiate between the *cis* and *trans* configuration of the double bonds is seldom made, the use of these oils in nutritional experiments may lead to wrong conclusions. Milk fat of ruminants also contains about 8% *trans* fatty acids due to transformation of part of the dietary unsaturated fatty acids by the bacteria of the rumen, unless this is prevented by special techniques to encapsulate the dietary fat (Nestel *et al.*, 1973).

Table 1A

Fatty acid composition (%) of the experimental fats used in Diets A

| Fatty acids | Diet | | |
|---|---|---|---|
| | A1 (high 18:1 *cis*) | A2 (high 18:1 *trans*) | A3 (high 16:0) |
| 12:0 | — | — | 0·3 |
| 14:0 | — | — | 1·2 |
| 16:0 | 11·3 | 10·9 | 43·4 |
| 18:0 | 2·6 | 3·2 | 5·3 |
| 20:0 | 0·5 | 0·6 | 0·6 |
| 16:1 *c* | 0·8 | 0·4 | 0·4 |
| *t* | | 0·4 | |
| 16:2 *c* | 0·2 | — | — |
| *t* | | 0·2 | |
| 18:1 *c* | 73·5 | 37·4 | 38·4 |
| *t* | — | 35·4 | — |
| 20:1 *c* | 0·4 | 0·3 | — |
| *t* | — | 0·2 | — |
| 18:2 *c*, *c* | 9·9 | 9·2 | 10·2 |
| *c*, *c* or *t*, *t* | — | 1·3 | — |

Composition of diet A is given as a liquid-formula diet (LFD) with 38% dietary energy provided by a fat having one of the fatty acid compositions mentioned in the table. Furthermore, the LFDs contained 21·5% dietary energy from milk proteins, 39·5% dietary energy provided by carbohydrates (of which about 85% simple sugars, such as lactose and maltodextrose) and 1% fat from sources such as dried skim milk powder and carbohydrates.

In addition to the cholesterol-free LFD, 9 out of 18 volunteers from group A1, 9 out of 18 from A2 and 9 out of 17 from A3 consumed one egg per day to provide about 250 mg cholesterol per day.

elaidic acid present in a "typical" American, cholesterol-rich diet, and those of Iongh *et al.* (1965) and of McOsker *et al.* (1962), who concluded that elaidic acid administered in combination with diets very low in cholesterol, or with cholesterol-free diets, had, respectively, only a very slight or no influence on serum cholesterol concentrations. From the results given in Fig. 1B it again appears that the influence of about 14 cal% elaidic acid on serum total cholesterol is like that of a saturated fatty acid and, in fact, is only slightly less active than a mixture of lauric and myristic acid consumed in equal amounts. Moreover, this

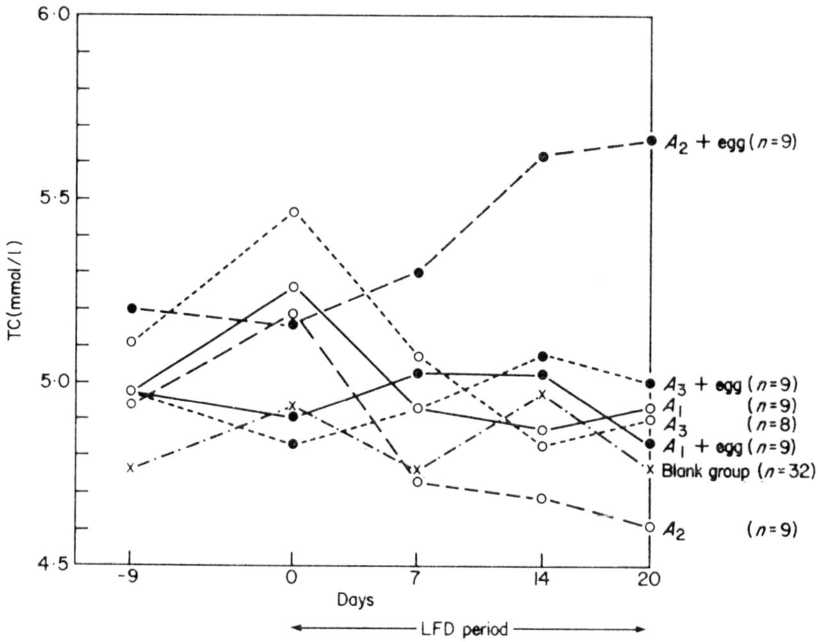


Fig. 1A. Average serum total cholesterol values (TC) of the 6 Liquid-formula diet (LFD) groups (Table 1A) during the 20-day LFD-period and the preceding 9-day period (base-line). From 32 volunteers living in the same monastery but not participating in the LFD experiment, fasting-blood samples were also taken on the days indicated. In this blank group, for unknown reasons, systematical ($p < 0{\cdot}10$) differences in the subsequent TC values occurred. None of the different diets induced systematic differences in TC level, but diet A2 (35·4% *trans* isomers of oleic acid) in the presence of dietary cholesterol caused, after 20 days, a difference in TC value with the A1 diet (olive oil) which is systematical (confidence level > 90%).

experiment shows that variations in polyunsaturated fatty acids cannot always be related to blood lipid concentrations; increasing the linoleic acid concentration in the liquid-formula diet containing 40 cal% fat (including 115 mg cholesterol/1000 kcal) from 10 to 34% (or, expressed differently, from 4 to 14 cal%) at the expense of oleic acid, did decrease the effect of 37% of a mixture of lauric and myristic acid (the main saturated fatty acids of the notoriously atherogenic coconut oil) on serum cholesterol concentration, but not the effect of 34% elaidic acid or of 36% oleic acid (the main fatty acids of hydrogenated soyabean oil and olive oil respectively). The pathophysiological consequences of these data are difficult to analyse, as we found that although serum total cholesterol concentration was not changed by an increase in the amount of linoleic acid in the diet, the fatty acid composition of the esterified

Table 1B

Fatty acid composition (%) of experimental fats used in Diets B

| Fatty acids | Diet | | | | | | Reference (safflowerseed) oil |
|---|---|---|---|---|---|---|---|
| | B1 | | B2 | | B3 | | |
| | low | high | low | high | low | high | |
| 12:0 | 27 | 27 | — | — | — | — | — |
| 14:0 | 10 | 10 | — | — | — | — | — |
| 16:0 + 18:0 | 12 | 12 | 13 | 12 | 14 | 13 | 10 |
| 18:1 *c* | 41 | 18 | 78 | 54 | 41 | 18 | 14 |
| 18:1 *t* | | | | | 35 | 35 | |
| 18:2 *c, c* | 10 | 34 | 10 | 34 | 10 | 34 | 76 |

Composition of diet B is given as a liquid-formula diet with 40% dietary energy provided by a fat of one of the fatty acid composition mentioned in the table, about 3% fat from other dietary components, 19% proteins (of which 90% milk proteins) and 38% carbohydrates (of which 60% simple sugars such as lactose, glucose and sacharose). Dried egg yolk was added to obtain an LFD containing 115 mg cholesterol per 1000 kcal (4·184 mJ). Average daily LFD consumption was about 1900 kcal (7·949 mJ). As reference diet a cholesterol-free LFD with 40% dietary energy provided from safflowerseed oil was used. For further technical details see Vergroesen and De Boer (1971).

cholesterol fraction (about 70% of total cholesterol) was definitely influenced by an increased linoleic acid content, as the cholesteryl oleate concentration decreased in both groups with increasing dietary linoleic acid concentration (Table 2).

It has been long recognized that atherosclerosis is characterized by a great accumulation of lipids, mainly cholesteryl esters, in the intima of the arterial wall. Smith and Slater (1972) concluded that the major part of the cholesteryl esters in the advanced atherosclerotic lesion originates directly from plasma lipoprotein and that only a small proportion accumulates as a result of local esterification of cholesterol. Comparison of the fatty acid composition of the cholesteryl esters in the athero-sclerotic lesion with that of plasma shows interesting differences. In experimental animals the lesion invariably shows a higher proportion of cholesteryl oleate and a lower proportion of cholesteryl linoleate than plasma. Similar results have been found in human studies, especially on comparison of fatty streaks with plasma. The cholesteryl ester composi-

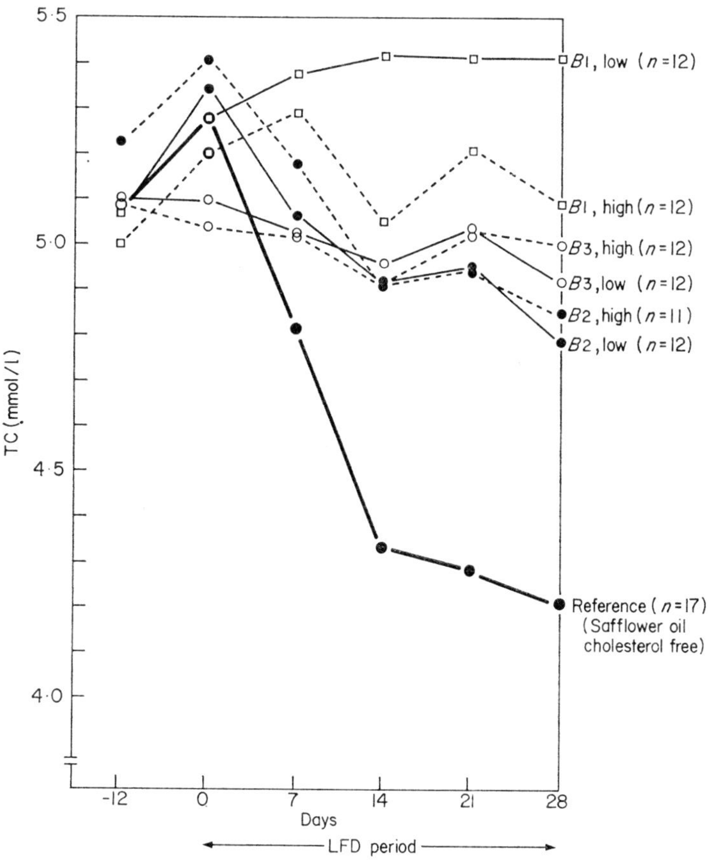


Fig. 1B. Course of the average serum TC levels during the 28-day LFD period and the preceding 12 days (base-line). The composition of the LFDs is described in Table 1B.

tion of human plaques has greater similarity to that of plasma. It has been suggested by Zilversmit and Newman (1966) that the compositional changes in the intima lipids during atherogenesis probably break down the metabolic or structural barrier to the entry of plasma lipoprotein which is present in the normal intima and which protects the arterial wall. The increased permeability of the arterial wall results in a greater deposition of plasma lipids. The greater entry of plasma lipoprotein will dilute the characteristic fatty acid pattern of the cholesteryl esters in the fatty streak which explains the greater similarity in cholesteryl ester fatty acid composition between advanced lesions and plasma.

These findings regarding the relationship between plasma cholesterol

Table 2

Average fatty acid compositions (% ± standard error) of serum cholesteryl esters after feeding the LFDs B2 (low and high 18:2) and B3 (low and high 18:2) for 28 days

| Fatty acids | Dietary fat: B2 low | B2 high | B3 low | B3 high |
|---|---|---|---|---|
| | 18:1 *cis* 78%<br>18:2 *cis,cis* 10% | 18:1 *cis* 54%<br>18:2 *cis,cis* 34% | 18:1 *trans* 35%<br>18:1 *cis* 41%<br>18:2 *cis,cis* 10% | 18:1 *trans* 35%<br>18:1 *cis* 18%<br>18:2 *cis,cis* 34% |
| 12:0 | 0·30 ± 0·11 | 0·41 ± 0·20 | 0·13 ± 0·07 | 0·30 ± 0·16 |
| 14:0 | 1·56 ± 0·19 | 0·81 ± 0·23 | 0·67 ± 0·13 | 1·24 ± 0·29 |
| 16:0 | 10·04 ± 0·87 | 11·46 ± 0·48 | 10·85 ± 0·39 | 10·72 ± 0·60 |
| 16:1 | 3·23 ± 0·28 | 2·86 ± 0·29 | 4·17 ± 0·27 | 3·14 ± 0·30 |
| 18:0 | 1·59 ± 0·17 | 1·41 ± 0·23 | 1·85 ± 0·32 | 1·43 ± 0·28 |
| 18:1 | 26·52 ± 0·42 | 18·33 ± 0·91 | 22·76 ± 0·45 | 13·89 ± 0·67 |
| 18:2 | 46·03 ± 1·42 | 58·63 ± 1·38 | 52·31 ± 1·01 | 61·39 ± 1·42 |
| 18:3 | 0·76 ± 0·12 | 0·33 ± 0·10 | 1·11 ± 0·25 | 0·73 ± 0·24 |
| 20:3 | 0·43 ± 0·11 | 0·09 ± 0·05 | 0·19 ± 0·09 | 0·30 ± 0·26 |
| 20:4 | 5·15 ± 0·36 | 3·78 ± 0·37 | 3·24 ± 0·29 | 3·87 ± 0·31 |

($n$ = 12, except B3 low: $n$ = 11.) For further information see Table 1B and Fig. 1B.

levels and degree of atherosclerosis suggest that elevated serum cholesterol levels cause the accumulation of cholesteryl esters in the arterial wall so resulting in atherosclerosis. The nature of the dietary fat influences the degree of atherosclerosis as well as the amount and composition of the plasma cholesteryl esters. The question arises whether only the total amount of cholesteryl esters circulating in the blood is important or whether composition of the cholesteryl esters also plays a role. In other words: whether individual plasma cholesteryl esters differ in atherogenic properties.

A low serum cholesterol level, induced by dietary fat, normally means a high proportion of linoleic acid and a low proportion of oleic acid in the serum cholesteryl esters, and vice versa: a high serum cholesterol level, induced by dietary fat, leading to atherosclerosis means a low proportion of linoleic acid and a high proportion of oleic acid in the serum cholesteryl esters in man (Thomasson *et al.*, 1967) and in experimental animals (Gottenbos and Thomasson, 1961; Moore, 1969). Such experiments do not answer the question whether the individual plasma cholesteryl esters differ in atherogenic properties.

A difference in atherogenic properties of individual cholesteryl esters can be caused by:

1. differential entry of plasma esters into the arterial wall or differential removal of the esters from the intima which will influence the total amount of cholesteryl esters in the lesion;
2. differential influence of the cholesteryl esters on the nature and/or severity of the atherosclerotic lesion. They may, for instance, determine the character of the local tissue reactions, which lead to a further progression of the lesion.

A combination of these mechanisms is, of course, also possible.

Differential entry of plasma cholesteryl esters into the progressing lesions seems unlikely if it is assumed that whole plasma lipoprotein enters the intima. No information is available about a differential efflux of cholesteryl esters from atherosclerotic lesions. If it is accepted that the fatty streak progresses to fibrous plaque and complicated lesion it can be postulated that cholesteryl oleate is the most atherogenic cholesteryl ester because it is the most abundant cholesteryl ester present in the early stage of the fatty lesion (Smith, 1965). However, the only experimental indication that the accumulated cholesteryl esters might differ in their influence on the nature of the progression of the atherosclerotic lesion is provided by the often quoted experiment of Abdulla *et al.* (1967). These workers studied the relative sclerogenic properties of cholesterol and its esters by assaying the tissue reactions after subcutaneous injection in the abdominal wall of rats. They found that these lipids could be ranked in the order (most $\rightarrow$ least sclerogenic) as follows: cholesteryl oleate $>$ free cholesterol $>$ cholesteryl palmitate $=$ cholesteryl linoleate $>$ cholesteryl arachidonate. If the extrapolation of these results to the connective tissues of the arterial wall is justified, it could then be concluded that the more polyunsaturated cholesteryl esters are less atherogenic and would cause less damage than cholesteryl oleate. Further research will be needed in order to test the validity of the hypothesis that the individual cholesteryl esters differ in atherogenic properties. Gottenbos (1974) discussed this subject and described an animal-experimental model which makes it possible to determine the atherogenic effect of individual cholesteryl esters.

If the differences between individual cholesteryl esters in atherogenic properties are found to be great, not only the total plasma cholesterol level but also the composition of the cholesteryl esters should be used as criteria for measuring the risk of atherosclerosis. It can be expected that in that case a high proportion of linoleic acid and a low proportion of oleic acid will be preferable. Vergroesen *et al.* (1970) showed that in order to induce the lowest possible plasma cholesterol level in man, a diet rich in fat containing a high percentage of linoleic acid acts much more favourably than a low-fat diet. Diets rich in linoleic acid also will induce a high proportion of linoleic acid and a low proportion of oleic acid in the plasma cholesteryl ester fatty acids. A low-fat diet not only will induce higher blood lipid levels than a diet rich in linoleic acid but also—due to the conversion of excess carbohydrates into oleic and palmitic acid—to an unfavourable cholesteryl ester fatty acid composition. Long-term experiments with rabbits (Gottenbos and Thomasson, 1961; Vles *et al.*, 1964) demonstrated that carbohydrate-rich diets are more atherogenic than diets high in linoleic acid which supports the above-mentioned concept.

Surprisingly little research has been done on the repair processes in the atherosclerotic areas. Adams (1970) and Zilversmit (1970) believe that an increased phospholipid synthesis in the atheromatous plaques might serve to dissolve the local cholesterol deposits. According to Adams, polyunsaturated lecithine in the blood and artery wall may play an important role as a substrate for plasma lecithin–cholesterol acyltransferase (LCAT) or a corresponding enzyme in the vascular tissue, leading to a transfer of linoleic acid from lecithin to cholesteryl linoleate which is subsequently mobilized. According to this hypothesis at least a partial cure of the atheromatous lesions can be expected due to the removal of the atherogenic factor, cholesterol. The recently published findings of Armstrong and Megan (1972) in monkeys, of Clarkson *et al.* (1973) in pigeons, and the older observations of Vles *et al.* (1964) in rabbits, support the concept that even serious atheromatous lesions can indeed regress to a less active and fatal stage.

To return to the discussion on the relative value of diets which lower blood lipids it is important to realize that in man the sum of the percentages of cholesteryl oleate and cholesteryl linoleate is fairly constant at between 70 and 80 % of total esterified cholesterol. As shown in Table 2, the increase of linoleic acid concentration in the diets containing elaidic acid clearly reduced the (atherogenic) cholesteryl oleate fraction and increased cholesteryl linoleate. These data suggest that, if the cholesteryl ester hypothesis is valid, a decreased atherogenic tendency caused by the increased linoleic acid concentration in the diet can be induced, although this is not always accompanied by a decrease in serum total cholesterol concentration.

From the results in Fig. 1B it follows that the same applies to oleic acid, as, again, an increase of linoleic acid from 4 to 14 cal % did not influence the serum total cholesterol concentration. Another example of experimental conditions in which predictive equations such as those of Keys or Hegsted do not hold has been found in one of our previous experiments (Vergroesen and De Boer, 1970; Vergroesen, 1972). In this study we observed that even extremely large amounts of linoleic acid—up to 95 % linoleic acid in a cholesterol-free liquid-formula diet containing 50 cal % fat—do not induce a greater reduction in blood cholesterol concentration than the 20–25 % reduction already obtainable with 35 cal % safflower oil containing 75 % linoleic acid and 10 % palmitic acid. In fact, the same 20–25 % reduction in blood cholesterol was observed in a group of about 100 adolescents consuming a "normal" Dutch diet (35–45 cal % fat and a daily intake of 200–500 mg cholesterol) in which margarine with 50–55 % linoleic acid and about 25 % saturated fatty acids, sunflowerseed oil for shallow and deep frying and a filled milk (3·5 % safflowerseed oil in skimmed milk) were substituted for butter, lard and milk with 3·5 % butter fat. During the period of high linoleic acid intake the children consumed daily 20–25 cal % of linoleic acid, which was apparently sufficient to compensate for the blood lipid increasing effect of about 10 cal % saturated fatty acids and dietary cholesterol. These results are in agreement with the conclusions drawn by Brown (1971) from her own, Keys' and Hegsted's dietary studies, which predicted that the maximum effect of linoleic acid on serum total cholesterol levels will manifest itself at 17 cal % given a daily intake below 500 mg cholesterol. Apparently, a rather narrow range exists (between 10–16 cal %) in which the effect of linoleic acid on serum cholesterol concentration changes from minimal to maximal.

To conclude this discussion of the effects of different fatty acid compositions on blood lipid concentrations we should like to stress the point that not only the cholesterol fraction, but also serum phospholipids and triglycerides, react in a similar qualitative way as the cholesteryl esters to dietary fat modifications. Quantitatively, the phospholipid concentration is less influenced (maximal about 15 % reduction is possible) than cholesterol, while triglyceride concentrations react more pronouncedly (a reduction of more than 50 % is obtainable—see, for instance, Vergroesen and De Boer, 1971). Even now, it is still not yet clear what roles phospholipid and/or triglyceride concentrations play in atherogenesis, although the type of atherosclerosis observed in hypertriglyceridaemic patients (types IV and V according to Fredrickson's classification) and in diabetics, which is predominantly localized in the smaller, peripheral arteries of the legs and eyes, for example, suggests a specific effect of raised triglyceride levels, possibly in relation to abnormal insulin concentrations (see Chapter 5).

## IV. ARTERIAL THROMBOSIS

The favourable influence of diets high in linoleic acid and low in saturated fat on the prevention or inhibition of atherosclerotic disease is commonly explained by their effect of lowering blood cholesterol. It seems reasonable to expect that prevention of the "normal" increase in blood lipoprotein levels with age, especially when combined with prevention of a rise in arterial blood pressure, will result in a real primary prevention of atherosclerosis if started sufficiently early in life. Nevertheless, we must still accept that most, if not all, adults living in the developed (prosperous) countries in which moderate-to-serious atherosclerosis is already prevalent, will respond only to a limited extent to dietary modifications, with only a partial regression of existing lesions. At the sites of these lesions, intra-arterial thrombotic processes will, in any case, play their secondary roles in the morbidity due to atherosclerosis by the formation of rapidly growing arterial platelet thrombi, thus occluding an already partially obturated artery. Furthermore, circulating blood platelets are thought to play an important part in the pathogenesis of atherosclerosis because they form small mural thrombi at sites of endothelial damage. Transformation of these thrombi into atheromatous tissue has been reported, but deviations in lipid composition between platelets, fresh mural thrombi and athermatous lesions strongly suggest that an additional metabolic mechanism is involved. In the formation of mural thrombi the tendency of the blood platelets to adhere to subendothelial tissue, to release prothrombotic material, and to aggregate is of primary importance. As is reviewed by Hornstra in Chapter 6, the type of dietary fat definitely influences the arterial thrombotic process, possibly by its effect on platelet aggregation: saturated fats enhance thrombus formation, whereas polyunsaturated fatty acids clearly diminish it. Results from clinical centres such as Sophia Children Hospital, Rotterdam, The Netherlands (Fernandez *et al.*, to be published), and the Atherosclerosis Research Group, Saint Vincents Hospital, Montclair, N.J., USA (Fleischman *et al.*, 1973) strongly suggest that platelet aggregation in hyperlipidaemic children, diabetics and postmyocardial infarction patients, will gradually decrease after diets high in linoleic acid have been substituted.

How this favourable effect of linoleic acid can be explained is still open to discussion. One possibility is a change in the fatty acid composition of the cellular membranes of endothelium and/or platelets, resulting in decreased thrombotic properties of these tissues. Furthermore, the diets high in linoleic acid will change the fatty acid composition of adipose tissue, which, in turn, will influence the types of fatty acids released into the blood under, for instance, the influence of high catecholamine concentrations. Hoak *et al.* (1970) have demonstrated *in vitro* that albumin-bound linoleic acid enhances platelet aggregation much less effectively than, for instance, albumin-bound oleic and palmitic acid. Another explanation might be sought in the possibility of an increased biosynthesis of prostaglandin $E_1$ ($PGE_1$), a very potent inhibitor of platelet adhesion and aggregation. In nearly all tissues $PGE_1$ can be synthesized in response to a nervous or hormonal stimulation of the organ from dihomo-$\gamma$-linolenic acid (20:3 *n*-6, 9, 12), an intermediate* fatty acid formed during the conversion of linoleic acid (18:2 *n*-6, 9) into arachidonic acid (20:4 *n*-6, 9, 12, 15). Both 20:3 *n*-6, 9, 12 and 20:4 *n*-6, 9, 12, 15 are present in the phospholipids of cell membranes and, after release by phospholipase $A_2$, can be converted by PG-synthetase into $PGE_1$ and $PGE_2$ respectively. $PGE_2$ does not inhibit platelet aggregation but has, in fact, a slightly stimulating effect. Since the feeding of increasing amounts of linoleic acid does not result in increasing concentrations of arachidonic acid in cell membranes, it is possible that the observed increased urinary excretion of PG metabolites resulting from diets high in linoleic acid (Van Stratum *et al.*, to be published), is indicative of a stimulated $PGE_1$ biosynthesis from 20:3 *n*-6, 9, 12 (Thomasson, 1969). However, because of analytical problems no quantitative relationship between the amounts of dietary linoleic acid and $PGE_1$ biosynthesis *in vivo* have so far been measured. Apart from the inhibiting effect of $PGE_1$ on platelet aggregation and adhesion, $PGE_1$ and $PGE_2$ have hypotensive effects, antagonize the hypertensive properties of adrenaline and angiotensin, are potent inhibitors of catecholamine-induced free fatty acid release from adipose tissue, increase natriuresis, especially after its inhibition by, for instance, vasopressin, decrease the influence of both sympathetic and parasympathetic nerve stimulation on myocardial tissue (see for a recent review Ramwell, 1973) and finally appear to have, in most circumstances, a very potent antiarrhythmic and inotropic activity on the myocardium (Zijlstra *et al.*, 1972; De Boer *et al.*, 1973).

## V. VITAMIN E

Except in cases of chronic fat malabsorption (which are discussed by K. Sickinger in Chapter 3) the function of dietary fat as a carrier of the

* It should be realized that, in the biochemical sequence of linoleic acid to arachidonic acid, dihomo-$\gamma$-linolenic acid is not an intermediate in its true sense because acyl CoA-esters, rather than the free fatty acids, are the substrates for desaturation and chain elongation—the various acyl CoA-esters being mainly involved in the biosynthesis of different types of complex lipids, whence the free fatty acids are derived by enzymic hydrolysis.

fat-soluble vitamins A, D, E and K is seldom critical in human nutrition. We therefore considered it outside the scope of this book to deal, for instance, with hypervitaminosis A and D caused by the consumption of liver tissue from polar bears, etc., or with hypovitaminosis A, D and K as observed in patients with chronic fat malabsorption, as these subjects are clearly the field of the specialized physician.

Although both hyper- and hypovitaminosis E are almost unknown human disease entities, the role of vitamin E in human nutrition is reviewed by F. C. Jager in Chapter 9, as it is claimed that an increase in the consumption of linoleic acid and other polyunsaturated fatty acids needs to be accompanied by an increase in vitamin E to prevent the development of fatty acid peroxides, which some investigators believe to be associated with premature ageing of tissues and cancer. Most of these suggestions are based on experiments performed *in vitro* in the absence of the natural antioxydants and radical scavengers such as glutathion, vitamin C and E, or on analytical observations in dead tissue where the problem of differentiating between cause and result is obvious. It should be realized that most oils rich in linoleic acid are the natural sources of vitamin E, while animal fats such as butter, lard, fish oils and some vegetable oils as cocoa butter and coconut oil have marginal vitamin E contents. In fact, it is impossible to induce vitamin E deficiency in any animal species without the prior "stripping" of the oils to remove the vitamin E. As explained by Jager, there is no reason to suppose that under normal conditions an increased intake of polyunsaturated oils will ever lead to unfavourable side effects *in vivo*. The many life-span or long-term studies on mice (Vles and Gottenbos, 1972a), rats (Alfin-Slater *et al.*, 1957, 1970, 1973; Vles and Gottenbos, 1972b), rabbits (Vles *et al.*, to be published), and man (Ederer *et al.*, 1972) did not reveal any increase in cancer frequency due to diets high in linoleic acid.

## VI. MISCELLANEOUS EFFECTS

The foregoing is not meant to suggest that the ingestion of natural or processed oils and fats never can lead to pathological changes. As already discussed, a high intake of the saturated fatty acids lauric, myristic, palmitic, and possibly also stearic acid will cause in many people an increase in lipoprotein levels in blood, especially of low density (beta) lipoprotein, with a concurrent increased risk of developing atherosclerosis. The nutritional aspects of heated and oxidized fats are receiving much attention, for shallow frying and continuous or intermittent deep frying of oils and fats is common practice in households, restaurants and industrial food processing. Extensive reviews of the many biological investigations in various species of animals fed heated and oxidized oils over prolonged periods are available. The most up-to-date ones are those of Artman (1969), Nolen (1972), Lang (1973), and Potteau (1973). Artman concludes that "there is ample evidence to show that used frying fats are harmless when consumed at realistic dietary levels, even over long periods of time." Potteau comes to the same conclusion, but recommends a proper choice of oils and fats (with a low content of fatty acids with three or more double bonds), a thermostatic control of the frying temperature ($<200°C$) and the regular discarding of used oils.

As mentioned before, the hydrogenation of edible oils is a common technological procedure for changing product properties. This practice should be limited to those cases where it is absolutely necessary, as it in any case results in a severe loss of linolenic and, more important, linoleic acids, which, as previously stated, are essential to human nutrition. The biological action of hardened oils in general and of the *cis/trans* isomers of oleic acid in particular have been extensively investigated and reviewed by Gottenbos and Thomasson (1965), Alfin-Slater *et al.* (1957, 1970), and Le Breton and Lemarchal (1969). These studies showed no adverse effects from feeding *trans* fatty acids or hydrogenated oils. To what extent the formed *cis–trans* and *trans–trans* isomers of linoleic acid might be responsible for specific effects under extreme conditions has not, as yet, been well-studied due to technological problems in the preparation of sufficient quantities needed to perform long-term studies. In practice this problem can be neglected for the time being as in the above-mentioned long-term or life-span studies with mice, rats and rabbits by Vles and Gottenbos (1972a and b) and Vles *et al.* (to be published) three differently hydrogenated soyabean oils were fed in high concentrations to the animals without any detectable macroscopic or microscopic change which could be attributed to the different oils. The only exception was formed by the most extreme hydrogenated soyabean oil, characterized by about 60% *trans* fatty acids and less than 1% linoleic acid (18:2 *n*-6, 9 *cis*, *cis*), which, as was to be expected, was responsible for a severe degree of atherosclerosis in rabbits, including two lethal myocardial infarctions after more than five years' feeding and more micro-infarctions in the other animals of this group.

A really serious problem has been caused by the rapid increase, since 1960, in the cultivation of rapeseed—one of the cruciferae species. The production of rapeseed is stimulated, mainly for economical reasons, especially in Canada and northwestern and central Europe. The presence of thioglucosides in rapeseed meal limits its use as a source of protein in animal feed. The oil is mainly used for human consumption as table and frying oil, shortenings and margarine. Rapeseed oil, mustardseed oil

Table 3

Fatty acid composition of fats originating from aquatic animals (salt and fresh water)

| SOURCE | SATURATED FATTY ACIDS | | | | | | | | | | | | | | | MONOUNSATURATED | | | | | | | | |
|---|---|---|---|---|---|---|---|---|---|---|---|---|---|---|---|---|---|---|---|---|---|---|---|---|
| | 4 | 6 | 8 | 10 | 12 | 14 | 15 | 16 | 17 | 18 | 19 | 20 | 22 | 24 | total | 14:1 | 16:1 | 17:1 | 18:1 | 20:1 | 22:1 | 24:1 | 19:1 | total |
| SALT WATER[1)] | | | | | | | | | | | | | | | | | | | | | | | | |
| PERCH (OCEAN) | | | | | | 4.6 | 0.6 | 12.6 | 1.0 | 3.6 | 0.8 | | | 0.5 | 23.7 | | 8.0 | | 22.0 | 8.0 | 8.7 | | | 46.7 |
| HERRING (PACIFIC) | | | | | | 7.6 | 0.4 | 18.3 | 0.5 | 2.2 | | | | | 29.0 | | 8.3 | | 16.9 | 9.4 | 11.6 | 0.9 | | 47.1 |
| HERRING (MENHADEN) | | | | | | 8.0 | 0.5 | 28.9 | 1.0 | 4.0 | 0.9 | | | | 43.3 | | 7.9 | | 13.4 | 0.9 | 1.7 | 0.9 | | 24.8 |
| PILCHARD | | | | | 0.1 | 7.3 | 0.6 | 15.6 | 0.8 | 3.5 | 0.1 | 0.3 | 0.1 | 0.1 | 28.5 | | 9.0 | | 10.4 | 1.5 | 1.5 | 0.7 | | 23.1 |
| COD (ATLANTIC) | | | | | | 1.8 | 0.5 | 33.4 | 0.9 | 4.0 | | | | | 40.6 | | 2.4 | | 11.8 | 1.6 | 0.7 | | | 16.5 |
| COD LIVER OIL | | | | | | 2.8 | 0.4 | 10.7 | 1.2 | 3.7 | 0.6 | | | | 19.4 | | 6.9 | | 23.9 | 8.8 | 6.4 | 0.5 | | 46.5 |
| OYSTER (PACIFIC) | | | | | | 2.7 | 0.9 | 21.4 | 1.4 | 4.0 | | | | | 30.4 | | 4.6 | | 8.5 | | 2.6 | | | 15.7 |
| MUSSEL | | | | | | 1.9 | 0.7 | 23.0 | 0.8 | 5.3 | 0.4 | | | | 32.1 | | 2.0 | | 5.2 | 1.7 | 0.2 | | | 9.1 |
| FISH OIL (PERUVIAN) | | | | | 0.1 | 7.5 | 0.6 | 17.5 | 0.6 | 4.0 | 0.1 | 0.3 | | | 30.7 | | 9.0 | | 11.6 | 1.6 | 1.2 | | | 23.4 |
| " (PORTUGESE) | | | | | 0.1 | 6.7 | 0.8 | 17.8 | 0.8 | 3.6 | 0.4 | 0.4 | 0.2 | 0.1 | 30.9 | | 6.0 | 0.3 | 13.0 | 4.3 | 3.8 | 0.6 | | 27.4 |
| " (SOUTH AFRICAN) | | | | | 0.2 | 8.0 | 0.4 | 15.7 | 0.8 | 3.7 | 0.2 | 0.6 | 0.2 | 0.2 | 30.0 | 0.2 | 8.5 | | 9.2 | 2.5 | 3.1 | | | 23.5 |
| SALMON (YOUNG) | | | | | | 3.4 | 1.0 | 10.2 | 1.6 | 4.4 | 0.7 | | | | 21.3 | | 5.0 | | 17.6 | 4.0 | 5.3 | 1.1 | | 33.0 |
| WHALE | | | | | 0.2 | 7.7 | 0.7 | 13.4 | 1.0 | 2.7 | 0.6 | 0.2 | 0.1 | | 26.6 | 0.8 | 10.5 | 0.3 | 27.6 | 6.8 | 2.4 | 0.3 | | 48.7 |
| HERRING (ENGLISH) | | | | | 0.1 | 6.1 | 0.4 | 10.8 | 0.4 | 1.4 | 0.2 | 0.1 | 0.1 | 0.2 | 19.8 | 0.2 | 7.3 | 0.3 | 10.3 | 13.4 | 21.2 | 0.8 | 0.1 | 53.6 |
| FRESH WATER[2)] | | | | | | | | | | | | | | | | | | | | | | | | |
| EEL | | | | | | 5.9 | 0.6 | 14.0 | 0.7 | 1.4 | | | | | 22.6 | 1.6 | 12.4 | 1.1 | 27.8 | 28.3 | | | | 71.2 |
| TROUT | | | | | | 2.1 | 0.8 | 11.9 | 1.5 | 4.1 | | | | | 20.4 | | 8.2 | | 19.8 | 3.0 | 3.4 | 0.7 | | 35.1 |
| BURBOT | | | | | | 1.1 | | 21.1 | 0.8 | 5.4 | | | | | 28.4 | | 7.8 | 0.9 | 19.5 | 1.0 | 0.5 | 4.2 | | 33.9 |
| PIKE | | | | | | 4.6 | 0.7 | 15.7 | | 2.6 | | | | | 23.6 | 0.5 | 15.2 | 1.5 | 11.6 | 2.6 | 0.9 | | | 32.3 |
| PIKE-PERCH | | | | | | 7.1 | 1.6 | 26.4 | | 2.0 | | | | | 37.1 | 0.7 | 17.0 | 1.5 | 17.8 | 1.3 | 0.9 | | | 39.2 |
| STURGEON | | | | | | 2.1 | | 21.5 | 0.9 | 2.3 | | | | | 26.8 | | 7.3 | 1.2 | 49.1 | 3.3 | 0.7 | | | 61.6 |
| SALMON | | | | | | 15.1 | | 15.3 | 1.5 | 3.8 | | | | | 35.7 | | 5.6 | 0.9 | 27.2 | 8.0 | 10.5 | | | 52.2 |

| SOURCE | UNSATURATED FATTY ACIDS | | | | | | | | | | | | | | | |
|---|---|---|---|---|---|---|---|---|---|---|---|---|---|---|---|---|
| | DIUNSATURATED | | | | | TRIUNSATURATED | | | | | | HIGHER UNSATURATED | | | | | |
| | 16:2 | 18:2 | 20:2 | 22:2 | total | 16:3 | 18:3 | 20:3 | 22:3 | 24:3 | total | 16:4 | 18:4 | 20 | 22 | 24 | total |
| SALT WATER[1] | | | | | | | | | | | | | | | | | |
| PERCH (OCEAN) | 0.9 | 1.5 | | | 2.4 | | 0.6 | | | | 0.6 | | 1.6 | 10.1 | 13.0 | | 24.7 |
| HERRING (PACIFIC) | 1.0 | 1.6 | | | 2.6 | | 0.6 | | | | 0.6 | | 2.8 | 9.0 | 8.9 | | 20.7 |
| HERRING (MENHADEN) | 0.8 | 1.1 | 0.5 | | 2.4 | | 0.9 | | | | 0.9 | | 1.9 | 11.4 | 15.1 | | 28.4 |
| PILCHARD | 2.0 | 2.0 | 0.5 | 0.1 | 4.6 | 1.8 | 1.2 | 1.2 | 0.2 | | 4.4 | 2.8 | 2.8 | 19.3 | 12.0 | | 36.9 |
| COD (ATLANTIC) | 0.6 | 1.2 | | | 1.8 | | 0.8 | 0.4 | | | 1.2 | | 1.2 | 15.6 | 22.5 | | 39.3 |
| COD LIVER OIL | 1.0 | 1.5 | 0.5 | | 3.0 | | 0.9 | 0.1 | | | 1.0 | | 2.6 | 9.0 | 16.0 | | 27.6 |
| OYSTER (PACIFIC) | 1.6 | 1.2 | | | 2.8 | | 1.6 | | | | 1.6 | | 4.3 | 23.4 | 21.7 | | 49.4 |
| MUSSEL | 0.5 | 0.6 | 0.5 | | 1.6 | | 0.3 | | | | 0.3 | | 1.8 | 25.8 | 28.7 | 0.6 | 56.9 |
| FISH OIL (PERUVIAN) | 1.2 | 1.9 | 0.7 | 0.1 | 3.9 | 2.0 | 1.3 | 1.2 | 0.2 | | 4.7 | 2.5 | 3.2 | 17.8 | 11.0 | 0.5 | 35.0 |
| " (PORTUGESE) | 1.0 | 1.7 | 0.4 | 0.1 | 3.2 | 0.6 | 1.3 | 1.0 | 0.2 | | 3.1 | 1.7 | 3.3 | 12.2 | 15.0 | 0.6 | 32.8 |
| " (SOUTH AFRICAN) | 2.0 | 1.5 | 0.7 | | 4.2 | 2.0 | 1.2 | 1.7 | 0.2 | | 5.1 | 3.2 | 2.2 | 20.1 | 9.3 | 0.5 | 35.3 |
| SALMON (YOUNG) | 1.7 | 1.6 | 0.6 | | 3.9 | | 1.1 | 0.1 | | | 1.2 | | 2.9 | 14.2 | 22.6 | | 39.7 |
| WHALE | 0.9 | 2.2 | 0.3 | | 3.4 | 0.3 | 1.2 | 0.8 | 0.3 | | 2.6 | 1.0 | 1.3 | 6.3 | 8.3 | | 16.9 |
| HERRING (ENGLISH) | 0.6 | 1.0 | 0.2 | 0.2 | 2.0 | 0.7 | 2.0 | 0.4 | | | 3.1 | 1.3 | 3.3 | 8.2 | 7.8 | | 20.6 |
| FRESH WATER[2] | | | | | | | | | | | | | | | | | |
| EEL | | 1.0 | | | 1.0 | | | | | | | | | 1.3 | 1.2 | | 2.5 |
| TROUT | 1.2 | 4.6 | 0.6 | | 6.4 | | 5.2 | 0.4 | | | 5.6 | | 1.5 | 7.2 | 22.2 | | 30.9 |
| BURBOT | | 4.5 | | | 4.5 | | 1.2 | | | | 1.2 | | | 18.1 | 10.1 | | 28.2 |
| PIKE | | 7.6 | | | 7.6 | | 7.0 | | | | 7.0 | | | 15.7 | 14.4 | | 30.1 |
| PIKE-PERCH | | 3.0 | | | 3.0 | | 2.7 | | | | 2.7 | | | 8.3 | 13.3 | | 21.6 |
| STURGEON | | 1.3 | | | 1.3 | | 0.9 | | | | 0.9 | | | 5.0 | 2.6 | | 7.6 |
| SALMON | | 1.5 | | | 1.5 | | 0.9 | | | | 0.9 | | | 3.9 | 3.2 | | 7.1 |

1 Analyses by Gruger *et al.* (1964).
2 Reichwald and Meizies (1973).

Table 4

Fatty acid composition of fats originating from terrestrial animals

| SOURCE | | SATURATED FATTY ACIDS | | | | | | | | | | | | | | | MONOUNSATURATED | | | | | |
|---|---|---|---|---|---|---|---|---|---|---|---|---|---|---|---|---|---|---|---|---|---|---|
| | | 4 | 6 | 8 | 10 | 12 | 14 | 15 | 16 | 17 | 18 | 19 | 20 | 22 | 24 | total | 14:1 | 16:1 | 18:1 | 20:1 | 22:1 | 24:1 | total |
| GOOSE[1)] | | | | | | | 0.4 | | 20.8 | | 6.6 | | | | | 27.8 | 0.5 | 2.4 | 58.1 | | | | 61.0 |
| GOAT | | | | | | 3.5 | 2 | | 25.5 | | 28 | | | | | 59.0 | | | 38.5 | | | | 38.5 |
| TURKEY | | | | | | ——— | ——— | 25.3 | ——— | ——— | ——— | | | | | 25.3 | | | 38.5 | | | | 38.5 |
| CHICKEN | | | | | | | 0.5 | | 25 | | 4 | | | | | 29.5 | | 7 | 42 | | | | 49.0 |
| RABBIT | TAME | | | | | 1.5 | 4 | | 30 | | 5 | | | | | 40.5 | 1.5 | 6 | 34 | | | | 41.5 |
| | WILD | | | | | — | 1.5 | — | 22 | | 6 | | 1 | | | 30.5 | 1.5 | 4.5 | 13 | | | | 19.0 |
| MILK FAT | SUMMER | 3 | 1.5 | 1 | 2 | 3 | 9 | | 25 | | 8 | | 1 | | 1 | 54.5 | 1 | 3 | 39 | | | | 43.0 |
| | WINTER | 3.5 | 1.5 | 1.5 | 3 | 5 | 10 | | 26 | | 12 | | 1 | | 1 | 64.5 | 1.5 | 4 | 33 | | | | 38.5 |
| HORSE | SUMMER WINTER | | | | | | 4 | | 26 | | 5 | | | | | 35.0 | 1 | 7 | 34 | | | | 42.0 |
| 3 TALLOW | | | | | | | 3 | | 29 | | 20 | | 1 | | | 53.0 | 0.5 | 2 | 42 | | | | 44.5 |
| SHEEP | | | | | | 1 | 2 | | 24 | | 27 | | 1 | | | 55.0 | 0.5 | 1 | 39 | | | | 40.5 |
| PIG | | | | | | | 1 | | 28 | | 13.5 | | | | | 42.5 | | 3 | 46 | | | | 49.0 |
| 4 BUTTER | | 3 | 2 | 1.5 | 3 | 4 | 12.1 | 1.5 | 25.0 | 1.0 | 11.1 | | 1.3 | | | 65.5 | 2 | 2.6 | 26.1 | 0.1 | | | 30.8 |

| SOURCE | UNSATURATED FATTY ACIDS | | | | | | | | | | | | | | | | |
|---|---|---|---|---|---|---|---|---|---|---|---|---|---|---|---|---|---|
| | DIUNSATURATED | | | | | TRIUNSATURATED | | | | | | HIGHER UNSATURATED | | | | | |
| | 16:2 | 18:2 | 20:2 | 22:2 | total | 16:3 | 18:3 | 20:3 | 22:3 | 24:3 | total | 16:4 | 18:4 | 20 | 22 | 24 | total |
| GOOSE[1] | | 9.7 | | | 9.7 | | | | | | | | | | | | |
| GOAT | | | | | | | | | | | | | | 2.5 | | | 2.5 |
| TURKEY | | 23.3 | | | 23.3 | | | | | | | | | | | | |
| CHICKEN | | 21 | | | 21 | | | | | | | | | | | | |
| RABBIT TAME | | 14 | | | 14 | | 2.5 | | | | 2.5 | | | 1.5 | | | 1.5 |
| RABBIT WILD | | 8 | | | 8 | | 42 | | | | 42 | | | 1.5 | | | 1.5 |
| MILK FAT SUMMER | | 5 | | | 5 | | 0.5 | | | | 0.5 | | | 1 | | | 1 |
| MILK FAT WINTER | | 3 | | | 3 | | 0.5 | | | | 0.5 | | | | | | |
| HORSE SUMMER | | 5 | | | 5 | | 17 | | | | 17 | | | | | | |
| HORSE WINTER | | 20 | | | 20 | | 2 | | | | 2 | | | | | | |
| TALLOW | | 2 | | | 2 | | 0.5 | | | | 0.5 | | | | | | |
| SHEEP | | 4 | | | 4 | | | | | | | | | 0.5 | | | 0.5 |
| PIG | | 6 | | | 6 | | 0.5 | | | | 0.5 | | | 2 | | | 2 |
| [4] BUTTER | | 3.4[2] | | | 3.4 | | 2.0 | | | | 2.0 | | | | | | |

Analyses by Unilever Research, Vlaardingen, unless otherwise stated.

1 Brixius and Treiber (1974).

2 *cis-cis* Linoleic acid content 0·8% only.

3 Bovine.

4 Spring.

## Table 5

## Fatty acid composition of various vegetable fats

| SOURCE | SATURATED FATTY ACIDS | | | | | | | | | | | | | | | MONOUNSATURATED | | | | | | | | |
|---|---|---|---|---|---|---|---|---|---|---|---|---|---|---|---|---|---|---|---|---|---|---|---|---|
| | 4 | 6 | 8 | 10 | 12 | 14 | 15 | 16 | 17 | 18 | 19 | 20 | 22 | 24 | total | 14:1 | 16:1 | 17:1 | 18:1 | 19:1 | 20:1 | 22:1 | 24:1 | total |
| GROUNDNUT OIL | | | | | | | | | | | | | | | | | | | | | | | | |
| INDIA | | | | | | | | 10.5 | | 3 | | | | | 18.5[2)] | | | | 50 | | | | | 50.0 |
| ARGENTINA | | | | | | | | 11.0 | | 2.5 | | | | | 19.5[2)] | | 0.5 | | 35.5 | | | | | 36.0 |
| NIGERIA[1)] | | | | | | | | 9.5 | | 3.6 | | 1.5 | 2.6 | 1.4 | 18.6 | | 0.6 | | 55.5 | | 1.3 | 0.1 | | 57.5 |
| VIRGINIA<br>WEST AFRICA | | | | | | | | 7.0 | | 4 | | | | | 17.0[2)] | | 0.5 | | 62 | | | | | 62.5 |
| COCOA BUTTER | | | | | | | | 26 | | 33 | | 1.0 | | | 60 | | 0.5 | | 35 | | | | | 35.5 |
| COCONUT FAT | | 0.5 | 8 | 6.5 | 47 | 20 | | 9 | | 3 | | | | | 94 | | | | 7 | | | | | 7.0 |
| COTTONSEED OIL | | | | | | 1 | | 25 | | 3 | | 0.5 | | | 29.5 | | 1 | | 18 | | | | | 19.0 |
| LINSEED OIL | | | | | | | | 6.5 | | 4.5 | | | | | 11.0 | | | | 21 | | | | | 21.0 |
| MAIZE OIL | | | | | | | | 13 | | 2.5 | | | | | 15.5 | | | | 28 | | 0.5 | | | 28.5 |
| OLIVE OIL | | | | | | | | 13.5 | | 3 | | | | | 16.5 | | 1 | | 71 | | 0.5 | | | 72.5 |
| PALM OIL | | | | | | 1 | | 45 | | 5 | | 0.5 | | | 51.5 | | 0.5 | | 38 | | | | | 38.5 |
| PALM KERNEL OIL | | | 3 | 3.5 | 47 | 16 | | 9 | | 2.5 | | | | | 81.0 | | | | 15 | | | | | 15.0 |
| RAPESEED OIL | | | | | | | | | | | | | | | | | | | | | | | | |
| EUROPE | | | | | | | | 4 | | 1 | | 0.7 | | | 5.7 | | 0.5 | | 14 | | 9 | 46 | | 69.5 |
| CANADA | | | | | | | | 3.5 | | 0.5 | | 0.5 | 0.5 | | 5.0 | | 0.5 | | 25 | | 11 | 31 | | 67.5 |
| CANBRA | | | | | | | | 4.5 | | 1.5 | | 0.5 | | | 6.5 | | 0.5 | | 55 | | 2 | 4 | | 61.5 |
| SAFFLOWERSEED OIL | | | | | | | | 7 | | 2.5 | | | | | 9.5 | | | | 14.5 | | | | | 14.5 |
| SESAME OIL | | | | | | 0.5 | | 9 | | 5 | | 0.5 | | | 15.0 | | 0.5 | | 40 | | 0.3 | | | 40.8 |
| SOYABEAN OIL | | | | | | 0.5 | | 11 | | 4.0 | | | | | 15.5 | | 0.1 | | 23 | | | | | 23.1 |
| SUNFLOWERSEED OIL | | | | | | | | 6.5 | | 4 | | 0.5 | 0.7 | | 11.7 | | | | 24 | | | | | 24.0 |

| SOURCE | UNSATURATED FATTY ACIDS | | | | | | | | | | | | | | | | |
|---|---|---|---|---|---|---|---|---|---|---|---|---|---|---|---|---|---|
| | DIUNSATURATED | | | | | TRIUNSATURATED | | | | | | HIGHER UNSATURATED | | | | | |
| | 16:2 | 18:2 | 20:2 | 22:2 | total | 16:3 | 18:3 | 20:3 | 22:3 | 24:3 | total | 16:4 | 18:4 | 20 | 22 | 24 | total |
| GROUNDNUT OIL | | | | | | | | | | | | | | | | | |
| INDIA | | 30 | | | 30 | | | | | | | | | | | | |
| ARGENTINA | | 43.5 | | | 43.5 | | | | | | | | | | | | |
| NIGERIA[1)] | | 23.0 | | | 23.0 | | | | | | | | | | | | |
| VIRGINIA | | 20 | | | 20 | | | | | | | | | | | | |
| WEST AFRICA | | | | | | | | | | | | | | | | | |
| COCOA BUTTER | | 4 | | | 4 | | | | | | | | | | | | |
| COCONUT FAT | | 2 | | | 2 | | | | | | | | | | | | |
| COTTONSEED OIL | | 51 | | | 51 | | 0.5 | | | | 0.5 | | | | | | |
| LINSEED OIL | | 14 | | | 14 | | 53 | | | | 53 | | | | | | |
| MAIZE OIL | | 55 | | | 55 | | 0.5 | | | | 0.5 | | | | | | |
| OLIVE OIL | | 10 | | | 10 | | 0.5 | | | | 0.5 | | | | | | |
| PALM OIL | | 10 | | | 10 | | | | | | | | | | | | |
| PALM KERNEL OIL | | 2.5 | | | 2.5 | | | | | | | | | | | | |
| RAPESEED OIL | | | | | | | | | | | | | | | | | |
| EUROPE | | 15 | | 0.5 | 15.5 | | 9 | | | | 9 | | | | | | |
| CANADA | | 17 | | 0.5 | 17.5 | | 10 | | | | 10 | | | | | | |
| CANBRA | | 20 | | | 20 | | 10 | | | | 10 | | | | | | |
| SAFFLOWERSEED OIL | | 75 | | | 75 | | | | | | | | | | | | |
| SESAME OIL | | 44 | | | 44 | | 0.5 | | | | 0.5 | | | | | | |
| SOYABEAN OIL | | 52 | | | 52 | | 8 | | | | 8 | | | | | | |
| SUNFLOWERSEED OIL | | 63 | | | 63 | | 0.5 | | | | 0.5 | | | | | | |

1 Analyses by Unilever Research, Vlaardingen, unless otherwise stated.
2 Comprising C20 and higher.

(mainly used in certain areas of India) and fish oil are characterized by the presence of very long chain fatty acids (more than 20 carbon atoms) which, as described by Vles in Chapter 10, are responsible for a series of undesirable biochemical and pathological changes in many tissues, including heart muscle, red muscle fibres, kidneys, liver, adrenals, etc., of all animal species so far studied. For obvious reasons, direct experiments on man are difficult to defend, but the few observations available strongly suggest that man is as sensitive in this respect as other animal species. As said before, rapeseed is an important crop in some countries and it is, therefore, a lucky development that the culture of rapeseed strains with a low to an almost zero content of these fatty acids is rapidly becoming feasible. This will be stimulated in near future as more countries are to follow the example of Sweden, Canada, The Netherlands and Italy where voluntary or officially imposed restrictions on the use of these oils in human food are accepted by the food industry. In the case of fish oil, there are no known possibilities of lowering the content of the same type of fatty acids. This is especially important in the case of hydrogenated fish oils, the only ones, that can be used for human consumption, as natural fish oil is notorious for the rapid development of rancid odours. For the time being over-fishing in the coastal waters of northwestern Europe and Peru, the main suppliers of fish oil as a by-product of the fish meal production for cattle fodder, has already reduced the amount of fish oil. Nevertheless, we consider it would be wise to revaluate in the near future the value of fish for direct human consumption. Although fish is an excellent source of protein, its initial efficiency in the breeding of animals for human consumption is only 10–30 %. The intake of oil per serving of fish is low, so that no potential danger to man exists, contrary to what occurs if the oils are first concentrated, hydrogenated and subsequently used for human food.

Finally, to facilitate the reading of the other chapters, in which the complete fatty acid composition and the cholesterol concentration of the relevant diets is not always specified, a summary of the available data on the more important fats and oils is given in Tables 3 to 5. This list can never act as a substitute for thorough chemical analysis, however, as many factors, including the average temperature during the cultivation of the oil-yielding plants, can greatly influence the fatty acid composition of the final products.

## REFERENCES

Abdulla, Y. H., Adams, C. W. M. and Morgan, R. S. (1967). The reaction of connective tissues to implantation of purified sterol, sterol esters, phosphoglycerides, glycerides and free fatty acids. *J. Pathol. Bacteriol.* **94**, 63–71.

Adams, C. W. M. (1970). Local factors in atherogenesis: an introduction. *In* "Atherosclerosis" (R. J. Jones ed.), pp. 28–34. Springer-Verlag Berlin, Heidelberg, New York.

Alfin-Slater, R. B., Wells, A. F., Aftergood, L. A. and Deuel, H. J. (1957). Nutritive value and safety of hydrogenated vegetable fats as evaluated by long-term feeding experiments with rats. *J. Nutr.* **63,** 241–261.

Alfin-Slater, R. B., Wells, P. and Aftergood, L. A. (1970). Longevity and multi-generation studies in rats fed hydrogenated fats of increasing polyunsaturated fat content. *J. Am. Oil Chem. Soc.* **47,** no. 7, Abstract 274.

Alfin-Slater, R. B., Wells, P., Aftergood, L. A. and Melnick, D. (1973). Dietary fat composition and tocopherol requirement: IV Safety of polyunsaturated fats. *J. Am. Oil Chem. Soc.* **50,** 479–484.

Anderson, J. T., Grande, F. and Keys, A. (1961). Hydrogenated fats in the diet and lipids in the serum of man. *J. Nutr.* **75,** 388–394.

Armstrong, M. L. and Megan, M. B. (1972). Lipid depletion in atheromatous coronary arteries in rhesus monkeys after regression diets. *Cir. Res.* **30,** 675–680.

Artman, N. R. (1969). The chemical and biological properties of heated and oxidized fats. *Adv. Lipid Res.* **7,** 245–330.

Astrup, P. (1972). Some physiological and pathological effects of moderate carbon monoxide exposure. *Brit. Med. J.* **4,** 447–452.

Brixius, L. and Treiber, H. (1974). *Fette Seifen, Anstrichmittel,* **76,** 83–86.

Brown, H. B. (1971). Food patterns that lower blood lipids in man. *J. Am. Diet Ass.* **58,** 303–311.

Burr, G. O. and Burr, M. M. (1929). A new deficiency disease produced by the rigid exclusion of fat from the diet. *J. Biol. Chem.* **82,** 345–367.

Chance, G. W., Albutt, E. C. and Edkins, S. M. (1969a). Serum lipids and lipoproteins in untreated diabetic children. *Lancet* **i,** 1126–1128.

Chance, G. W., Albutt, E. C. and Edkins, S. M. (1969b). Control of hyperlipidaemia in juvenile diabetes. Standard and corn-oil diets compared over a period of 10 years. *Brit. Med. J.* **3,** 616–618.

Clarkson, T. B., King, J. S., Lofland, H. B., Feldner, M. A. and Bullock, B. C. (1973). Pathologic characteristics and composition of diet-aggravated atherosclerotic plaques during "regression". *Exp. Mol. Pathol.* **19,** 267–283.

Constandinides, P. (1965). "Experimental Atherosclerosis." Elsevier, Amsterdam.

De Boer, J., Houtsmuller, U. M. T. and Vergroesen, A. J. (1973). Inotropic effects of prostaglandins, fatty acids and adenosine phosphates on hypodynamic frog hearts. *Prostaglandins,* **3,** 805–825.

De Haas, J. H. (1973). Primary prevention of coronary heart disease, a socio-pediatric problem. *Hart Bull.* **4,** 3–11.

De Iongh, H., Beerthuis, R. K., Hartog, C. den, Dalderup, L. M. and Spek, P. A. F. van der (1965). Biblth. "Nutr. Dieta", Fasc. 7, pp. 137–152.

Ederer, F., Leren, P., Turpeinen, O. and Frantz, I. D. Jr. (1971). Cancer among men on cholesterol-lowering diets. Experience from five clinical trials. *Lancet* **ii,** 203–206.

Eggen, D. A., Strong, J. P. and Newman, W. P. (1969). Experimental atherosclerosis in primates: A comparison of selected species. *Ann. N.Y. Acad. Sci.* **162,** 110–119.

Fleischman, A. I., Simpkins, H. and Bierenbaum, M. L. (1973). Beneficial effect of increased dietary linoleate upon in vivo platelet function in man. *Circulation* **48,** suppl. 4, p. 55.

Fredrickson, D. S. (1972). Introduction to symposium: Factors in childhood that influence the development of atherosclerosis and hypertension. *Amer. J. Clin. Nutr.* **25,** 221–223.

Fredrickson, D. S. and Levy, R. I. (1972). Familial hyperlipoproteinaemia. *In* "The Metabolic Basis of Inherited Disease" (ed. 3) (J. B. Stanbury, J. B. Wijngaarden and D. S. Fredrickson, eds.), pp. 545–614. McGraw-Hill, New York.

Glueck, C. J. and Tsang, R. C. (1972). Pediatric familial type II hyperlipoproteinemia: Effects of diet on plasma cholesterol in the first year of life. *Am. J. Clin. Nutr.* **25,** 224–230.

Glueck, C. J., Fallat, R., Buncher, C. R., Tsang, R. and Steiner, P. (1973). Familial combined hyperlipoproteinemia: Studies in 91 adults and 95 children from 33 kindreds. *Metab. Clin. Exp.* **22,** 1403–1428.

Golubjatnikov, R., Paskey, T. and Inhorn, S. L. (1972). Serum cholesterol levels of Mexican and Wisconsin schoolchildren. *Am. J. Epidemiol.* **96,** 36–39.

Gottenbos, J. J. and Thomasson, H. J. (1961). Aorta atheromatosis in rabbits on feeding cholesterol or fats. *Colloq. Int. Cent. Nat. Rech.* No. 99, 221–239.

Gottenbos, J. J. and Thomasson, H. J. (1965). The biological action of hardened oils. Biblth. "Nutr. Dieta", Fasc. 7, pp. 110–129.

Gottenbos, J. J. (1974). IFMA Symposium 1974 (to be published).

Gruger, E. H. Jr., Nelson, R. W. and Stansby, M. E. (1964). Oils from 21 species of fish. *J. Am. Chem. Soc.* **41,** 662–667.

Haust, M. D. (1970). Injury and repair in the pathogenesis of atherosclerotic lesions. *In* "Atherosclerosis" (R. J. Jones, ed), pp. 12–20. Springer-Verlag, Berlin, Heidelberg, New York.

Hegsted, D. M., McGandy, R. B., Myers, M. L. and Stare, F. J. (1965). Quantitative effects of dietary fat on serum cholesterol in man. *Amer. J. Clin. Nutr.* **17,** 281–295.

Hegsted, D. M., McGandy, R. B., Myers, M. L. and Stare, F. J. (1968). Effects of specific fatty acids on serum cholesterol in man: Studies with semisynthetic materials. *In* "Symposium Dairy Lipids and Lipid Metabolism, Chicago 1967". (M. F. Brink and D. Kritchevsky, eds).

Hoak, J. C., Spector, A. A., Fry, G. L. and Warner, E. D. (1970). Effect of free fatty acids on ADP-induced platelet aggregation. *Nature* **228,** 1330–1332

Holman, R. T. (1971). Essential fatty acid deficiency. *In* "Progress in the Chemistry of Fats and other Lipids" (R. T. Holman, ed.), Vol. IX, pp. 275–348. Pergamon Press, Oxford.

Kannel, W. B. and Dawber, T. R. (1972). Atherosclerose as a pediatric problem. *J. Pediat.* **80,** 544–554.

Keys, A., Anderson, J. T. and Grande, F. (1965). Serum cholesterol response to changes in the diet. IV Particular saturated fatty acids in the diet. *Metab. Clin. Exp.* **14,** 776–787.

Kingsbury, K. J., Morgan, D. M., Stovold, R. and Brett, C. G. (1969). The relationships between plasma cholesteryl polyunsaturated fatty acids, age and atherosclerosis. *Postgrad. Med. J.* **45,** 591–601.

Kingsbury, K. J., Brett, C., Stovold, R., Chapman, A., Anderson, J. and Morgan, D. H. (1974). Abnormal Fatty Acid Composition and Human Atherosclerosis. *Postgrad. Med. J.* **50,** 425–440

Kritchevsky, D. (1969). Experimental atherosclerosis in primates and other species. *Ann. N.Y. Acad. Sci.* **162,** 80–88.

Kritchevsky, P. O., Levy, R. I. and Fredrickson, D. S. (1970). Early detection and treatment of familial type II hyperlipoproteinemia. *Circulation* **42,** suppl. III, p. 11.

Kwiterovich, P. O., Levy, R. I. and Fredrickson, D. S. (1970). Early detection and treatment of familial type II hyperlipoproteinemia. *Circulation* **42,** suppl. III, p. 11.

Lang, K. K. (1973). Die physiologische Wirkungen erhitzter Fette, imbesondere der Frittierfette, *Fette Seifen, Anstrichmittel* **75,** 73–76.

Le Breton, E. et Lemarchal, P. (1969). Indérêt biochimique et biologique de l'acide elaïdique et des acides gras trans. *Cah. Nutr. Diet.* **4,** suppl. 2, 11–26.

Lloyd, J. K. (1966). Control of dietary fat in relation to diabetic complications in children. *Proc. Nutr. Soc.* **25,** 74–83.

McOsker, D. E., Mattson, F. H., Sweringer, H. B. and Kligman, A. M. (1962). The influence of partially hydrogenated dietary fats on serum cholesterol levels. *J. Am. Med. Ass.* **180,** 380–385.

Malmros, H. (1969). Dietary prevention of atherosclerosis. *Lancet* **ii,** 479–484.

Moore, J. H. (1969). The effect of diets containing different proportions of butterfat and maize oil on plasma lipids and aortic atherosis in rabbits. *Brit. J. Nutr.* **23,** 125–134.

Nestel, P. J., Havenstein, N., Whyte, H. M., Scott, T. J. and Cook, L. J. (1973). Lowering of plasma cholesterol and enhanced sterol excretion with the consumption of polyunsaturated ruminant fats. *New Engl. J. Med.* **288,** 379–382.

Nolen, G. A. (1972). Effects of fresh and used hydrogenated soybean oil on reproduction and leratology in rats. *J. Am. Oil Chem. Soc.* **49,** 688–693.

Paulsrud, J. R., Pensler, L., Whitten, C. F., Stewart, S. and Holman, R. T. (1972). Essential fatty acid deficiency in infants induced by fat-free intravenous feeding. *Am. J. Clin. Nutr.* **25,** 897–904.

Portman, O. W. (1970). Arterial composition and metabolism: Esterified fatty acids and cholesterol. *Adv. Lipid. Res.* **8,** 41–114.

Potteau, B. (1973), Huiles chauffées: IV Evaluation de la qualité des corps gras de friture aspects nutritionnels. *Rev. Fr. Corps Gras* **20,** 471–480.

Ramwell, P. (ed) (1973). "The Prostaglandins", Plenum Press, New York, London.

Reichwald, I. and Meizies, A. Die fettsäuren der lipide im fleisch von süsswasserfischen und seefischen. *Z.f. Ernährungswissen* **72,** 1, 86–91.

Roberts, J. C. and Strauss, R. (eds) (1965). "Comparative Atherosclerosis." Hoeber Medical Division, Harper and Row, New York.

Sietz, F. G. (1969). *Fette Seifen, Anstrichmittel,* **71,** 446–451.

Sinclair, H. M. (1956). Deficiency of essential fatty acids and atherosclerosis, etcetera. *Lancet* **i,** 381–383.

Smith, E. B. (1965). The influence of age and atherosclerosis on the chemistry of aortic intima. *J. Atheroscler. Res.* **5,** 224–240.

Smith, E. B. and Slater, R. S. (1972). Relationship between low-density lipoprotein in aortic intima and serum-lipid levels. *Lancet,* **i,** 463–469.

Söderhjelm, L., Wiese, H. F. and Holman, R. T. (1971). The role of polyunsaturated acids in human nutrition and metabolism. *In* "Progress in the Chemistry of Fats and Other Lipids" (R. T. Holman, ed.), Vol. IX, pp. 555–585. Pergamon Press, Oxford.

Thomasson, H. J. (1962). Essential fatty acids. *Nature,* **194,** 973.

Thomasson, H. J., De Boer, J. and De Iongh, H. (1967). Influence of dietary fats on plasma lipids. 9th Int. Soc. Geograph. Path., Leyden. *Path. Microbiol.* **30,** 629–647.

Thomasson, H. J. (1969). Prostaglandins and cardiovascular diseases. *Nutr. Dieta* **11,** 228–240.

Vergroesen, A. J., De Boer, J. and Thomasson, H. J. (1970). Influence of three dietary fats given at three caloric levels on serum lipids in man. *In* "Atherosclerosis;

Proceedings of the Second International Symposium" (R. J. Jones, ed.), pp. 452–455. Springer-Verlag, New York.
Vergroesen, A. J. und De Boer, J. (1971). Quantitative and qualitative Effekte mehrfach ungesättigter und anderer Fettsäuren in der menschlichen Diät. *In* "Wissenschaftliche Veröffentlichungen der Deutschen Gesellschaft für Ernährung" Band 22, "Polyenfettsäuren", pp. 76–89. Dr. Dietrich Steinkopff Verlag, Darmstadt.
Vergroesen, A. J. (1972). Dietary fat and cardiovascular disease: possible modes of action of linoleic acid. *Proc. Nutr. Soc.* **31,** 323–329.
Vles, R. O., Büller, J., Gottenbos, J. J. and Thomasson, H. J. (1964). Influence of type of dietary fat on cholesterol-induced atherosclerosis in the rabbit. *J. Atheroscler. Res.* **4,** 170–183.
Vles, R. O. and Gottenbos, J. J. (1972a). Long-term effects of feeding butterfat, coconut oil and hydrogenated or non hydrogenated soyabean oil. 1. Eighteen-month experiment in mice. *Voeding* **33,** 428–433.
Vles, R. O. and Gottenbos, J. J. (1972b). Long-term effects of feeding butterfat, coconut oil and hydrogenated or non hydrogenated soyabean oil. 2. Life-span experiments in rats. *Voeding* **33,** 455–465.
Weis, E. E. and Wilcox, E. B. (1972). Serum cholesterol from pre-adolescence through young adulthood. *J. Am. Diet. Ass.* **61,** 155–158.
Wissler, R. W. and Vesselinovitch (1968). Comparative pathogenetic patterns in atherosclerosis. *Adv. Lipid Res.* **6,** 181–206.
Zilversmit, D. B. and Newman, H. A. I. (1966). Does a metabolic barrier to circulating cholesterol protect the arterial wall? *Circulation* **33,** 7.
Zilversmit, D. B. (1970). Metabolism of arterial lipids. *In* "Atherosclerosis" (R. J. Jones, ed.), pp. 35–41. Springer-Verlag, Berlin, Heidelberg, New York.
Zijlstra, W. G., Brunsting, J. R., Ten Hoor, F. and Vergroesen, A. J. (1972). Prostaglandin $E_1$ and cardiac arrhythmia. *Eur. J. Pharmacol.* **18,** 392–395.

# APPENDIX I

# DIET AND CORONARY HEART DISEASE

*A Joint Statement of The Food and Nutrition Board Division of Biology and Agriculture*
*National Academy of Sciences—National Research Council and the Council on Foods and Nutrition American Medical Association*
*July, 1972*

## A. Notice

This statement was developed under the aegis of the National Research Council, whose institutional responsibilities were discharged in the following manner.

The members of the authoring committee were selected for their individual scholarly competence and judgment with due consideration for the balance and breadth of disciplines. Responsibility for all aspects of this statement rests with the committee, to whom we express our sincere appreciation.

Although reports are not submitted for approval to the Academy membership nor to the Council, each is reviewed according to procedures established and monitored by the Academy's Report Review Committee. Such reviews are intended to determine, *inter alia*, whether the major questions and relevant points of view have been addressed and whether the reported findings, conclusions, and recommendations arose from the available data and information. Distribution is approved, by the President, only after satisfactory completion of this review process.

## B. Diet and Coronary Heart Disease

Coronary heart disease is the major public health problem in the United States and in many other countries. In 1970, for example, some 666,000 Americans, of whom about 171,000 were under the age of 65, died of coronary heart disease (CHD) and many more were disabled by the same disorder. It is particularly disturbing that many relatively young Americans in their most productive years are killed or incapacitated by this disease.

Epidemiologic, experimental, and clinical investigations have identified a number of "risk factors" associated with susceptibility to CHD that can be manipulated. These include an elevation in plasma lipids, especially plasma cholesterol; high blood pressure (hypertension); heavy cigarette smoking; obesity; and physical inactivity. The evidence is not sufficient to quantitate the benefits that may be expected to come from modifying these various risk factors, but the seriousness of the situation demands that all reasonable means be used to reduce the conditions that contribute to risk of CHD.

There is abundant evidence that the risk of developing CHD is positively correlated with the level of cholesterol in the plasma. This risk, independent of other risk factors mentioned above, is relatively small at levels less than 220 mg/100 ml but increases progressively with each increment in plasma cholesterol above this level. Approximately one-third of American men, and a less definitely known proportion of women, consuming their usual diets maintain plasma cholesterol levels at or below 220 mg/100 ml. There is extensive evidence that the level of cholesterol in the plasma of most people can be lowered by appropriate dietary modification. Generally, such lowering can be achieved most practicably by partial replacement of the dietary sources of saturated fat with sources of unsaturated fat, especially those rich in polyunsaturated fatty acids, and by a reduction in the consumption of foods rich in cholesterol. Preliminary evidence suggests that faithful and continued consumption of a cholesterol-lowering diet over a period of years can reduce the coronary attack rate in middle-aged men. As would be expected in dealing with a chronic disease of this kind, early intervention appears to be more effective than intervention after the disease is evident.

Elevation of other plasma lipids (plasma triglycerides) also imposes an increased risk of CHD. The elevation of plasma triglycerides is often, but not always, associated with an elevation of plasma cholesterol. Plasma triglycerides can also be modified by dietary intervention. Although there are as yet no satisfactory epidemiologic data to support the conclusion that triglyceride-lowering diets can reduce the occurrence of CHD in persons with hypertriglyceridaemia, the inference from clinical studies that such a reduction can be anticipated is strong.

In summary, the average level of plasma lipids in most American men and women is undesirably elevated. The importance of lowering the plasma cholesterol in any individual depends in large part upon his usual plasma cholesterol concentration.

The evidence now available is sufficient to discourage further temporizing with this major national health problem. Therefore the Food and Nutrition Board and the Council on Foods and Nutrition recommend that:

1. measurement of the plasma lipid profile, particularly plasma cholesterol, become a routine part of all health maintenance physical examinations. Such measurements should be made in early adulthood, when coronary heart disease is still rare, and

repeated at appropriate intervals. The potential impact of other risk factors should also be periodically assessed;

2. persons falling into "risk categories" on the basis of their plasma lipid levels be made aware of this and receive appropriate dietary advice. Such advice may vary somewhat with the nature of the blood lipid profile [Fredrickson, Levy, and Lees (1967). *N. Eng. J. Med.* **276,** 34; Lees and Wilson (1971). *N. Eng. J. Med.* **284,** 186; Report of Inter-Society Commission for Heart Disease Resources, Circulation XLII: A55 (1971); American Health Foundation Position Statement on Diet and Coronary Heart Disease, *Preventive Medicine* **1,** 255 (1972)]. As indicated above, Americans should be advised to maintain a desirable body weight by an appropriate combination of physical activity and calorie intake. In "risk categories" it is important to decrease substantially the intake of saturated fat and to lower cholesterol consumption. In practice, this entails substituting polyunsaturated vegetable oils for part of the saturated fat in the diet.
3. care be taken to assure that the dietary advice given does not compromise the intake of essential nutrients. Desirable intakes of nutrients are indicated in the Recommended Dietary Allowances (NAS Publ. No. 1694, 1968);
4. since the foregoing recommendations will be effective only if they can be accomplished with relative ease, modified and ordinary foods useful for this purpose be readily available on the market, reasonably priced, and easily identified by appropriate labelling. Any existing legal and regulatory barriers to the marketing of such foods should be removed;
5. high priority be given to the conduct of studies that will determine reliably the extent to which the modification of plasma lipids, by dietary or other means, as well as modification of other risk factors, can reduce the risk of developing coronary artery disease.

# APPENDIX II

# RECOMMENDATIONS ON AMOUNT AND NATURE OF DIETARY FATS

*Netherlands Nutrition Council** (*May, 1973*)

## Introduction

The actual causes of atherosclerosis are only partly known. As a result, its prevention is still connected with many uncertainties and, therefore, the quantitative effect of the correction of only one of the causal factors—namely incorrect eating habits—is difficult to predict. Relevant investigations are still in progress. Although some of the conclusions from the results obtained are not unanimous and sometimes even controversial, there are very strong indications of a useful contribution to the prevention of atherosclerosis by dietary modifications—in addition to other measures—because a certain number of nutritional factors are known to contribute considerably to an increase in cholesterol and other lipid levels in the blood, the correlation of which with atherosclerosis and in particular with its complications, is generally accepted. By influencing these factors, it is possible to restrict the severity of the disease and its disastrous complications.

Among the particularly important factors promoting atherosclerosis and its complications, are the changes in the way of life and eating habits over the past decades which, in many cases, have led to disorders in the glucose and/or fat metabolism. The disorders concerned play, for instance, a causal role in the etiology of atherosclerotic cardiovascular diseases. In addition, other abnormalities frequently occurring, for example, obesity, hypertension and diabetes, can be the cause as well as result of the disorders mentioned.

Beside obesity, hypertension, diabetes, increased serum cholesterol and other lipid levels, other risk factors which can be modified are for instance: lack of physical exercise, smoking (particularly inhaling smoke) and psycho-social tensions. Unfortunately, it is not yet possible to quantify the effect of each risk factor but the severity of the situation requires that we should make use of all conceivable means which might possibly lead to a decrease in the incidence of cardiovascular diseases.

The advice of the Nutrition Council is purposely only concerned with desiderata regarding the *nutrition* of the Dutch population—without underestimating the causal influence of the other factors although the Nutrition Council is of the opinion that atherosclerosis and its complications in the Western world can only be greatly decreased if

* English translation of the official report of the Netherlands Nutritional Council (Chairman Professor C. den Hartog) (1973), *Voeding*, **34**, 552–557.

the other causal factors are also fought in an effective way. We may expect that a nutritional pattern as recommended below will have a favourable effect on the disease and its complications. The Council arrives at this expectation on the basis of investigations carried out by a number of members of the Committee on "Polyunsaturated fatty acids", as well as on the basis of a vast body of literature referred to in the work of Dr van Schaik and Dr Dalderup. The nutritional recommendations given below are for all the "healthy" population. For the formulation of these recommendations, the Council took into account the following facts:

1. that in the working male population over 30 years of age in Holland, many groups of people, roughly 25–30%, have high to very high cholesterol and/or lipid levels in the blood—as a consequence of high sensitivity towards saturated fat and/or some sugars and that these levels imply clearly an increased risk with respect to the progress of atherosclerotic changes;
2. there are no reasons to assume that corresponding findings in adult women will not give rise to similar and other complications;
3. that the results of descriptive and experimental epidemiological investigations show a clear effect of normalizing the fat metabolism and this will show even more clearly if these measures are taken at an earlier age, and applied for a longer period.

The foregoing points favour a clear primary prevention by means of nutritional measures destined for the whole population. As a result of these measures people who do not (yet) show/or hardly show the metabolism abnormalities mentioned, would be protected for a long time, while for those who have already advanced atherosclerotic changes, the development of accompanying complications could be checked.

Somewhat different and also stricter and more individual guidelines will of course hold for persons with pathological changes in glucose and/or fat metabolism (whether detected within the framework of a group investigation or not). The fact that this category in the Netherlands is alarmingly large, underlines the necessity of taking primary preventive measure other than those which can be realized through dietary modifications. The nutritional advice has been divided by the Council as follows:

A. recommendations on dietary composition for the "healthy" population.
B. guidelines for promoting the desired change in the diet of the Dutch population.

## A. Recommendations on Dietary Composition for the "Healthy" Population

*1. Calories*

The Council is of the opinion that the caloric intake of the greater part of the Dutch population is too high in relation to its physical activity. The result is that many people are overweight as a result of too much body fat. The total caloric intake should be regulated individually so that the "normal" body weight will be achieved or maintained. The "normal" body weight is connected with the height and build (muscle mass and frame development), as well as with age and sex. Overweight caused by too large an amount of body fat gives rise to disturbances of glucose and fat metabolism, as a result of which decreased glucose tolerance, diabetes and possibly atherosclerotic heart disease may also occur. In addition, hypertension often aggravated by obesity, means an extra burden for the cardiovascular system.

*2. Fats*

The majority of the Council is of the opinion that an effort should be made to restrict the consumption of fat in such a way that the dietary fats will supply 30 to maximum 40% of the total amount of calories instead of the average of more than 40%, which means that more than half the population consumes a diet too rich in fat.

For practical reasons, the Council thinks it advisable to try and achieve a decrease to about one-third of the total amount of calories: as to the nature of the fats, restriction of the use of saturated fat in particular is recommended.

Although our current knowledge does not enable us to give a quantitative norm for the optimal ratio between the different saturated and mono- and polyunsaturated fatty acids in the diet for the whole population, the Council is of the opinion that particularly in cases of an increased or increasing serum cholesterol level, a calorie-balanced diet, and also a replacement of saturated fatty acids by a considerable amount of polyunsaturated fatty acids in the diet will contribute to a decrease of the cholesterol and lipid levels in the blood. This means that the diet should contain a higher amount of linoleic acid than the average diet has at present. In this way, one of the risk factors for atherosclerosis and its complications will decrease. The Council holds the view that this can be achieved by choosing carefully from the range of normal foods available.

According to the majority of the members of the Council it is justified to expect that if high blood lipid levels are induced by a high percentage of dietary fat calories and an insufficient physical activity, polyunsaturated fats will only decrease effectively the cholesterol and lipid levels in the blood, if about one-third of the total amount of fatty acids is present as linoleic acid. This means in practice that for these cases, roughly doubling the present average amount of polyunsaturated fatty acids seems desirable (10–13 % of the total caloric intake).

The Committee recognizes it will not be easy—and certainly not so in the short term—for the whole population to put this into effect without making great changes in the food pattern. There are indications—based on epidemiological investigations but involving conditions such as more physical exercise, diets relatively low in calories and less smoking than in our present society—that a diet in which the saturated fat has been replaced by "basic foods" such as bread, rice and other cereals, may also restrict the development of atherosclerosis and its vascular complications. The preventive effect of such a low fat diet has not yet been confirmed by experimental investigations of man living in Western style.

*3. Proteins*

With regard to the protein content of the diet, the guidelines given by the "Norms" Committee of the Nutrition Council may be adopted; the recommendation is 10–12 % of the total caloric intake of which 30–50 % is animal protein.

*4. Carbohydrates*

The remaining calories will mainly be supplied by carbohydrates. Preferably, these should originate from whole cereal products and pulses and as little as possible from sugar.

*5. Cholesterol*

The amount of exogenous cholesterol should, on average, not exceed 250–300 mg/day per person.

## B. Recommendations which may Help to Promote the Desired Change in the Diet of the Dutch Population

1. The population should be informed of the basic principles of sound nutrition, as mentioned in previous recommendations 1–5 by capable people, media and authorities. These general guidelines should be further transformed into practical advice. According to the Council it is now possible to attain important improvements by a better choice of available foods.

a. With regard to the prevention of overweight by excess body fat, the use of a number of foods and beverages should be restricted. In its report "Obesity" (November 8, 1972) the Council extensively advised the Minister of Public Health that slimming is generally acceptable as long as a varied diet of a balanced composition is maintained.

In this connection it is important to recommend:

restriction of certain fat-rich foods;
restriction of sugar-rich foods;
restriction of the use of alcoholic drinks, and snacks.

b. The measures already mentioned above (Section A) will also partly contribute to a shift within the fatty acid pattern, because most margarines, butter, animal fat, baking and frying fat, fat in meat, fat in bakery products, cream, cream cheese and chocolate contain mainly saturated fatty acids and little amounts of polyunsaturated fatty acids. The preferable dietary fats should be relatively rich in polyunsaturated fatty acids. These are, besides certain (dietary) margarines and oils with a high content of linoleic acid*, some halvarines, fat from cereals and fat from some nuts and that of most fish and some poultry. The expectedly higher vitamin E requirement as a result of this increase in linoleic acid content, may be met by using sufficient amounts of wholemeal bread and vegetables. Most oils with a high linoleic acid content are, naturally, vitamin E sources.

c. Replacement of saturated fatty acids in the diet and the modification of the fatty acid pattern, should not be at the cost of protein-rich foods. Adequate although not too excessively large amounts of meat and meat products should therefore be maintained as animal protein sources. All fish and poultry are good protein sources and contain also relatively slight amounts of saturated fat. Milk, milk products and cheese contain, it is true, saturated fat but also various important nutrients. For this reason, the use of low-fat milk and skim-milk products and cheese is encouraged.

d. The carbohydrate portion of the calories will have to be derived from bread (preferably wholemeal bread not "enriched" by fat addition), wholemeal cereal products, such as rolled oats and similar cereal products, macaroni, rice, potatoes and pulses. These products also contribute greatly to a balanced diet as sources of vegetable proteins and a wide variety of other nutrients.

e. Limitation of the use of eggs to 2–3 per person per week on average,

* Most vegetable oils naturally contain much linoleic acid. Until a short time ago, linoleic acid disappeared for the greater part during the process of margarine production. Over the past few years, the process has been modified in such a way that a much larger amount of linoleic acid remains intact.

and limitation of the use of animal organ products, such as liver, kidney, etc.

2. The public advised in this way, should be helped to choose good foods with a low content of saturated fat, cholesterol and sugar. This can be promoted in the following ways:

if such food products, the fat of which may be enriched with linoleic acid, are easily obtainable at a reasonable price and easily recognizable by a clear labelling;
by removing legal barriers with regard to the production and sale of such products;
by increasing and intensifying information via the press. radio and TV, so helping people to make an adequate choice of foods;
by providing suitable meals to the Armed Forces, in hospitals, in canteens of Government and private enterprises and bodies and the hotel and catering trade, etc.;
by modernized instructions at all types of schools, higher professional schools and other professional training schools, as well as by integration of the science of nutrition in the curriculum of Medical faculties of Universities etc.

The Council realizes that the observance of its recommendations with regard to supplying information through all possible media, will require an objective supply of information and, in particular as far as a number of sectors of the food supply is concerned, will demand a great effort in the field of technological research and practical application. However, the Council is of the opinion that in connection with the importance of public health, it is necessary and justified to point clearly to these measures and insist upon their implementation.

2

# Epidemiological Data on Dietary Fat Intake and Atherosclerosis with an Appendix on Possible Side Effects

S. HEYDEN

*Department of Community Health Sciences, Duke University Medical Center, Durham, North Carolina, U.S.A.*

## I. INTRODUCTION

Epidemiological data on the relationship between dietary fat consumption and atherosclerosis have been presented in thousands of articles in medical journals, hundreds of medical textbooks and several prospective long-term studies in the United States. In order to gain an overall view of new developments in the field of research on hyperlipidaemia and clinical manifestations of atherosclerosis, it is necessary to discuss the hyperlipoproteinaemias first. However, since no prospective data are available on the relationship between specific types of hyperlipoproteinaemia and clinical manifestations of atherosclerosis, this chapter then discusses the well studied relationship of serum cholesterol concentration, dietary fat intake and the development of ischemic heart disease.

> "Few controversies have divided the medical community so sharply for such a long time as has the sterol hypothesis. The separation between two points of view has become so extreme that, on the one hand, there are respected scientists who believe that the evidence is already so convincing that further clinical testing is unnecessary, financially wasteful and actually unethical; and, aligned against them, are equally respected scientists who believe that the total weight of evidence accumulated over the many years is too slight to justify further work along these lines. The opinion of onc of thcsc groups may very well be substantiated eventually. On the one hand, evidence in favor of the hypothesis is inadequate to persuade the medical profession to place itself solidly behind an attempt to lower the plasma cholesterol level of the general population. On the other hand, the evidence is sufficiently suggestive to prevent the scientific community from discarding the hypothesis. In fact, a large share (probably more than half) of the research now in progress in the field of atherosclerosis is concerned with some aspect of the hypothesis." (Frantz and Moore, 1969.)

Later in the chapter the subject of dietary intervention is divided into two categories: primary prevention of ischemic heart disease (Section VII) where four internationally known trials will be covered and secondary prevention in patients with ischemic heart disease (Section VIII) where seven studies from several countries will be presented first, followed by four trials conducted in England with negative results.

## II. HYPERLIPOPROTEINAEMIA AND ATHEROSCLEROSIS

Only two manifestations of atherosclerosis have been associated with specific types of hyperlipoproteinaemia: coronary heart disease and peripheral vascular disease. There is no report to date of a relationship between cerebral vascular disease and any type of hyperlipoproteinaemia; however, a negative association between cerebrovascular disease and hypercholesterolaemia has been reported in several long-term prospective studies.

The hyperlipoproteinaemias can be classified in different types, (Fredrickson *et al.*, 1967) of which, type II, type III and type IV have been associated with atherosclerosis and its manifestations in several retrospective studies. In patients with the very uncommon type I syndrome no manifestations of coronary artery disease have been found. Type V patterns are also rare, and evidence of accelerated atherosclerosis in either patients or their families has not been striking.

Table 1

Hyperlipoproteinaemia in recent studies of patients with ischemic heart disease, and controls

| | | Per cent distribution of hyperlipoproteinaemia | | | | |
|---|---|---|---|---|---|---|
| No. of patients with IHD | | Normal | II | III | IV | V |
| | (5 studies) | | | | | |
| 126 | Boston/Bethesda[a] | 46 | 29 | 0 | 25 | 0 |
| 70 | Buffalo, N.Y.[b] | 26 | 44 | 0 | 30 | 0 |
| 108 | Aalborg, Denmark[c] | 22 | 43 | 11 | 16 | 8 |
| 105 | Drammen, Norway[d] | 43 | 31 | 0 | 26 | 0 |
| 100 | Göteborg, Sweden[e] | 41 | 24 | 13 | 22 | 0 |
| | Average | 36% | 34% | (5%) | 24% | – |

| | | Per cent distribution of hyperlipoproteinaemia | | | | |
|---|---|---|---|---|---|---|
| No. of "normal" persons | | Normal | II | III | IV | V |
| | (4 studies) | | | | | |
| 66 | Boston/Bethesda[a] | 89 | 3 | 0 | 8 | 0 |
| 11 | Buffalo, N.Y.[b] | 64 | 18 | 0 | 18 | 0 |
| 109 | Aalborg, Denmark[c] | 78 | 7 | 4 | 10 | 1 |
| 76 | Göteborg, Sweden[e] | 75 | 12 | 1 | 9 | 3 |
| | Average | 77% | 10% | (1%) | 11% | (1%) |

[a] Heinle *et al.* (1969).
[b] Falsetti *et al.* (1970).
[c] Dyerberg *et al.* (1970).
[d] Enger and Ritland (1970).
[e] Werkö (1971).

Prevalence of hyperlipoproteinaemia in the general population was estimated by one author to amount to only 5 % of Americans (Connor, 1970). More precise estimates will be forthcoming from the present Hyperlipoproteinaemia Prevalence Study, conducted by the National Heart and Lung Institute (NHLI). Preliminary analysis of available data would place this percentage considerably higher. Table 1 shows the per cent distribution of the hyperlipoproteinaemias in different parts of the United States and Scandinavia among patients with ischemic heart disease (IHD) and among those believed to be free of it.

More than one-third of patients with ischemic heart disease had a normal lipid electrophoresis according to these investigations published in 1969, 1970 and 1971. As expected, the most frequently observed type of hyperlipoproteinaemia in patients with ischemic heart disease was type II (34 % of all patients), followed by hyperlipoproteinaemia type IV (24 % of all patients). Since in some instances the "control population" was selected from hospitalized patients (with illnesses other than ischemic heart disease), the per cent distribution of hyperlipoproteinaemias in these populations are not indicative of the prevalence of hyperlipoproteinaemias in the general population. But it is interesting that 77 % of all subjects without ischemic heart disease were found to have a normal electrophoresis, only 10 % showed hyperlipoproteinaemia type II and 11 % hyperlipoproteinaemia type IV. Prospective data concerning the risk of ischemic heart disease or peripheral vascular disease in relation to lipoprotein types are non-existent.

### *Type II*

Hyper-$\beta$-lipoproteinaemia studied by Slack (1969) in male patients was associated with a mean age (at onset of ischemic heart disease) of 43 years and among female patients of 48 years. In the study by Jensen *et al.* (1967) the mean age at death from coronary disease in men with hyperlipoproteinaemia type II was 56 years, and the mean age at death in women was 58 years. The age at onset of, and age at death from, ischemic heart disease therefore is clearly much younger than the average age of onset and mean age of death from ischemic heart disease in the general population, when not associated with hyperlipoproteinaemia II.

Arteriosclerotic-type plaques have been observed in major pulmonary arteries in type II patients who have had no evidence of pulmonary hypertension. In addition, Roberts *et al.* (1970) described a peculiar valvular disease in five patients with hyperlipoproteinaemia II. The finding of extensive plaquing in the ascending aorta and proximal coronary artery in these young subjects who had no histories of rheumatic or congenital cardiac disease suggests an atherosclerotic etiology of the valvular disease. The finding of cholesterol clefts and foam cells in the aortic valve cusps is also strongly suggestive of an unusual etiology of valvular heart disease, namely atherosclerosis.

A surprisingly low frequency of peripheral atherosclerosis associated with familial hypercholesterolaemia (type II) was found by Harlan *et al.* (1966).

> "Two explanations may be offered. Arterial disease may develop early and follow a constantly progressive course which initiates parallel development of collaterals and minimizes the effect of arteriosclerotic narrowing. Alternatively, hypercholesterolaemia is not associated with a severe arteriosclerotic process in the peripheral arteries. The fact that arteriosclerosis obliterans is more frequently associated with abnormal glucose tolerance than hypercholesterolaemia is consistent with this last hypothesis. Glucose tolerance was normal in familial hypercholesterolaemia."

Widmer *et al.* (1969) were surprised not to find any difference in cholesterol levels and specifically hypercholesterolaemia among patients with peripheral atherosclerotic disease and healthy persons. The frequency of hypercholesterolaemia in patients with intermittent claudication was 20·5%, and the frequency of hypercholesterolaemia among the healthy persons without intermittent claudication was 16%. However, $\beta$-lipoprotein concentration was found significantly higher among the patients than among the healthy persons. Thirty-nine per cent of patients with intermittent claudication had elevated $\beta$-lipoproteins, whereas only 17·5% of the healthy persons had elevated $\beta$-lipoprotein levels. Unfortunately pre-$\beta$-lipoproteins were not measured. This finding is most unusual and contrary to several other investigations, the most recent one by Greenhalgh *et al.* (1971). Only 5% of their patients with peripheral vascular disease had hyper-$\beta$-lipoproteinaemia, whereas 30% had hypertriglyceridaemia with normal cholesterol levels. Electrophoresis, in most cases, showed increased pre-$\beta$-lipoprotein levels.

### *Type III*

> "Occlusive vascular disease is a serious and frequent accompaniment of type III. In the samples observed by us, occlusive peripheral vascular disease, especially of femoral and popliteal vessels with severe claudication, has been at least as frequent as coronary atherosclerosis." (Fredrickson *et al.*, 1967.)

Slack reported that in men with types III, IV and V hyperlipoproteinaemia, the risks were lower for ischemic heart disease than with type II, but the risk of peripheral vascular disease was increased. In his study the age of onset of ischemic heart disease seemed to be later in both men and women with types III, IV and V hyperlipoproteinaemia than with type II. There was also a notable absence of death from ischemic heart disease among patients with hyperlipidaemia associated with hypertriglyceridaemia. He concluded

> "The absence of deaths and the incidence of peripheral vascular disease among patients with types III, IV and V hyperlipoproteinaemia, suggests that there may be a real difference in the type of atheromatous lesion which develops compared with the more lethal disorder of type II hyperlipoproteinaemia."

In a detailed study of the peripheral circulation (Zelis *et al.*, 1970) nine out of twelve patients with hyperlipoproteinaemia type III showed subnormal values of the peak reactive hyperaemia blood flow. No significant differences in the peak reactive hyperaemia blood flow were demonstrable in patients with type II or type IV disorder in comparison to control persons.

Through combined use of drug and dietary treatment, patients with type III disease were considerably improved. The authors concluded that the "vascular cholesterol" in type III patients may be very labile. Combination therapy may have afforded a significant resorption of atherosclerotic plaques followed by increase of the arterial lumen with subsequent improved blood circulation.

According to Roberts *et al.* (1970) patients with type III are particularly susceptible to the development of peripheral arterial disease,

> "and objective improvement in peripheral blood flow also can occur with this medical regime."

Greenhalgh *et al.* (1971) suggested

> "that increased pre-$\beta$-lipoprotein levels might predispose to atherosclerosis with a predilection for arteries supplying the lower limbs, is an intriguing possibility."

### *Type IV*

> "Premature coronary arterial narrowing frequently occurs . . . over 40% have hyperuricaemia." (Roberts *et al.*, 1970.)

Levy and Fredrickson (1970) emphasized the accelerated coronary vessel disease in type IV patients. Fredrickson *et al.* (1967) pointed out that in patients with the primary form of hyperlipoproteinaemia IV, excessive body weight and abnormal glucose tolerance are extremely common. In their experience, the incidence of abnormal glucose tolerance in those with familial type IV patterns exceeded 90%. In a later study by the same group (Heinle *et al.*, 1969), 70% of patients with a type IV electrophoretic pattern demonstrated abnormal glucose tolerance. Schreibman *et al.* (1969) warned that the frequent finding of type IV hyper-pre-$\beta$-lipoproteinaemia in restrospective studies of patients selected because of coronary artery disease should not be interpreted as a possible risk of this lipid disorder. The risk may not be severe if obesity and diabetes mellitus do not co-exist even when onset of hyperlipoproteinaemia occurred in childhood.

> "A careful screening for this disorder in the pediatric group may furnish the material for a prospective study large enough to define this possibility further."

## A. Is Lipoprotein Electrophoresis Necessary?

Two answers are available to this question, one methodological, one epidemiological. According to the study by Schatz (1969) lipoprotein electrophoresis was not necessary for the identification of any of the 75 patients with type II and most (67 out of 71) patients with type IV hyperlipoproteinaemia. These two groups represent a majority (68·2%) of patients in his series. In only half of the twelve patients with phenotype III was the identification possible without electrophoresis. The very rare phenotype V could not be diagnosed without lipoprotein electrophoresis. In this particular series, none of the twelve patients with previously classified V pattern could be placed into this category. However, the detection of a wide chylomicron band on paper electrophoresis could be replaced by the simple observation of the plasma after keeping it overnight in the cold. In this situation, chylomicrons appear as a cream layer at the top. Schatz, therefore, concluded that

> "lipoprotein electrophoresis is not necessary for the proper identification of most patients with types II and IV hyperlipoproteinaemia, but may be of some benefit in separating patients with type III disease."

Harlan (1969) criticized that the lipoprotein electrophoretogram is a qualitative rather than a quantitative assessment, and, therefore, does not lend itself to quantifying the differences between individuals or the changes induced by therapy. In contrast, he writes,

> "measurements of cholesterol and triglyceride are quantitative, more readily available and usually furnish sufficient information to type the hyperlipidaemia."

The second answer represents the epidemiological viewpoint. Kannel *et al.* (1971) reported on the risk of coronary heart disease over 14 years in Framingham where $\beta$-lipoprotein, pre-$\beta$-lipoprotein and cholesterol levels were examined in 2282 men and 2845 women.

> "The mean level of each of the major serum lipids and lipoproteins was higher at the initial examination in those who went on to develop coronary heart disease than in cohorts who remained free of clinical manifestations of the disease over the 14-year period of observation. The risk for the development of coronary heart disease was proportional to the concentration of each lipid. The risk of ischemic heart disease proved proportional to the antecedent serum cholesterol level in men of all ages studied. Even after excluding persons with hypertension, diabetes, ECG abnormalities and the cigarette habit, a distinct gradient of risk proportional to the cholesterol concentration can be demonstrated. This tends to brand the lipid, not associated variables as the culprit . . ."
>
> "When risk of coronary heart disease was examined according to pre-$\beta$-lipoprotein concentration, adjusting for cholesterol, no residual risk gradient remained in men and younger women. In women over 50 years of age, however, pre-$\beta$-lipoprotein was superior to cholesterol levels in discriminating potential coronary heart disease cases."

Kannel *et al.* therefore concluded that in men

> "knowledge of the serum lipoprotein levels and the cholesterol concentration appears to provide no better discrimination of potential coronary victims than can be deduced from an accurate serum cholesterol value alone. Any one of the lipids or lipoproteins examined and by inference, a triglyceride as well can be used effectively for assessing vulnerability to coronary heart disease. None, however, would appear superior to the more convenient cholesterol determination for this purpose. In women, the picture appears to be somewhat different. In women under the age of 50, as in men, high cholesterol values and not pre-$\beta$-lipoprotein appeared to be associated with an increased risk. In older women, on the other hand, cholesterol appears to have no predictive value, and pre-$\beta$-lipoprotein actually appears to be superior to cholesterol for estimating."

The excellent predictability of an elevated cholesterol level for the development of myocardial infarction has been demonstrated in several long-term epidemiologic prospective studies, among others in our own Evans County Study (1971). We found over an eight- to nine-year observation period that for men with cholesterol levels of 260 mg% and above, the risk of developing ischemic heart disease was twice as high as for men with cholesterol levels below 220 mg %. Similarly, an excellent agreement between levels of serum cholesterol and significant arterial lesions observed in coronary angiography was found by Welch *et al.* (1970). Among 169 men with cholesterol levels less than 200 mg %, only 20 % had significant lesions. Among 186 men with levels more than 275 mg %, 81 % had significant lesions. There was a gradual increase in the percentage of significant lesions for each serum cholesterol level concentration, reaching almost 100 % in those men with cholesterol levels above 350 mg %. It is noteworthy that all men examined were under 40 years of age.

From the therapeutic standpoint, it should be recalled that over the past 15 years all dietary studies as means of primary prevention of ischemic heart disease or in the secondary prevention of reinfarction, concentrated on and were directed towards lowering of cholesterol levels. Although almost none of these studies were conducted in a double blind fashion with strictly comparable control persons, the trends in the results of both primary and secondary prevention studies seemed to favour the effect of a diet low in cholesterol and relatively high in polyunsaturated fatty acid to prevent ischemic heart disease and reinfarction. The conclusion, therefore, is justified that the measurement of the serum cholesterol concentration in an attempt to assess the risk of a man or woman (below the age of 50) for the development of ischemic heart disease as well as the treatment of hypercholesterolaemia would contribute significantly to the early detection and prevention of this epidemic disease. Additional assessment of the triglyceride levels would certainly be of help since a different dietary approach is indicated, and this might be a valuable contribution in the prevention of ischemic heart disease particularly in women above age 50, according to the Framingham data. The relative ease with which dietary changes produce complete normalization of abnormal hyperlipoprotein patterns (III, IV) and serum cholesterol as well as serum triglyceride concentrations should be encouraging to practising physicians. One cannot but be impressed by the fact that an appropriate dietary management of a cooperative and motivated patient can in most cases take the place of drug therapy. Notable exceptions to this statement are type I and IIa.

The importance of dietary influences on hyperlipoproteinaemias was demonstrated again by the study of plasma lipid and lipoprotein pattern in Greenlandic West Coast Eskimos (Bang *et al.*, 1971). The food of this population is very rich in protein, the quantity of carbohydrates is extremely small (estimated to be only 54 g per day) and a high animal fat intake of sea animals containing a large amount of polyunsaturated fatty acids. The levels of serum cholesterol and triglycerides as well as serum $\beta$-lipoprotein and pre-$\beta$-lipoprotein were substantially higher in Danish controls than in the Greenlandic Eskimos. A most striking observation was the near absence of pre-$\beta$-lipoproteins on the electrophoretic strips. Both plasma cholesterol and $\beta$-lipoprotein concentrations were at a very low level. The level of these lipids did not increase with advancing age—as was the case in Danish males. The low lipid levels were associated with a very low incidence of ischemic heart disease and with a near absence of any case of diabetes mellitus.

## B. Progress Report on Lipoprotein Phenotyping 1973

In 1954 the technical group of a Commission on "Lipoproteins and Atherosclerosis" came to the conclusion that the measurement of lipoprotein-concentrations is not superior to the simple measurement of serum cholesterol levels in its predictive power for ischemic heart disease. Almost 20 years later, a new trend seems to have evolved postulating that the measurement of cholesterol and triglyceride concentrations in the serum may be sufficient to give a valuable prediction for ischemic heart disease. Lipoprotein electrophoresis, according to some investigators, may not improve the predictive power of the combined measurement of cholesterol and triglycerides (Kannel *et al.*, 1971; Stamler, 1973). During almost two decades between these two statements lipoprotein electrophoresis has received wide attention although this typing system has undergone some criticism.

Pries *et al.* (1968) demonstrated the questionable reproducibility of the lipoprotein electrophoresis. Several investigators reported on intra-individual changes of types in multiple determinations which were hard to explain, e.g. type V converting into type IV under caloric restriction (Brunzell *et al.*, 1971); type V may convert temporarily into type II before complete normalization under isocaloric carbohydrate-reduced diet (personal observation, unpublished); type IV patients may convert under drug treatment with Atromid in some cases into type II (Strisower *et al.*, 1970). Hazzard *et al.* (1973) reported that

> "in many instances a small quantitative change in the level of either LDL-cholesterol or whole plasma triglyceride caused qualitative differences in lipoprotein phenotypes, especially in individuals with familiar combined hyperlipidaemia, who showed variable expression (types IIa, IIb, IV or V)."

These investigators examined the relationship between lipoprotein phenotypes and genetic lipid disorders in 156 genetically defined survivors of myocardial infarction. The lipoprotein phenotype of each survivor was determined primarily by measurement of his plasma triglyceride and low density lipoprotein (LDL)–cholesterol concentrations; his genetic disorder was identified by analysis of whole plasma cholesterol and triglyceride levels in relatives.

> "On an individual basis no lipoprotein pattern proved to be specific for any particular genetic lipid disorder; conversely, no genetic disorder was specified by a single lipoprotein pattern."

These drawbacks in the interpretation of the results of the lipoprotein electrophoresis make it difficult at the present time to find a classification of lipid abnormalities which would satisfy everybody. The latest (although certainly not last) suggestion comes from the Seattle Group (University of Washington), Goldstein *et al.* (1973), differentiating five distinct lipid disorders.

*1. Familial Hypercholesterolaemia*

This was characterized by the finding of pathological cholesterol levels in relatives of patients with myocardial infarction—all relatives had normal triglyceride levels. The cholesterol distribution was found to be bimodal and segregation analysis suggested autosomal dominant inheritance. The criterion which distinguished this disorder from other familial hyperlipidaemias was the nearly complete expression of hypercholesterolaemia in affected children.

*2. Familial Hypertriglyceridaemia*

This was characterized by the occurrence, in relatives of patients with myocardial infarction, of a normal cholesterol distribution but apparently bimodal triglyceride distribution. Segregation analysis in siblings again was consistent with autosomal dominant inheritance; however, hypertriglyceridaemia was not completely expressed in affected children (the study of offspring of affected subjects revealed that hypertriglyceridaemia was only expressed in about 13% of young relatives at risk).

*3. Familial Combined Hyperlipidaemia*

This was characterized by variability in expression of lipid levels among affected relatives of patients with myocardial infarction. Any combination of elevation in LDL-cholesterol and very low density lipoprotein (VLDL)-triglyceride or both, were observed among affected relatives. Affected individuals with this disorder manifested any one of four lipoprotein phenotypes: type IIa, IIb, IV or V patterns.

Dr Carlson commented at the 3rd Atherosclerosis Symposium in Berlin (October 24–28, 1973)

> "IIb or not IIb—that is here the question, a direct quotation from Shakespeare."

Dr Fredrickson (personal communication, 1973) said the

> "great issue in the wind now is that of type IIb or combined hyperlipidaemia representing a muddle of confusion which will have to be clarified before the value of having a fairly precise measure of LDL can be determined."

Nikkila and Aro (in Goldstein, 1973) independently reported that the most common form of familial hyperlipidaemia in survivors of myocardial infarction is one in which multiple lipoprotein types are observed among about 50 % of the first-degree relatives. These observations thus confirm the hypothesis by Goldstein *et al.*

*4. Polygenic Hypercholesterolaemia*

Neither hereditary nor identifiable environmental factors could be implicated. This disorder affected about 6 % of survivors.

*5. Sporadic Hypertriglyceridaemia*

Inheritance factors did not play a direct role in the pathogenesis of hyperlipidaemia in the survivors. The authors therefore designated them as "sporadic" cases in the non-genetic sense.

In October 1973, one of the original designers of the method for separating lipoproteins by electrophoresis, Dr Lees, summarized the present situation with the words

> "The qualitative lipoprotein methods of ten years ago have served us well and are still of value. However, it is increasingly apparent that classification schemes based on these methods do not fully describe the clinical and genetic spectrum of the hyperlipidaemias. It is now time to perfect the quantitative techniques mentioned above, and to develop new ones, so that we can define phenotypes that reflect more accurately the inherited biochemical defects that underlie the primary hyperlipidaemias."

Lees offered the following new classification

> "This table serves as a convenient means of display of the available data, and hopefully, as a guide, during the confusing period in which old concepts are breaking down and new ones are being formulated."

Present status of lipoprotein phenotyping

| Present nomenclature | Fredrickson-Lees phenotype | Plasma concentration of Cholesterol | Glycerides | LDL protein | Presumptive kinetic defect |
|---|---|---|---|---|---|
| Familial fat-induced lipaemia | I | Normal or high | Very high | Low | Impaired chylomicron removal |
| Familial hypercholesterolaemia | II (IIa, IIb) | High | Normal or high | High | Impaired β-lipoprotein removal |
| Broad-β-disease | III | High | High | Normal | Faulty conversion of pre-β to β-lipoproteins |
| Combined hyperlipidaemia | II, IIb or IV | Normal or high | Normal or high | Unknown | Unknown |
| Familial hyperglyceridaemia | IV | Normal | High | Normal | Impaired pre-β-lipoprotein removal |
| Mixed hyperlipaemia | V | High | High | Normal | Impaired removal of chylomicrons and pre-β-lipoproteins |

## III. SEASONAL CHANGES IN SERUM CHOLESTEROL CONCENTRATIONS

A discussion of epidemiolological data on the relationship between dietary fat consumption and influences on serum cholesterol would, of course, be incomplete if seasonal changes were not mentioned.

In the report of the National Diet-Heart Study (1968) it was stated that

> "there have been suggestions in the literature that serum cholesterol concentrations may show seasonal changes, with values in the winter being somewhat higher than in the summer. This would parallel the common finding that people gain weight during the winter and lose it in summer and could possibly be related thereto."

However, the results were rather inconclusive. Analysis of the data

> "does not prove that there is no significant seasonal trend in serum cholesterol, whether this be related to seasonal change in diet or to any other factor—for example endocrine changes. It does show that any possible seasonal effect does not greatly disturb the comparison between baseline values and average values for the whole period on prescribed diet."

Our own experience in this regard is quite different and we feel that there is indeed a powerful seasonal influence on cholesterol levels which may present a major difficulty in the analysis of data from persons placed on diets. In our Hypertension Intervention Study in overweight, hypertensive individuals (Heyden *et al.*, 1973b) in Evans County, Georgia, 63 persons were placed on a low-sodium weight reduction programme and 64 persons who were not given dietary advice, were charted for blood pressure measurements regularly. The baseline examination was done in August of 1971 during the peak of the heat and humidity characteristic for the summer season in Georgia. Cholesterol levels were comparable in both groups—mean level 211 mg% in the experimental and 212 mg% in the control group. Repeat cholesterol determination was done five months later during an unusual cold wave in January 1972, after an average weight loss of 8·0 kg (17·5 lb) in the experimental group and only 2·27 kg (5 lb) in the control group. It revealed a definite increase in cholesterol levels of an average 32 mg% in the experimental and an average of 35 mg% in the control group. In the experimental group, 38% remained at the baseline level ±20 mg% but 58% increased in serum cholesterol concentrations more than 20 mg%. In the control group, 29% remained at their initial cholesterol levels ±20 mg% but 69% increased more than 20 mg%. It is remarkable that in this obese, hypertensive population regardless of weight stability or weight loss after profound dietary changes, a definite increase in cholesterol levels was observed and that only two persons in the experimental group and only one person in the control group had decreased cholesterol levels by more than 20 mg% in five months.

Massek *et al.* (1962) reported important seasonal variations in cholesterol levels

> "with a marked drop in summer and autumn . . . based on extensive epidemiological investigations, comprising all age groups from newborn infants up to people above the age of 80 years . . . in the Czech population."

Chapman and Massey (1964) found that the highest mean values in the Los Angeles Heart Study occurred among persons examined in January and February; the lowest among August and September examinees.

Doyle *et al.* (1965) followed 52 men over a 12-month period.

> "Amost 50% of the group had a maximum difference of at least 50 mg%. No person had a difference of less than 20 mg% and two had differences in excess of 100 mg%."

The lowest levels were reached in July, while two peaks occurred in October/November and January/February.

Thorp (1963) emphasized that the amplitude and frequency of this variation differs according to location of the study and with the occupation, age and diet of the subjects studied.

> "If the annual variation of serum cholesterol of individuals is examined, a great majority show two peaks, which generally occur in the spring and autumn . . . 65% of the seasonal patterns are

dicyclic, and only 28% monocyclic. Yet when the results are averaged the predominant impression is of a monocyclic pattern, with a maximum in winter and a minimum in summer."

Data presented by Paul *et al.* (1963) showed a consistent seasonal variation in cholesterol levels in 2107 middle-aged men. The highest serum–cholesterol concentrations were encountered during the winter, the lowest in the spring or summer. In four consecutive years (1958–61) the values obtained in the autumn were definitely higher than those in spring or summer but never reached the peak values of winter time. The cholesterol determinations were not made per man per season. The procedure was, rather, to use the data procured from annual examinations to find the mean for each season. The magnitude of the variations (10–30 mg% from the lowest to the highest difference) has previously been assessed by others, e.g. by Thomas *et al.* (1961) in 25 prisoners during monthly determinations for one year. Higher cholesterol levels tended to prevail in December of 1958 and in January and November 1959; lower values were more prevalent in warmer months. A sharp decline was seen from March to May, when the lowest point of the year was reached.

Thomas observed differences up to 50 mg% in the mean values of 16 young men, similarly to Doyle's report. Physical activity did not seem to be of any importance in lowering the cholesterol levels in the warmer season, since only a few prisoners took advantage of the opportunity of some increased outdoor activity. Thomas has collected information from the literature pertaining to this problem of seasonal changes and found conflicting reports, among others one from Japan, showing seasonal variations in activity of the thyroid gland with highest BMR in winter and lowest in summer.

The following section is a summary statement on the potential influence of weight reduction on cholesterol metabolism. By the nature of a reducing diet, fat intake is usually drastically reduced except in the so-called high-protein diets promoted by Dr Stillman and Dr Atkin which practically eliminate carbohydrate intake. My own findings with several obese patients on a fat-restricted diet (25 g fat, 60 g carbohydrates, 60 g protein) providing roughly 700 kCal per day will follow (see pp. 68–69).

## IV. CHANGES OF CHOLESTEROL LEVELS DURING ACTIVE WEIGHT REDUCTION

Moses (1963) reported that a substantial drop in cholesterol occurs with weight loss followed after a few months at this weight level by a gradual return to control values in almost all subjects. Bierenbaum *et al.* (1963) on the other hand, found a permanent reduction of the cholesterol level in weight-reducing men. Galbraith *et al.* (1966) reviewed the confusing and conflicting reports on this problem in the literature. However, three possible trends for cholesterol levels following weight reduction seem to emerge—a decrease (five reports), no change (three reports), an increase (two reports). In the study by Galbraith *et al.* of nine very obese people, a drastic average decrease of 54 mg% (from a normal baseline of 198 mg%) after the first three weeks of active weight reduction was followed by a subsequent increase in every individual. Unfortunately, this was designed as a short-term experiment and long-term results from obese patients have been rarely reported in the literature.

This last experiment is mentioned because of the perhaps surprising observation that the nine excessively obese subjects with an average weight of 158 kg (348 lb) had normal cholesterol levels. Hartmann (1965) commented that "extreme obesity (overweight by 50% or more) is mostly accompanied by relatively low serum lipids". Connor and Connor (1972) wrote that physicians are often surprised that the heavy overweight subjects (135–270 kg: 300–600 lb) show a low cholesterol level (140–160 mg%). However, this was frequently seen in their practice in Iowa.

A typical example was the heaviest man ever seen in my clinic, a 36-year-old weighing 273 kg (601 lb). Both he and his friend, a 56-year-old man weighing 174 kg (384 lb), had cholesterol levels below 180 mg% on repeat examinations.

The National Diet-Heart Study (1968) reported a different finding

> "There is a tendency for hypercholesterolaemia to be more common as relative weight increases and the relationship appears to be approximately linear on the relative weight decile scale. Roughly, the 10% of participants with highest relative weights were grossly hypercholesterolaemic about twice as frequently as the 10% men with the lowest relative weight."

It may very well be that the National Diet-Heart Study was not concerned with grossly obese persons such as one is most likely to encounter in a special obesity clinic. In the experience of Van Houte and Kesteloot (1971) "cholesterol increases with weight up to 100 kg, but decreases at higher weight" in an epidemiological cardiovascular study of 42,804 military subjects. Schreibman *et al.* (1971) and Nestel *et al.* (1973) concluded from metabolic ward observations of eight obese patients that obese patients may double their cholesterol synthesis rate and cholesterol storage depot without increasing plasma cholesterol content: "In spite of increased synthesis and increased body cholesterol content, plasma cholesterol is not elevated". These authors found a rise in plasma cholesterol specific activity following weight reduction. This observation was consistent in all "labelled" patients even though plasma cholesterol itself sometimes rose and sometimes fell (personal communication, Schreibman, 1972).

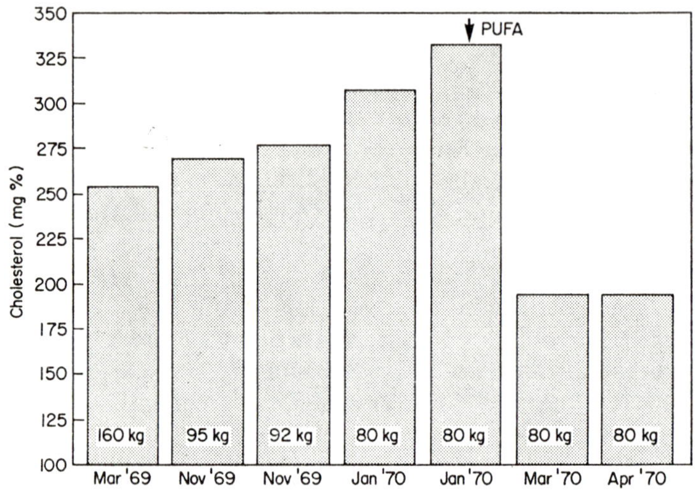


Fig. 1. Result of drastic weight reduction on cholesterol levels.

Figure 1 demonstrates the result of weight reduction on cholesterol levels in a 41-year-old man. He reduced his weight from 160 kg (352 lb), 3/1/69, to 80 kg (176 lb) by 12/31/69 (10 months) while continuing his profession as paint salesman without hospitalization and without any drug therapy to suppress his appetite. The cholesterol increased from 255 mg% at the beginning of his weight reduction programme to 335 mg% by the time he had reached his maintenance weight of 80 kg (176 lb) in January 1970. At this point we urged the patient to use polyunsaturated fat in the form of margarine for frying purposes and corn oil to be used in salads. By March 1970, the cholesterol had decreased predictably to 185 mg% and remained at this level during the following months. The remarkable fall of the cholesterol level can not simply be explained by the addition of polyunsaturated fatty acids to his diet. At the same time, between January and March, a seasonal effect has to be taken into account. The previous increase of the cholesterol level during active weight reduction in this patient is representative for a number of excessively obese persons; however, another reaction has been observed just as frequently.

In the past few years, we have seen many patients who were concerned about their slightly elevated cholesterol levels and who were disappointed to find out that in spite of drastic weight reduction, the cholesterol level did not change at all.

In moderately obese subjects, weight reduction more often seems to cause a drop in cholesterol, in our present experience at least, more frequently than an increase in cholesterol levels. The lability of vascular cholesterol in hyperlipoproteinaemia type III is well known. It is, therefore, not surprising that patients with this lipid disorder always, without exception, show a large decrease in cholesterol levels during weight reduction.

It is obvious that these so far unpredictable changes in cholesterol levels during and after weight reduction must be studied more systematically, classifying obese persons in "mild", "moderate" and "excessive" cases, analysing the data separately by sex and by age.

## V. CHANGES IN LIPOPROTEIN ELECTROPHORETIC PATTERN IN TYPES IV AND V DISORDERS WITHOUT AND/OR DURING WEIGHT REDUCTION

Strisower *et al.* (1970) suggested that

> "in type IV disease, the effect of Atromid-S should be monitored with serial paper electrophoretic strips to allow a careful comparison of the intensity of the beta band. If the intensity of this band increases, an undesirable lipoprotein shift has taken place and Atromid-S should be stopped. Ultracentrifugal studies have shown that severe forms of type IV disorders frequently respond to Atromid-S with a marked increase in the beta lipoprotein concentration; this may be considered equivalent to the iatrogenic conversion of a type IV to a type II disorder. Since type II disorders are the most malignant disturbances in terms of association with severe coronary atherosclerosis, the substitution of a type II disorder disturbance for a type IV disorder is most likely deleterious to the patient. The type IV to type II lipoprotein shift is generally unimportant if the type IV disturbance is mild or moderate; if it is severe, a significant shift occurs in nearly all cases."

We have in our files a case of a conversion into type II pattern in a patient with previous type IV pattern.

J.F.M., a 42-year-old self-employed feed mill farmer presented himself on 7/9/71 for diet counselling weighing 149 kg (328 lb). (Aged 17 his weight had been 100 kg: 220 lb.) The 12-hr fasting serum was cloudy, cholesterol level was 320 mg%, triglyceride level 615 mg%, $\beta$-lipoproteins slightly increased, pre-$\beta$-lipoproteins increased. This was diagnosed as consistent with phenotype IV. The patient was placed on a strict weight reduction programme with frequent intermittent fasting days. After nine weeks, his weight was reduced to 131 kg (289 lb) a weight loss of 18 kg (40 lb). He had worked continuously during this time and reported feeling well. His blood pressure had dropped from 180/125 mmHg to 110/88 mmHg. Lipid electrophoresis on 9/16/71 revealed the serum to be clear. Cholesterol had increased to 442 mg% while the triglycerides had markedly decreased to 252 mg% β-Lipoprotein which was only slightly increased in the previous lipoprotein analysis was this time reported increased and pre-β-lipoprotein was, again, increased. The data were consistent with phenotype II. It is possible to explain this remarkable shift by the changes which took place in his thyroid function. On the day of his first lipid electrophoresis the thyroid-function tests, T3 and T4 as well as free thyroxine were reported to be at a low normal level. After hyperlipoproteinaemia type IV had cleared under weight reduction, he became increasingly myxedematous and the hyperlipoproteinaemia changed to type II. After three days of TSH-stimulation the I-131 uptake at 24 hours was less than 1%, a pattern consistent with primary hypothyroidism. After adequate treatment with Synthroid, his lipid electrophoresis revealed a return to type IV pattern (January 10, 1972: Cholesterol 297 mg%, triglycerides 302 mg%, serum slightly cloudy, β-lipoprotein normal, pre-β-lipoprotein increased).

Strisower *et al.* (1970) also stated that no untoward lipoprotein shift occurs in type III disorders but they do not mention the possible changes in type V disorders. We have not seen any lipoprotein shift in type III disorders but have seen one in type V pattern:

Mrs G.H. was 62 years old and had diabetes mellitus, treated by Orinase and a history of myocardial infarction in September 1969. Her weight was considered normal at 64 kg (141 lb). On 2/15/70 she had a routine lipid electrophoresis which showed a serum cholesterol concentration of 303 mg% and triglycerides 485 mg%. The patient showed chylomicronaemia and hyper-pre-β-lipoproteinaemia, consistent with phenotype V. At the second lipid evaluation (3/23/70), one month after institution of a low-carbohydrate diet, emphasizing lean meats, fish and the use of polyunsaturated fatty acids, the cholesterol level was still elevated with 279 mg%, triglycerides had decreased to a normal level of 122 mg%. The phenotype V was changed into type II with hyper-β-lipoproteinaemia. Because of the obvious conversion of a type V to a type II disorder, the patient was followed closely without any changes in the dietary regime. This resulted in a decrease of the cholesterol to 256 mg%, further decrease of triglycerides to 98 mg% and eventually a normal lipoprotein pattern.

We would not have known anything about her transient hyper-β-lipoproteinaemia had we not examined the blood at this particular time. The recommendation by Strisower *et al.* of serial paper electrophoretic strips of patients undergoing drug therapy may, therefore, be extended to patients undergoing dietary treatment in order to gain more insight into the problem of iatrogenic conversions of one hyperlipoproteinaemia type into another.

## VI. CHANGES IN β-LIPOPROTEINS IN CASES OF HYPERLIPOPROTEINAEMIA TYPE II DURING WEIGHT REDUCTION

It is generally agreed that most cases of hyperlipoproteinaemia type II are more resistant to dietary changes than any other type of hyperlipoproteinaemia. Again, there are only very few reports in the literature. Wilson *et al.* (1971) stated that adherence to the American Heart Association (AHA) diet by 59 non-obese individuals caused a slight decrease in serum cholesterol concentrations of 9·7 % by the end of the first month but only a slight further decline during the remaining five months in this experiment. On the other hand, serum β-lipoprotein levels fell rapidly, reaching a mean of 12·6 % below baseline at one month and subsequently declined further to 17·3 % below the initial mean level at the end of the sixth month. Among eight individuals with type II disorder the cholesterol level decreased 13·3 % whereas the β-lipoprotein level decreased 20·5 %. This indicates a greater reponsiveness of the β-lipoproteins to dietary changes compared to serum cholesterol concentrations. The following three personal observations are added to clarify some of the problems involved in the dietary treatment of patients with hyperlipoproteinaemia type II.

*First Case Report* (Fig. 3)

J.B.P., a 53-year-old physician came to our clinic on 3/4/70 grossly obese. His weight was 92 kg (202 lb); his height was 175 cm. The lipoprotein analysis showed β-lipoprotein increased, pre-β-lipoprotein increased, hypercholesterolaemia—336 mg % and hypertriglyceridaemia—335 mg %. The data were consistent with hyperlipoproteinaemia type II. On 6/4/70, three months after the initial diagnosis, the weight had been reduced by 16 kg (36 lb) and the lipoprotein analysis revealed pre-β-lipoprotein still increased. β-Lipoproteins were normal, cholesterol—250 mg %, triglycerides—normal with 118 mg %. On 9/11/70, the β-lipoproteins and pre-β-lipoproteins were reported as "normal" although cholesterol was again increased to 310 mg %, triglycerides stayed normal with 120 mg %. At this third examination, the weight had been reduced to 68 kg and a seasonal effect on the cholesterol level must be taken into account with a lower level in June and an increase again during the fall.

After normalization of his weight to 67 kg (147 lb) the patient was reexamined on 11/24/70. The β-lipoprotein and pre-β-lipoprotein again were reported "normal"; the cholesterol remained elevated at 330 mg % whereas the triglycerides had further decreased to 85 mg%. The last lipid analysis was done in March, 1972. With weight maintenance at 67 kg (147 lb) the $\beta$-lipoproteins and pre-$\beta$-lipoproteins were again reported "normal"; serum cholesterol still elevated with 280 mg% and triglycerides normal with 83 mg%.

The clinical significance of the apparent reversal from hyper-$\beta$-lipoproteinaemia to a "normal" lipoprotein pattern, as judged by electrophoresis, reported from two different laboratories, remains

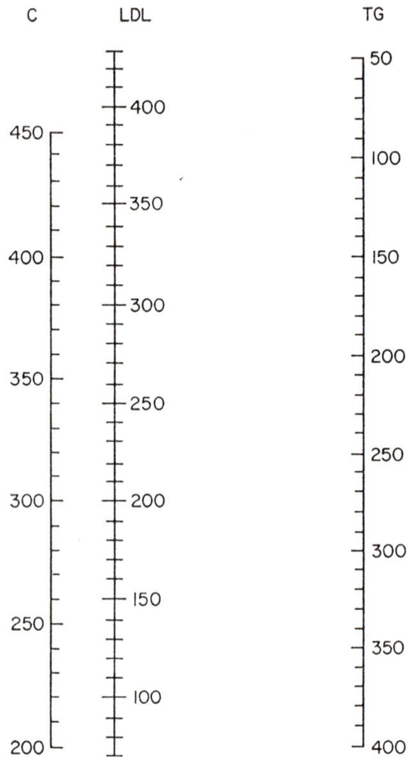


Fig. 2. Nomogram for estimation of plasma LDL concentration (in terms of mg/100 ml of cholesterol in this lipoprotein). This was derived from the equation LDL = C − (TG/5 + HDL) where HDL is assumed to be 45. (Fredrickson and Levy, 1972; Fredrickson, 1972.)

dubious in view of the abnormal low density lipoprotein according to the nomogram recommended by Dr Fredrickson (see Fig. 2). From the dietary standpoint, no further decrease of the cholesterol serum concentration can be expected while continuation of the low-carbohydrate and restricted-fat diet will guarantee the maintenance of a normal triglyceride level in the serum. The cholesterol in the food is limited to

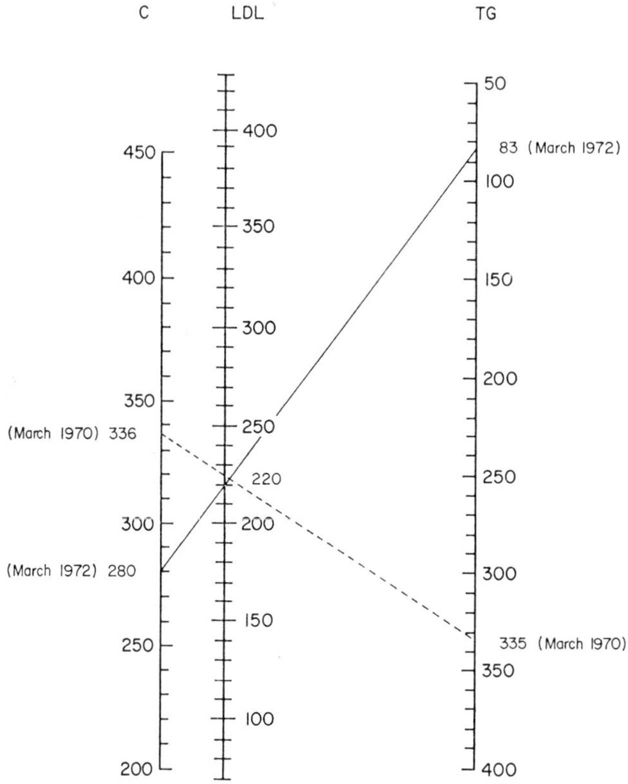


Fig. 3. First case report: Dr J.B.P. aged 53. Low density or $\beta$-lipoproteins are practically unchanged between March, 1970 and March, 1972. The desirable levels are 220 mg% or less for cholesterol and 140 mg% or less for triglycerides, connected with an LDL of 140–170. During weight reduction, the excess VLDL was metabolized to LDL which disappears more slowly. Technically, this represents a conversion from type IIb to type IIa.

less than 300 mg, the calories derived from fat amounts to 35% of the caloric intake and a major portion of it consists of polyunsaturated fatty acids.

*Second Case Report* (Fig. 6)

Mr A.L., aged 57 years (height 182 cm, weight 127 kg: 280 lb) came on 1/6/72 for the treatment of severe essential hypertension (on several occasions 190/110 and 180/130 for the past 10 years). At the age of 17 years his weight had been normal at 74 kg (162 lb).

Within two months, his blood pressure dropped under weight reduction to 150/115, 145/100, 140/95, 135/95, 142/92, 138/90, 134/88, 128/86 mmHg after losing 26 kg (58 lb). On 3/6/72 his weight was 109 kg (222 lb), on 5/29/72, 87 kg (192 lb), remaining at this level until 2/5/73.

Lipid electrophoresis prior to the start of the weight reduction programme on 1/6/72 revealed hyperlipoproteinaemia, type II. This normalization was aided by adhering to a 700 calorie diet consisting of 25 g fat, 60 g carbohydrates and 60 g protein. Weight reduction was aided by weekend fasting from Friday night until Monday morning permitting only non-caloric liquids ad libitum.

Lipoprotein analysis

| | 1/6/72 | 3/6/72 | 5/29/72 | 2/5/73 |
|---|---|---|---|---|
| Cholesterol, total | 358 | 249 | 253 | 220 |
| Triglycerides | 100 | 180 | 112 | 113 |
| Serum observation | clear | clear | clear | clear |
| Chylomicrons | absent | absent | absent | absent |
| β-Lipoprotein | increased | normal | normal | normal |
| Pre-β-lipoprotein | normal | normal | normal | normal |
| α-Lipoprotein | normal | normal | normal | normal |
| Data consistent with phenotype | II | normal | normal | normal |

Lipoprotein analysis

| | Results |
|---|---|
| Cholesterol, total | 358 |
| Triglycerides | 100 |
| Serum observation | CLEAR |
| Lipoprotein electrophoresis | |
| CHYLOMICRONS | ABSENT |
| BETA LIPOPROTEIN | INCREASED |
| PRE-BETA LIPOPROTEIN | NORMAL |
| ALPHA LIPOPROTEIN | NORMAL |
| Data consistent with phenotype according to Fredrickson | II |

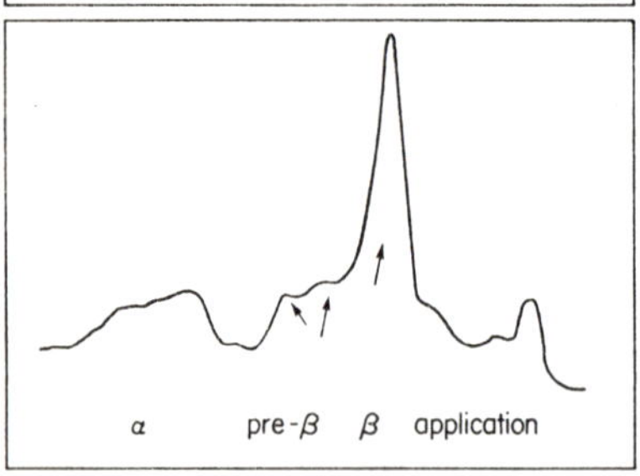


Fig. 4.

Lipoprotein analysis

| | Results |
|---|---|
| Cholesterol, total | 249 |
| Triglycerides | 180 |
| Serum observation | CLEAR |
| Lipoprotein electrophoresis | |
| CHYLOMICRONS | ABSENT |
| BETA LIPOPROTEIN | NORMAL |
| PRE-BETA LIPOPROTEIN | NORMAL |
| ALPHA LIPOPROTEIN | NORMAL |
| Data consistent with phenotype according to Fredrickson | NORMAL |

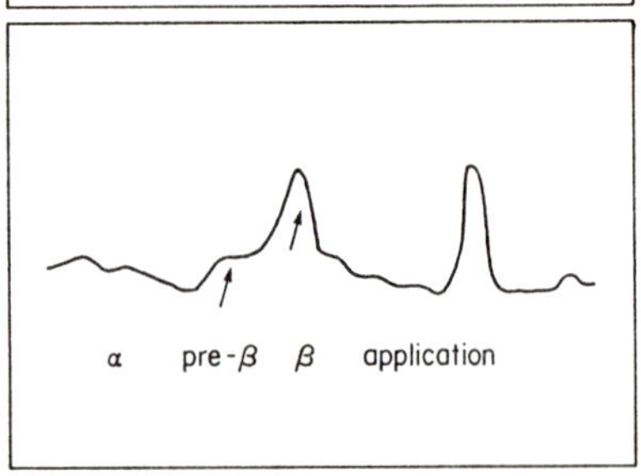


Fig. 5.

The patient frequently ate fish and chicken in larger quantities and therefore on several days each week would eat only approximately half the amount of fat permitted (15 g) and instead increase his protein intake from 60–100 g.

His total intake, however, would never exceed 735 calories per day (100 g protein = 400 calories). The remarkable reversal from a highly abnormal lipoprotein pattern to a normal lipid electrophoresis (see Figs 4 and 5) within the short period of two months is most unusual. The nomogram according to Fredrickson showed a normal low density protein after the weight became normal (see Fig. 6).

Weight maintenance and strict adherence to a 1600 kCal diet, with polyunsaturated fatty acids amounting to $>10\%$ of his total caloric intake, resulted in a further drop of the cholesterol concentration to a normal level (Feb. 1973).

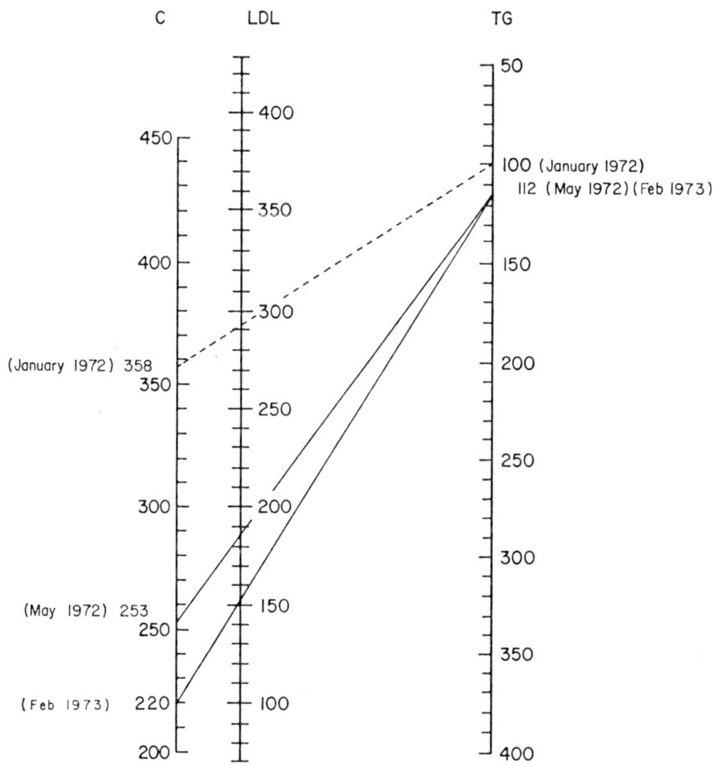


Fig. 6. Second case report: Mr A.L. aged 57. After 40 kg (90 lb) weight loss, LDL decreased from 292 to 185 within five months, after one year LDL was normal.

*Third Case Report* (Fig. 7)

Mrs M.G., aged 44 years, had known about her hypercholesterolaemia for many years and had been treated with thyroid medication for 24 years and, in addition, with nicotinic acid for one year. Since she had developed rhythm abnormalities shown by ECGs we discontinued the thyroid medication. The nicotinic acid was stopped because it had no apparent effect on her cholesterol level. Since the age of 20 she had gained approximately 31 kg (68 lb) and her present weight of 84 kg (184 lb) was regarded as at least 21 kg (46 lb) overweight (12/2/70).

The lipoprotein analysis revealed cholesterol—315 mg%, triglycerides—280 mg%, β-lipoproteins increased and the pre-β-lipoproteins increased, consistent with phenotype II. Within five months, the weight was lowered to 64 kg (141 lb) and the triglycerides decreased to 80 mg%. The cholesterol level

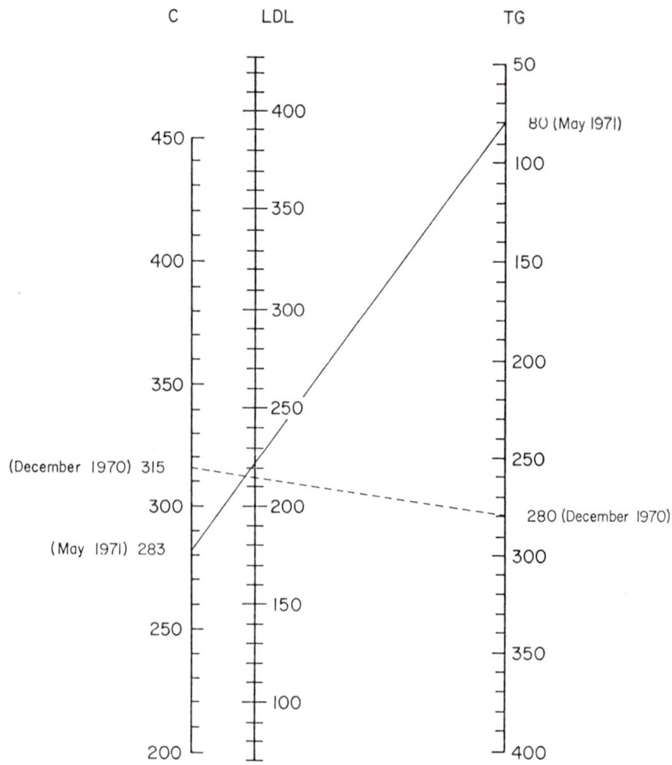


Fig. 7. Third case report: Mrs M.G. aged 44. LDL remained practically unchanged although cholesterol decreased slightly and triglycerides became normalized after 19 kg (42 lb) weight loss.

had only slightly decreased to 283 mg% (5/1/71). However, the possibly misleading electrophoretic finding, which was again confirmed at a later lipid electrophoresis on 7/26/71, was that β-lipoproteins were "normal", pre-β-lipoproteins were normal and the data were consistent on both occasions with a "normal phenotype". With the weight reduction of 19 kg (42 lb) and adherence to a diet low in fat and extremely low in cholesterol (less than 200 mg), the abnormal phenotype II supposedly had changed into a "normal pattern". The decrease in the serum cholesterol concentration between December 1970 and summer of 1971 could be solely explained by the seasonal changes. One must keep in mind, however, the presently used method of analysing lipid patterns. According to the nomogram by Dr Fredrickson the patient has not changed the $\beta$-lipoprotein level at all (see Fig. 7).

## VII. PRIMARY PREVENTION OF ISCHEMIC HEART DISEASE

1. The primary prevention of ischemic heart disease with dietary intervention has been investigated by a Finnish medical team (Turpeinen *et al.*, 1971). Three hundred and thirteen mental patients without overt ischemic heart disease, in one mental institution, were treated with a diet low in cholesterol, high in polyunsaturated fatty acid, whereas mental patients in another hospital were used as control persons without dietary intervention. Among the 313 dieters without ECG evidence of ischemic heart disease, 17 developed such evidence* (annual incidence rate per 1000 was 14·4). Among 241 control persons without evidence of ischemic heart disease by ECG, a total of 30 developed ischemic heart disease* (annual incidence rate per 1000 was 33·0). The difference in new development of ischemic heart disease in the two groups was significant with $P < {\cdot}01$. The first study lasted from 1958 to 1965. In March 1965, the study protocol called for a switch-over in the experiment, changing the control hospital into the experimental hospital with dietary intervention and leaving the mental patients in the former experimental hospital as controls. Cholesterol levels decreased immediately in the new experimental hospital and increased in the control hospital with a difference of 30 mg %. By 1971, more cases of ischemic heart disease were diagnosed by ECG in the control hospital than in the experimental hospital but at that point in time, the number of new cases was still too small to reach a statistically significant difference (see also p. 322).

2. The Anti-Coronary Club in New York was initiated in 1957, inventing the Prudent Diet with a P/S ratio 1·25–1·50 (usual American Diet P/S ratio 0·3/0·4), 400 mg dietary cholesterol, total fat intake 33 % and 1·6 g dietary sodium. Archer (reported by Stamler, 1971) recorded in 1969 the incidence of new coronary events: during the 3954 person-years of active experience, accumulated by the 941 experimental subjects, 37 new coronary events occurred. This represents an overall incidence rate of 6·8 per 1000 person-years of experience. The 457 men of the control group, in comparable age categories, have accumulated 3122 person-years of experience and 51 new coronary events, resulting in an age-adjusted incidence of 13·4 per 1000 person-years of experience.

* This includes deaths from coronary heart disease (CHD).

Interestingly, an inactive experimental group (532 men) evolved, shifting from active to inactive status. The observed incidence rate was 7·8 per 1000 person-years of experience, representing 42 new coronary events, predictably a rate between the active experimental and the control group. Total observation time was 12 years.

As expected by the lower total fat intake and the rather drastic restriction of dietary sodium, the number of obese subjects and hypertensive subjects in the experimental group declined at the same time when the main thrust was lowering of cholesterol levels (Rinzler, 1968). After four years of observation, the percentage of obese persons in the experimental group declined from 56% to 18%, the percentage, of hypertensives from 26% to 10%. In contrast, the control group had 45% obese at entry and after four years still 44%. Among the control persons, 11% were hypertensive at entry into the study and after four years 13% were hypertensive. Hypercholesterolaemia (260 mg% or more) was found among 43% of the experimental group at entry and declined to 20% after four years. In the control group, 38% were defined as hypercholesterolaemics and after four years, 32% still belonged to this group. After initial weight reduction, the maintenance diet contained 23% protein, 47% carbohydrates, 30% fat, less than 300 mg cholesterol.

3. The only dietary study under double blind conditions was conducted in an elderly male population, living at a Veterans' Administration Centre in Los Angeles (Pearce and Dayton, 1971). In an eight-year controlled clinical trial of a diet high in polyunsaturated vegetable oils and low in saturated fat and cholesterol, 846 men were assigned randomly to a conventional diet (422) or to one similar in all respects, except for a substitution of vegetable oils for saturated fat (424). Fatal atherosclerotic events were more common in the control group (70 versus 48; $P<0·05$). It is noteworthy that in Leren's dietary trial and in the second report from the British Medical Research Council (1968) no difference was found in the rates of sudden death between experimental dietary and control groups, whereas sudden death in this Veterans' Administration Study was observed in 27 controls and in 18 men of the dietary group. Also, cerebral infarction occurred more often in controls: 22 versus 13. However, total mortality was similar in the two groups: 178 controls versus 174 "dieters" demonstrating an excess of non-atherosclerotic deaths in the experimental group.

The conclusions of these authors concerning the potential co-carcinogenic influence of this type of dietary changes will be discussed in a later section.

4. A preliminary analysis of the results after seven years of dietary intervention in the Chicago Coronary Prevention Evaluation Program

(C.P.E.P.) in 519 men aged 40–59 years with several risk factors but free of ischemic heart disease, was presented by Stamler (1971). It is important to note that other risk factors such as hypertension, obesity, cigarette smoking and physical inactivity, besides hypercholesterolaemia, were influenced at the same time—a multiple risk factor intervention. Among 377 men at high risk who adhered to a low-fat, low-cholesterol diet, a seven year cumulative age corrected coronary mortality rate of 5 per 1000 was found (2 CHD deaths occurred among 377 adherers). The same analysis revealed an age adjusted coronary mortality rate of 27 per 1000 among the 142 drop-outs (4 actual cases within the same observation period).

The *coronary mortality* rates of adherers and drop-outs were compared with 2916 men from the "Pooling Project", matched for age, medical and risk factor criteria. The Pooling Project combines the experience of six prospective long-term epidemiological studies of 6640 middle-aged (30–59 years old) men over a ten-year period, i.e. followed without intervention. The coronary mortality rate was 20/1000 (59 actual cases), i.e. similar as the rate of the drop-outs. The rates for sudden death were 2/1000 among C.P.E.P. adherers, 10/1000 among drop-outs and 15/1000 among matched men from the Pooling Project. Death rates combined from all causes were recorded: 27/1000, 36/1000 and 50/1000, respectively.

The author concluded:

> "For 377 continuing active participants in the C.P.E.P. . . . total mortality at seven years is 46% lower compared with the experience of 2916 Pooling Project men; CHD mortality and sudden death mortality are 75% and 86% *lower*, respectively."

These primary prevention studies—the New York Anti-Coronary Club, the Finnish Mental Hospital Study and the Chicago Coronary Prevention Evaluation Program, with the exception of the Los Angeles Veterans' Administration Domiciliary Center Study—have not been designed as double blind group studies and are, therefore open to criticism. But the combined findings indicate that change in living habits, particularly diet, is associated with decreased incidence or mortality, or both, from ischemic heart disease.

## VIII. SECONDARY PREVENTION OF ISCHEMIC HEART DISEASE

1. The first dietary intervention study for patients with myocardial infarction (MI) was conducted by Lyon *et al.* (1956). One hundred and fifty-five patients adhered to a low-fat, low-cholesterol regimen

(a maximum of 50 g fat, 200 mg cholesterol per day) whereas 125 patients without dietary intervention were followed. Both groups had comparable β-lipoprotein levels at the onset of the study. Diet intervention caused a significant decrease in these β-lipoprotein levels, whereas no change occurred in the control group.

The treatment lasted three years and eight months in the experimental group, with 15 re-infarctions, in contrast to 51 re-infarctions in the control group followed for four years and two months. After an average follow-up period of about four years the treated group had a statistically significant lower fatality rate: 2·6 versus 10·0 % mortality rate due to recurrent myocardial infarction.

Several authors have criticized that the investigators failed to give any information concerning the criteria of admission to the study, the criteria for the diagnosis of re-infarction and for the methods of judging adherence to the diet (Oliver, 1966; Stamler, 1967). While it is true that in the 1970s a study without this additional information would not be acceptable to medical journals it should be remembered that, back in 1956, somebody had to first conceive the idea of dietary therapy. It is felt that this pioneer work definitely has its place in the history of dietary intervention trials.

2. Another secondary prevention trial was reported during the same year (1956, and last report 1965) by Nelson, with a follow-up of 88 diet-adhering and 154 non-dieting patients with myocardial infarction (a total of 100 patients with previous MI were forced to eat in restaurants and were, therefore, unable to follow the dietary instructions and 54 patients did not adhere to the diet). These two groups, 100 and 54 patients (mean age 58) were used as controls to the 88 patients (mean age 56) adhering and responding to the diet—50–60 g fat/day with emphasis on polyunsaturated fatty acid intake with cholesterol levels decreasing (in two-thirds of diet-adherers, the serum cholesterol concentration was lowered more than 10 %). No objection can be raised to the use of non-adherers as controls, since the two groups were comparable in age, sex, heart size, ECG abnormalities and patients with normalized ECG.

In the experimental treatment group, only 31 CHD deaths occurred during 10–13 years of observation (mortality of 35 %). In contrast, the mortality from atherosclerotic heart disease in the control group was much higher: 122 (=79 %). Thus at the end of the 10–13 years of observation period, 57 of the 88 diet-adherers and 32 of the 154 non-adherers were still alive.

3. Morrison (1960) used the same approach, a low-Wat, low-cholester diet containing about 1600 calories daily with 20–25 g fat and 50–70 mg cholesterol, 225 g carbohydrates, 120 g protein for 50 patients with

myocardial infarction. It is necessary to remind oneself that the increased use of polyunsaturated fatty acid in dietary therapy was introduced only in the late 1950s and had not been common knowledge among all investigators at that time. However, this approach of a low-fat, low-cholesterol diet, again, led to a sizeable decrease in serum cholesterol concentrations from a mean of 312 mg % to 220 mg %.

Likewise, total lipids and neutral fats declined markedly. Unfortunately, a few uncooperative patients were dropped from the original treatment group and new cases were added, possibly introducing a degree of bias.

The mortality experience was quite different from that of a control group of 50 patients who were left with their own dietary habits. After eight years, survival rates were 56 % for the treatment group and 24 % for the control group. After 12 years, the mortality was 62 % in the dietary group and 100 % in the control group. Oliver (1966) objected to the study design and execution since there was a marked weight reduction in the treatment group and no weight loss in the control series. Furthermore, he criticized that the study was not conducted in a double blind fashion and the degree of surveillance of the treatment group was greater than that for the control group. We feel that it was just this particular aspect, the intensive guidance through a dietary programme for the 50 patients in the experimental group which led to the success not only in the most important aim, the reduction in mortality compared to a control group, but also in the other objective measurements—weight loss and decrease in cholesterol levels. If the control group had been followed similarly with some dietary control, they too would have lost weight and they might also have decreased cholesterol levels and would not have constituted a control group as such. Studies conducted under double blind procedures are extremely expensive and are hard to manage in the free-living population. Even in an institutionalized population group as observed by Dayton and co-workers (1969b), a sizeable proportion of the experimental group did not adhere to the dietary intervention.

4. For three years, Koranyi (1963) followed survivors of myocardial infarction who were treated with a low-fat diet (35–40 g per day) and control patients without dietary restrictions. The serum lipids were not measured but the mortality after three years of observation showed marked differences: 8·6 % in the dietary group and 19·7 % in the control group.

5. Hood *et al.* (1965) from Sweden reported a retrospective study over a 17-year observation period. A group of 112 patients with previous myocardial infarction or angina pectoris or with essential hypercholesterolaemia was compared with a control group. The 112 control

patients were matched by sex, age, blood pressure, degree of vascular symptoms and cholesterol levels. In the control group there had been either none, minor, or inconsistent dietary alterations. Both groups consisted of 61 women and 51 men.

The management of the treated group incorporated a low-fat, low-cholesterol diet with the addition of 50–60 g of oils high in polyunsaturated fatty acids. Mean serum cholesterol concentrations were reduced by 20% in the diet group and 6% in the control group in women. Among the dieters, four women died and among the control group 18 women died during the observation period. The favourable mortality experience in females was also observed in males. There were 21 males in the diet group who previously had a myocardial infarction and two of them died. Of the 21 males with myocardial infarction in the control group, 12 died. However, the mean serum cholesterol concentration decrement in the diet group was only 7%, whereas in the control group it was 14%. There is no apparent explanation for the discrepancy in the findings among male and female patients as far as cholesterol levels are concerned.

6. A study by Leren (1970) in Norway dealt with 412 men, aged 30–64 years, randomized into two groups one to two years after their first myocardial infarction. For the experimental group a diet low in saturated fats and cholesterol (264 mg/day) and high in polyunsaturated fats (soyabean oil) was recommended. Fat comprised 39% of the total calories and contained 55 g (52·7%) polyunsaturated fatty acid and 22 g (21·6%) saturated fatty acid with a P/S value of 2·4. After five years the incidence of fatal and non-fatal myocardial reinfarction was found to be significantly reduced. Sudden death was uninfluenced. Major coronary heart disease relapses, including fatal and non-fatal events (myocardial infarction), were significantly less ($P = 0{\cdot}05$) among the 206 men placed under dietary management compared to the control group.

After 11 years, death from all causes had occurred in 101 of the original dieters and 108 controls. A significantly reduced myocardial infarction mortality in the original diet group was found (32 versus 57, $P = 0{\cdot}004$). The total number of coronary deaths (fatal myocardial infarction and sudden death) was 79 in the diet group and 94 in the control group ($P = 0{\cdot}097$).

The CHD mortality was correlated with age, serum cholesterol level, blood pressure, body weight, smoking habits, and a combination of these risk factors. When combining data from both groups, a three-fold greater CHD mortality rate was demonstrable among the hyper-cholesterolaemic, hypertensive smokers than among those in whom these factors were low or absent.

7. Bierenbaum *et al.* (1973) presented data of a 10-year observation

period with dietary therapy. One hundred men, 30–50 years old, with documented coronary artery disease and past myocardial infarction, were placed under dietary management with a 28% of cal. fat diet. One hundred men whose diets were not managed were matched with regard to age at entry to the study, age at infarction, number of infarctions, blood pressure level, degree of angina, and serum cholesterol level among other factors. Over a period of five years the diet-managed group experienced and maintained a significant reduction in serum cholesterol level which the non-diet-managed group did not.

> "Over a period of 10 years there were significant reductions in serum-lipids in the diet-managed group compared with the control group. In this predominantly lipoprotein-phenotype IV group, using a diet containing less than 9% of calories as saturated fats and less than 400 mg exogenous cholesterol daily, the degree of unsaturation of the diet did not appear to influence either serum–lipid values or mortality rates. After 10 years, the diet-managed group had a 17% greater survival-rate than the control group (in comparison to the control group $P<0{\cdot}05$!). This is especially true of the younger men, who were under 45 years when they entered the study. In this under 45-group, incidence was over twice as high in the control group as in the study group. Even in the over-45 group, the incidence in the control group was one-third higher than in the study group . . . Dietary change instituted after 45 may still be beneficial."

The authors repeatedly mention the importance of weight reduction in the study group. After weight normalization, the study group was on approximately 2000 calories, 20·4% derived from protein (102 g), 27·8% derived from fat (61·8 g) and 51·8% from carbohydrates. It seems particularly remarkable that all individuals in this study were followed up for 10 years. No subject was lost to the study for any reason except death. To enable the men to adhere more easily to the prescribed diet for protracted periods, specially prepared frozen dinners, including pies, and ice-cream substitute, and oil, were obtained from a project store at reduced prices.

The following four studies constitute the only dietary intervention trials in the world literature which did not demonstrate the influence of dietary intervention: they were all conducted in England. The first was a four-year study of patients with myocardial infarction; after three years of treatment with corn oil (60 g daily) the "cholesterol level decreasing effect became weaker". The mortality rate among 28 patients within two years was 14·3% which was reportedly slightly higher than in a control group of male patients also with myocardial infarctions under anticoagulant therapy (Watson, 1963).

The second study (with dietary intervention) (Rose *et al.*, 1965) lasted only two years and was conducted in three small groups (28, 26 and 26 patients). An 80 g "oil cocktail" was given daily which, in many patients, led to the discontinuation of oil intake because of development of diarrhoea, nausea and distaste. The experimental group was placed on corn oil, the control group on olive oil and the second control group was left without advice on dietary fats.

Of the 28 patients in the corn oil supplemented diet group, 52% remained free of re-infarctions after two years. Of the 26 patients in the olive oil supplemented control group, 57% remained free of reinfarction and of the 26 patients in the second control group without dietary intervention, 75% remained free of re-infarctions. The interpretation by the investigators was that under the

> "circumstances of this trial, corn oil cannot be recommended as a treatment of ischemic heart disease; it is most unlikely to be beneficial, and it is possibly harmful."

This conclusion is not warranted from a short-term investigation with such small numbers of patients involved. There is no question that the statistical design of the study was sound. However, the only conclusion permissible is that it was a valuable pilot study for a future project, employing a different method of application of the use of oils in cooking and baking, as well as enlarging the number of subjects to be studied.

During the same year (1965) the British Medical Research Council published the results of a study of 252 patients with myocardial infarction (123 in the dietary group and 129 control patients without dietary therapy). The follow-up extended from 1957 through 1963. Already after one year, the cholesterol levels in the experimental group and the control group were no longer significantly different. The patients in the control group, without dietary advice, may have been influenced by the general trend in public education programmes and decreased their fat consumption. The method of this experimental design must have encouraged the control patients to pay more attention to their dietary habits since all patients, including the controls, had to record the foods eaten during the first seven weeks on a certain day each week and later always on the first day of each month, including weighing foods to be consumed. In addition, regular interviews of dietary habits were conducted and the weight was measured.

After five years, the final results were not different in the two groups: the experimental group experienced (among 123 patients) 46 re-infarctions and 10 deaths from myocardial infarction. Among the control group (129 patients), 48 experienced re-infarctions and 12 died of myocardial infarction.

The fourth study in male patients under the age of 60, again conducted by the British Medical Research Council (1968) also used "oil cocktails" (43 g daily plus 42 g of soyabean oil for cooking). Among the 199 patients in the dietary experimental group cholesterol levels decreased from a mean of 272 mg % to 213mg %. Sixty-two men had a re-infarction (31 %). The 194 patients in the control group, without dietary advice, showed cholesterold level decreases from a mean of 273 mg% to 259 mg%, 74 patients had re-infarctions (38 %).

The authors expressed surprise that their results did not show the same beneficial effect of a diet low in cholesterol, high in polyunsaturated fatty acid in the treatment of patients with myocardial infarction as had been reported by Dr Leren from Oslo. The main difference in the selection of patients was that the Norwegian patients had stabilized their myocardial infarction according to the study protocol at least 20 months prior to entry into the study. In contrast, the British study admitted patients after an average of 36 days following the acute event. It is well known that the re-infarction rate is highest during the first year and diminishes progressively during subsequent years. Another difference between the two studies is that less than 50 % of the patients in London continued the experiment for four years whereas all patients in Oslo adhered to the regime for five years, except, of course, those who died. Therefore, a great number of patients in London were unable to possibly benefit from the long-term use of polyunsaturated fatty acids as was the case in the Oslo study. This last report by the British Research Committee (1968) concluded:

> "There is no indication that this type of diet affects mortality. The combined evidence, however, suggests that a proportion of non-fatal re-infarctions might be prevented, though more evidence is required to confirm this effect."

In view of the cancer mortality reported from the study by Pearce and Dayton (1971) it is interesting to note that in the experimental dietary group after seven years of observation one cancer occurred (= 0·5 %) whereas six cases of fatal carcinoma were observed in the control group (3 %)—another proof that the long-term use of polyunsaturated fatty acid diets is most unlikely to cause or favour carcinogenesis.

## IX. THE PRESENT SITUATION IN THE COMMUNITY OF EVANS COUNTY (U.S.A.)

After countless clinical studies and investigations under metabolic ward conditions showing unequivocally positive results of a diet low in cholesterol, high in polyunsaturated fatty acid in lowering cholesterol levels, the major concern at this time is how to bring about the decrease of serum cholesterol levels in the community. We have investigated this problem during seven to nine years of observation in the Evans County Study in Georgia. Many epidemiologic studies have been concerned with the relationship of hypercholesterolaemia to the development of ischemic heart disease based on the level of hypercholesterolaemia at the intake examination. Relatively little attention has been directed towards epidemiologic study of those individuals in the community who had elevated baseline serum cholesterol concentrations and who subsequently have decreased to normal values.

The purpose of our study in Evans County was two-fold. The first was to define the percentage of people in the total population examined twice (1960–62 and 1967–69) who significantly decreased their cholesterol level. The second goal was to investigate the possible relationship between decreases of cholesterol level and changes in dietary habits in persons remaining free of vascular disease.

Cholesterol levels were determined during *both* examinations in a total of 2272 persons. Of these 1507 were white, 711 white males and 796 white females. The black sample consisted of a total of 765 persons: 321 black males and 444 black females. This sample white to black ratio represents the racial distribution of the total community very closely.

Hypercholesterolaemia was arbitrarily defined as a level of 240 mg/100 ml or above. Changes in cholesterol levels were compared from the intake examinations (1960–62) to the second round of examinations (1967–69). Significant decreases were defined as those occurring in persons who had a baseline serum cholesterol concentration of 240 mg/100 ml or higher which in 1967 had decreased at least 40 mg/100 ml. Persons with decreases of serum cholesterol concentrations were matched for race, sex and age ($\pm$3 years) with control individuals who either remained at their baseline level or had increased levels.

We interviewed each healthy person with significant decreases who remained free of heart disease or strokes, and one control person in order to evaluate reasons for decreases. There were only two refusals. A small number of people had migrated but were known to be alive and healthy. Interviews were conducted in the homes. The questionnaire comprised 26 items, covering major changes in the person's diet between the first and second examination (1960–62 and 1967–69). Medication as a factor in lowering cholesterol levels could be dismissed. We were interested mainly in dietary habits and particularly in changes in the consumption of visible fat and types of meat.

As will be seen, only a few subjects actually decreased cholesterol levels to a significant degree and remained free of vascular diseases.

## A. Results

Hypercholesterolaemia (≥240 mg/100 ml) at the baseline examination was found almost twice as frequently in females as in males of both races, i.e. 19 % in white males but 31 % in white females and 13 % in black males but 23 % in black females (Table 2).

Table 2

Distribution of cholesterol ≥240 mg/100 ml by age in race–sex groups, 1960–62

| | White males | | White females | | Black males | | Black females | |
|---|---|---|---|---|---|---|---|---|
| Age (yr) | Par | Cases | Par | Cases | Par | Cases | Par | Cases |
| 15–24 | 118 | 2 | 108 | 2 | 81 | 0 | 91 | 3 |
| 25–34 | 109 | 15 | 110 | 11 | 43 | 3 | 54 | 2 |
| 35–44 | 167 | 35 | 189 | 43 | 79 | 11 | 111 | 18 |
| 45–54 | 259 | 61 | 239 | 79 | 171 | 33 | 167 | 45 |
| 55–64 | 175 | 42 | 182 | 93 | 89 | 13 | 129 | 44 |
| 65–74 | 110 | 25 | 131 | 71 | 68 | 10 | 90 | 32 |
| 75+ | 9 | 3 | 13 | 6 | 6 | 2 | 4 | 2 |
| TOTAL | 947 | 183 | 972 | 305 | 537 | 72 | 646 | 146 |

Per cent with cholesterol ≥ 240 mg/100 ml

| Age (yr) | White males | White females | Black males | Black females |
|---|---|---|---|---|
| 15–24 | 1·7 | 1·9 | 0 | 3·3 |
| 25–34 | 13·8 | 10·0 | 7·0 | 3·7 |
| 35–44 | 21·0 | 22·8 | 13·9 | 16·2 |
| 45–54 | 23·6 | 33·1 | 19·3 | 26·9 |
| 55–64 | 24·0 | 51·1 | 14·6 | 34·1 |
| 65–74 | 22·7 | 54·2 | 14·7 | 35·6 |
| 75+ | 33·3 | 46·2 | 33·3 | 50·0 |
| TOTAL | 19·3 | 31·4 | 13·4 | 22·6 |

For white males there is a steady increase in percentage of hypercholesterolaemic individuals up to the age of 55–64 years followed by a slight decrease in the age group 65–74. For white females there is a sharp increase in the prevalence of hypercholesterolaemia at age of menopause (at the ages of 45–54 years, the prevalence is higher than in males of the same age) and a further increase of hypercholesterolaemic subjects after menopause (twice as many females as males of the same age group). For black males except at the age of 45–54 years, there is no sizeable increase in percentage of hypercholesterolaemic subjects at each age. There is a higher prevalence of hypercholesterolaemia in the white than the black with increasing age. The age relationship for black females is similar to that among white persons.

In view of the known relationship of incidence of ischemic heart disease and hypercholesterolaemia in general, the lowering of cholesterol levels was, of course, considered of potential benefit. Fifty-seven white males and females with hypercholesterolaemia in 1960 died prior to re-examination. Of 458 white male and female survivors with hypercholesterolaemia (as defined at the baseline examination) and re-examination in 1967–69, only 34 showed a decrease of cholesterol levels ≥40 mg/100 ml and were found free of vascular disease. An additional 23 persons (5%) also had a decrease of cholesterol levels but were diagnosed with vascular disease. It is interesting to note, therefore, that of the total white population with hypercholesterolaemia only 7·4% had significant reductions in serum cholesterol concentrations and were healthy after an average 87-month period.

Among the black males and females, 24 individuals with hypercholesterolaemia died prior to re-examination. Of the 196 survivors with hypercholesterolaemia, only nine persons (5·6%) had a decrease in cholesterol levels ≥40 mg/100 ml during the same observation time. In 1967 through 1969 an additional nine black persons (5·6%) also had a decrease of cholesterol levels but were diagnosed as having vascular disease. Table 3 shows the status of the subjects in August of 1970 when an attempt was made to locate all persons with decreases of serum cholesterol level for interviews.

In the hope of eliciting reasons for lowering of cholesterol levels in the general community (where no drug intervention or any other effort had

Table 3

All persons with hypercholesterolaemia (≥240 mg/100 ml) at intake examination who survived to the second examination and whose cholesterol values decreased ≥40 mg/100 ml

| Status, August 1970 | 57 Whites | 18 Blacks |
|---|---|---|
| Vascular disease | 23 | 9 |
| Migration, alive and well | 6 | 1 |
| Interviewed, alive and well | 27 | 7 |
| Not interviewed, alive and well | 1 | 1 |

been directed toward hypercholesterolaemia) we examined the dietary habits among this group (Table 4).

To make the dietary interview meaningful, control persons with high cholesterol levels who either had remained hypercholesterolaemic or

Table 4

Dietary changes—comparison of subjects with decreased cholesterol levels and controls with increased serum cholesterol concentrations[a]

| Hypercholesterolaemia | 27 White males and females | 27 Controls |
|---|---|---|
| Dietary changes | 25 (93%) | 17 (63%)[b] |
| Average no. of changes | 3 | 2 |
| Diabetes mellitus with dietary changes | 4 | 5 |
| Diabetes mellitus without dietary changes | 0 | 1 |
| Medication (thyroid hormones) | 4 | 1 |
| Gastrectomy | 1 | 0 |

[a] White subjects only.
[b] Probability significant at the 5% level.

increased further were asked the same questions. Quite marked differences in changes of dietary habits appeared between the "decreasers" (93%) and controls (63%) among whites, whereas numbers among blacks were too small to permit any conclusion. Specific dietary changes are enumerated in Table 5.

The table indicates that more than twice as many persons with decreases of cholesterol levels eliminated certain food items from their diets than persons whose cholesterol levels remained at the same level or increased. These changes are particularly interesting in view of the drastic cholesterol reductions among the 27 white persons interviewed. The mean level in 1960–62 was 293 mg/100 ml and in 1967–69, 220 mg/100 ml; the 27 control individuals started at a mean level of 260 mg/100 ml with a subsequent increase in 1967–69 to 289 mg/100 ml (+29 mg/100 ml).

Table 5
Number of individuals who changed dietary habits

| Food items eliminated | "Cholesterol decreasers" | "Cholesterol increasers" |
|---|---|---|
| Fried foods | 16/27 | 4/27 |
| Eggs | 11/27 | 4/27 |
| Hard fat | 10/27 | 5/27 |
| Desserts | 10/27 | 5/27 |
| Pork | 12/27 | 8/27 |

As expected, dietary changes were encountered mainly in diabetics with hypercholesterolaemia regardless of whether they belonged to the "decreasers" or to the controls: out of ten diabetics nine reported several alterations in dietary customs.

## B. Comment

McDonough *et al.* (1965) reported from the prevalence examination in Evans County that blacks "have significantly more calories in the diet" than whites, but that black males weighed less. "Significant differences were noted in animal fat intake", providing more saturated fatty acids and less linoleic acid in the average diet of blacks. In spite of these differences, the cholesterol levels in 1960–62 were significantly higher in whites. The re-examination in 1967–69 revealed essentially the same differences in dietary intake and again fewer black persons with high cholesterol levels than white persons, though not at a significant level.

The conclusion seems unavoidable that cholesterol levels are less influenced by the life-long fat intake among blacks and that once serum cholesterol concentrations are in the high range they do not carry the same high risk as in whites.

The causes of hypercholesterolaemia are still shrouded with uncertainties as to which are more important in an individual case, genetic or environmental (i.e. dietary) factors. However, the influence of diet on hypercholesterolaemia, e.g. dietary manipulation by reducing cholesterol intake and increasing polyunsaturated fatty acids is well documented and has been discussed previously. One purpose of this study was to find the possible effects of dietary influences on hypercholesterolaemic individuals in the community. The number of individuals free of vascular disease displaying a significant decrease of cholesterol levels was distressingly small, leaving only 27 white and 7 black individuals for analysis. It is felt that this small percentage of the hypercholesterolaemic segment of the total community becoming normocholesterolaemic

(7·4% whites, 5·6% blacks) is in itself interesting for the planning of future intervention studies.

As far as one can judge from the small numbers involved, changes in dietary customs among the white hypercholesterolaemic subjects who were interviewed might indeed have contributed to the significant reduction of the serum cholesterol level from an initial mean value of 293 mg/100 ml to a desirable mean value of 220 mg/100 ml. We were able to rule out seasonal variations. In only four cases was the first blood sample taken during the winter and the second during the summer. In all other cases, sampling time was identical as far as season is concerned and, therefore, reductions beyond 40 mg/100 ml as cut-off point in this study could not be explained by either seasonal variations nor by intra-individual changes which in reliable laboratories are reported to amount to between ±5 and ±20 mg/100 ml.

Age is another factor influencing cholesterol levels in the community. Generally speaking, after a steep increase of cholesterol levels from the age of 20 to 50 years, the serum cholesterol concentrations level off without further increase. This was shown in the prevalence study by McDonough *et al.* However, a decrease after the age of 50 to account for almost 70 mg/100 ml in the 27 white persons who were interviewed has not been reported in any population study. In addition it should be noted that these men and women were spread over the entire age range of the population.

The results of our study may lead one to ask whether it would be desirable or even necessary to change the dietary habits of the black community. We have documented definite overall changes in nutrition in Evans County with the preferential use of vegetable oil and margarine among the white community, whereas the black community still adheres to the traditional way of eating and heavy use of animal fat, in particular salt-rich bacon drippings and lard.

If neither the incidence of cerebrovascular disease nor the incidence of ischemic heart disease—as demonstrated in other publications from this study—is markedly influenced by the cholesterol concentration in the serum of blacks, one might well concentrate on other dietary aspects in blacks. Undoubtedly, the salt content of the diet among black men and women would be a more important target for intervention as a contributing factor in the control of hypertension. Likewise, among blacks the considerably higher carbohydrate and total caloric intake would require dietary advice among the large numbers of black women with decreased glucose tolerance. On the other hand, among whites the results from this study certainly are suggestive of the value of more wide spread use of dietary treatment of hypercholesterolaemia.

## X. THE OBLIGATION FOR THE FUTURE OF THE COMMUNITY

Epidemiologic research must now be converted into applied epidemiology on the community level. It seems significant to us that the American Heart Association and the National Heart and Lung Institute are the agencies who have alerted the medical profession and have given fresh impulses to the necessity for profound dietary changes in the American nutrition. Cardiologists and internists, nurses and physician's associates find themselves more and more in the role of health educators. The motivation of potential patients without causing anxiety, the education towards self-responsibility for one's own health without sounding evangelistic and the power of persuasion without overwhelming the patient with scientific facts, is an art. It is predictable that this art, in the years to come, will be a very important quality of the physician in the field of prevention of chronic diseases. Modern medicine is facing two major obligations with regard to hyperlipidaemia: firstly, the finding of asymptomatic patients in the community similar to the case finding of new diabetics and secondly, the motivation of these "healthy" individuals for long-term therapy.* The bridging of the gap between our capacity to treat hyperlipidaemias effectively and the presently insufficient and ineffective application of this knowledge is the task for the future. The National Heart and Lung Institute has recently issued a number of relevant questions to research institutions throughout the United States which we shall try to answer in the following sections.

### A. What Educational Programmes can be Developed for Individuals and Groups of Patients with Different Learning Abilities and Backgrounds

In my experience, the best results—regardless of learning ability and background—can be expected from a combination of individual instruction and group therapy. Individual instruction ideally includes family members. Group therapy alone does not seem to be very effective and group therapy in our use of the word should be limited to a free exchange between different members of the same peer group. Individual instruction must be maintained over a long period of time with regular weekly short meetings of ten minutes duration during which the dietary diary is being reviewed with the patient. In the past, many patients have expressed the desire for continuation of keeping a diary, although we felt they did not need to do so any longer. However, the psychological effect of checking one's own dietary intake must be recognized. Review of the diary does not take more than a few minutes. Patients who are

* See also Appendixes I and II of the introductory chapter (pp. 33 and 36).

unable to write are being taught to fill out a diary by simple drawings, e.g. fruits or in case they have used egg whites, drawing the number of eggs they have consumed. If the main dish is fish, a simple F will suffice, if chicken or pork C or P respectively.

We also gave patients, who were unable to write, a postage scale for weighing meat and fish portions. They were taught to watch for three numbers on the postage scale: 12 oz of Haddock fish equals approximately 6 oz of chicken or 3 oz of sirloin roast in caloric value. They were instructed to write these numbers, 12, 6 or 3, down in their diary and this way learn to judge by eyesight how much fish they could consume in comparison to pork or chicken. In summary, the most important part of the educational programme is an individualized regular teaching programme, whereas the free exchange among members of a peer group is of secondary importance. Each individual must be taught to fill out a dietary diary and to use a dietary scale.

In addition to giving out a one page table showing the cholesterol content of certain food items (see Table 6 for example) the dieters

Table 6

Cholesterol content (mg%) in $3\frac{1}{2}$ oz selected foods (limit of cholesterol intake per day: 300 mg)

| | | | |
|---|---|---|---|
| Dairy products | | Seafood | |
| Egg yolk ($3\frac{1}{2}$ oz) | 1400 | Oysters | 326 |
| Egg (1 yolk) | 300 | Caviar | 300 |
| Butter | 300 | Lobster | 208 |
| Cream | 140 | Crab | 145 |
| Cheddar cheese | 100 | Shrimp | 125 |
| Ice cream | 45 | Sardines | 70 |
| Whole milk (1 cup) | 35 | Salmon | 60 |
| Cottage cheese | 15 | Halibut | 60 |
| Skim milk (1 cup) | 1 | Herring | 58 |
| Egg white | 0 | Cod | 50 |
| | | Trout | 50 |
| Meats | | Miscellaneous | |
| Brains | 2000 | Vegetable oils | 0 |
| Liver | 250–600 | Margarine | 0 |
| Kidney | 400 | Cereals | 0 |
| Beef | 100 | Fruits | 0 |
| Pork | 100 | | |
| Veal | 90 | | |
| Chicken | 75 | | |
| Turkey | 75 | | |
| Lamb | 70 | | |

should be instructed, simply, how to limit the total intake of cholesterol to less than 300 mg per day, and to increase the polyunsaturated fatty acid intake to more than 10 % of the total caloric intake. A person with normal weight and a daily intake of 2000 calories, should consume at least 22 g polyunsaturated fatty acids in order to achieve the 10 % level of intake of polyunsaturated fatty acids. However, in a person who needs to reduce weight, e.g. on a 1000-calorie diet, the same prescription would give the patient 20 % of his total intake in the form of polyunsaturated fatty acid.

## B. How Can Patients be Stimulated to Follow Diet Modifications for Extended Periods of Time?

Any diet modification de-emphasizing animal fat but emphasizing the use of fresh fruits, salads, vegetables, skim milk products and lean meats and fish will produce a general feeling of well being. This, in our experience, has been the most powerful stimulant to follow the diet modifications for extended periods of time. In other patients it may be the discontinuation of drugs which will encourage the patient more than anything else; in another group of patients it is the close participation of the patient in the follow-up of his own laboratory studies, be it cholesterol, uric acid, glucose, blood pressure levels or, as exemplified in two cases, ECG changes over a relatively short period of time.

The first patient was a 49-year-old white male who was informed about negative T waves in his chest leads (the only abnormal finding in an extensive endocrinologic work-up). His weight was 164 kg (360 lb) when the first ECG was taken. The second cardiogram was taken after a weight loss of 13·6 kg (30 lb) and the third ECG was taken after losing a total of 31·8 kg (70 lb) (Fig. 8). He was referred to us by the Vocation and Rehabilitation Service since he was unable to find a job due to Pickwick Syndrome. His regained mental alertness and the knowledge that abnormalities in his ECG had disappeared during weight reduction made him a most cooperative patient. (See pp. 88–89: note T wave changes from left to right.)

The second ECG was done on a 39-year-old black female whose weight on 10/9/70 was 173 kg (381 lb). On 9/19/70 after her weight had been reduced to 163 kg (358 lb) the ECG showed definite improvements in her T waves and on 11/13/70 when she had reduced her weight to 154 kg (339 lb) the abnormalities from the first ECG had been eliminated (Fig. 9). This patient, who was unable to read or write, was more impressed by the negative and, later, positive T waves than by the fact that she had chemical diabetes mellitus. The diabetes disappeared when she weighed 127 kg (280 lb).

Other patients are more influenced by family history and by observation of the same disorder among friends and relatives. In summary, it is the time involvement of the physician, his willingness to let the patient—regardless of his background—participate in the laboratory and ECG studies which bring about the best stimulation for patients to follow diet modifications for extended periods of time. It is, in short, the physician's concern and personal interest which leads to the patient's recognition of his own responsibility for his health.

## C. What are the Characteristics of Individuals with Good and Poor Adherence? How can this Information Assist in Planning Patient Nutrition Programmes?

Obvious candidates for poor diet adherence are patients with psychiatric histories, alcoholism and nicotine addiction. It is our personal experience that the group with the poorest prognosis for diet adherence is the group of white, female cigarette smokers. The fact that all other race/sex groups are able to quit smoking when requested seems to be a good indicator of future diet adherence. We also agree with the finding by Stamler (personal communication, 1972) that patients weighing over 136 kg (300 lb) are a relatively poor risk for future success in any dietary programme. Another important factor is the cooperation of members of the patient's family. Ideally, all members involved in buying and preparing food should be instructed at the time of the first instruction of the patient. It is often possible from the first interview to assess the willingness of the family to cooperate with dietary changes. It is equally important to realize that in a female patient with lipid abnormalities, the full understanding of the problem is required from her husband. However, if he shows no interest in dietary changes in his household, the entire programme may be jeopardized (Heyden *et al.*, 1973).

At the time of the first interview it is, therefore, valuable to ask a few questions, regarding past history of psychiatric disorders, alcoholism, cigarette smoking habit, weight history and maximum weight in the past, and the expressed assurance of interest of family members in the dietary changes of the patient. The distance from the clinic and mode of transportation to and from the clinic, and the working hours of the patient in relation to clinic hours also need to be taken into consideration.

## D. How Can the Programme be Evaluated by the Patient, Nutritionist and Physician?

The most objective evaluation of a successful dietary programme is, of course, the improvement or normalization of the laboratory result. Laboratory results, however, may not always be influenced by the dietary changes suggested and adhered to by the patient. Two other possibilities are the weekly follow-up with a dietary diary composed by

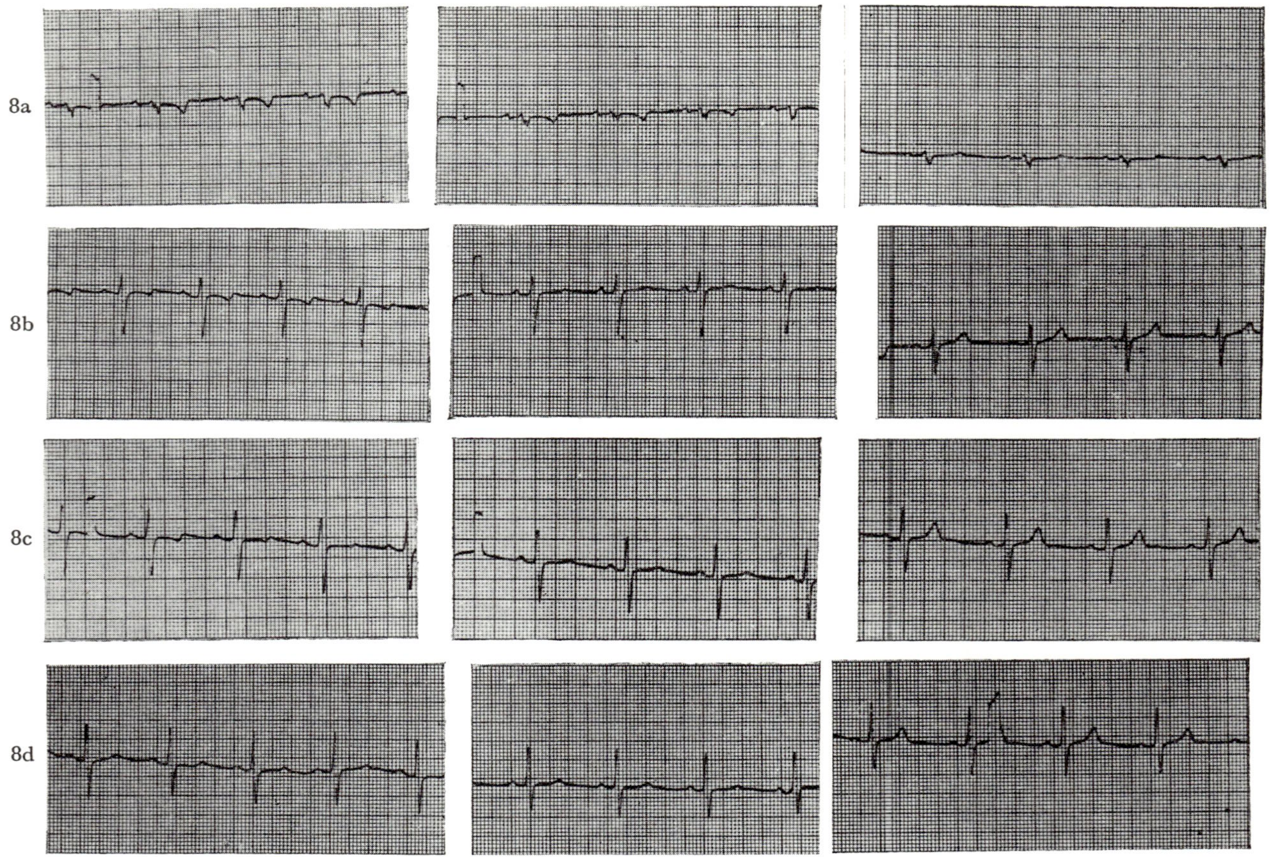


Fig. 8. ECG changes after weight loss from 164 kg (360 lb) to 150 kg (330 lb) to 132 kg (290 lb).

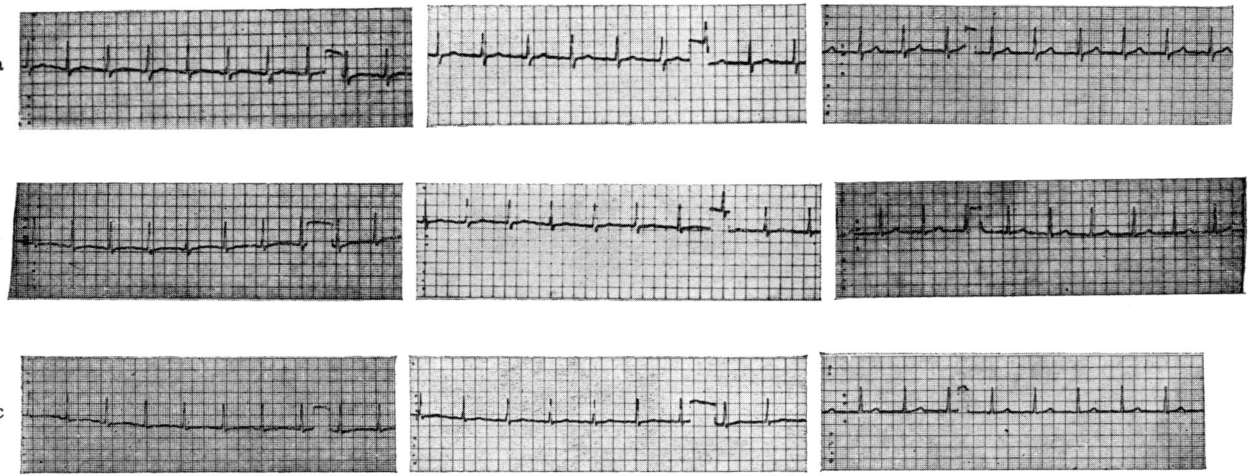


Fig. 9. ECG changes after weight loss from 173 kg (381 lb) to 163 kg (358 lb) to 154 kg (339 lb).

the patient and/or a visit by the nutritionist or nurse to the home of the patient at unannounced times, e.g. dinner or lunch time, checking the ingredients and weighing the food portions to be consumed.

## E. How Can the Educational Programme be Taught to Nutritionists?

It has been customary in our institution that a dietetics intern follows the physician in the Cardiac Rehabilitation Clinic held once a week in the afternoon, observing the individual instruction of a patient and his or her spouse. Since dietary habits are uniformly rather poor, common dietetic errors in persons with abnormal lipid values may be brought out in several interviews from past dietary habits. The preoccupation of some nutritionists with various vitamin deficiencies of diets at a time when multi-vitamin capsules are available in a great number of different preparations needs to be replaced by a concern for the hidden sources of cholesterol, of animal fat and of "empty" calories. These individual training sessions with only a few patients probably do more for the education of a nutritionist than classroom lectures. Ideally, they should be followed by placing a single patient into the responsibility of a dietetic's intern under the supervision of the physician.

## F. What Knowledge Does the Nutritionist Need in Order to Work Effectively with Physicians Concerning the Patient's Nutritional Needs?

The modern nutritionist must have a definite knowledge of the cholesterol content of beef, chicken, seafood and fish, e.g. in three-ounce units in order to assess quickly the total cholesterol intake of a daily menu and whether more than 300 mg of dietary cholesterol has been consumed in one day. She needs to know the definite advantage of corn, sunflower and safflower oil versus peanut oil and coconut oil and their effect on cholesterol levels rather than the vitamin concentration in certain vegetables and fruits. She must know how to apply polyunsaturated fatty acids in margarine and vegetable oils into calorically restricted and calorically unrestricted diets, e.g. stressing the different caloric values of a tablespoon of vegetable oil versus a tablespoon of margarine. She ought to be prepared to suggest recipes for skim milk "milk shakes", for sherbets with the use of egg whites without cream or whole milk, etc. All this requires a rather limited knowledge which can be taught within a few hours, but the nutritionist also needs to be thoroughly informed about the major diseases which may be effectively prevented by treatment of certain risk factors through nutritional habits and dietary changes (hyperlipoproteinaemia, hypercholesterolaemia, hypertriglyceridaemia, hypertension, hyperglycaemia and hyperuricaemia). This latter part may need considerably more time.

## G. What Efforts Can be Made to Increase the Exchange of Information Between Nutritionist and Physician?

Diets must be ordered in a similar fashion as a medical prescription of drugs with an accompanying explanation as to what can be expected from a particular change and possible side effects. The dietitician–nutritionist should be given more detailed information in disease processes. It is insufficient simply to give her an order for a specific diet. An increase of the exchange of information between the nutritionist and physician can only be expected by mutual respect and is best taught on an individual basis following and cooperating with a single patient. The nutritionist has to learn how to search for hidden sources of cholesterol and animal fat in a patient's regular diet which may enable the nutritionist to advise the patient about the necessary changes. Questions regarding the past dietary habits must go into great detail (and must include such questions as to the occasional use of cashew and macadamia nuts, must bring out the differences between buttermilk, whole milk drinks, dried whole milk, evaporated milk, condensed milk, sweet or sour cream, and dried non-fat milk, evaporated skim milk, cream substitutes or the use of baked products known for their high animal fat composition, packaged dinners, desserts, etc.).

## H. What Factors Enhance or Impede the Physician's Use of Diet Counseling Services? How May this Information be Used?

The physician's use of dietary counseling services depend on his personal interest and authority in the problems involved. If he does not personally attend to the details of a prescribed diet, he will not succeed. Those physicians who are willing to spend time in letting the dieticians participate in the medical and laboratory results of prescribed dietary changes will be most successful in the use of diet counseling services. This makes the dietician or nutritionist an active participant in the health delivery team rather than a passive bystander whose technical advice is being used occasionally without any responsibility for follow-up.

## I. In What Roles can Personnel Other than Nutritionists be Used in the Dietary Programme? What Training Do They Need?

It is obvious that patients who have gone through a dietary programme themselves could be the best potential teachers for other patients. In the past, we have used the experience of a physician's associate who for three months went through our programme and became a very good teacher to others; we have used the services of a registered nurse who, upon completion of her own dietary programme for severe hypertension was able to help us greatly in our diet instructions of other patients on a part-time basis. In the Hypertension Intervention Study in Evans County, Georgia (Heyden *et al.*, 1973) we have trained a housewife who had undergone the prescribed weight reduction and salt restriction, reduced her weight to a normal level and at the same time brought her hypertensive blood pressure levels under control. She subsequently observed our diet programme at the Department of Community Health Sciences for four days. Thereafter she successfully managed the weekly supervision of 63 obese, hypertensive individuals including detailed dietary advice about caloric values, fat content, the value of protein in low-caloric diets and the elimination of sodium rich foods. We feel that the training of a non-professional in a Nutrition Education Programme is best accomplished by having this particular person go through the programme herself and then supervising her on her instruction of patients, placing increased responsibilities into her hands. No formal education in nutrition or dietetics is required in our opinion.

## REFERENCES


Bang, H. O., Dyerberg, J. and Nielsen, A. B. (1971). Plasma lipid and lipoprotein pattern in Greenlandic west-coast Eskimos. *Lancet* (June 5), 1143.

Bierenbaum, M. L., Fleischman, A. I., Raichelson, R. I., Hayton, T. and Watson, P. B. (1973). Ten-year experience of modified-fat diets on younger men with coronary heart disease. *Lancet* (June 23), p. 1404.

Brunzell, J. D., Porte, D., Jr. and Bierman, E. L. (1971). Evidence for a common saturable removal system for dietary and endogenous triglyceride in man. *J. Clin. Invest.* **50,** 15a (Abstr.).

Chapman, J. M. and Massey, F. J. (1964). The interrelationship of serum cholesterol, hypertension, body weight and risk of coronary disease; results of the first ten years follow-up in the Los Angeles Heart Study. *J. Chron. Dis.* **17,** 933.

Connor, W. E. (1970). Diet and coronary heart disease. *Mod. Med.* **38,** 85.

Connor, W. E. and Connor, S. L. (1972). The key role of nutritional factors in the prevention of coronary heart disease. *Prev. Med.* **1,** 28.

Dayton, S. *et al.* (1969a). *Circulation* **40,** Suppl. 2.

Dayton, S., Pearce, M. L., Hashimoto, S., Dixon, W. J., and Tomiyasu, U. (1969b). A controlled clinical trial of a diet high in unsaturated fat. *Am. Heart Ass. Monograph* 25. AHA, Inc. New York.

Doyle, J. T., Kinch, S. H. and Brown, D. F. (1965). Seasonal variation in serum cholesterol concentration. *J. Chron. Dis.* **18,** 657.

Dyerberg, J., Bang, H. O. and Nielsen, J. A. (1970). Plasma lipids and lipoproteins in patients with myocardial infarction and in a control material. *Acta Med. Scand.* **187,** 365.

Enger, S. Chr. and Ritland, S. (1970). Serum lipoprotein pattern in myocardial infarction. *Acta Med. Scand.* **187,** 365.

Evans County Incidence Study, Symposium (1971). (J. C. Cassel, ed.) *Arch. Int. Med.* **128,** 883–990.

Falsetti, H. L., Schnatz, J. D., Greene, D. G. and Bunnell, I. L. (1970). Serum lipids and glucose tolerance in angiographically proved coronary artery disease. *Chest* **58,** 111.

Frantz, I. D., Jr. and Moore, R. B. (1969). The sterol hypothesis in atherogenesis. *Am. J. Med.* **46,** 684.

Fredrickson, D. S. (1972). A physician's guide to Hyperlipidemia. *Mod. Conc. Cardiovasc. Dis.* **41,** 31.

Fredrickson, D. S., Levy, R. I. and Lees, R. S. (1967). Fat transport in lipoproteins—an integrated approach to mechanisms and disorders. *N. Engl. J. Med.* **276,** 32.

Fredrickson, D. S. and Levy, R. I. (1972). Familial hyperlipoproteinemia. *In* "The Metabolic Basis of Inherited Disease", 3rd edition (J. B. Stanbury, J. B. Wyngaarden and D. S. Fredrickson, eds), pp. 531–614. McGraw-Hill, New York.

Galbraith, W. B., Connor, W. E. and Stone, D. G. (1966). Weight loss and serum lipid changes in obese subjects given low-calorie diets of varied cholesterol content. *Ann. Int. Med.* **64,** 268.

Goldstein, J. L., Schrott, H. G., Hazzard, W. R., Bierman, E. L. and Motulsky, A. G. (1973). Hyperlipidemia in coronary heart disease: II. Genetic analysis of lipid levels in 176 families and delineation of a new inherited disorder, combined hyperlipidemia. *J. Clin. Invest.* **52,** 1544.

Greenhalgh, R. M., Lewis, B., Rosengarten, D. S., Calnan, J. S., Mervart, I. and Martin, P. (1971). Serum lipids and lipoproteins in peripheral vascular disease. *Lancet* (October 30), 947.

Harlan, W. R., Jr., Graham, J. B. and Estes, E. H., Jr. (1966). Familial hypercholesterolemia, a genetic and metabolic study. *Medicine* **45,** 77.

Harlan, W. R., Jr. (1969). A nomogram for determining types of hyperlipidemia. *Arch. Int. Med.* **124,** 64.

Hartmann, G. (1965). Gibt es eine Prophylaxe der Arteriosklerose? *Schw. Med. Wschr.* **95,** 555.

Hazzard, W. R., Goldstein, J. L., Schrott, H. G., Motulsky, A. G. and Bierman, E. L. (1973). Hyperlipidemia in coronary heart disease. *J. Clin. Invest.* **52,** 1569.

Heinle, R. A., Levy, R. I., Fredrickson, D. S. and Gorlin, R. (1969). Lipid and carbohydrate abnormalities in patients with angiographically documented coronary artery disease. *Am. J. Cardiol.* **24,** 178.

Heyden, S. (1969). Epidemiology. *In* "Atherosclerosis" (F. G. Schettler and G. S. Boyd, eds), pp. 587–631. Elsevier, New York.

Heyden, S., Walker, L., Hames, C. G. and Tyroler, H. A. (1971). Decrease of serum cholesterol levels and blood pressure in the community. *Arch. Int. Med.* **128,** 982.

Heyden, S., DeMaria, W., Barbee, S. and Morris, M. (1973). Weight reduction in adolescents. *Nutr. Metabol.* **15,** 295.

Heyden, S., Tyroler, H. A., Hames, C. G., Bartel, A., Thompson, J. W., Krishan, I. and Rosenthal, T. (1973b). Diet treatment of obese hypertensives. *Clin. Sci. Mol. Med.* **45,** 209.

Hood, B., Sanne, H., Örndahl, G., Ahlström, M. and Welin, G. (1965). Long-term prognosis in essential hypercholesterolemia. The effect of strict diet. *Acta Med. Scand.* **178,** 161.

Jensen, J., Blankenhorn, D. H. and Dornerup, V. (1967). Coronary disease in familial hypercholesterolemia. *Circulation* **36,** 77.

Kannel, W. B., Castelli, W. P., Gordon, T. and McNamara, P. M. (1971). Serum cholesterol, lipoproteins and the risk of coronary heart disease. *Ann. Int. Med.* **74,** 1.

Koranyi, A. (1963). Prophylaxis and treatment of coronary syndrome. *Ther. Hung.* **12,** 17.

Lees, R. S. (1973). A progress report on lipoprotein phenotyping (Editorial). *Lab. Clin. Med.* **82,** 529.

Leren, P. (1970). The Oslo diet-heart study. *Circulation* **42,** 935.

Levy, R. I. and Fredrickson, D. S. (1970). The current status of hypolipidemic drugs. *Postgrad. Med.* **47,** 130.

Lyon, T. P., Yankley, A., Fogman, J. W. and Strisower, B. (1956). Lipoproteins and diet in coronary heart disease. *Calif. Med.* **84,** 325.

Masek, J., Krikava, L. and Osancova, K. (1962). Epidemiological survey of cholesterolaemia and its significance. *Rev. Czech. Med.* **8,** 186.

McDonough, J. R., Hames, C. G., Stulb, S. C. and Garrison, G. E. (1965). Coronary heart disease among Negroes and Whites in Evans County, Ga. *J. Chron. Dis.* **18,** 443.

Medical Research Council (1965). Low-fat diet in myocardial infarction. *Lancet* (Sept. 11) **501.**

Medical Research Council (1968). Controlled trial of soya-bean oil in myocardial infarction. *Lancet* **ii,** 693.

Morrison, L. M. (1960). Diet in coronary atherosclerosis. *J. Am. Med. Ass.* **173,** 884.

Moses, C. (1963). "Atherosclerosis, Mechanisms as a Guide to Prevention". Lea and Febiger, Philadelphia.

The National Diet-Heart Study (1968). Final Report. *Am. Heart Ass. Monograph* 18, AHA, Inc. New York.

Nelson, A. M. (1956). Treatment of atherosclerosis by diet: I. Results in patients followed from 36–72 months. *Northwest Med.* **55,** 643.
II. Common errors preventing effective cholesterol and phospholipid changes. *Northwest Med.* **55,** 792.
III. Selection and management of patients. *Northwest Med.* **56,** 874.

Nelson, A. M. and Douglas, C. (1965). Influence of a fat-controlled diet in patients with coronary heart disease (German). *Med. Welt* (Sept. 4), 2063.

Nestel, P. J., Schreibman, P. H. and Ahrens, E. H. (1973). Cholesterol metabolism in human obesity. *J. Clin. Invest.* **52,** 2389.

Oliver, M. F. (1966). Control of hyperlipidaemia. *In* "Modern Trends in Pharmacology and Therapeutics" (W. F. M. Fulton, ed.). Butterworths, London.

Paul, O., Lepper, M. H., Phelan, W. H., Dupertuis, G. W., MacMillan, A., McKean, H. and Park, H. (1963). A longitudinal study of coronary heart disease. *Circulation* **28,** 20.

Pries, C., Van Gent, C. M., Baes, H., Polano, M. K., Hulsman, H. A. M. and Querido, A. (1968). Primary hyperlipoproteinemia: the clinical classification of the most common types. *Clin. Chim. Acta* **19,** 181.

Roberts, W. C., Levy, R. I. and Fredrickson, D. S. (1970). Hyperlipoproteinemia, a review of the five types with first report of necropsy finding in type III. *Arch. Path.* **90,** 46.

Rose, G. A., Thomson, W. B. and Williams, R. T. (1965). Corn oil in treatment of ischaemic heart disease. *Brit. Med. J.* **1,** 1531.

Schatz, I. J. (1969). Classification of primary hyperlipidemia, observations on 214 patients. *J. Am. Med. Ass.* **210,** 701.

Schreibman, P. H., Wilson, D. E. and Arky, R. A. (1969). Familial type IV hyperlipoproteinemia. *N. Engl. J. Med.* **281,** 981.

Schreibman, P. H., Nestel, P. and Ahrens, E. H., Jr. (1971). Cholesterol metabolism in obesity. *Circulation* (Suppl. II) **43** and **44,** 1.

Slack, J. (1969). Risk of Ischemic heart disease in familial hyperlipoproteinemic states. *Lancet* (December 27), 1380.

Stamler, J. (1967). "Lectures on Preventive Cardiology", p. 434. Grune and Stratton, Inc., New York, London.

Stamler, J. (1971). Acute myocardial infarction—progress in primary prevention. *Brit. Heart J.* **33** (Suppl.), 145.

Stamler, J. (1973). Epidemiology of coronary heart disease. *Med. Clin. N. Amer.* **57,** 5.

Strisower, E. H., Adamson, G. and Strisower, B. (1970). Treatment of hyperlipidemic states. *Med. Clin. N. Amer.* **54,** 1599.

Tech. Group, Comm. on Lipoproteins and Atherosclerosis (1954). Evaluation of serum lipoprotein and cholesterol measurements as predictors of clinical complications of atherosclerosis: Appendix A. *Circulation* **14,** 725.

Thomas, C. B., Holljes, H. W. D. and Eisenberg, F. F. (1961). Observations on seasonal variations in total serum cholesterol level among healthy young prisoners. *Ann. Int. Med.* **54,** 413.

Thorp, J. M. (1963). Seasonal variations of lipids. *In* "The Control of Lipid Metabolism" (J. K. Grant, ed.). Academic Press, New York.

Turpeinen, O., Miettinen, M., Karvonen, M. J., Roine, P., Pekkarinen, M., Lehtosuo, E. J. and Alivirta, P. (1971). Diätetische Praevention von Herzgefaessererkrankungen. *In* "Fettstoffwechselstoerungen" (G. Schettler, ed.). G. Thieme, Stuttgart.

Van Houte, O. and Kesteloot, H. (1971). Epidemiological cardiovascular study of 42,804 military subjects. *Circulation* (Suppl. II) **43** and **44,** 236.

Watson, W. C. (1963). Long-term administration of corn oil in management of patients with acute myocardial infarction: a four-year study. *Brit. Med. J.* **2,** 1366.

Welch, C. C., Proudfit, W. L., Sones, F. M., Jr., Shirley, E. K., Sheldon, W. C. and Razavi, M. (1970). Cinecoronary arteriography in young men. *Circulation* **42,** 647.

Werkö, L. (1971). Can we prevent heart disease? *Ann. Int. Med.* **74,** 278.

Widmer, L. K., Hartmann, G., Duchosal, F. and Plechl, S. Ch. (1969). Risk factors in arterial occlusions of the limbs. *Dtsch. Med. Wschr.* **94,** 1107.

Wilson, W. S., Hulley, S. B., Burrows, M. I. and Nichaman, M. Z. (1971). Serial lipid and lipoprotein responses to the American Heart Association fat-controlled diet. *Am. J. Med.* **51,** 491.

Zelis, R., Mason, D. T., Braunwald, E. and Levy, R. I. Effects of hyperlipoproteinemias and their treatment on the peripheral circulation. *J. Clin. Invest.* **49,** 1007.

## APPENDIX: POSSIBLE SIDE EFFECTS OF DIETARY FATS

### A. Multiple Sclerosis

It is not surprising that many epidemiological hypotheses regarding multiple sclerosis, which still evades precise etiology, have been brought forward, tested and either disproved or left unproven. The incidence of this disease appears to be lower in warmer latitudes. It has been mentioned by several investigators that it is extremely difficult to study a low-incidence disorder like multiple sclerosis systematically. It is reported to occur more frequently in females, although this has not been found in all studies; in some studies there is an excess of males among older patients with multiple sclerosis. A viral etiology (Brody *et al.*, 1971) has been suspected as in many other chronic degenerative diseases. Even the type of tooth filling has come under suspicion. The disease supposedly occurs more frequently in higher socio-economic groups but proposed urban–rural differences in the incidence are not well documented (Bernsohn and Stephanides, 1967). The observation of a low familial occurrence is thought (not proven) to be associated with environmental rather than genetic factors. Another hypothesis concerns the epidemiological similarities between multiple sclerosis and Hodgkin's disease. The age of clinical onset is the same as in Hodgkin's disease. Newell (1970) also reported that the geographic distribution of mortality from multiple sclerosis in the United States is similar to the geographic distribution of Hodgkin's disease mortality among young adults in countries of the Western civilization. Both diseases are said to be rare in Japan.

A recent editorial in the *British Medical Journal* (6/5/71) mentioned the dietary hypothesis and listed several promotors of this theory. A few authors have drawn attention to the high incidence of multiple sclerosis in some parts of the world where diets generally tend to be rich in saturated fatty acids. In at least one retrospective study of patients with multiple sclerosis and control persons this hypothesis was not borne out.

The study of the dietary intake of non-hospitalized persons with multiple sclerosis by Witschi *et al.* (1970) revealed that the amount of total fat and the proportion of animal fat were lower than in studies of other investigators. Fat in the average daily diet of the male patients with multiple sclerosis ranged from 32–125 g (mean 73 g). Animal fat contributed 67% and 62% of the total fat for men and women respectively (19–109 g for men 19–93 g for women).

In comparison, Browe's (1967) group of healthy men (1514 civil service employees) showed a daily intake of 124 g of fat of which 74% was from animal sources. In the study of Boston-Ireland brothers,* the dietary calculations of interviews from 85 pairs of brothers showed the Bostonians to have a mean fat intake of 158 g of which 86% was from animal sources. 70 dietary histories calculated by the Framingham study** showed an average fat intake of 154 g for men and 106 g for women, of which 75% came from animal sources. Davidson *et al.* (1962) obtained dietary records from 42 men and 62 women, all of whom were apparently healthy ageing persons and reported that animal fat provided over 70% of the total dietary fat for nearly three-quarters of the subjects. Studies of Benedictine monks, whose diet is comparable with that of the average American indicate that they derive 75% of their fat from animal sources.

It has been suggested that modification of the diet for patients with multiple sclerosis (reduction of total fat, inclusion of greater amounts of polyunsaturated fatty acids) may improve the patient's functional condition and reduce the relapse rate (Swank, 1961; Swank and Bourdillon, 1960). We agree with the editorial from the *British Medical Journal* that adding either sunflower seeds or corn oil to the normal diets of patients suffering from multiple sclerosis will do no harm. This eventually may turn out of importance to some patients, particularly in view of a more recent chemical investigation of the levels of linoleate and oleate levels of the serum lipids of patients suffering from multiple sclerosis and of controls (see Editorial, *Brit. Med. J.*, 1971). The percentage of linoleate in the patients with multiple sclerosis was lower than in the controls, while that of oleate was higher. The two groups of patients were then fed with linoleate supplements (emulsion of sunflower seed oil). In both groups the percentage of the linoleate levels rose strikingly, but it seemed to fall rather more rapidly in the patients with multiple sclerosis after termination of the dietary experiment. The low linoleate levels in multiple sclerosis patients are difficult to explain. Since the absorptive mechanism is unimpaired the suggestion was made that the rate of loss or of utilization of linoleate may be abnormally high in patients with multiple sclerosis.

In summary, the two facts, namely the diversity of etiological hypotheses in multiple sclerosis with contradictory statements from credible investigators and the—as yet unexplained but interesting—findings of an abnormally high utilization of linoleate or an abnormally high rate of loss of linoleate in patients with multiple sclerosis make it impractical to go beyond these speculations. However, it is felt that the dogmatic assertion that multiple sclerosis is the result of a dietary deficiency of polyunsaturated fatty acids is unwarranted at this time (see Bernsohn and Stephanides, 1967).

* Trulson *et al.* (1964). ** Mann *et al.* (1962).

## B. Carcinogenesis

The question of undesirable side effects from the long-term use of a low-cholesterol diet with the emphasis on the polyunsaturated fatty acids briefly developed into a major public concern after the publication of an article in the *Lancet* on 3/6/71, "Incidence of cancer in man on a diet high on polyunsaturated fat" by Pearce and Dayton. In their eight-year controlled clinical trial of a diet high in polyunsaturated vegetable oils and low in saturated fat and cholesterol, 174 deaths were noted in the experimental group and 178 deaths in the control group. In the experimental group 31 of the 174 deaths were due to cancer as opposed to 17 out of 178 deaths in the control group. The authors unfortunately concluded from their findings that it is "premature to make a blanket prescription of a diet high in polyunsaturated fat for the entire population", implying that their data could mean that the polyunsaturated fatty acid diet might have had a co-carcinogenic effect in the experimental group. However, a review of the table showing adherence to diet in patients with fatal carcinomas during the diet phase clarifies the situation and removes any doubt that the diet high in polyunsaturated fatty acids and low in cholesterol might have had anything to do with carcinogenesis or co-carcinogenesis. Not less than 12 cases of fatal carcinoma were found in persons who adhered less than 20 % of the time to the experimental diet (see Table 7)

Table 7

Adherence to diet in patients with fatal carcinoma during the diet phase[a]

| Adherence(%) | Control group | Experimental group |
|---|---|---|
| 0–10 | 2 | 10 |
| 10–20 | 1 | 2 |
| 20–30 | 1 | 3 |
| 30–40 | 0 | 0 |
| 40–50 | 3 | 3 |
| 50–60 | 3 | 3 |
| 60–70 | 0 | 4 |
| 70–80 | 2 | 2 |
| 80–90 | 4 | 1 |
| 90–100 | 1 | 3 |
| | 17 | 31 |

[a] Adherence, calculated from attendance records, is expressed as a percentage of the maximum number of meals which could have been taken in the study dining-hall.

$x^2 = 10{\cdot}26$; $P > 0{\cdot}3$.

Only 19 persons from the experimental group, thus, died with cancer and adhered to the prescribed diet between 20 and 100% during the eight year observation period. Therefore, any statistical significance is being automatically removed between the control and the experimental group since people in the experimental group who did not adhere to the diet can hardly be called dieters. It was, therefore, not surprising that another group of four investigators (Ederer *et al.*, 1971) found that the results of their studies "are consistent with the hypothesis that the cholesterol-lowering diets do not influence cancer risk".

## C. Breast Cancer

In considering dietary fat intake and breast cancer, we are probably not even dealing tangentially with a causal relationship. Animal experiments in rats in the hands of one group of investigators (Carroll and Khor, 1971) showed that semi-synthetic diets containing 10% and 20% (by weight) of corn oil produced more mammary adenocarcinomas after treatment with a single oral dose of DMBA than in a group of rats on diets containing only 0·5% or 5% corn oil. The same investigators reported that experiments with ten different fats and oils fed at the 20% level indicated that unsaturated fats enhance the yield of adenocarcinomas more than saturated fats. In addition, it was found that the diet high in corn oil enhanced the tumour yield when it was fed only after administration of the carcinogen but not when it was fed only before. This suggested to these authors that the effect was related to development of the tumours rather than to distribution and metabolism of the carcinogen or other factors concerned with tumour initiation. Reviewing other animal studies (Carroll and Khor, 1971), it appears that edible oils such as olive oil, Crisco and lard can enhance mammary carcinogenesis in the rat. The incidence of spontaneously occurring mammary tumours in rats was independent whether the fats were heat treated or untreated. The level of α-tocopherol was increased in another rat experiment containing 20% corn oil and the result was a decrease in tumour yield in rats treated with DMBA.

Carroll and co-workers (1968) admitted that their findings with corn oil in animals did not support the epidemiologic observations by Lea. Lea had suggested that there was a positive correlation between consumptions of fats and oils and death rates from malignant neoplasm of the breast relating this to the cholesterol and cholesterogenic content of certain dietary fats. However, the example of the American black female with a definitely lower incidence of breast cancer in comparison to the white counterpart in the United States provides a good example of the irrelevance of this fat hypothesis in carcinogenesis of the breast. Black females are known to have used in the past (and are still using at the present time) more animal fats in their diets than white females. There are more powerful environmental and sociological influences involved in the development of breast cancer than dietary factors, among others the age at first pregnancy, the number of pregnancies, cancer family history breast feeding versus non-breast feeding, the age at menarche, the age at menopause or artificial menopause, the presence or absence of benign cystic disease or treatment with oestrogen-containing hormones. For each one of the factors cited one can show great differences between white and black females and between Japanese women and American white females. The mortality from breast cancer is believed to be nine times higher among American whites than among Japanese women. However, environmental and sociological factors change drastically in Japanese immigrating to the United States west coast and Hawaii. With these changes, significant increases in breast cancer are being reported among first and second generation Japanese women.

Disregarding for the moment the isolated experimental finding of corn oil as co-carcinogenic in breast cancer development, one is more impressed by the several laboratory studies revealing that increasing the level of fat in general in the diet increases the yield of mammary tumours in laboratory animals. The higher incidence of spontaneous breast carcinoma in mice fed a high-fat diet has been reported as early as 1945. Other workers observed that rats develop more mammary fibroadenomas when fed on high-fat diets regardless of the type of fat used. On the other hand, there is ample evidence from animal experiments that underfeeding and caloric restriction decrease the incidence of a variety of tumours, including breast tumours. The literature on this subject has been summarized by Tannenbaum (1959).

However, this finding of an increase in breast cancer in overfed animals cannot be confirmed from human experience. Body weight and incidence of breast cancer cannot be correlated in available studies. The topic has been well reviewed in the German literature by Borneff and Fabian (1966) and by Schettler and Wagener (1965).

## D. Colon Cancer

A report by the Research Committee of the World Health Organization (1966) assumed a positive association between the mortality from colon cancer and arteriosclerotic heart disease (ASHD). However, a negative correlation between the mortality from gastric and colon cancers suggested opposing etiological factors.

"The negative correlation of colon to gastric cancer, the positive association of colon cancer to arteriosclerotic heart disease and the relatively high rate of colon cancer among Jews in New York City may be related to a dietary pattern, possibly high in terms of saturated fats. The low rate of colon cancer, particularly in Japan, is also consistent with this view." (Report of the Research Committee WHO on Gastroenterology, 1966.)

What does not fit into this apparent relationship between colon cancer and arteriosclerotic heart disease is the sex ratio of colon cancer. Rectum cancer is a predominantly male disease; however, in contrast, cancer of the colon generally has a slight predominance of women which of course is not true for ASHD in women in Western countries. Table 8

Table 8

Age-standardized rates[a] of mortality from cancer of specified gastro-intestinal sites, at ages 0–74 years, for Japanese in Japan and Japanese and Caucasians in California

| | Japan[b] | | California[c] | | | | | |
|---|---|---|---|---|---|---|---|---|
| | (Japanese) | | Foreign-born | | U.S. born | | Caucasian | |
| | Men | Women | Men | Women | Men | Women | Men | Women |
| Stomach (151) | 58·4 | 30·9 | 29·9 | 13·0 | 11·7 | 11·3 | 8·0 | 4·0 |
| Colon (153) | 1·9 | 2·1 | 6·1 | 7·0 | 6·3 | 10·4 | 7·9 | 8·3 |
| Rectum (154) | 3·3 | 2·8 | 4·0 | (4·0) | (3·1) | (2·0) | 4·2 | 2·8 |
| TOTAL (151, 153–4) | 63·6 | 35·8 | 40·0 | 24·0 | 21·1 | 23·7 | 20·0 | 15·1 |

From Ackerman, 1972.

[a] Age-standardized with direct method, using Segi's common standard as adopted by the working party of World Health Organization of Gastroenterology. See *Gut* 5, 196 (1964).

[b] Average annual rates for 1960–61 in Japan.

[c] Average annual rates for 1957–64 for Japanese in California and 1959–61 for Caucasians in California. Rates in parentheses are based on fewer than 10 deaths.

reflects the slightly higher age-standardized mortality rate for Caucasian women with colon cancer and a markedly lower mortality rate for Caucasian women with cancer of the rectum. The same applies to non-white females in the United States. It is important to keep this discrepancy in mind when one tries to interpret the marked decline of gastric cancer and sharp increase of colon cancer for American born Japanese, and Japanese living in California. Wynder and Shigematsu choose to interpret the increase of colonic cancer among the Japanese migrants to the United States "a most important epidemiologic clue, that can best be accounted for by dietary changes" (Wynder and Shigematsu, 1967). These authors pointed out correctly (as was also shown by Ackerman, 1972: Table 8) that colon and rectum cancer is very rare in Japanese in their home country. In the Japanese diet only a small percentage of calories eaten is fat which is mostly polyunsaturated in contrast to 40–44% fat in the American diet, nearly half of which is saturated. Second generation Japanese in Hawaii also obtain about 40% of their calories from fat and their blood cholesterol levels are similar to those of the continental United States population. It is certainly tempting to correlate these two observations, the changes in the quality of dietary fat, the increase in total fat intake and the increase in colon cancer but proof is missing so far. Ackerman (1972) has contributed some laboratory observations to this hypothesis.

> "Bacteriological studies of faeces in subjects from Britain and America have shown highly increased counts of bacteroides and a higher concentration of steroids than in Ugandans or Japanese. Furthermore, the steroids were degraded to potentially carcinogenic agents. We would expect a low fat vegetarian diet to be associated with reduced levels of neutral steroids and of bile salt degradation products in the faeces."

In the study just mentioned by Wynder and Shigematsu (1967) patients with colon cancer and control persons consumed eggs, milk, butter, cheese and meat in the same quantities. In three more studies no consistent relationships were found between cancer of the large bowel and fried food or milk consumption. Similarly, Pernu (1960) did not find any positive relationship between the development of cancer and animal meat and fat consumption. Higginson (1966) also reported no significant differences in any dietary intake between cases with cancer of the large bowel and control subjects.

After unsuccessful attempts to blame carcinogenesis of the colon on fats, recent research has turned to carbohydrates and roughage in the diet particularly after comparing data between South African Bantus and industrialized nations. The diet of the South African with his bulky stools and rapid transit is made up of high roughage and unrefined carbohydrates. The Western diet has low bulk with refined sugar and flours. This results in a longer transit time, decreased frequency of defaecation, faecal stasis and prolonged contact of any potential carcinogen with the mucosal surface (Ackerman, 1972 and Editorial–*Medical World News*, 1971). It may be relevant that most retrospective studies of patients with cancer of the colon and control persons revealed a higher degree of constipation in the past history of the cancer patients. In contrast, the Bantu is obsessed with the idea that he must not be constipated. His concept of constipation differs from the Western concept. He feels that if he does not have three or four bowel movements per day he is already constipated and he remedies this situation by frequent enemas. The Bantu produces huge bulky stools and the faeces have a rapid transit. The rapid transit has been well documented by radiopaque markers and fluoroscopy (Ackerman, 1972). It would, therefore, seem appropriate to lay the fat hypothesis (as etiological factor in colon cancer) to rest.

Professor Rose (London) along with distinguished epidemiologists like Professors Keys, Blackburn, Taylor, Kannel, Paul and Reid as well as Professor Stamler recently published (Rose *et al.*, 1974) a study of 90 cases of colon cancer whose initial levels of blood-cholesterol were found surprisingly to be lower than expected. Rose and co-workers chose to interpret their data with the (I believe) unwarranted opinion that the patients with colon cancer were individuals with lower levels of blood cholesterol who tended to form more bile salts

> "perhaps in part as a result of their higher intake of polyunsaturated fatty acids. This would increase the amount of substrate available for the carcinogen-forming bacteria, and hence increase also the risk of colon cancer. The negative association between blood cholesterol level and colon cancer risk might arise if in some individuals the intestine were more extensively colonised with bile-degrading bacteria, perhaps as a result of a higher intake of polyunsaturated fat or a lower intake of fibre. . . . There is need for further study of the relation in individuals between carcinogen producing faecal bacteria and the dietary intake of polyunsaturated fat and fibre."

There is an uneasy feeling that this paper may have created the wrong impression that polyunsaturated fatty acids might be implicated in the development of colon cancer. Professor Rose kindly provided me with the actual number of patients who had their cholesterol determination within five years prior to death from colon cancer. As it turned out there were 48 patients, that is more than 50% of the total number of colon cancer patients, who died within five years of the cholesterol determination. In view of the importance of this question, we take a look at the five-year cancer survival rates published in the 1974 *Cancer Facts and Figures* of the American Cancer Society; we find colon and rectum cancer together. The five-year cancer survival rates are quoted as 69% in localized cases and 39% in cases with regional involvement. The chances to survive early diagnosis of colon cancer and surgery (and/or radiation therapy) are pretty good. We therefore can assume that people dying within five years of their last cholesterol determination must have had either regional involvement or widespread metastatic disease.

The second question which I raised, was also answered by Professor Rose: 30 of the 90 individuals with colon cancer were 55 years and older. From the epidemiological literature it is a well-known observation that men above the age of 55 do have lower cholesterol levels or remain at a plateau compared to younger men whose cholesterol levels on the average rise from 180 mg% at 18 to 245 mg% at 50. Those 30 men in my opinion would have to be excluded from any further analysis of an

Table 9

| Interval from screening to death (years) | No. of cases | % with cholesterol level "below expectation" |
|---|---|---|
| <2 | 13 | 77 |
| 2–3 | 20 | 60 |
| 4–5 | 15 | 53 |
| 6–7 | 11 | 82 |
| 8–9 | 5 | 40 |
| >10 | 26 | 62 |
| | 90 | 63 |

| Age at screening (years) | No. of subjects | % with cholesterol level "below expectation" |
|---|---|---|
| <45 | 13 | 54 |
| 45–54 | 47 | 70 |
| 55–64 | 27 | 59 |
| >65 | 3 | 67 |
| | 90 | 63 |

*Note:* in none of the 90 patients was even an attempt made to assess retrospectively the consumption of polyunsaturated fats and oils.

alleged association between low cholesterol and development of cancer of the colon. Professor Rose in a personal communication added that

> "the cholesterol deviation to lower levels is greater when the interval from screening to diagnosis is short, i.e. in sick men. If we take out the men found within one year to have cancer, there is not in the remainder any correlation between cholesterol deviation and interval to diagnosis."

An editorial of the *British Medical Journal* (1973) came to the conclusion "No convincing case has been made that PUFA cause either premature ageing or cancer". A recent study, presenting the 13-year experience of the Diet and Heart Disease Study conducted by Singman *et al.* (1973), similarly concluded: "Our observations lend no confirmation to the alleged association between excess cancer mortality and high PUFA diets". This study was mentioned earlier. In brief, 1764 men, 40–59 years of age, have come under long-term observation: a control group of 533 men, an active experimental group of 378 men keeping a relatively high PUFA diet and an inactive experimental group of 853 men who were once active subjects but now limit their participation to appearance at the study facilities annually for physical examination to ascertain the status of study end-points were also included. The results of the 13-year observation period are presented in Table 10.

Table 10

Number of deaths in study group, by cause as of September 1970

| Cause | Experimental | | Control |
|---|---|---|---|
| | Active | Inactive | |
| Heart disease[a] | 30 | 58 | 10 |
| Cancer | 6 | 15 | 10 |
| Other | 5 | 12 | 5 |
| Total | 42 | 85 | 25 |
| Person-years of observation | 5903 | 6156 | 4372 |

[a] Includes the group of subjects who entered the study with prior overt coronary heart disease. These subjects have never been included in prior reports since they could not add to the experience concerning new coronary heart disease. However, they have been included here since they can contribute to cancer experience (Singman *et al.*, 1973).

Regarding the specific question raised by Rose and co-workers, the following table (Table 11) does not lend support to the hypothesis advanced by Rose *et al.*

Obviously, the lowest number of deaths from cancer was encountered in the active experimental group with only one case of colon cancer! Table 12 reveals the expected and actual number of deaths from cancer. In the age group 40–49 years not a single case of cancer was observed

Table 11

Number of deaths in study group from cancer, June 1957 to September 1970

| Site | Experimental | | Control |
|---|---|---|---|
| | Active | Inactive | |
| Esophagus | 1 | | |
| Stomach | | | 3 |
| Colon | 1 | 3 | 1 |
| Rectum | | 1 | |
| Pancreas | 1 | 1 | |
| Liver | | 1 | 1 |
| Larynx | | 1 | |
| Lung | 1 | 3 | 1 |
| Prostate | | 1 | |
| Spine | 1 | | |
| Brain | 1 | 1 | 1 |
| Lymphosarcoma | | 2 | 2 |
| Leukemia | | | 1 |
| General peritoneal | | 1 | |
| Total | 6 | 15 | 10 |

[a] Cases of cancer in inactive subjects developing within six months of becoming inactive have been charged to the active group (Singman *et al.*, 1973).

Table 12

Expected and actual number of deaths from cancer

| Group | Age at entry to study group | | | |
|---|---|---|---|---|
| | 40–49 | | 50–59 | |
| | Observed | Expected | Observed | Expected |
| Experimental | | | | |
| Active | 0 | 1·6 | 6 | 23·3 |
| Inactive | 0 | 3·1 | 15 | 19·7 |
| Total | 0 | 4·7 | 21 | 43·0 |
| Control | 2 | 3·6 | 8 | 13·2 |

From Singman *et al.* (1973).

in the active or inactive experimental group; however in the age group 50–59 years the observed deaths from cancer in the active experimental group was four times lower than expected. In the inactive experimental group and in the control group the observed deaths from cancer were much closer to the expected number of deaths. The evidence thus presented exculpates polyunsaturated fatty acid diets from causing cancer.

## E. Gastric Cancer

At present it is safe to state that any evidence, from animal experiments and from a few retrospective studies of human cancer patients, for cancer induction by dietary fats is of purely academic interest.

O'Gara *et al.* (1969) concluded from animal studies that "corn oil appears to contain either more of the carcinogen or a more potent one than hydrogenated fat". He therefore suggested that it would be "advisable to avoid the excessive re-use of cooking fats in the preparation of foods for human consumption". On the other hand, two retrospective studies of stomach cancer patients and controls did not show any difference in the use of fat. Graham *et al.* (1967) applied the questionnaire method to 188 males with cancer of the stomach and 800 control patients without neoplastic diseases and found no significant differences in the type of fats used for frying. Higginson (1966) stated that patients with gastric cancer showed a dietary pattern indicating an increased use of animal fats, cooked fats, fried foods, bacon, and a decreased use of dairy products in comparison to control persons. However, the differences between patients and controls were not statistically significant. Gastric cancer patients had a slight increase in daily use of pork, sausage and bacon, and a slightly increased consumption of fried potatoes, fried foods for breakfast and fried meats. Furthermore, in patients with gastric cancer a modestly increased use of lard and collected fats was demonstrated. They used predominantly animal fat in cooking as compared to the controls. A higher proportion also re-used their fats but the answers were open to doubt because a social stigma is attached to re-use of fat. Higginson concluded that the degree of increased use of homemade lard, bacon drippings, collected fats and/or of reduced use of refrigeration among the gastric cancer patients was insufficient to support a causal relationship between fat and gastric cancer.

> "Thus, while heated or animal fats would appear unlikely as major carcinogenic or co-carcinogenic agents in gastric carcinoma, our findings would suggest that they cannot be completely excluded as

> of etiological significance, since they are widespread dietary items in many communities with a high frequency of gastric carcinoma."

Evidence from both animal experiments and from the retrospective studies just quoted would, however, not pertain to the findings in Japan where there is the highest stomach cancer morbidity and mortality in the world. The diet of the Japanese is known to be low in fat and the majority of the fat stems from vegetable oils. Even more important are the rapidly changing age standardized rates of mortality from gastric cancer in Japanese men and women moving to Hawaii and the west coast of the United States. As can be seen in Table 8 (p. 101), stomach cancer mortality decreases almost by half in the foreign born Japanese living in Hawaii and the United States and a further decline occurs in American born Japanese approximating the rates of the host country.

An interesting hypothesis has been advanced by Stukonis and Doll (1969). They confirmed the well known relationship between gastric cancer and low social class in England. In their hypothesis, they went one step further and compared the physical activity and caloric expenditure at work of men in low and high social groups. They found that a banker, for example, would expand only 2850 kCal per day whereas a miner may expand as many as 4030 kCal per day.

> "Men, whose work involved expenditure of a large amount of physical activity, require to consume more food and, if carcinogens in foods are responsible for the production of gastric cancer, men who eat more will be more at risk for developing the disease. The mean calorie intake of housewives (2100 kCal) was lower than that for any of the groups of employed males and it is possible that differences in the amount of food eaten could be largely responsible for the fact that the incidence of gastric cancer is almost universally 50 to 100% higher in men than in women."

The authors concluded that differences in dietary habits between men in different social classes were likely to be important. Among them, carcinogens may be present in greater concentration in cheap foods than in expensive foods. However, no detailed analysis was made in the amount of fat consumed in these two groups. The standardized mortality ratio for gastric cancer for men in England (1949–53) in occupations requiring light physical activity was 84, in occupations requiring intermediate activity 106 and in occupations requiring heavy physical activity 147.

Wynder and Shigematsu (1967) mentioned that death rates for colon cancer have a strong negative correlation with those of gastric cancer. A negative correlation was also found between gastric cancer mortality and arteriosclerotic heart disease mortality.

## F. Cholelithiasis

The so-called AHA- (American Heart Association) diet, or Prudent Diet or PUFA-Diet has produced some unexpected side effects. For example, the effect of long-term ingestion of a diet low in cholesterol and saturated fat, and high in unsaturated fat on cholelithiasis has been evaluated. Autopsy records from the Los Angeles Veterans Administration clinical trial on the prevention of coronary heart disease were reviewed (Sturdevant *et al.*, 1972). Subjects in the trial were male veterans over 54 years old. During the eight-year study, 351 deaths occurred; 187 autopsy records were classifiable for presence or absence of gallstones. Stones were found in 23 out of 92 (25 %) of autopsied subjects who had eaten the experimental diet, and in 14 out of 92 (15 %) autopsied subjects who had eaten the control diet ($P = 0{\cdot}12$). Stratification on adherence to diet with elimination of the lowest-adhering third showed that 20 out of 61 (33 %) experimental subjects and 9 out of 64 (14 %) controls had stones ($P = 0{\cdot}02$). Of those who ate more than 500 meals during the study, 19 out of 63 (30 %) experimental subjects and 11 out of 70 (16 %) controls had stones ($P = 0{\cdot}08$).

Mean weight at entry to study was significantly greater in subjects with gallstones at autopsy:

| | Weight of men with gallstones | Weight of men without gallstones | *P* |
|---|---|---|---|
| Experimental | 75 kg (165 lb) | 67 kg (147 lb) | 0·01 |
| Control | 77 kg (169 lb) | 69 kg (152 lb) | 0·02 |

Of those subjects who were more than 15 % over desirable weight, 15 out of 49 (31 %) had stones, as did 22 out of 136 (16 %) of the non-obese subjects ($P = 0{\cdot}06$). The authors specifically stated that weight loss was not related to the finding of gallstones. In addition, only very few persons lost any appreciable amount of weight.

> "Mean serum cholesterol at entry, and mean change in serum cholesterol during the study, were not related to presence or absence of stones."

> "These data suggest that long-term consistent ingestion of the experimental diet predisposed to gallstone formation in these men. An adequate biochemical explanation of this hypothesis is not available. Population studies of prevention of atherosclerosis by similar diets should include investigations of cholelithiasis."

This reviewer still feels that the weight of an individual and the degree of obesity may be a more important factor than dietary fatty acid composition. Unfortunately, the gallstones were not analysed. This would have been interesting in the light of animal experiments (Dam, 1971), showing that the incorporation of soyabean oil and cod liver oil in the diet increases the tendency to produce amorphous pigmented gallstones. On the other hand (also in animals), fats containing polyunsaturated fatty acids counteract the formation of cholesterol gallstones! The same author demonstrated the difference in the effects of a butter fat diet and a diet of 40 % linoleic acid containing margarine: with butter fat, 60 % of the animals had cholesterol gallstones, whereas with the margarine diet only 4·6 % had cholesterol gallstones. The incidence of amorphous pigmented gallstones was low with both types of fat.

## G. Unexplained Effects on Blood Pressure, Cigarette Smoking and Uric Acid Concentration

Drastic dietary changes are followed by unexplained effects on several parameters. In the National Diet–Heart Study, the emphasis was on lowering serum cholesterol concentrations but blood pressure was also found to be lower than prior to the trial. In addition, cigarette smoking habits changed since more people had quit smoking cigarettes at the end of the two-year trial in comparison to those who had started smoking cigarettes during these two years of observation. Rinzler (1968) reported from the Anti-Coronary Club that among persons adhering to the so-called Prudent Diet, the percentage of hypertensives was decreased within four years, from 25·9 % to 9·9 %, in contrast to control persons where the percentage of hypertensives increased from 10·9 % to 13·1 % within the same time. In this particular study, cigarette smoking did not change significantly in the experimental group. In a study of 59 non-obese, normal and hyperlipidaemic men, reported by Wilson *et al.* (1971), adherence to the American Heart Association diet produced, within six months, a slight increase of uric acid values. All mean values during the diet period were higher than baseline values. The difference between baseline and the peak value was statistically significant. Only a minor difference between the weight at the intake examination and at the end of this six months observation period was noted (minus 0·6 kg: 1·4 lb). No significant change was noted in systolic and diastolic blood pressure during these six months.

Obviously, the unexplained effects of dietary changes on several parameters should be studied more systematically. It is evident that we must defferentiate the effect of dietary changes in initially overweight and initially normal weight subjects.

## CONCLUSIONS

From the material presented, several conclusions seem to be justified.

1. Any association, alleged to exist between the use of polyunsaturated fatty acid and the development of cancer in several organs can be dismissed. Evidence brought forward in favour of this hypothesis has been examined and evidence contrary to the assumed relationship has been presented.

2. The relationship between polyunsaturated fatty acids and multiple sclerosis needs further evaluation. The correlation found between dietary fat intake and the disease under study may be purely circumstantial but it is felt that it is definitely worthwhile to pursue the hypothesis further in larger groups of patients, both in retrospective studies of dietary habits of patients and controls and as therapy in comparison to a group of patients treated without any dietary intervention.

3. The advantage shown in several prospective studies of a diet low in cholesterol, high in polyunsaturated fatty acid for the prevention of major coronary events and the prevention of recurrence of myocardial infarction and death from myocardial infarction is substantial. Beneficial effects of such a dietary regime have been shown in all trials with the notable exception of the investigations reported from the United Kingdom. Reasons for this discrepancy are not clear. On the other hand, it seems inescapable that all these studies have been started with subjects at a rather late age, resulting in a definite decrease of atherosclerotic heart disease but not altering the overall mortality in the post-dietary phase of several trials. An increasing number of investigators in the field of atherosclerosis research feel that the whole question of development of the disease, and prevention of it, is a pediatric problem and we, therefore, may only see a major impact on this epidemic by starting dietary intervention at school age. Recognition of this important aspect and actual institution of dietary changes on a population-wide basis may take several years. In the meantime, we are faced with the problem of changing dietary habits among the adolescent and middle-aged population in Western countries who need to be educated, persuaded and motivated to accept the dietary changes on a life-long basis.

## REFERENCES

Ackerman, L. V. (1972). Some thoughts on food and cancer. *Nutrition Today* **7,** 2.

Bernsohn, J. and Stephanides, L. M. (1967). Aetiology of multiple sclerosis. *Nature* **215,** 821.

Borneff, J. und Fabian, B. (1966). Kanzerogene Substanzen in Speisefett und -oel. *Arch. Hyg. Bakt.* **150,** 485.

Brody, J. A., Sever, J. L. and Henson, T. E. (1971). Virus antibody titers in multiple sclerosis patients, siblings and controls. *J. Am. Med. Ass.* **216,** 1441.

Browe, J. H., Morlley, D. M., Logrillo, V. M. and Doyle, J. T. (1967). Diet and heart disease in the Cardiovascular Health Center: III. Dietary intake and physical activity of male civil service employees. *J. Am. Diet. Ass.* **50,** 376.

Carroll, K. K. and Khor, H. T. (1971). Effects of level and type of dietary fat on incidence of mammary tumors induced in female Sprague-Dawley rats by 7,12-dimethylbenz-anthracene. *Lipids* **6,** 415.

Carroll, K. K., Gammal, E. B. and Plunkett, E. R. (1968). Dietary fat and mammary cancer. *Canad. Med. Ass. J.* **98,** 590.

Dam, H. (1971). Determinants of cholesterol cholelithiasis in man and animals. *Am. J. Med.* **51,** 596.

Davidson, C. S., Livermore, J., Anderson, P. and Kaufman, S. (1962). The nutrition of a group of apparently healthy aging persons. *Am. J. Clin. Nutr.* **10,** 181.

Dayton, S., Pearce, M. L., Hashimoto, S., Dixon, W. J. and Tomiyasu, U. (1969). A controlled clinical trial of a diet high in unsaturated fat. *Am. Heart Ass. Monograph,* 25. AHA Inc., New York.

Ederer, F., Leren, P., Turpeinen, O., Frantz, I. D., Jr. (1971). Cancer among men on cholesterol-lowering diets. Experience from 5 clinical trials. *Lancet* (July 24) 203.

Editorial (1971). Fats and multiple sclerosis. *Brit. Med. J.* (June 5).

Editorial (1971). Is roughage the key to colon cancer? *Med. World News* (Jan. 29), p. 14.

Editorial (1973). Are PUFA harmful? *Brit. Med. J.* (October 6), No. 58831.

Graham, S., Lilienfeld, M. and Tidings, J. E. (1967). Dietary and purgation factors in the epidemiology of gastric cancer. *Cancer* **20,** 2224.

Higginson, J. (1966). Etiological factors in gastrointestinal cancer in man. *J. Natn. Cancer Inst.* **37,** 527.

Lea, A. J. (1965). *Brit. Med. J.* **1,** 488.

Lea, A. J. (1966a). *Lancet* **ii,** 322.

Lea, A. J. (1966b). *Nature, Lond.* **209,** 57.

Lea, A. J. (1967). *Ann. Roy. Coll. Surg.* **41,** 432.

Mann, G. V., Pearson, G., Gordon, T. and Dawber, T. R. (1962). Diet and cardiovascular disease in the Framingham study: I. Measurement of dietary intake. *Am. J. Clin. Nutr.* **11,** 200.

The National Diet-Heart Study (1968). Final Report. *Am. Heart Ass. Monograph,* 18, AHA, Inc. New York.

Newell, G. R. (1970). Etiology of multiple sclerosis and Hodgkin's disease. *Am. J. Epidem.* **91,** 119.

O'Gara, R. W., Stewart, L., Brown, J. and Hueper, W. C. (1969). Carcinogenicity of heated fats and fat fractions. *J. Natn. Cancer Inst.* **42,** 275.

Pearce, M. L. and Dayton, S. (1971). Incidence of cancer in men on a diet high in polyunsaturated fat. *Lancet* **i,** 464.

Pernu, J. (1960). An epidemiological study on cancer of the digestive organs and respiratory system. A study based on 7078 cases. *Ann. Med. Int. Fenn.* **49,** 33.

Report. WHO Research Committee on Gastroenterology (1964). *Gut,* **5,** 196.

Rinzler, S. H. (1968). Primary prevention of coronary heart disease by diet. *Bull. N.Y. Acad. Med.* **44,** 936.

Rose, G., Blackburn, H., Keys, A., Taylor, H. L., Kannel, W. B., Paul, O., Reid, D. D. and Stamler, J. (1974). Colon cancer and blood cholesterol. *Lancet* **i,** 181.

Schettler, G. und Wagener, H. (1965). Krebs und Fettstoffwechsel. *Med. Welt* (Sept. 18) No. 38, 2135.

Singman, H. S., Archer, M. and Bergner, L. (1973). Cancer mortality and polyunsaturated fatty acids. *Mount Sinai J. Med.* **15,** 677.

Stukonis, M. and Doll, R. (1969). Gastric cancer in man and physical activity at work. *Int. J. Cancer* **4,** 248.

Sturdevant, R. A. L., Dayton, S. and Pearce, M. L. (1972). Effect of low cholesterol, high unsaturated fat diet on cholelithiasis: Abstract, Cardiovascular Disease Epidemiology Conference (AHA) Tampa, Florida 2/28 and 29, 1972.

Swank, R. L. (1961). "A Biochemical Approach to Multiple Sclerosis." Springfield, Ill., U.S.A.

Swank, R. L. and Bourdillon, R. B. (1960). Multiple sclerosis: assessment of treatment with a modified low-fat diet. *J. Nerv. Ment. Dis.* **131,** 468.

Tannenbaum, A. (1959). Nutrition and cancer. *In* "The Physiopathology of Cancer", 2nd ed., p. 517, Paul B. Hoeber, Inc., Medical Book Department of Harper and Brothers, New York.

Trulson, M. F., Clancy, R. E., Jessop, W. J. E., Childers, R. W. and Stare, F. J. (1964). Comparisons of siblings in Boston and Ireland. Physical, biochemical and dietary findings. *J. Am. Diet. Ass.* **45,** 225.

Wilson, W. S., Hulley, S. B., Burrows, M. I. and Nichaman, M. Z. (1971). Serial lipid and lipoprotein responses to the American Heart Association fat-controlled diet. *Am. J. Med.* **51,** 491.

Witschi, J. C., Littell, A. S., Houser, H. B. and Sorensen, A. I. (1970). Dietary intake of non-hospitalized persons with multiple sclerosis. *J. Am. Diet. Assoc.* **56,** 203.

Wynder, E. L. and Shigematsu, T. (1967). Environmental factors of cancer of the colon and rectum. *Cancer* **20,** 1520.

3

# Clinical Aspects and Therapy of Fat Malassimilation with Particular Reference to the Use of Medium-chain Triglycerides

K. SICKINGER

*Krankenhaus Waldshut, Germany*

## I. INTRODUCTION

Malassimilation involves all conditions which accompany disturbances in digestion and absorption. Both the digestion and absorption of food take place almost exclusively in the small intestine, one of its specific functions being the assimilation of fat. The small intestine can only fulfil this function with the aid of other organ systems, in particular that of the stomach and the pancreas, the liver and the functional complexes of the autonomic nervous system and hormones.

In the sections which follow only the physiology, pathophysiology of fat digestion and absorption and the therapy of fat malassimilation will be discussed. In this context, the term fats refers primarily to triglycerides. These are the glycerine esters of long-chain, saturated and unsaturated fatty acids whose chain length is mainly $C_{14}$ to $C_{18}$. In terms of quantity and calories they constitute the major proportion of food fat. In Europe the daily fat intake is approximately 80–140 g, there being wide fluctuations depending on geographical location and on the individual. The quantity of cholesterol and phospholipids, in comparison, is of little significance. The absorption capacity of the small intestine for cholesterol is, for example, very low. At maximum it is only approximately 2–3 g per day and, moreover, is dependent on the intake of triglycerides (Goodman, 1965; Treadwell and Vahouny, 1968; Bloomstrand and Ahrens, 1958).

It is not only for didactic reasons that disturbances in fat digestion and absorption are to be discussed separately: with the exception of extremely specific or selective disorders of the intestinal mucosa, e.g. primary dissacharidase deficiency, primary glucose–galactose malabsorption or other disturbances, fat malassimilation is usually the preliminary and main symptom of digestive disorder. Triglyceride maldigestion or triglyceride malabsorption is generally the main symptom of a secretory pancreatic insufficiency or sprue. Both maldigestion and malabsorption of triglycerides lead to steatorrhoea. Steatorrhoea is not only the sole symptom of malassimilation specific to the small intestine, but also the only symptom which is constant, easy to detect clinically and measurable in terms of quantity. Another reason why particular significance is attached to the physiology and pathophysiology of fat malassimilation is the high calorie content (9·3 cal/g) of triglycerides. A faecal fat excretion of 100 g/day, which is not uncommon in the case of severe pancreatic insufficiency, accordingly represents an energy loss of >900 cal.

The human body is mainly an aqueous system. However, about 40 %

of the calories taken are in the form of triglycerides which are completely insoluble in water. So for the assimilation of triglycerides there must be mechanisms present which change the insoluble triglycerides, temporarily at least, in such a way that they are made compatible with the aqueous phase of the small intestine. This involves complex processes of triglyceride splitting, solubilization in the small intestine, absorption in the intestinal epithelial cells, resynthesis of triglycerides from these epithelial cells and their removal from the cells. This multi-stage operation is extremely prone to disturbances. In clinical terms this gives rise to some important aspects of differential diagnosis, forming the basis for the appropriate therapy.

The decisive question for the success of therapy for any severe malassimilation syndrome is always the extent to which it is possible to restore fat assimilation. There are two basic approaches: either the disturbance is removed, e.g. by diet in the case of gluten-intolerant sprue or normal digestion or absorption is restored by symptomatic measures. One of these measures in the therapy of maldigestion in the case of a pancreatic insufficiency is, for example, replacement therapy using pancreatic enzymes. Another, much more universal, symptomatic treatment in cases of maldigestion and malabsorption consists in replacing long-chain triglycerides by medium-chain triglycerides with a chain length of only 6–10 C-atoms. The different physical properties of medium-chain triglycerides give rise to interesting physiological and therapeutic aspects. By way of an introduction to the problems of fat malassimilation the physiological aspects of the digestion and absorption of long-chain triglycerides will now be discussed.

## II. PHYSIOLOGY OF TRIGLYCERIDE DIGESTION AND ABSORPTION

The overall process of triglyceride digestion and absorption can be divided into approximately seven individual stages (Fig. 1). This division is very schematic because the individual stages form a continuous process and are greatly dependent one upon the other. We can, however, make a basic distinction between the intraluminal phase and the intracellular phase.

### A. Intraluminal Phase of Fat Digestion

#### *1. Emulsification and Hydrolysis*

Triglycerides enter the stomach with the food and here the fat is reduced

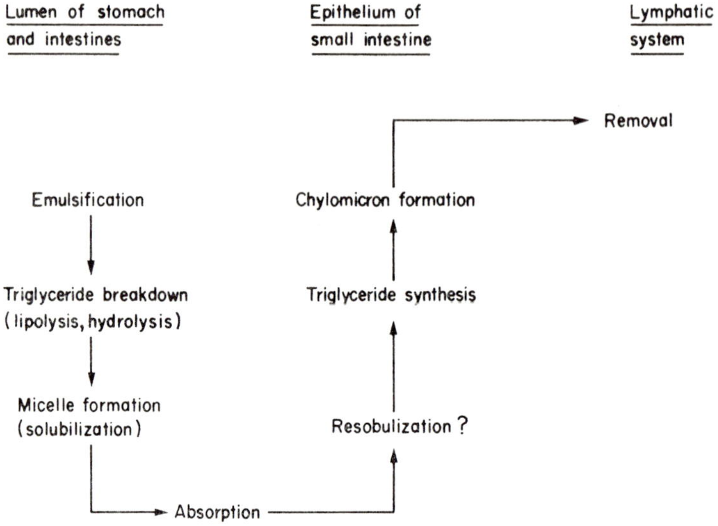


Fig. 1.

to smaller and smaller particles by mechanical action and the action of gastric lipase. At the same time the food entering the stomach and the duodenum stimulates the secretion of enteric hormones such as cholescystokinin, enterogastrone, pancreozymin, secretin and possibly enterocrinin. The complexities of this hormonal secretion will not be detailed here (Sheehy and Floch, 1964).

Peristaltic action in the stomach and upper jejunum breaks down the triglyceride droplets into minute particles. Bile salts reduce the interfacial tension at the oil/water interface only a little and are thus poor emulsifiers on their own (Dasher, 1952; Dreher *et al.*, 1967). However, in conjunction with extremely polar lipids—lecithin, monoglycerides and free fatty acids, i.e. including products of hydrolysis, the bile salts effect a greatly increased reduction of the interfacial tension. The combination of bile salts and polar lipids thus has a much greater emulsifying effect than the bile salts on their own. This fact alone demonstrates the interaction of the various processes concerned in intraluminal triglyceride digestion. The size of the fat particle resulting from emulsification is around $0{\cdot}6\mu$. The relative surface of the triglyceride particles is thus increased by a factor of about 10,000.

Triglyceride splitting, i.e. hydrolysis, starts in the stomach. The gastric lipase is, however, not identical to the pancreatic lipase. Gastric lipase acts primarily on short- and medium-chain triglycerides (Schonheyder and Volqvartz, 1946). It has been more closely characterized by Cohen *et al.* and differs from pancreatic lipase in its lower molecular weight and a pH optimum of 4–7. It is therefore acid-stable up to a pH of 2. As gastric lipase is also able to hydrolyse the fats contained in milk in the absence of bile acids, it is likely that it contributes towards milk fat digestion in infants. The physiological effect of gastric lipase in adults is a matter of controversy because the pH optimum is considerably higher than the normal pH in the stomach and gastric lipase develops only about 10% of its maximum activity in adults. It does, however, have a certain pathophysiological and therapeutic significance in the therapy of triglyceride digestion and absorption disorders using medium-chain triglycerides (Cohen *et al.*, 1971).

The importance of hydrolysis in the small intestine by means of pancreatic lipase was realized many years ago (Artoum and Reale, 1935; Frazer and Sammons, 1945). It was not until 1952 however that Mattson *et al.* were able to prove the specificity of pancreatic lipase in the hydrolysis of triglycerides. They demonstrated that the main split products of triglycerides are $\beta$-monoglycerides and free fatty acids. The latter result from splitting the $\alpha$- or $\alpha^1$-esters of the triglycerides, i.e. the 1- and 3-esters of the triglycerides. Later Hofmann showed that the $\beta$-isomer of the monoglycerides occurs in the lumen of the small intestine almost without exception only after the administration of triglycerides.

Pancreatic lipase acts at the interface of the emulsified triglyceride particles (Sarda and Desnuelle, 1958). The greater the surface of the triglyceride particles, the greater its activity. Although on the one hand a specificity of splitting the $\alpha$- and $\alpha^1$- (or 1- and 3-) position of the triglyceride molecule was demonstrated in purified pancreatic lipase, on the other hand the speed of splitting of these two positions depends on the chain length of the fatty acids. For example, in the case of synthetic triglycerides having butyric acid with four C-atoms in the $\alpha$-position and palmitic acid with 16 C-atoms in the $\alpha^1$-position, the butyric acid is split $2\frac{1}{2}$ times more quickly by pancreatic lipase than palmitic acid (Entressangles *et al.*, 1961). However, the difference in splitting speed is unimportant unless there is a considerable difference in the chain length of the fatty acids. There are no stereo-specific differences between the $\alpha$- and $\alpha^1$- (1- and 3-) positions (Tattrie *et al.*, 1958). Where short- or medium-chain fatty acids predominate in the $\beta$-position the $\beta$-ester is also split by the pancreatic lipase (Benzonana *et al.*, 1964). The same authors were also able to demonstrate that short- and medium-chain monoglycerides are isomerized more quickly than monoglycerides with long-chain fatty acids. This may mean that the more rapid splitting of short- and medium-chain triglycerides occurs via a more rapid isomerization of the fatty acids to the α-position.

Pancreatic lipase is activated not only by the surfactant effect of conjugated bile acids in the emulsification of triglycerides; for example conjugated bile salts also move the pH optimum of the pancreatic lipase from 8–9 to 6–7 which corresponds to the pH in the lumen of the small intestine (Borgström, 1954). Brief mention should be made here of the considerable importance of pancreatic bicarbonate as regards the consistency of the pH in the small intestine, because it is the pancreatic bicarbonate which neutralizes the hydrochloric acid of the stomach, thus creating the prerequisite conditions for triglyceride hydrolysis and the concurrent solubilization of the triglyceride split products.

Basically, in the first stage of hydrolysis one β-monoglyceride molecule and two fatty acid molecules are produced from one triglyceride molecule. During later stages a secondary hydrolysis can occur after isomerization to α-monoglyceride. The final result is, besides free fatty acids, only 72% β-monoglycerides, 6% α-monoglycerides and 22% free glycerol. Thus the triglyceride hydrolysis has two basic split products—monoglycerides and free fatty acids. The water-insoluble triglycerides have given rise to monoglycerides and fatty acids which also are not readily soluble in water. However, unlike triglycerides, monoglycerides and fatty acids are polar substances, i.e. they have a polar arrangement of hydroxyl groups hydrophilic in character. The water-solubility of monoglycerides and fatty acids is, nevertheless, so slight that they could only be absorbed very slowly by the intestinal epithelium via an aqueous phase. Under such circumstances the increasing concentration of split products would cause hydrolysis to cease immediately, i.e. through the action of the pancreatic lipase there would soon be a balance between hydrolysis and re-esterification (Hofmann, 1966, 1968). This is averted by the so-called micellar solubilization or micelle formation.

### 2. *Micelle Formation*

Borgström and later, above all, Hofmann demonstrated the varying behaviour of triglycerides and their split products in the presence of bile salts in numerous experiments (Borgström, 1960; Hofmann, 1963a, b, 1964, 1965). Bile acids are $C_{24}$-carboxylic acids with a steroid nucleus containing hydroxyl groups (Haslewood, 1964). They are produced in the liver from cholesterol via numerous enzymatic processes. The bile salts are secreted by the liver conjugated to glycocoll (glycine) or taurine in a ratio of about 3:1. Unlike cholesterol, the bile acids, in particular because of the hydroxyl groups and the conjugation with glycine and taurine, are more polar and more water-soluble (Hofmann, 1965). Conjugated bile salts with a lower pH have greater water-solubility than their unconjugated precursors (Hofmann and Small, 1967). As to the location of synthesis an initial distinction is made between the primary bile acids, cholic acid and chenodeoxycholic acid and the secondary bile acids.

The primary bile acids are synthesized in the liver direct from cholesterol. The secondary bile acids, desoxycholic acid and lithocholic acid in particular, are produced from cholic acid or from chenodeoxycholic acid via dehydroxylation by chiefly anaerobic intestinal bacteria. This dehydroxylation takes place in the lower ileum and mainly in the colon. Deconjugation, i.e. splitting-off of glycine or taurine, is a prerequisite condition for dehydroxylation. Lithocholic acid has very low water-solubility and there is therefore no significant re-absorption either in the terminal ileum or in the colon. Deoxycholic acid, however, is re-absorbed in the ileum and in the colon, conjugated again in the liver with glycine or taurine and re-secreted with the bile (Lack and Weiner, 1967; Weiner and Lack, 1968; Hofmann, 1966, 1967, 1968). The specific physiology and pathophysiology of the bile acid metabolism will be discussed in the chapters on "enteric bile acid loss syndrome" and "bacterial deconjugation" (summarized description Hofmann, 1967, 1972; Weiner and Lack, 1968). The primary bile acids, cholic acid and chenodeoxycholic acid, predominate in human beings and in most mammals, each making up about 40 %. Most of the remainder consists of deoxycholic acid (Sjövall, 1960).

It is the hydrophobic steroid nucleus, ending with a hydrophilic carboxyl group, which accounts for the polarity of the bile salts. As already mentioned, polarity is increased by conjugation with glycine and taurine. Polar lipids of these types are termed amphipaths. They are concentrated at the water/oil interface. The hydrophobic parts of the molecule are oriented towards the oil phase, the hydrophilic parts towards the aqueous phase.

Bile salts are water-soluble, i.e. in a low concentration they form molecular solutions. Some of the bile salt molecules form a monolayer at the interfaces (oil/water or water/air). This reduces interfacial tension. When the bile acid concentration reaches a certain "critical" level, the result is polymolecular aggregates which are termed micelles. This concentration is known as the "critical micellar concentration". This process takes place only at a definite temperature, the "critical micellar temperature". The critical micellar concentration and the critical micellar temperature are constants for the individual bile salts.

The triglyceride split products and the fat-soluble substances take part in this micellar solubilization in all fat digestion processes in the small intestine (Hofmann, 1967). It was stressed at the beginning that the basic triglyceride split products are monoglycerides and fatty acids. However, under the conditions prevailing in the small intestine three fatty acids are also immediately ionized, i.e. salts are formed. If we arrange these three split products in order of ascending polarity, the fatty acids are seen to have the weakest polarity, followed by the monoglycerides, the ionized fatty acids having the strongest polarity. The same order applies to solubility in the bile salt micelle. Even lower than the solubility of non-ionized fatty acids is the micellar solubilization of cholesterol. These split products of varying polarity, however form so-called mixed micelles with the bile salts. These are aggregates of polar bile acids with lipids of varying polarity. Figure 2 shows two different models of micelles, i.e. spherical and discoid micelles. The centre in each case is formed by the hydrophobic-hydrocarbon chains of the lipids or their split products.

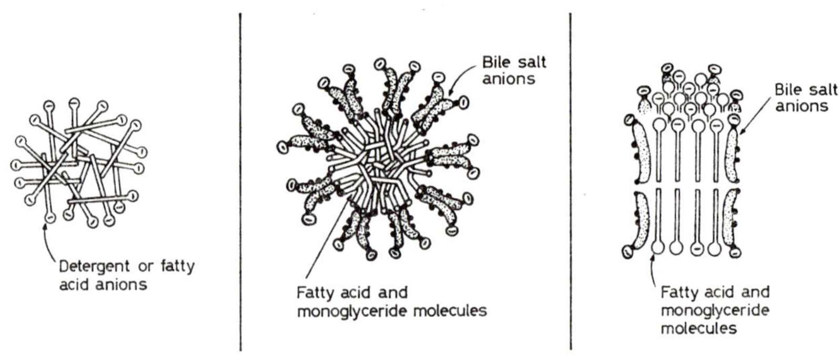


Fig. 2. Molecular arrangement of a typical soap or anionic detergent micelle (left) contrasted to two proposed models for the bile salt-polar lipid micelle (centre and right). From Hofmann, A. F. (1968). In "Medium Chain Triglycerides" (E. Senior, ed.), University of Pennsylvania Press, U.S.A.

Mixed bile acid micelles have an advantage over straight micelles, which consist only of bile acids and non-ionized fatty acids for example, in that the critical micellar concentration and the critical micellar temperature are lower. Mixed micelles are also larger than straight bile salt micelles. Substances which have a low polarity or no polarity, such as triglycerides, diglycerides and cholesterol can be solubilized in small quantities in the hydrophobic centre of the micelles. The critical micellar concentration is also dependent on the degree of saturation of the fatty acids. Unsaturated fatty acids and monoglycerides with an unsaturated fatty acid require a lower bile acid concentration for micellar solubilization than saturated fatty acids and their monoglycerides. Finally the bile acids also have different critical micellar concentrations. For dihydroxy-bile acids, e.g. chenodeoxycholic acid, it is 0·5–2 mM, for trihydroxy-bile acids, e.g. cholic acid, it is 4–5 mM.

In the small intestine the bile acid concentration is 4–10 mM and the temperature (37°C) is always well above the critical micellar temperature. Micellar solubilization is thus possible under these conditions. Understandably enough, micelle formation is also dependent on the pH factor. This applies in particular to free fatty acids which show better micellar solubilization in their ionized form. The ionization of three fatty acids diminishes below a pH of 6·5 and—besides hydrolysis being impaired—the micellar solubilization is also disturbed. So we may also speak of a critical micellar pH. Micelle formation is only possible within a range of pH 5·6–pH 7·0. The mixed bile acid micelles consist of about 85 bile salt molecules. The diameter of the entire micelle is about 40–50 Å (Borgström, 1965). The particle sizes have been reduced by a factor of about 100 in comparison with an emulsion and the relative surface has increased 10,000 times. This means that $1 \times 10^6$ micelles can be formed from one emulsion particle. Unlike emulsions micellar solutions are clear.

Hofmann and Borgström (1962) used ultracentrifugation to demonstrate that an oily and an aqueous micellar phase are present during fat digestion. The oily phase consists mainly of triglycerides, diglycerides and other lipids which are non-polar or only slightly polar. In the micellar phase monoglycerides and fatty acids predominate in the mixed micelles. There is an active exchange of individual molecules between the two phases. For this reason we must regard the micelle more as a physical state lasting less than 1 millisecond. Thus in the oily phase ionized fatty acids for example are also present and, as already mentioned, diglycerides, triglycerides and cholesterol in the micelle. The ionization of the fatty acids and their micellar solubilization together with the monoglycerides prevents re-esterification. Absorption takes place from the micellar solution phase.

## B. Absorption

The triglyceride split products are absorbed primarily as monoglycerides and free fatty acids (Mattson and Volpenheim, 1964). The individual processes are for the most part still unexplained. It is supposed that the micelles pass the solubilized lipid molecules to the microvilli either by the molecular exchange process already mentioned or that the bile acids make direct contact with the microvilli and act themselves as a type of conveyance (Hofmann and Borgström, 1962). There are at least indications that taurodeoxycholate is absorbed by the epithelium of the jejunum. The physiological significance of this process is, however, not yet clear (Johnston, 1968). The fat-solubility of the diglyceride split products obviously plays a major part in penetrating the membrane (Hogben, 1960). In recent years considerable doubt has again been expressed concerning the transport of entire lipid globules in the form of pinocytosis. (Dobbins, 1968; Rubin, 1966). The entry into the epithelial cells of the small intestine is however certainly a passive process which is independent of temperature and the inactivation of the enzymes by heat or antimetabolites (Johnston, 1968; Borgström, 1964; Strauss, 1966).

As no details are known of the entry of fat into the cell we do not know either which is the limiting step in the interluminal phase of fat absorption. It may be the transition from emulsion to the micellar phase but it may also be the passage of the micellar phase into the epithelium (Hofmann, 1967).

## C. Intracellular Resynthesis of Triglycerides

Unlike absorption, the resynthesis of monoglycerides and fatty acids to triglycerides is an energy-consuming process. The process as such was described as early as 1884 (Munk, 1884). There are two paths for this process in the epithelial cells of the small intestine; both require fatty acids activated to coenzyme A derivatives.

In the monoglyceride synthesis pathway absorbed monoglyceride serves as an acceptor for fatty acids. This is the decisive pathway in terms of quantity. In the other—the $\alpha$-glycerophosphate synthesis path—$\alpha$-glycerophosphate is formed from free glycerol and then acts as a fatty acid acceptor. The phospholipids are also synthetized via this pathway. With the aid of ATP and Mg-ions the free fatty acids are bonded to coenzyme A by fatty acyl coenzyme-A lipase (fatty acid thiokinase or acyl coenzyme-A synthetase). This is a microsomal enzyme which reacts specifically only with long-chain fatty acids (Senior and Isselbacher, 1960).

In the monoglyceride synthesis pathway fatty acid activated by monoglyceride transacylase (fatty acyl coenzyme A) are transferred chiefly to $\beta$-monoglycerides. However, the enzyme also reacts with $\alpha$-monoglycerides. Further acylation is effected by the diglyceride acylase (Clark and Hübscher, 1960). In the $\alpha$-glycerophosphate synthesis pathway glycerol is first phosphorylated to α-glycerophosphate. The glycerol need not be a glycolytic decomposition product of glucose in the epithelial cells (Dawson and Isselbacher, 1960); free, e.g. absorbed glycerol may be used in small quantity. The epithelial cells of the small intestine contain the glycerokinase necessary for this selection (Clark and Hübscher, 1962; Haessler and Isselbacher, 1963).

α-glycerophosphate reacts with two molecules of activated fatty acid, the result being phosphatidic acid. This is the common metabolite of the synthesis of triglycerides and phospholipids. The 1-α-phosphatidate phosphohydrolase splits off the phosphate group and a diglyceride is formed. The triglyceride is formed by the addition of a further activated fatty acid (Johnston, 1968). The phospholipids which are built up via the α-glycerophosphate synthesis pathway differ greatly from nutritional diglycerides in their composition and the distribution of the fatty acids. In contrast, the fatty acid composition of the triglycerides synthesized via the monoglyceride pathway shows a striking similarity to the nutritional triglycerides. This confirms the view that the monoglyceride synthesis pathway predominates in the resynthesis of triglycerides (Johnston, 1968). According to the calculations of several authors 85% of triglycerides are synthesized via the monoglyceride pathway and only 15% via the α-glycerophosphate pathway (Paris and Clement, 1968; Kern and Borgström, 1965).

In the epithelial cells of the small intestine there is also found a lipase which splits the intercellular monoglycerides into fatty acids and glycerol (Senior and Isselbacher, 1963). The physiological significance of this monoglyceride lipase probably consists in a regulating function in triglyceride synthesis. If there is an excess of free fatty acids the triglyceride resynthesis takes place via the monoglyceride synthesis pathway. However, if the ratio of free fatty acids to monoglycerides deviates substantially from the normal 2:1, the monoglyceride lipase can compensate this lack of fatty acids. About 18% of the β-monoglycerides absorbed are split intracellularly in this way (Paris and Clement, 1968).

## D. Transport From the Epithelial Cells of the Small Intestine (Formation of Chylomicrons)

The long-chain nutritional triglycerides are not transported from the epithelial cells until chylomicrons have been formed. These are about 86% triglycerides, 8·5% phospholipids, 3% cholesterol and cholesterol ester and 2% protein. The protein is most probably a β-lipoprotein (Isselbacher and Budy, 1963). The synthesis of this protein can easily be prevented by means of protein synthesis inhibitors such as puromycin, acetocycloheximide or ethionine (Sabesin and Isselbacher, 1965). Thus administration of puromycin results in a build-up of triglycerides in the epithelial cells of the small intestine with no increase of triglycerides in the blood. A similar disturbance occurs as in the case of acanthocytosis which accompanies an a-$\beta$-lipoproteinaemia.

The synthesis of the $\beta$-lipoproteins in the epithelial cells occurs, as does resynthesis in the microsomal fraction. The synthesized triglycerides probably remain in contact with the multi-enzyme complex of the triglyceride synthetase until a critical triglyceride concentration is reached. The triglycerides are then passed to a protein acceptor, the chylomicron being spontaneously formed (Johnston, 1968). The mechanism whereby the chylomicrons are passed from the cells into the lymphatic system has not yet been fully explained. It is probably a type of reverse pinocytosis (Palay and Karlin, 1959; Strauss, 1968). The formation of chylomicrons again allows the transportation of large quantities of water-insoluble triglycerides in an aqueous phase, e.g. in the lymph and in the blood.

## E. Medium-chain Triglycerides

### *1. Composition and Main Properties*

Medium-chain triglycerides are those with a fatty acid chain length of 6–10 C-atoms. The triglycerides occurring mainly in food have a chain length of 12–18 C-atoms (Fig. 3). Some naturally occurring oils, e.g. palm kernel oil and coconut oil, contain approximately 48% lauric acid (C 12:0) and up to 15% fatty acids with even shorter chain length.

Medium-chain triglycerides are obtained by distilling fatty acids (Fig. 4). Steam-hydrolysis of coconut oil produces a mixture of fatty acids. From this, by means of distillation, the fraction with the major proportion of capric (C 10:0) and caprylic acid (C 8:0) is obtained. This fraction of the medium-chain fatty acids is then re-esterified by

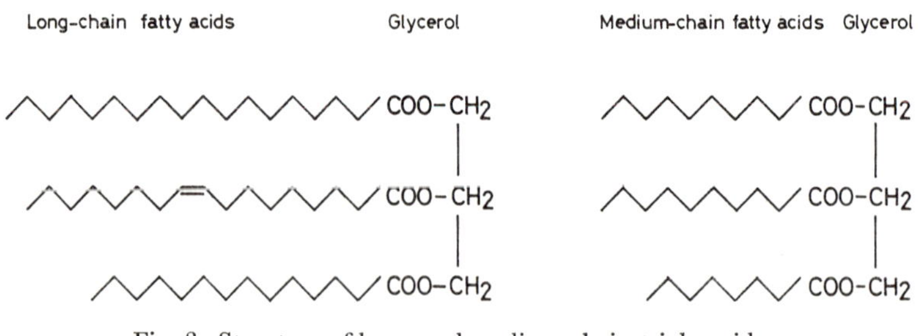


Fig. 3. Structure of long- and medium-chain triglycerides.

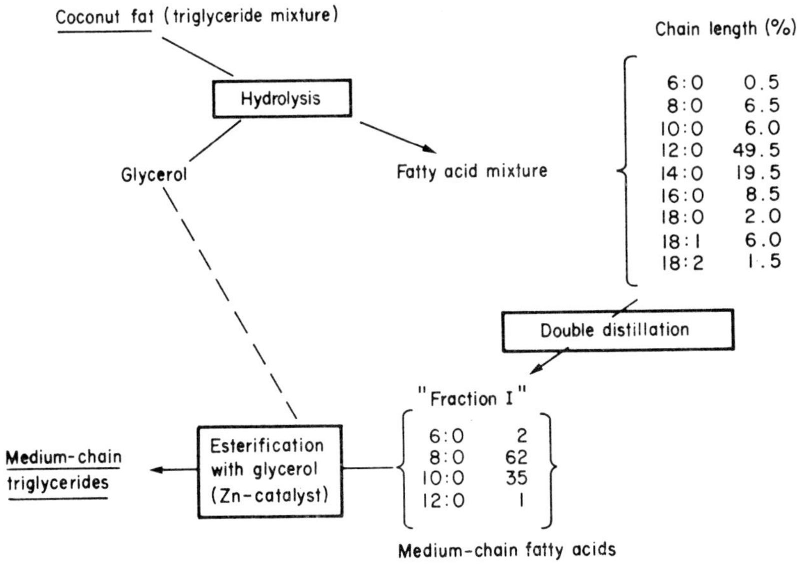


Fig. 4.

means of a finely distributed zinc catalyst with glycerol to medium-chain triglyceride. The melting and boiling points of these saturated medium-chain fatty acids and their triglycerides are much lower than those of the long-chain nutritional triglycerides. Medium-chain triglycerides are liquid at room temperature. By virtue of the smaller molecular size the water-solubility of medium-chain fatty acids is 100 times that of the long-chain fatty acids (see Table 1) (Ralston and Hoerr, 1942). The small molecular size and greater water-solubility of medium-chain fatty acids or their triglycerides give rise to their different behaviour during digestion, absorption, transport from the epithelial cells of the small intestine and in intermediate metabolism.

Table 1

Principal physical properties of long- and medium-chain fatty acids

| | Palmitic acid (C 16:0) | Octanoic acid (C 8:0) |
|---|---|---|
| Melting point (°C) | 63·1 | 16·7 |
| Solubility in water at 20°C (mg/100 ml) | 0·72 | 68 |

## F. Digestion and Absorption

### *1. Lipolysis*

Medium-chain triglycerides are hydrolysed more rapidly and more completely than long-chain triglycerides both *in vitro* and *in vivo* (Entressangles *et al.*, 1961; Desnuelle and Savary, 1963; Greenberger *et al.*, 1966). If $C^{14}$-tricaprylate, a medium-chain triglyceride with fatty acid chain lengths of 8 C-atoms is introduced into the small intestine of a rat, 92% of the triglyceride is hydrolysed in 15 minutes, whereas in a control experiment with tripalmitin only 29% is hydrolysed. If the intestinal loops are irrigated before the experiment to remove the pancreatic lipase this reduces the hydrolysis of the long-chain triglycerides considerably more than that of the medium-chain triglycerides (Greenberger *et al.*, 1966). The reason for this difference has not yet been fully explained. It is certain that medium-chain $\beta$-monoglycerides isomerize more rapidly than the $\beta$-monoglycerides of long-chain fatty acids (Desnuelle and Savary, 1963; Entressangles *et al.*, 1964).

A hydrolysis of medium-chain triglycerides in the stomach has also been described by several authors. This is effected by a gastric lipase which has since been detected in animals (Engstrom *et al.*, 1968; Clark *et al.*, 1969) and in human beings (Cohen *et al.*, 1971). It is located in the microsomal fraction and can be distinguished from pancreatic lipase on various points. It is still stable at a pH of 2 and has a pH optimum of 6·3–7. The molecular weight, being 40–50,000 is much lower than that of pancreatic lipase (>500,000). As regards the specificity of splitting the $\alpha$-positions and the rapid hydrolysis of medium-chain triglycerides there is no difference to the long-chain triglycerides. The physiological significance of this gastric lipase has not yet been completely explained. In infants it probably effects a more rapid hydrolysis of milk triglycerides. Because of its lower activity as regards long-chain triglycerides its physiological significance for normal fat digestion is but slight (Cohen *et al.*, 1971).

### *2. Absorption*

The peculiar behaviour of medium-chain triglycerides in the intestinal lumen and in absorption is primarly due to the greater water-solubility of triglyceride and its split products. The lower interfacial tension of the smaller triglyceride molecule with water alone, facilitates emulsification. Micellar solubilization is not necessary. This later point was demonstrated by Clark and Holt in experiments on rats (Clark and Holt, 1968). During a constant infusion of medium-chain $C^{14}$-trioctanoin the absorption over a longer period was 1560 $\mu$moles fatty acid/hr. After preparation of an external biliary fistula the intraluminal hydrolysis was somewhat reduced, bile now being completely absent, yet absorption was unchanged. Under these conditions the fatty acid concentration in the epithelial cells of the small intestine also remain constant (20 $\mu$moles fatty acid/g wet weight) as did the "turnover time" of 44 min. When not only the bile, but also the pancreatic juice, was diverted by a fistula the absorption rate dropped to 510 $\mu$moles fatty acid/hr—i.e. to about one-third of the initial value. When the pancreatic fistula was retained and the bile re-diverted into the small intestine absorption did not improve. Neither was the fatty acid concentration in the epithelial cells reduced in animals without pancreatic lipase. The "turnover time" was, however, significantly longer than in the control period. These findings prove that the penetration of the triglyceride trioctanoin is disturbed when no pancreatic lipase is present. Lack of pancreatic lipase is thus of greater significance than the absence of micellar solubilization due to lack of bile salt.

Analysis of the intestinal mucosa showed that after administration of medium-chain triglycerides, e.g. $C^{14}$-trioctanoin, under normal conditions the triglycerides are present in the form of free fatty acids. If however absorption takes place in the absence of pancreatic lipase the medium-chain triglyceride absorbed in the epithelial cells is present mainly as unsplit triglyceride (Greenberger *et al.*, 1966; Clark and Holt, 1968; Playoust and Isselbacher, 1964). This means that where pancreatic lipase is absent medium-chain triglycerides are also absorbed unsplit. The step which limits the rate of absorption of medium-chain triglycerides is always the penetration into the epithelial cells of the small intestine. Under normal conditions the penetration of free fatty acids and monoglycerides takes place more rapidly than that of the unsplit triglycerides in the absence of pancreatic lipase.

If medium-chain triglycerides are present in the small intestine at the same time as long-chain triglycerides the absorption of long-chain triglycerides is no longer maximal in comparison to a control in which long-chain triglycerides alone are present. However, the total of triglycerides absorbed under these conditions is greater than the maximum absorption of long-chain triglycerides or medium-chain triglycerides (Clark and Holt, 1968, 1969). The mechanism by which medium-chain fatty acids are absorbed has not yet been fully explained. It is possible that, unlike long-chain fatty acids and their monoglycerides, they are actively absorbed. Under the electron microscope the absorbed medium-chain fatty acids appear as clear droplets in the endoplasmic reticulum of the epithelial cell of the small intestine. These droplets do not reduce osmium however. They are probably only a small proportion of the absorbed medium-chain fatty acids which have undergone chain lengthening and then behave in a similar way to long-chain fatty acids (Greenberger *et al.*, 1965; McKay *et al.*, 1967; Reeve and Franks, 1968).

Because of their smaller molecular size and other physical properties connected with this (in particular their greater water solubility) medium-chain triglycerides are also absorbed in the colon (Valdivieso and Schwabe, 1966; Pihl *et al.*, 1966). Absorption depends on concentration. The maximum absorption of medium-chain fatty acids in the colon of dog is about 25% of the absorption in the jejunum (Pihl *et al.*, 1966). But the entry of medium-chain fatty acids into the epithelium is not necessarily equivalent to absorption. Numerous tissues, e.g. stomach, jejunum, caecum and pancreas, can oxidize up to eight times more medium-chain fatty acids (Chalfin and Holt, 1966).

*3. Metabolism in the Epithelial Cell of the Small Intestine*

In contrast to long-chain fatty acids, medium-chain fatty acids, absorbed mainly as free fatty acids under normal conditions, are activated to coenzyme A thiolester only to a slight extent (Senior and Isselbacher, 1960). In the epithelial cells the monoglycerides of medium-chain fatty acids are rapidly hydrolysed by a glycerol monoester hydrolase (monolipase) (Senior and Isselbacher, 1963). Finally the medium-chain triglyceride absorbed unsplit is hydrolysed by another intracellular lipase. Playoust and Isselbacher (1964) demonstrated that these intracellular lipases differ from pancreatic lipase not only in their substrate specificity but also in other parameters. The intracellular lipase effects complete hydrolysis of medium-chain triglycerides absorbed unsplit.

Only a minute proportion of the medium-chain fatty acids is resynthesized to triglyceride in the epithelial cell. About 9% of the radioactivity of $C^{14}$-caprylic acid can be detected in fatty acids with a chain length of 10–20 C-atoms. It is surmised that either the $C^{14}$-caprylic acid is broken down to $C^{14}$-acetate and then incorporated in long-chain fatty acids or that the $C^{14}$-caprylic acid undergoes a direct chain lengthening. The second possibility seems to be the more likely (Reeve and Franks, 1968).

*4. Transport of Medium-chain Fatty Acids from the Epithelial cells of the Small Intestine*

As early as 1913 Raper ascertained that short-chain fatty acids, in comparison to long-chain triglycerides, were not re-discovered in the thoracic duct of dog in the same proportion as they were administered (Raper, 1913).

In 1950 and 1951 Bloom *et al.* demonstrated precisely that $C^{14}$-caprylic acid (C 8:0) is transported mainly via the portal vein (Bloom *et al.*, 1951; Kiyasu *et al.*, 1952). These experiments and others performed by Borgström later support the hypothesis that, depending on the fatty acid chain length, long-chain triglycerides leave the epithelial cells of the small intestine as triglycerides via the lymphatic system, but medium- and short-chain triglycerides as free fatty acids via the portal vein (Borgström, 1955). It was then proved, in quantitative investigations on dogs, that 98% of the $C^{14}$-tricaprylate is transported in the form of free fatty acids via the portal vein (Hashim *et al.*, 1964; Hashim, 1968). The formation of chylomicrons is not necessary here. For this reason protein synthesis inhibitors, e.g. puromycin, cycloheximide and ethionine, have no or only a minimal adverse effect on the transport of medium-chain fatty acids from the epithelial cells (Sabesin and Isselbacher, 1965; Greenberger *et al.*, 1966). As medium-chain triglycerides are not transported via the lymphatic system, or only in small quantities, the lymph flow increases only slightly during the absorption of medium-chain triglycerides or only at the start of absorption. The reason for this initial increase of the intestinal lymph flow measured in the thoracic duct is not yet known. The daily lymph flow in the thoracic duct is reduced to half by the administration of medium-chain triglycerides in comparison to long-chain triglycerides (Simmonds, 1955; Lee *et al.*, 1968).

### *5. Conclusion*

To sum up we may say that medium-chain triglycerides are split more rapidly in the small intestine by pancreatic lipase and possibly also by one of the gastric lipases in addition (see Table 2). The result is almost

Table 2

Causes of improved splitting (hydrolysis) and absorption of medium-chain triglycerides

| | |
|---|---|
| 1. | Complete hydrolysis even at reduced pancreas lipase level |
| 2. | Possible additional effect of a stomach lipase |
| 3. | Micelle formation in the small intestine not necessary |
| 4. | Direct absorption of non-hydrolysed medium-chain triglycerides (breakdown of triglycerides in epithelium of small intestine) |

exclusively free fatty acids. Lipolysis, solubilization in the small intestine and thus absorption also are not affected by bile-salt deficiency. Pancreatic lipase deficiency however, leads to a moderate disturbance of hydrolysis and absorption. Under conditions comparable to pancreatic lipase deficiency medium-chain triglycerides are however still hydrolysed and absorbed much more rapidly than long-chain triglycerides. Under these conditions medium-chain triglycerides are absorbed unsplit and intracellular hydrolysis takes place. Medium-chain triglycerides are transported from the epithelium of the small intestine via the portal vein as free fatty acids. When medium-chain triglycerides are administered the intestinal lymph flow increases to a lesser extent than in the case of long-chain triglycerides.

## G. Metabolism of Medium-chain Triglycerides and Medium-chain Fatty Acids

During metabolism medium-chain triglycerides and their fatty acids also behave in a different way from long-chain triglycerides. Here however we shall discuss only those essential differences necessary to the understanding of various indications for a diet containing medium-chain triglycerides. Numerous experiments have demonstrated that 10–15 times more long-chain triglycerides than medium-chain triglycerides are incorporated in hepatic lipids. Medium-chain triglycerides, on the other hand, are broken down to $CO_2$ to a far greater extent and very much more rapidly. About 15–20 % of the carbon taken in as medium-chain triglyceride is expired in 50 min as $CO_2$. Only a small proportion of the carbon was detected in the hepatic lipids (Schwabe *et al.*, 1964; Scheig, 1968; Hashim, 1968). The medium-chain fatty acids are transported to the liver via the portal vein. Their main metabolites—$CO_2$, ketone bodies and acetate—then appear in the hepatic vein. Only a small proportion of the medium-chain fatty acids undergo a conversion to long-chain fatty acids and are esterified to triglycerides (Hashim, 1968).

As early as 1917 Embden demonstrated that acetoacetic acid is formed when the rabbit liver is perfused with caprylic acid. Using gaschromatography Freund and Weinsier detected acetone in the expiratory air after the administration of medium-chain triglycerides. The maximum acetone expiration was six hours. When the dose of medium-chain triglycerides was increased the formation and expiration of acetone also increased. This effect was reproduced. The simultaneous administration of saccharose halted the expiration of acetone. For this reason these authors suggest that, for example, the susceptibility to ketosis in diabetes should be examined by means of medium-chain triglycerides (Freund and Weinsier, 1966). The reason for hyper-ketonuria after the administration of medium-chain triglyerides is the rapid absorption and the rapid breakdown of medium-chain fatty acids to short-chain metabolites.

The effect of medium-chain fatty acids on insulin secretion is not yet fully known. It is assumed on the basis of numerous experiments on animals that medium-chain fatty acids stimulate the $\beta$-cells of the pancreas, in particular in dogs (Sanbar *et al.*, 1965; Sanbar and Martin, 1967; Horino *et al.*, 1968). In man it is only the combined intraduodenal instillation of medium-chain fatty acids with glucose which leads to a greater increase of serum insulin as compared to the instillation of glucose alone (Linscheer *et al.*, 1967). It is not yet known whether this increase is due to the direct effect of medium-chain fatty acids on the $\beta$-cells of the pancreas or to an increase of pancreozymin or glucagon in the duodenal mucosa. In patients with decompensated cirrhosis of the liver and portacaval shunts, either spontaneous or surgical, the intraduodenal administration of medium-chain fatty acids leads to a much higher titre of medium-chain fatty acids in the peripheral circulation than in non-cirrhotic patients (Linscheer *et al.*, 1966). An increase in serum insulin was also observed in these patients when only small doses of medium-chain triglycerides were administered (Greenberger *et al.*, 1968a). However it must be reasoned that it is not only the greater increase of medium-chain fatty acids in the peripheral blood which is the cause of the increase of insulin secretion but also that the decompensated cirrhosis of the liver with spontaneous or surgical shunts binds or breaks down the insulin formed to a lesser extent. Larger doses of medium-chain triglycerides (1·0 g/kg) lead to a measurable increase in serum insulin in normal persons also (Tamio *et al.*, 1968).

It has also been suggested that medium-chain fatty acids have a direct influence on glucose metabolism (Randle *et al.*, 1963). An increase in free fatty acids is said to inhibit glucose metabolism (Nestel *et al.*, 1964). However, when medium-chain triglycerides are administered orally in a dose of 1 g/kg body weight glucose utilization is increased (Tantibhedhyangkul *et al.*, 1967). It is difficult to decide whether this is perhaps only the result of the increase in serum insulin already discussed.

The behaviour of the serum triglycerides after administration of medium-chain triglycerides is, however, of practical significance. Serum triglycerides hardly increase, or not at all, after the administration of medium-chain triglycerides as the latter are transported from the intestine as free fatty acids. This behaviour was demonstrated in a metabolic disturbance, which accompanies lipoprotein-lipase deficiency, the rare, fat-induced hypertriglyceridaemia, hyperlipoproteinaemia type I (Furman, 1968). Owing to lipoprotein-lipase deficiency the long-chain triglycerides are not hydrolysed at the adipose tissue and the result is hypertriglyceridaemia. If these patients are given medium-chain triglycerides instead of long-chain triglycerides no more chylomicrons are formed and the medium-chain fatty acids are transported in the portal blood as free fatty acids. The high serum triglyceride level is lowered or normalized (Furman *et al.*, 1965; Reissell, 1966; Frederickson *et al.*, 1967).

In the case of carbohydrate-induced hypertriglyceridaemia (type IV), on the other hand, not such a good result is obtained by replacing carbohydrates by medium-chain triglycerides as by long-chain triglycerides. If 40 to 70% of the total calorie intake is replaced by medium-chain triglycerides, i.e. if most of the carbohydrates are exchanged for medium-chain triglyceride, the serum triglyceride is only reduced in some cases. It is only when medium-chain triglyceride supplies over 70% of the calories that an improvement can be achieved in carbohydrate-induced hypertriglyceridaemia. In contrast, even small proportions of long-chain triglycerides are sufficient to inhibit endogenous triglyceride synthesis (Furman *et al.*, 1965; Frederickson *et al.*, 1967). By replacing long-chain dietary triglycerides by medium-chain triglycerides the nutrition of patients with maldigestion or malabsorption can be improved. Under these circumstances the low or even extremely low serum triglyceride level could rise or become normal.

According to Kuo and Huang children, given medium-chain triglycerides because of pancreatic insufficiency due to cystic fibrosis of the pancreas, showed a slight to moderate increase in serum triglyceride. This too is probably only the result of the nutritional status returning to normal and not a specific effect of medium-chain triglycerides. The palmitic acid (C 16:0) content of the adipose tissue rose slightly (Kuo and Huang, 1965).

The influence of medium-chain triglycerides on the cholesterol metabolism in both animals and man has been examined in numerous experiments (Furman, 1968). In practically all investigations the replacement of long-chain saturated triglycerides by medium-chain triglycerides led to a drop in the serum cholesterol level both when the cholesterol content of the diet was normal and when a greater quantity of cholesterol was ingested (Grande, 1962; Kritchevsky and Tepper, 1965). Only in hens did the serum cholesterol increase on administration of medium-chain triglycerides (Fisher and Kaunitz, 1964). The mechanism of this cholesterol-reducing effect is not yet fully known. As the administration of medium-chain triglycerides leads to increased fat conversion in the liver, acetate may be removed from cholesterol synthesis (Kritchevsky and Rabinowitz, 1966).

## III. CLINICAL ASPECTS OF MALASSIMILATION

The term "malassimilation" covers both maldigestion and malabsorption syndromes (Haemmerli and Ammann, 1963; Jeffries *et al.*, 1964;

Kalser, 1964; Ammann *et al.*, 1968; Haemmerli, 1970). Maldigestion consists in a disturbance of the intraluminal hydrolysis, i.e. in the case of fat digestion, incomplete splitting of triglycerides. Defective lipase secretion, i.e. lipase deficiency, is not the only cause of maldigestion however. A bile acid deficiency can impair the hydrolysis of the triglycerides indirectly via disturbances in the micellar solubilization. If triglyceride split products cannot undergo micellar solubilization which renders them absorbable, the resulting concentration of split products also causes lipolysis to cease. This means that the intraluminal fat digestion can be disturbed by the disease of various organ systems. Maldigestion can therefore be subdivided into gastrogenous, pancreatogenous, and hepatobiliary maldigestion. Malabsorption (impaired fat absorption) is on the other hand always caused by a disturbance in the small intestine itself. Malabsorption syndromes are therefore specific to the small intestine. The malassimilation syndromes can therefore be classified according to the cause of the disturbance (Kalser, 1964; Booth, 1966; Jeffries *et al.*, 1969; Haemmerli, 1970). However this may also be done according to the site of the disturbance (Sleisinger, 1969). The latter course will be followed here (Table 3).

Malassimilation syndromes are divided into those with a disturbance in the intraluminal phase (maldigestion), those with a disturbance of the intestinal mucosa transport (malabsorption) and finally those connected with intestinal lymph drainage disturbances. There is another group where the cause of impaired digestion or absorption cannot be clearly classified. This classification also shows that it is not always possible to distinguish precisely between maldigestion and malabsorption. In the case of primary or secondary disaccharidase deficiency, for instance, there is maldigestion in the true sense of the term but due to the site of the disturbance, i.e. at the brush border of the epithelial cell of the small intestine, malabsorption is present too. There are, on the other hand, numerous conditions of primary, but in particular secondary malabsorption complicated by bacterial growth in the upper small intestine which can lead to an additional disturbance of the intraluminal phase of fat digestion by deconjugation and dehydroxylation of the bile acids.

With few exceptions steatorrhoea is a symptom of the malassimilation syndrome. It is clinically manifest in most cases, especially severe secretory pancreatic insufficiency, and so typical then, that special examination methods are not essential. In typical primary malabsorption, e.g. in coeliac disease (sprue) steatorrhoea is also usually present and can be clinically classified. But in some malassimilation syndromes steatorrhoea is but slight, i.e. not clinically manifest. So in these diseases

Table 3

Classification of malassimilation syndromes according to site of disturbance (Sleisinger 1969, modified)

I. Disturbances of the intraluminal phase (maldigestion)
   (a) incomplete lipolysis: pancreas insufficiency, maximum hyperchlorhydria (Zollinger–Ellison syndrome), gastric resection or functional impairment.
   (b) impairment of micelle formation (insufficient, conjugated bile acids): maximum hyperchlorhydria (Zollinger–Ellison syndrome), diseases of the bile ducts and the liver, increased loss of bile acids ("enteral loss of bile acids" in the case of ileitis terminalis or iliac resection or impairment, distal resection of the small intestine, cholestyramine therapy), bacterial deconjugation of the bile acids ("syndrome of the blind loop", diverticulosis of the small intestine, etc.).

II. Disturbances of the intestinal transport of mucosa (malabsorption)
   (a) primary malabsorption ("primary sprue"): gluten-induced sprue (adult celiaca), tropical sprue, unclassifiable sprue (idiopathic sprue).
   (b) secondary malabsorption (secondary sprue): regional enteritis, irradiation lesions, allergic (eosinophilic) enteritis, lambliasis, coccidiosis, generalized mastocytosis (urticaria pigmentosa), amyloidosis, scleroderma, drugs, impaired arterial circulation, proximal resection of the small intestine.
   (c) specific and selective impairment: primary disaccharidase deficiency (lactase, saccharase-isomaltase deficiency) secondary disaccharidase deficiency (lactase deficiency), relative disaccharidase deficiency, primary glucose-galactose malabsorption, abetalipo-proteinaemia, cystinuria, Hartnup syndrome, vitamin-$B_{12}$ malabsorption.

III. Impairment of intestinal lymph transport
   (a) primary intestinal lymphedema (primary exudative enteropathy).
   (b) secondary intestinal lymphedema.

IV. Unclassifiable impairment
   Diabetic enteropathy (diabetic steatorrhoea and diarrhoea), hypoparathyroidism, hyperthyrosis, dysgammaglobulinaemia.

---

we must distinguish between (1) general symptoms resulting from malassimilation, primarily steatorrhoea and (2) specific symptoms caused by the basic disease.

Although we shall be dealing chiefly with triglyceride malassimilation brief mention will be made of the basic methods of examination which are of practical importance and which serve to detect malassimilation and aid further clinical differentiation.

## A. Methods of Diagnosis and Differential Diagnosis of Fat Malassimilation

Many methods for the diagnosis and differential diagnosis of malassimilation syndromes have been described. Some of them, however, are of but little significance although they are routine practice in many hospitals. Here only a few well-tried tests and their significance will be described: stool weight, faecal fat excretion, $J^{131}$-triolein test, pancreatic function tests, D-xylose test, X-ray and biopsy of small intestine. The determination of faecal nitrogen (Table 4) should also be mentioned.

Table 4

Methods for the diagnosis and differential diagnosis of fat maldigestion and malabsorption

Differential diagnosis of steatorrhoea

| Methods | Maldigestion | Malabsorption |
|---|---|---|
| Stool weight | increased | increased |
| Fat excretion in stool | increased | increased |
| Tiolein test ($J^{131}$) | pathological | pathological |
| Pancreas efficiency test (secretin-cholecystokinin test; determination of lipase after test meal) | pathological | normal |
| D-xylose-test | normal | pathological |
| Biopsy of the small intestine | normal | pathological |
| Radiography of the small intestine | normal (sometimes pathological) | pathological |
| Stool nitrogen | pathological | pathological |

*1. Stool Weight*

A precise, quantitative record of stools forms the basis for all quantitative stool analyses. One essential precondition for the diagnostic value of the stool weight and that of other quantitative stool analyses is regular intake of food, the diet supplying 80–100 g fat and the same amount of protein every 24 hr. Nevertheless it is necessary to collect stools in 24-hr portions over a period of at least 3–4 days or, where there is considerable irregularity, over 72–96 hr. If the stool weight is under 150 g/24 hr further quantitative analyses are usually superfluous. In the case of maldigestion or pancreatic insufficiency the stool weight rises to 1000 g/24 hr. Stool weights are similarly high in coeliac disease. Subtotal resection of the small intestine can lead to stool weights of up to 2500 g and over (Sickinger, 1973).

*2. Faecal Fat Determination*

Quantitative faecal fat determination is the only direct method, and the most reliable, of detecting maldigestion or malabsorption. The standard method today is van de Kamer's faecal fat determination by titration or a modification of it (van de Kamer *et al.*, 1949; Frazer, 1952). Normally faecal fat excretion does not exceed 5 g/24 hr (Frazer, 1952) or 7 g/ 24 hr (Kramer *et al.*, 1962). On a general consensus of opinion steatorrhoea is assumed at a faecal fat excretion of over 7 g/24 hr. In the case of developing coeliac disease it rises to 20–30 g or over (Wilson and Dietschy, 1971). It is at its highest in excretory pancreatic insufficiency where it can reach up to 100 g/day, depending on fat intake. The faecal fat determination method allows no distinction to be made between maldigestion and malabsorption. Van de Kamer himself had realized that in attempts at fatty acid extraction by petroleum ether from an aqueous–alcohol mixture only 40–60 % of the medium-chain triglycerides with a fatty acid chain length of C 8 to C 12 would be dealt with (van de Kamer *et al.*, 1949; Saunders, 1967). In computing triglycerides by van de Kamer's titration method a mean molecular weight of 284 is assumed for the long-chain dietary fatty acids. As however the mean molecular weight of medium-chain triglycerides is 158 and only about half of this the incomplete extraction of medium-chain fatty acids is compensated by the over-estimation of the molecular weight (Senior, 1968; Sickinger and Hannemann, 1968) (Table 5). This possible error is of minor importance in practice because medium-chain triglycerides are so much better absorbed than long-chain triglycerides, even in the case of fat malassimilation, that only 1–4 % of the faecal fat consists of medium-chain triglycerides (Smits *et al.*, 1968).

Table 5

Relationship between molecular weights of fatty acids and recovery after a single extraction with light petroleum (Sickinger and Hannemann, 1968)

| | Medium-chain fatty acids | Long-chain fatty acids | |
|---|---|---|---|
| Mean molecular weight | 158 (= 56) | 284 (= 100) | (van de Kamer) |
| Recovery (%) | 57 | 100 | (Saunders) |
| | 63 | 100 | (own results) |

Nevertheless some authors have modified van de Kamer's method in such a way that medium-chain fatty acids can also be completely extracted (Braddock *et al.*, 1968; Jeejeebhoy and Kozak, 1970; Kelleher, *et al.*, 1970). However, these modifications do make the quantitative faecal fat determination more difficult as the composition, i.e. the mean molecular weight of the faecal fatty acids, is not known in each case. When medium-chain triglycerides are being administered, therefore, other authors recommend basic modification of the formerly prevalent method of faecal fat determination after wet extraction with ethanol and petroleum ether (Friedner and Moberg, 1967; Jeejeebhoy and Kozak, 1970) or with ethanol and toluol (Cohen *et al.*, 1969). Senior computed the faecal fat content by glycerol determination before and after decomposition. He believes that in this way it is simple to differentiate between maldigestion in the case of pancreatic insufficiency and malabsorption (Senior, 1965). Wolochow *et al.* measure the change in capacity of a condenser under the influence of a previously prepared faecal fat suspension (Wolochow *et al.*, 1965; Willig *et al.*, 1970). Odourless, clean processing of small quantities of faeces is unfortunately not yet possible. Recourse must therefore often be made to auxiliary methods. These are microscopic faecal fat determination and the $J^{131}$-triolein or $J^{131}$-olein test.

### *3. Microscopic Analysis of Faecal Fat*

This method has been somewhat unjustly discredited as it is usually employed by personnel who are more or less indifferent or who have had insufficient training. For many doctors and numerous hospitals it is often not only the only practicable method of detecting steatorrhoea but is a valuable screening test for the practising gastro-enterologist (Brooks, 1972). For practical purposes it is advisable to stain the stool sample not only with Sudan III solution but also to add a preparation of 30% acetic acid and heat over a Bunsen burner. There will usually be a marked fat concentration at the edge of the heated cover plate.

Reference is made to literature as regards details of technique and semi-quantitative analysis (Drummey *et al.*, 1961; Rothmann and Katz, 1964; Moore *et al.*, 1971). Chemically proven steatorrhoea can also be detected microscopically in about 69% of the cases. It is always easier to detect steatorrhoea microscopically in case of maldigestion especially in secretory pancreatic insufficiency than in the case of primary malabsorption, e.g. coeliac disease. In cases where steatorrhoea is only slight microscopic detection is successful in only about 40% of the cases (Moore *et al.*, 1971).

### *4. $J^{131}$-triolein Test*

After oral administration of $J^{131}$-triolein the excretion of $J^{131}$ in the faeces and the increase of radioactivity in the blood are measured. If the excretion of $J^{131}$ is lower than 5% or if the maximum in the blood remains below 5% of the dose given this is evidence of a disturbance in fat digestion or fat absorption. A differential diagnosis of maldigestion and malabsorption cannot be made with the $J^{131}$-triolein test. The result is often normal where steatorrhoea is slight. For this reason its diagnostic significance is limited (Pimparkar *et al.*, 1961).

*5. Pancreatic Function Tests*

*a. Secretin pancreozymin test.* After the introduction of a twin duodenal probe, which also allows the gastric juice to be withdrawn, pancreatic secretion is first determined fasting. There follows maximum stimulation of the pancreatic function with secretin and later with pancreozymin, the dose being one clinical unit per kg body weight, intravenously. After the secretion volume has been measured in 20-minute fractions the bicarbonate content and activity of chymotrypsin, trypsin, amylase and possibly lipase is determined. If a pancreatic carcinoma is suspected a cytological examination can also be made of the duodenal secretion (Lagerlöf, 1972; Dreiling and Janowitz, 1957; Creutzfeldt, 1964; Rick, 1971).

Functional disturbances of the pancreas can affect the various parameters of the exogenous pancreatic function in various ways: (1) isolated enzyme deficiencies, e.g. an isolated trypsin or lipase deficiency; (2) a disassociated reduction of pancreatic secretion and (3) a complete or even reduction of secretion or output of all substances tested (Rick, 1971).

*b. Stimulation by test drink (Lundh test).* The pancreatic function is stimulated by a drink composed of corn oil, skim-milk powder, glucose and possibly polyethylene glycol. The duodenal contents are then collected in four 30-minute fractions or as a total quantity over a period of two hours and the trypsin and possibly lipase content determined. If the pancreatic secretion is disturbed the total volume and the trypsin or lipase are significantly reduced. This test is much simpler than the secretin-pancreozymin test but not quite so reliable (Lundh, 1962; Stalder and Kayasseh, 1972).

*c. Faecal enzyme activity determination.* There are satisfactory correlations between the intraduodenal excretion of chymotrypsin and trypsin and the residual activity in the faeces. Chymotrypsin or trypsin is determined by titration with the aid of specific substrata (Haverback *et al.*, 1963). The normal chymotrypsin activity in the faeces is over 120 $\mu$g/g faeces; allowing for errors and limitations chymotrypsin determination is a valuable screening test in the diagnosis of pancreatic insufficiency (Ammann, 1970; Ammann and Filipini, 1967).

*6. D-xylose Test*

D-xylose is a pentose, a monosaccharide which is resorbed in the upper small intestine via a similar sodium-dependent process but which is only incompletely metabolized in the liver. For this reason after administration of 25 g/500 ml $H_2O$, with normal intestinal functioning, 5 g (20% of the dose) is excreted in the urine in the next 5 hr. Over 90% of patients with steatorrhoea resulting from malabsorption show reduced D-xylose absorption and excretion in urine. The result of the test is normal in the case of steatorrhoea resulting from maldigestion. Thus the D-xylose test has a greater significance as regards differential diagnosis (Benson *et al.*, 1957; Sickinger, 1965).

### *7. Biopsy of Small Intestine*

This has become a safe routine method. There are numerous biopsy probes available today, most of which work on the principle of the "aspiration biopsy". The mucous membrane of the small intestine is drawn in through a side opening; as suction increases a spring mechanism is released which acts on a rotating blade and the membrane is guillotined (Crosby and Kugler, 1962). Modern, hydraulically driven probes allow biopsies be taken *ad lib.* which are then carried upwards by water via a special tube (Brandborg *et al.*, 1959; Loder *et al.*, 1964). Quite simple apparatus is available, however, which is less suceptible to breakdowns (Choudhoury *et al.*, 1964; Maratka and Sedka, 1964; also Ammann, 1971).

Biopsy of the small intestine can be performed today on outpatients without much risk (Ammann, 1971). The only contra-indication is haemorrhagic diathesis. The failure rate is 6–12 %; the complication rate is, on the whole, low but depends on the type of probe used and the experience of the operator (Rubin and Dobbins, 1965; McPherson, 1970; Ammann, 1971). The previously familiar difficulties in the pylorus passage of probes can be eliminated by i.v. injection of 10–20 mg Metoclopramide (Sickinger *et al.*, 1965). Use of a Camus probe (Jeynard and Co., Paris), which can be stiffened with a wire, also facilitates the passage of the pylorus (Ayulo, 1970; Classen, 1968).

The biopsy is subjected to examination by microscope or stereo-microscope and then to an histological examination. Biochemical analyses, e.g. determination of dissacharidase activity are also possible. A biopsy of the small intestine allows primary malabsorption, i.e. coeliac disease, to be ascertained or excluded as the cause of steatorrhoea. Disturbances of the intestinal lymph flow also give a characteristic stereo-microscopic and histological picture. A biopsy is indispensable for the diagnosis of Whipple's disease. It is more or less normal in typical cases of maldigestion, e.g. pancreatic insufficiency.

### *8. Radiography of Small Intestine*

Fractionated X-ray examination of the small intestine is a very valuable method for the differential diagnosis of maldigestion and malabsorption. In the case of primary malabsorption (coeliac disease; sprue) typical, if non-specific changes are to be observed, in particular marked hypotonia of the intestinal loops, a coarsening of the fold contours and diffusion or accumulation of contrast. However, it is not always possible to exclude the possibility of coeliac disease by means of X-ray examination (Isbell *et al.*, 1969). This method also provides valuable diagnostic aids in the case of the enteric protein loss syndrome (exudative enteropathy), which may also be accompanied by steatorrhoea (Wagner *et al.*, 1968). Fractionated radiography is also imperative for the detection of impeded passage, blind sacks, stenoses and interior fistulae and of pathological changes, e.g. in regional enteritis, sclerodermia or amyloidosis. These processes can all cause steatorrhoea. This is usually a case of increased bacterial conjugation of bile salts—"the blind loop syndrome" (Seliger *et al*, 1971; Prevot, 1966).

## B. Disturbances in the Intraluminal Phase (Maldigestion)

### 1. *Incomplete Lipolysis*

*a. Pancreatic insufficiency.* Table 6 shows the various causes of pancreatic insufficiency. We can make a basic distinction between the several

Table 6

Causes of secretory pancreatic insufficiency (according to H. Schmidt, 1971)

1. Chronic and chronically recurrent pancreatitis
2. Acute and recurrent acute pancreatitis
3. Pancreatic carcinoma, papillary carcinoma
4. Pancreatectomy
5. Benign impairment of the flow of the pancreatic secretion
6. Primary atrophy and lipomatosis of the pancreas
7. Mucoviscidosis
8. Pancreatic cysts
9. Pancreatic insufficiency and chronic neutropenia syndrome
10. Isolated congenital enzyme defects
11. Protein deficiency in the diet (Kwashiorkor)
12. Impairment of pancreas function as a result of diseases of other organs of the gastrointestinal tract
13. Reduced digestive efficiency of pancreatic enzymes at a normal level of pancreatic secretion

mechanisms which may lead to an exocrine pancreatic insufficiency:

i. a reduced supply of enzymes, pancreatic lipase in particular, through atrophy or damage to the glandular parenchyma resulting from protein deficiency or rare, genetic enzyme defects, e.g. isolated lipase deficiency;

ii. impaired enzyme secretion in the case of organic stenoses in the region of the pancreatic excretory duct or insufficient endogenous stimulation of pancreatic secretion;

iii. reduced activity of pancreatic enzymes secreted in normal quantities, especially lipase, resulting from a drop in the pH of the duodenum and upper jejunum, e.g. in the Zollinger–Ellison syndrome;

iv. finally, combinations of two different mechanisms are possible. For example an organic stenosis in the pancreatic duct leads gradually to atrophy of the preceding glandular sections.

In connection with the various causes of pancreatic insufficiency we must make a distinction between:

i. specific symptoms of the primary disease, e.g. in the case of chronic pancreatitis or carcinoma of the caput pancreatis and

ii. general symptoms of maldigestion.

The specific symptoms will not be gone into here. Reference is made to specialist literature, e.g. Schmidt (1971).

The general symptoms of maldigestion are caused by the passage of undigested, unabsorbed food components into the lower sections of the small intestine and into the colon. This leads to a secondary overgrowth of bacteria causing putrefaction and fermentation processes. The result is an increased formation of gases, meteorism and a great deal of offensive flatulence. The individual stools become larger and the number of motions increases. Extremely watery diarrhoea is not typical. The stools are light in colour and, typically, show oily exudation. This liquid oil, which is pathognomonic for maldigestion in the case of pancreatic insufficiency as compared to steatorrhoea in the case of malabsorption, e.g. coeliac disease, is of importance in differential diagnosis. One recurrent striking point is that even patients with an extreme reduction of pancreatic function do not necessarily show any typical symptoms of maldigestion (Schmidt, 1971). In the case of marked steaorrhoea which is always the chief symptom of maldigestion there is a typical drop in body weight as steatorrhoea increases. A steatorrhoea of 100 g/day means an energy loss of 900 calories. Patients attempt to make up this loss of calories by increasing food intake. In some patients, especially those with chronic calcifying pancreatitis, there is often a fear of food which sometimes leads to severe pains in the epigastric region. Pancreatic insufficiency in early childhood leads to developmental disturbance.

Protein deficiency symptoms such as hypalbuminaemia, oedema, ascites and anaemia are sometimes to be observed.

*2. Laboratory Diagnosis*

It is only when pancreatic secretion is greatly reduced that food utilization is disturbed, i.e. the stool weight rises to over 200 g/day. There is then always an increased faecal fat excretion of over 7 g/day. There are great fluctuations in food utilization even in total or nearly total loss of pancreatic secretion. For instance, in total pancreatectomy with a constant fat intake of 80–100 g/day faecal fat excretion can fluctuate between 35 and 107 g (Whitfield *et al.*, 1965). On the other hand steatorrhoea does not occur until the lipase in the duodenum drops to below 25% of the normal level (Dornberger *et al.*, 1948; Müller-Wieland, 1962). Faecal nitrogen excretion shows a similar pattern. It rises above the upper normal limit of 0·5 g/day. In the case of total pancreatectomy it is between 5·5 and 10·9 g/day (Whitfield *et al.*, 1965).

For the early diagnosis of a secretory pancreatic insufficiency the secretin–pancreozymin test must be performed (Creutzfeldt, 1964) or trypsin and lipase in the duodenal fluid are determined by the Lundh test after a test meal. Finally, chymotrypsin and possibly trypsin activity can also be determined in 24-hr stool collections.

*3. Specific Diagnosis of Pancreatic Diseases*

The most frequent cause of exocrine pancreatic insufficiency is chronic recurring pancreatitis and chronic pancreatitis. Abuse of alcohol is top of the list of aetiological factors with 36·6%, followed by diseases of the biliary tract in 27·2% of cases. The cause is unknown in the remaining 36·2% (Creutzfeldt *et al.*, 1970). In keeping with the alcohol factor the male sex predominates, above all in the lower age groups, the ratio being about 3:1. Severe pains in the epigastric region with nausea and vomiting recurring over a period of months and years are the decisive clinical symptoms. In 75% of the patients there is a drop in body weight but a clinically manifest maldigestion develops at a comparatively late stage. For this reason the laboratory diagnosis outlined above must be employed as far as possible in the early stages. The calcification in the pancreatic region (Fig. 5) to be detected by X-ray of the epigastrium without contrast medium confirms the diagnosis. The frequency of occurrence of this calcification, chiefly in the ducts, varies greatly. In the South of France it is 94% (Sarles *et al.*, 1965; Sarles, 1971), whereas in Ireland it has been observed in only 9% of the cases. In southern Germany the figure is also high.

By definition, acute pancreatitis heals without reduction of the pancreatic function. It is only recurrent, acute pancreatitis that destroys the pancreatic tissue. Scar strictures of the pancreatic duct or intrapancreatic cysts are often to be observed here.

Carcinoma of the pancreas predominates in the upper age group. The mean age is 60–65 years. It is rare in patients under 40. The male sex also predominates here, the ratio being 3:2. In 70% of the cases

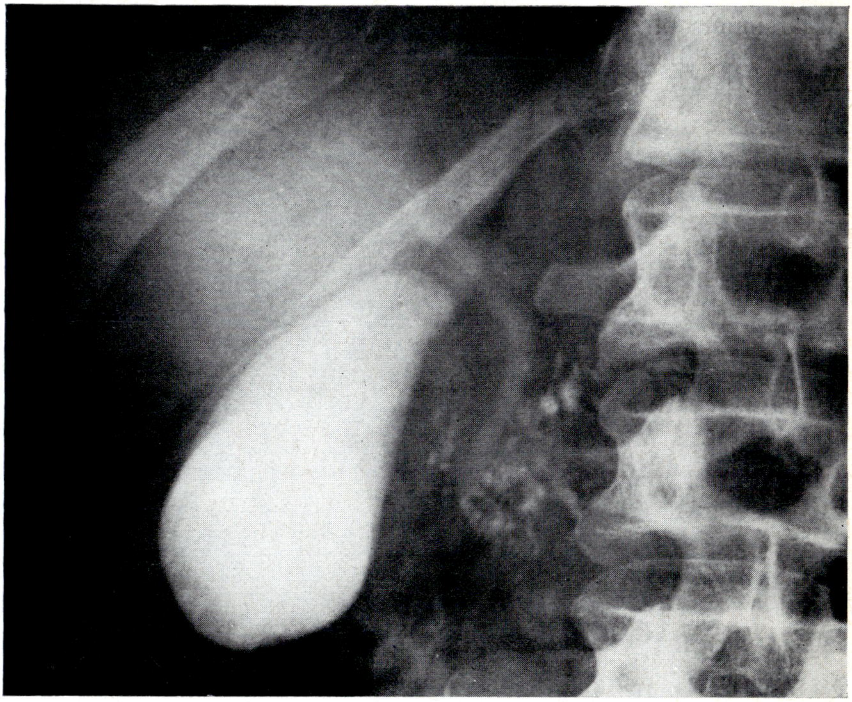

Fig. 5. Calcification in the pancreatic region by calcifying chronic pancreatitis.

the carcinoma is at the head of the pancreas. The causes include as yet unknown factors, abuse of alcohol and nicotine. It is seldom that pancreatic carcinoma is preceded by chronic pancreatitis (Moldow and Connelly, 1968; Paulino-Netto *et al.*, 1960; Lundh and Nordenstam, 1970). The symptoms are generally determined by the tumour. Colicky pains in the upper abdomen radiating into the back therefore play a prominent part. Tumour and maldigestion lead to a very rapid loss of weight and general wasting. By compressing the pancreatic duct, a carcinoma at the head of the pancreas can lead to maldigestion at an early stage, whilst lesions of the cauda pancreatis do not usually give rise to symptoms until an advanced stage. Then more uncharacteristic digestive complaints predominate—sensation of fullness, nausea and flatulence. Constipation often occurs. An obstructive jaundice often occurs where the common bile duct is compressed. Subclinical or clinical diabetes mellitus occurs when the pancreatic tissue is destroyed, chiefly when the cauda pancreatis is effected. Patients with carcinoma of the pancreas tend towards recurrent thromboses. In 25% pulmonary embolisms are the cause of death. The most reliable method of detecting a carcinoma of the pancreas is an exploratory laparotomy. Neither radiological methods, in particular hypotonic duodenography and caeliography nor laparoscopy allow a reliable early diagnosis to be made.

After therapeutic total pancreatectomy, which is seldom possible, maldigestion occurs to a varying extent. Diabetes mellitus is a consequence (Creutzfeldt *et al.*, 1961). Steatorrhoea does not occur after a partial distal resection for chronic pancreatitis unless more than 75% has been removed. Resection of the head of the pancreas, however, the tail remaining, maldigestion occurs earlier whilst diabetes does not develop until later (Kalser *et al.*, 1968). The clinical symptoms and diagnosis of other pancreatic diseases will not be explored here. They generally play but a secondary role in practice. Reference is made to literature on the subject (e.g. Schmidt, 1971).

*a. Therapy of secretory pancreatic insufficiency.* The therapy of the primary disease will not be dealt with here. It is only when pain is the predominant symptom in the case of chronic pancreatitis that surgery may be necessary. An attempt should be made to halt the progress of chronic pancreatitis by elimination of causative noxae (e.g. diseases of bile ducts or abuse of alcohol). If a stenosis is present in the pancreatic duct the pancreatic function can recover after surgery.

In the majority of cases the therapy of secretory pancreatic insufficiency can only be symptomatic. Priority must be given to replacement therapy with pancreatic ferments. Dietary measures will also be necessary in most cases. Allowance must be made in the diet for the accompanying diabetes mellitus which often does not become manifest or more severe until the pancreatic insufficiency has been well compensated.

In substitution therapy with pancreatic ferments allowance must be made for the fact that the preparations used have a high enzyme content. Their lipase content is the decisive factor. This often differs greatly (Berndt and Müller-Wieland, 1969; Müller-Weiland and Berndt, 1969). The galenic form is also of prime importance. Preparations with a high enzyme content, a high proportion of lipase in particular, may not have the desired effect if the enzymes are released incompletely or too late

(Grözinger *et al.*, 1972). Approximately 100 dragees would be required to replace the total quantity of pancreatic lipase. This corresponds to a volume of pancreatic secretion of 1·51 per day. About 20% of this dose is normally sufficient. It is often impossible to eliminate the residual steatorrhoea in the case of pancreatic insufficiency even with large doses (Creutzfeldt *et al.*, 1961; Schultis and Wagner, 1968). There may be various reasons for this:

the pancreatic ferments do not become fully effective. If they are administered in the form of powder or granulate, for instance, they are irreversibly inactivated by the acid pH of below 3 in the stomach;

so activity losses of 40–60% must be expected (Iber, 1968). For this reason pancreatic ferments in the form of powder or granulate are only of use when the gastric juice is achlorhydric and, in particular, there is simultaneous acceleration of passage, e.g. partial gastrectomy and duodenopancreatectomy. Loss of bicarbonate secretion in the upper small intestine will cause the pH to drop to below 7. This inhibits lipase activity. The optimum pH for micellar solubilization will not be present either. Although additional doses of sodium bicarbonate can normalize digestion in such cases, this form of therapy requires 20–30 g of sodium bicarbonate/day. This is not practicable in the long term. Finally pancreatic insufficiency is often accompanied by an increase in bacteria in the middle and upper small intestine. Mainly anaerobic intestinal bacteria deconjugate the bile acids. The "blind loop syndrome" thus also develops. It is therefore advisable to disinfect the small intestine with, for example, tetracyclines from time to time, at least when therapy is started (see also p. 163);

the effectiveness of the pancreatic ferments can be influenced but negligibly by the way in which they are administered (Drube, 1963; Iber, 1968; Jordan and Grossman, 1959). Although an hourly dose of pancreatic ferments is more effective it is usually impracticable. What is decisive is that the total calorie intake and the fat intake should be divided amongst 5 to 7 small meals for the better utilization of the pancreatic secretion still taking place.

### *4. Diet in the Case of Pancreatic Insufficiency*

A special diet is not essential in uncomplicated cases of secretory pancreatic insufficiency (Bircher and Haemmerli, 1967). Food should have a high calorie content. To guarantee a sufficiently high calorie intake there must be an adequate proportion of fat because even in the case of pancreatic insufficiency the more fat is ingested, the more is absorbed (Wollaeger *et al.*, 1948). A residual steatorrhoea of up to 20 g/day can be tolerated. This does not usually give rise to any clinical symptoms. Fat tolerance must be ascertained from case to case. It can be between 50 and 150 g/day. However, if despite adequate and regular substitution the clinical signs of fat maldigestion such as meteorism, flatulence and a high stool weight of over 300 g/day occur, the fat intake must be reduced or the long-chain nutritional triglycerides replaced by medium-chain triglycerides which may, of course, be included in the regimen from the start. It is advisable, particularly for residual steatorrhoea to counteract occasional vitamin-deficiency symptoms by regular parenteral administration of fat-soluble vitamins A, D, E and K (e.g. Adek-Falk[R]), possibly also vitamin $B_{12}$ at intervals of 1–4 weeks.

With secretory pancreatic insufficiency medium-chain triglycerides are hydrolysed more rapidly and more completely than long-chain triglycerides (Table 7). Complete splitting is therefore possible even when the concentration of pancreatic lipase is reduced. The additional effect of one of the gastric lipases is the subject of discussion. The greater

Table 7

Differences between long- and medium-chain triglycerides during Digestion, Absorption and Transport from the epithelial cells of the small intestine

| Long-chain triglycerides | Medium-chain triglycerides |
|---|---|
| DIGESTION (intraluminal) | |
| 1. Emulsification | quicker and more readily |
| 2. Lipolysis (pancreas lipase) | quicker and more complete |
| 3. Micelle formation (conjugated bile acids) | not necessary |
| ABSORPTION | |
| 1. Passage into the cell | quick, also possible as the unsplit triglyceride |
| 2. Triglyceride synthesis | not necessary |
| Chylomicron formation | intracellular lipolysis |
| TRANSPORT | |
| via the lymphatic system | hardly any, medium-chain fatty acids are transported via the Vena portal |

water solubility makes micelleformation unnecessary and the medium-chain triglycerides or their split products are transported to the epithelial cells of the small intestine more quickly and more completely even when micellar solubilization is disturbed. Finally, where pancreatic lipase is deficient medium-chain triglycerides are also absorbed unsplit by the epithelial cells.

In treating pancreatic insufficiency visible fat is replaced in part or in its entirety by medium-chain triglycerides. Substitution therapy with pancreatic ferments continues where pancreatic insufficiency is severe. It may be possible to reduce substitution whilst medium-chain triglycerides are being administered. Where pancreatic insufficiency is slight and if therapy is necessary at all, substitution may sometimes be dropped completely if dietetic therapy includes medium-chain triglycerides. Patients for whom therapy with medium-chain triglycerides would appear most suitable are those with, for example, occlusion of the duodenal papillae and bile acid deficiency in the small intestine (Pinter *et al.*, 1964; Holt *et al.*, 1965; Kuo and Huang, 1965; Kistler, 1967; Erdmann, 1968; Beck *et al.*, 1968; Sickinger, 1968a, b; Gracey *et al.*, 1969).

The combined therapy of pancreatic insufficiency with pancreatic ferments and medium-chain triglycerides will be demonstrated by means of an example: in a 60-year-old patient pancreatic insufficiency was caused by carcinoma of the papilla. The obstructive jaundice was eliminated by means of choledochoduodenostomy. There was a steatorrhoea of 24 g and an increased stool weight of 410 g/day (Table 8). After replacing visible fat by medium chain triglycerides (70 g/day) the faecal fat excretion dropped to 7 g/day. When the pancreatic ferment

Table 8

Therapy of excretory pancreatic insufficiency by pancreatic enzymes and medium-chain triglycerides

H. Sch. male(s), 60-years-old — *Diagnosis:* papillary carcinoma, pancreatic insufficiency

| Diet | | Long-chain triglycerides 100 g/day | | Medium-chain triglycerides 70 g/day | |
|---|---|---|---|---|---|
| Nutrizym® | | — | 6 pills | 6 pills | — |
| Stool weight | g/d | 410 | 280 | 120 | 150 |
| Stool fat | g/d | 24 | 14 | 7 | 13 |

therapy was dropped, the substitution of medium-chain triglycerides being retained, the faecal fat rate rose to 13 g (Sickinger, 1969b).

The efficacy of therapy with medium-chain triglycerides can be demonstrated particularly well in patients with total pancreatectomy. In such cases the residual steatorrhoea is reduced by about half (Beck *et al.*, 1968; Kümmerle *et al.*, 1969) (Fig. 6).

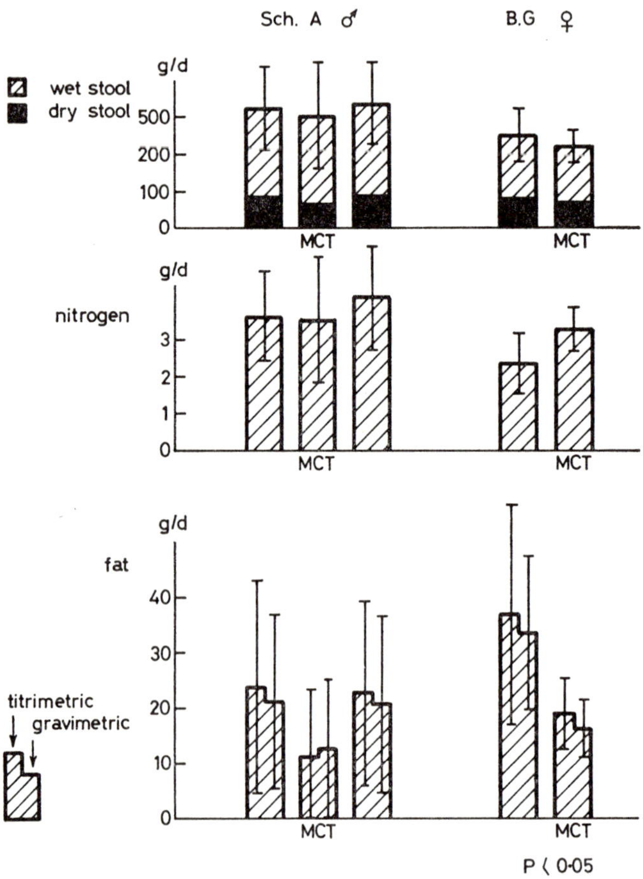


Fig. 6. Therapy of maldigestion after total pancreatectomy with pancreatic enzymes and medium-chain triglycerides (Beck *et al.*, 1968).

*5. Zollinger–Ellison Syndrome*

The maximum stimulation of gastric acid secretion by a gastrine-producing tumour in the pancreas causes the pH in the upper small intestine to drop. This reduces the activity of the pancreatic enzymes, lipase in particular. If the pH drops to below 3, the pancreatic lipase is irreversibly inactivated. The therapy for such conditions is surgery. The pancreatic tumour is resected where possible, even a total pancreatectomy may be performed. However, as such tumours are generally malignant and multiple duodenal or gastric ulcers dominate in the clinical picture, total gastrectomy is usually unavoidable (Vogel *et al.*, 1967; Shimoda and Rubin, 1968; Creutzfeldt *et al.*, 1970). In the interim, however, steatorrhoea can be treated by substituting medium-chain triglycerides for the nutritional fat. A disturbance in micellar solubilization also plays a part in the pathogenesis of this steatorrhoea (see pp. 123 and 154).

*a. Steatorrhoea after partial gastrectomy.* In 13–74% of cases partial gastrectomy is followed by loss of weight (Corsini *et al.*, 1966; Wall *et al.*, 1967). This is most frequenty caused by insufficient food intake and not by impaired food utilization (Drube, 1963; McKay, 1970; Ross, 1971). Steatorrhoea is present in 60–70% of the patients (Corsini *et al.*, 1966; Welbourn, 1967). In the majority of cases it is but slight. It is more often a "chemical" than a clinical steatorrhoea (Drube, 1963; Corsini *et al.*, 1966). The more extensive the gastrectomy, the greater the likelihood that steatorrhoea will occur. It increases in about the following order: gastroenterostomy $<$ Billroth I $<$ oesophagoduodenostomy $<$ Billroth II $<$ oesophagojejunostomy.

The pathogenesis is complex. Impaired lipolysis is not the only factor. There are several which contribute—either in isolation or in combination—towards steatorrhoea after partial gastrectomy.

### *6. Gastrogenous Factors*

The emptying of the residual stomach is accelerated after partial gastrectomy (Lundh, 1958; Corsini *et al.*, 1966). Emptying is more rapid when the duodenum plays no part. This means that the digestion phase, i.e. fat emulsification in the stomach, is abbreviated and disturbed. The acid and pepsin secretion of the stomach is also reduced by gastrectomy. The hyperosmolar chyme passes direct into the upper jejunum. The loss of the pylorus means not only that there is no well-dosed emptying of the stomach, the "jet effect" which furthers emulsification is also absent.

### *7. Pancreatic Factors*

The pancreatic function is impaired in various ways by gastrectomy. Loss of the duodenum also means that the pancreatic secretion is no longer stimulated by secretin or that it is stimulated too late. Pancreatic secretion is also limited even in the presence of exogenous secretin and pancreozymin (Wagner, 1967; Hillman, 1968).

### *8. Enteric Factors*

Today it is generally thought that gastric resection does not damage the structural function of the epithelial cells to such an extent as to result in malabsorption. Localized changes can be compensated by the lower small intestine (Drube, 1963; Corsini *et al.*, 1966; Wagner, 1967; Hillman, 1968). Thus steatorrhoea after partial gastrectomy is caused primarily by a disturbance in the intraluminal phase, i.e. maldigestion. Patients in whom gastric resection gives rise to a gluten-intolerant enteropathy (coeliac disease; sprue) with marked steatorrhoea, are an exception (Hedberg *et al.*, 1966; Binder, 1970). The most frequent disturbance after elimination of the duodenum is insufficient mixing of chyme with bile and pancreatic secretion. Triglycerides are but poorly emulsified in such cases; lipolysis is incomplete and the micellar solubilization disturbed, leading to insufficient fat digestion and absorption.

Bacterial overgrowth in the small intestine can lead to a disturbance in the intraluminal phase of fat digestion. Stagnation of chyme in the afferent loop after gastric resection provides favourable conditions for the growth of atypical bacteria. Extreme proliferation of intestinal bacteria occurs in gastrojejunocolonic fistulae (Wirts, 1963; Bishop, 1965).

*a. Diagnosis.* Steatorrhoea occurring after gastric resection should be further investigated by differential diagnosis. The possibility of coeliac disease must be eliminated by means of biopsy of the small intestine. Pancreatic insufficiency can be excluded by means of the secretin-pancreomyzin test or the Lundh test. As these procedures are not completely reliable where the duodenum is eliminated, chymotrypsin determination in the faeces may be used. It is only in special clinics that the qualitative and quantitative bacteriological examination of the small intestine and the $C^{14}$-respiration test can be performed (see section on "blind loop syndrome"). Finally, a precise, fractionated examination of the passage of the small intestine will be carried out in any case to exclude an afferent loop syndrome and a gastrojejunocolonic fistula. Other diagnostic information is given in the section on the "blind loop syndrome" (p. 163).

*b. Therapy.* Where there is a specific cause of steatorrhoea the appropriate therapy must be introduced, i.e. in the case of coeliac disease gluten-free diet, in pancreatic insufficiency the administration of pancreatic ferments and in the case of bacterial overgrowth in the afferent loop disinfection of the small intestine by means of antibiotics. If despite detailed diagnosis no specific cause is found, only non-specific measures can be taken. These include giving several small meals instead of one or two large meals. This makes allowance for the reduced capacity of the stomach. In order to stimulate the pancreatic function Drube also recommends a preparatory meal to be taken half an hour before the main meal.

One method of covering the complex pathogenesis of steatorrhoea after gastric resection is to replace nutritional fat by medium-chain triglycerides. These are digested in cases of both bile acid and pancreatic lipase deficiency and adequately absorbed even if there is atrophy of the intestinal mucosa. Surgery is indicated in cases of gastrocolic fistula, gastroileostomy or obstruction of the afferent loop. Surgical intervention will also be necessary if the conservative measures mentioned above do not lead to an improvement. The aim will generally be surgery in the form of a Billroth I type of stomach.

Table 9

Therapy of diarrhoea and steatorrhoea following partial gastrectomy and vagotomy by replacement of nutritional triglycerides by medium-chain triglycerides

H. Wi (female), 53-years-old — *Diagnosis:* gastric resection, "dumping syndrome" following vagotomy

| Dietary fat | | Long-chain triglycerides 70 g/day | Medium-chain triglycerides 70 g/day |
|---|---|---|---|
| Diarrhoea | | +++ | — |
| Stool weight | g/day | 720 | 240 |
| Fat content | g/day | 25 | 8 |

In a small percentage of cases vagotomy, truncular vagotomy in particular, leads to severe diarrhoea with occasional steatorrhoea. The following case is an example of the author's own experience in treating such complications with medium-chain triglycerides (see Table 9).

A Billroth I partial gastrectomy had been performed on a 53-year-old female patient three years previously to remove a tumour of the cardia. Truncular vagotomy was inevitable. The patient had since suffered from extremely severe diarrhoea with up to 20 motions daily. There was also steatorrhoea. The D-xylose test, biopsy of the small intestine and secretory pancreatic function were completely normal. A "dumping syndrome" was diagnosed, carbohydrate intake reduced and frequent small meals given. There was no improvement. Subsequently the nutritional triglycerides were replaced by medium-chain triglycerides. The diarrhoea ceased immediately. The stool weight dropped and the moderate steatorrhoea became normal. On this therapy the patient has now been free of symptoms for four years.

*c. Defective micelle formation.* Micelle formation is an essential stage in intraluminal fat digestion. This requires, *inter alia*, a correct bile acid concentration of 2mM ("critical micellar bile acid concentration"). It is only possible however under certain physical conditions: the "critical micellar pH" of 6·5 is essential. Finally only conjugated bile acids can form micelles. There are therefore various conditions leading to impaired micelle formation and thus defective triglyceride digestion and absorption:

1. a drop in pH in the upper small intestine;
2. disturbance of the bile acid synthesis and secretion;
3. increased bile acid loss;
4. increased deconjugation of bile acids in small intestine.

### *9. Drop in pH in Upper Small Intestine (Zollinger–Ellison Syndrome)*

Diarrhoea and steatorrhoea occur in about half the patients with the Zollinger–Ellison syndrome (Soergel, 1969; Creutzfeldt, 1969). Hyperacidity in the jejenum is the cause of steatorrhoea (GO). This does not only result in inactivation of the pancreatic lipase but also in a relative disturbance of micellar solubilization caused by a drop in pH below the "critical micellar pH" and finally in precipitation of glycin-conjugated bile acids. After withdrawal of the gastric juice diarrhoea and steatorrhoea cease immediately (Summerskill, 1959) as happens after suppression of gastric acid secretion by large doses of atropin and after total gastrectomy without removal of tumour (Vogel *et al.*, 1967; Shimoda and Rubin, 1968). In many cases of the Zollinger–Ellison syndrome changes in the mucosa of the upper jejunum is an attendant cause of steatorrhoea (Shimoda and Rubin, 1968; Mansbach *et al.*, 1968). See p. 175 for therapy.

### *10. Disturbance in Bile Acid Synthesis and Secretion*

Bile acid concentration in the small intestine is reduced if secretion is disturbed as in intra- and extrahepatic obstructive jaundice, e.g. also in primary biliary cirrhosis. The pathogenesis of steatorrhoae in cases of liver cirrhosis has not been definitively determined (Losowsky and Walker, 1969; Marin *et al.*, 1969) as only 30–60% of liver cirrhotic patients have steatorrhoea (Baroana *et al.*, 1962; Beck and Gnauck, 1962; van Goidsenhoven *et al.*, 1963; Linscheer, 1970). However this is usually a chemical steatorrhoea with an average faecal fat excretion of 10 g/day; it rarely rises above 30 g (Beck and Gnauck, 1962; Sickinger, 1964; Linscheer, 1970; Sun *et al.*, 1967).

The secretory pancreatic function is limited after submaximum or maximum stimulation in about 40% of patients with cirrhosis of the liver but this is not connected with the extent of the stearorrhoea (Creutzfeldt and Widmann, 1956; Baraona *et al.*, 1962; van Goidsenhoven *et al.*, 1963; Zieve and Mulford, 1967; Marin *et al.*, 1969). Some authors succeeded in reducing or eliminating steatorrhoea by giving pancreatic ferments, sometimes in large doses (Sun *et al.*, 1967; Földes *et al.*, 1966; Eisenburg *et al.*, 1969).

In other investigations steatorrhoea in the case of cirrhosis of the liver could not be influenced by pancreatic ferments (Beck and Gnauck, 1962; Sickinger, 1964). More recent investigations have shown that in the case of liver cirrhosis it is not only the transfer of cholic acid from the blood into the liver which is impaired (Blum and Spritz, 1966) but that cholic acid synthesis from cholesterol in the liver is also reduced to about 25% of the normal. This reduces the bile acid pool to about half (1·3 g compared to a normal 2·4 g) and leads to a drop in the bile acid concentration in the small intestine (Vlahcevic *et al.*, 1970, 1971, 1972). We may thus assume that defective micellar solubilization may be the main cause or one of the causes of steatorrhoea in non-alcoholic and alcoholic cirrhosis (Badley *et al.*, 1969; Linscheer, 1970; Hofmann, 1971).

Examination of carbohydrate absorption in the small intestine by the D-xylose test in patients with cirrhosis of the liver produces normal results (Oberhauser *et al.*, 1962; Sickinger, 1965; Marin *et al.*, 1968). Spuriously positive results were observed only in patients with ascites (Baraona *et al.*, 1962; Friedmann and McEvan, 1963; Marin *et al.*, 1968).

A biopsy of the small intestine shows pathological changes in about half the patients with cirrhosis of the liver. These include degeneration of the basement membrane, connective tissue in the stroma, changes in the villous capillaries and slight villous oedema (Astaldi and Stroselli, 1960). These histological changes are slight and completely uncharacteristic. Their pathogenetic significance is not yet completely clear. They are probably the results of portal hypertension and an increased pressure in the lymphatic system. Impaired fat transport by the lymph is therefore also a subject of discussion.

Bile acid deficiency is the chief cause of steatorrhoea in cases of obstructive jaundice or primary biliary cirrhosis. In such cases steatorrhoea is generally much more marked and occurs earlier than in cirrhosis of the liver.

*As therapy* substitution with bile acids is contra-indicated because both in obstructive jaundice and primary biliary cirrhosis and in cirrhosis of the liver a reduced bile acid secretion and/or synthesis is the chief cause of steatorrhoea. It is thought possible that the pancreatic function is disturbed in alcoholic cirrhosis at least. Thus if therapy is indicated at all attempts should be made at treatment with pancreatic ferments. It is only when there is pancreatic lipase and bile acid deficiency that medium-chain triglycerides are better hydrolysed and absorbed than long-chain nutritional triglycerides especially as micelle formation is not necessary for medium-chain triglycerides (Holt *et al.*, 1965; Holt, 1967; Linscheer *et al.*, 1966; Sickinger, 1968b; Beck *et al.*, 1968). A combined therapy with pancreatic ferments and medium-chain triglycerides is possible.

Linscheer (1970) recommends small quantities of fat between 40 50 g/day, distributed over 4–6 meals in the treatment of steatorrhoea in metabolically decompensated cirrhosis of the liver, using medium-chain triglycerides instead of nutritional fats in order to avoid side effects such as temporary diarrhoea and intestinal cramp which he observed in 10% of patients with liver cirrhosis on a diet containing medium-chain triglycerides. When such small doses are given there is no marked rise in the medium-chain fatty acids in the cerebrospinal fluid even in patients with advanced metabolically decompensated liver cirrhosis (Linscheer *et al.*, 1968).

### *11. Increased Loss of Bile Acid (Cholereic Enteropathy)*

*a. Pathogenesis.* Inlike other water-soluble substances conjugated bile acids are absorbed to but a small extent in the jejunum but selectively and actively in the ileum (Von Tappeiner 1878; Fröhlicher, 1936; Borgström *et al.*. 1963; Lack and Weiner, 1967; résumé see Dowling, 1972). Numerous investigations in the past ten years have shown that an elimination of the ileum, e.g. in resection of an extensive ileitis terminalis caused by damage to the ileum from X-ray therapy or detour anastomosis, can partly or fully interrupt the enterohepatic bile acid circulation (Austad *et al.*, 1967; Hardison and Rosenberg, 1967; Hofmann, 1967; Playoust *et al.*, 1965; Berk and Scay, 1972). All conditions resulting from ileal resection, elimination of the ileum and loss of function therefore come under the heading of cholereic enteropathy, steroid-wasting syndrome or Sickinger syndrome (Hofmann, 1967; Meihoff and Kern, 1968; Sickinger, 1969a).

*b. Pathophysiology and clinical aspects.* One facultative symptom of this syndrome is triglyceride malabsorption, i.e. steatorrhoea. It is caused by a drop in the bile acid concentration below the critical micellar concentration of 2mM. If the bile acid absorption in the terminal ileum, which is normally 95–97% sinks to 80%, the daily bile acid synthesis, normally 300–400 mg rises to a maximum of 3000 mg (Fig. 7). The enteric bile acid loss is compensated by an increase in the rate of synthesis. If, however, the bile acid loss exceeds the maximum possible rate of synthesis, the bile acid pool, normally 3–4 g, is reduced. Despite recirculating 6–8 times in 24 hr, the bile acid concentration in the jejunum is too low for micelle formation and triglyceride splitting and absorption is disturbed (Hardison and Rosenberg, 1968; Hofmann, 1965, 1967, 1972; Stanley and Nemchausky, 1966; Carey and Small, 1972; Small *et al.*, 1972).

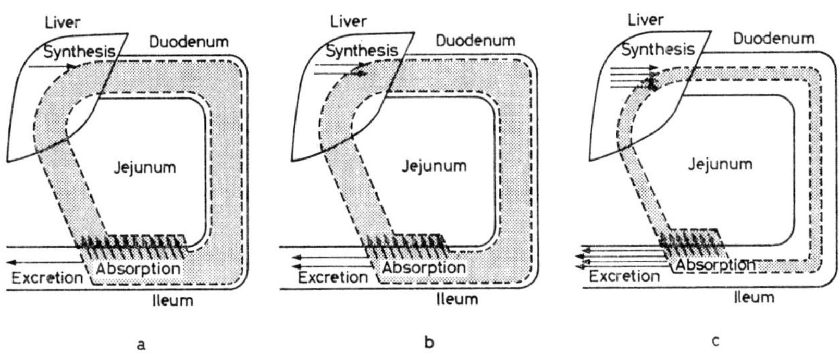


Fig. 7. Enterohepatic bile-acid circulation and bile-acids pool:
(a) normal bile acids synthesis and absorption;
(b) reduced absorption. By increasing the synthesis of bile acids the normal size of the pool (dotted area) is maintained (compensated loss of bile acids);
(c) strongly reduced absorption. Even with the maximum, individually varying increase in the synthesis, the size of the pool is reduced (decompensated loss of bile acids). (According to Hofmann, 1967, as modified by Sickinger, 1969.)

When bile acid reabsorption in the ileum is normal far less than 1 g of bile acid reaches the colon daily. The compensatory increase in bile acid synthesis in the liver after the reabsorption in the ileum has been interrupted leads to an increased bile acid excretion in the faeces. This can be as much as 3 g/day depending on the rise in synthesis in the liver. Bile acids act on the colonic mucosa in the same way as contact laxatives of the bisacodyl type. Patients with enteric bile-acid loss form less desoxycholic acid in the large intestine than normal persons. Thus the primary bile acids, cholic acid and chenodesoxycholic acid, predominate. Chenodesoxycholic acid in particular stimulates peristalsis in the large intestine (Galapaux *et al.*, 1938; Bergmann, 1952) and inhibits electrolyte and water absorption (Forth *et al.*, 1966; Mekhjian *et al.*, 1968, 1971; Hofmann, 1972). Where extensive portions of the ileum are out of action or have been removed, i.e. a loss of more than 100 cm, the compensatory increase in bile acid synthesis is inadequate (Fig. 7). This results additionally in increased stool weight or diarrhoea and considerable steatorrhoea with a faecal fat excretion of between 30 and 60 g/day. The enteric bile acid loss is decompensated.

*c. Increased decon gation of bile acids in small intestine.* In cases of cholereic enteropathy the ratio of glycine conjugates to taurine conjugates, normally 2–3, rises to 15–20. This is caused by two factors: taurine is not absorbed as well as glycine in the small intestine. This means that more taurine is lost in the faeces than glycine. Moreover, unlike taurine, glycine is synthesized in the liver whilst the taurine in the taurine conjugates is derived from food only. The taurine pool thus diminishes rapidly (Admirand, 1972; Wilson and Dietschy, 1972).

Hyperoxaluria develops in about 75 % of patients with ileal resection. 10–20 % of these patients develop nephrolithiasis (Hofmann *et al.*, 1970a, b; Dowling *et al.*, 1971; Admirand *et al.*, 1971; Admirand, 1972; Smith *et al.*, 1972). There are two possible causes of this hyperoxaluria:

a. metabolism of the glycine re-absorbed in the small and large intestines to oxalic acid in the liver. This is possible but of little significance in quantitative terms;
b. increased absorption of oxalic acid in the small intestine. This is most likely the cause of hyperoxaluria and nephrolithiasis after ileal resection.

There are three possible ways of treating this hyperoxaluria and thus of preventing nephrolithiasis: cholestyramine (Questran[R], Quantalan[R], Quemid[R]) and ion exchanger resin, binds the bile acids and thus obviously prevents increased conjugation. Peroral administration of taurine in a dose of approximately 9 g/day replenishes the taurine pool and reduces the endogenous synthesis of glycine. Finally tetracycline may be used to reduce deconjugation by influencing the intestinal flora and thus ameliorating or completely eliminating secondary hyperoxaluria (Hofmann *et al.*, 1970a, b; Dowling *et al.*, 1971; Admirand *et al.*, 1971; Smith *et al.*, 1972; Admirand, 1972).

*d. Diagnosis.* Characteristic chologenous diarrhoea develops immediately after an ileal resection or bypass (Rowe, 1967; Sickinger, 1969a, b; Hofmann and Poley, 1969; Bahls, 1970) (Table 10). The connection is more difficult to assess clinically where there is loss of ileal function, e.g. in extensive ileitis terminalis or conditions following X-ray treatment of the lower abdomen (Austad *et al.*, 1967). One important symptom for differential diagnosis may be tenesmus of the large intestine arising from increased motility caused by the bile acids. It is also characteristic that

Table 10

Diagnosis of chologenic diarrhoea

A. Clinical

1. Occurrence of diarrhoea immediately after ileum resection, impairment or irradiation; terminal ileitis (often only recurrent diarrhoea or only increased stool weight).
2. Tenesmes.
3. Decrease of diarrhoea in the second half of the day.
4. Strongly increased stool weight in the absence of, or with only slight, steatorrhoea. Strong steatorrhoea after ileum resection indicates that no real chologenic diarrhoea is involved.
5. Decrease of diarrhoea and stool weight after a tentative administration of cholestyramine.
6. Exclusion of other causes: irradiation, biopsy of the small intestine, test to determine the functioning of the small intestine and pancreas; hyperthyrosis, Verner–Morrison syndrome.

B. Laboratory

1. Hypocholesterinaemia (further decrease under the influence of cholestyramine. In case of extremely decreased values usually no occurrence of diarrhoea).
2. Impaired vitamin $B_{12}$ absorption; Schilling test gives pathological result.
3. Direct detection of enteral loss of bile acids by the isotope dilution method or cumulative stools method (not yet available as routine tests).
4. $^{14}$C-glycocholic acid breath test.
5. Hyperoxaluria.

tenesmus and diarrhoea are most severe in the forenoon, i.e. after the first meal, and diminish in the afternoon. During the night, when no food is taken, diarrhoea ceases completely (Sickinger, 1969a, b). The reason for this is that the bile acid pool is replenished overnight and therefore the bile acid concentration is higher in the colon too in the morning. In the course of several incomplete recirculation cycles the bile acid pool diminishes as does the bile acid concentration in the small and large intestines (Van Deest *et al.*, 1968). Ileal resection is not followed by chologenous diarrhoea in every case. In patients having undergone lesser ileal resection however an increase in stool weight is sometimes to be observed (Sickinger, 1969a, b). The more extensive the resection or inactivation of the ileum the sooner steatorrhoea develops in addition to diarrhoea. This is the result of decompensation of the enteric bile acid loss. In cases of extensive ileal resection of over 1 m the faecal fat loss is 30–60 g/day.

A low serum cholesterol level is characteristic of cholereic enteropathy.

Cholesterol is the main precursor or basal substance of bile acid synthesis. As cholesterol synthesis and absorption is limited in man the serum cholesterol level drops in cases of cholereic enteropathy (steroid-wasting syndrome) (Meihoff and Kern, 1968). Since vitamin $B_{12}$ is also absorbed selectively in the terminal ileum (Booth and Mollin, 1957), the vitamin $B_{12}$ absorption is also disturbed immediately after ileal resection, i.e. the Schilling test also shows pathological results. Nygaard *et al.* (1970) demonstrated that vitamin $B_{12}$ absorption increases significantly a year after ileal resection, there apparently having been a process of adaptation. Oxalic acid excretion is increased in 75% of patients with ileal resection. Oxalic acid determination in urine is comparatively simple compared to other methods yet to be discussed.

It is possible to determine enteric bile acid loss direct by means of $C^{14}$-labelled bile acids using the isotope dilution method (Lindstedt, 1957; Hardison and Rosenberg, 1967) or by means of the cumulative faecal excretion (Lindstedt and Norman, 1956; Stanley and Nemchausky, 1967). However, these methods have attained no practical importance as yet.

The isotope breath test developed in recent years can be used for the indirect measurement of increased bacterial deconjugation of the bile acids, which usually accompanies an enteric bile acid loss: after peroral administration of approximately 10 $\mu c$ $C^{14}$-glycine cholate in a 300 ml test meal the $CO_2$ exhaled is absorbed over 2- to 4-min periods and the relative proportion of ${CO_2}^{14}$ determined in a scintillation counter after 2 and 4 hr (possibly also after 6 hr and later). The proportion of radioactive ${CO_2}^{14}$ is raised when the bile acid deconjugation in the intestine is abnormally high. This test is simple and cheap to perform and can be done on outpatients. The determination of $C^{14}$ in the faeces can also be used for the same purpose. In cases of enteric bile acid loss the faecal excretion over 24 hr is over 7% of the $C^{14}$ administered (Fromm and Hofmann, 1971).

Labelling the cholic acid, i.e. the steroid molecule, with $H^3$ (tritium) is a more suitable method for the direct detection of enteric bile acid loss. This double-labelling method is somewhat more complicated but produces more reliable results. In this case the pathological value is over 20% of the $H^3$ administered/24 hr. This method can be used to determine exactly the extent of the increased bile acid deconjugation in the intestine and the enteric bile acid loss. In cases where this loss is only slight, and where the intestinal passage is rapid Fromm recommends additional labelling with a non-absorbable radioactive substance, e.g. $Cr^{51}$-chromous chloride (Fromm and Hofmann, 1971; Fromm, 1972). A rise in the glycine-taurine quotient in the duodenal bile above a maximum normal figure of 4·5 to 10–20 is also a more exact indication of an enteric bile acid loss than, for example, a pathological vitamin $B_{12}$ absorption test (Schilling test) (Bruusgaard, 1972).

*e. Therapy of diarrhoea and steatorrhoea in cholereic enteropathy.* Firstly cholereic enteropathy leads to a reduction, or a tendency to reduction, of the bile acid concentration in the jejunum; secondly the increased bile acid synthesis in the liver and incomplete re-absorption in the ileum give rise to a raised bile acid concentration in the colon. The former is the cause of steatorrhoea, the latter of chologenous diarrhoea. Both must be taken into account in therapy. Although substitution therapy with conjugated bile acids reduces steatorrhoea, the typical diarrhoea accompanied by tenesmus is increased (Hardison and Rosenberg, 1966; Hofmann and Grundy, 1965). The administration of other non-absorbable and non-laxative detergents, e.g. Tween$^{R}$, may normalize fat digestion yet the diarrhoea remains unaffected. Cholestyramine, a non-absorbable ion exchanger which binds bile acids in exchange for chlorine ions has a favourable effect on the diarrhoea (Table 11).

Table 11

Therapy of diarrhoea and steatorrhoea in the case of enteral loss of bile acids

A. Chologenic diarrhoea without steatorrhoea
 (with limited ileum resection, resection less than 50 cm)
 "compensated enteral loss of bile acids".
 Cholestyramine 4–16 g/day
  dose as low as possible
  to be administered chiefly in the morning.
 In case of provocation of a distinct steatorrhoea, use therapy B.

B. Chologenic diarrhoea with some steatorrhoea
 (with extensive ileum resection, up to 90 cm, or with reduced capacity to synthesize bile acids)
 Initial "decompensation of the enteral loss of bile acids".
 1. Cholestyramine 4–16 g/day
 2. Replacement of dietary triglycerides by medium-chain triglycerides.

C. Pronounced steatorrhoea with diarrhoea
 (extensive ileum resection, more than about 90 cm)
 "decompensated enteral loss of bile acids".
 Replacement of dietary triglycerides by medium-chain triglycerides.
 Cholestyramine only if diarrhoea persists in spite of substitution.
 If required, disinfection of the intestine with antibiotics.

In normal persons cholestyramine therapy, by binding the bile acids in the small intestine, does not cause any steatorrhoea worthy of note unless the dose is around 25 g/day (Hashim *et al.*, 1961). In cases of compensated enteric bile acid loss steatorrhoea can be caused by smaller doses if an appreciable increase in bile acid synthesis is no longer possible. For this reason the dose of cholestyramine used in the therapy of chologenous diarrhoea should be as low as possible. Experience has shown that it should be between 4 and 16 g/day. Cholestyramine is taken before meals. If this gives rise to considerable steatorrhoea or if steatorrhoea is already present, the long-chain nutritional triglycerides should be replaced as far as possible by medium-chain triglycerides. Their water solubility is about 100 times better and they are well-absorbed even if micellar solubilization is no longer possible owing to bile acid deficiency (Zurier *et al.*, 1965).

Steatorrhoea may be the main symptom in cases of extremely extensive ileal resection, e.g. over 100 cm. Replacing nutritional triglycerides by medium-chain triglycerides is of the utmost importance here (Hofmann and Poley, 1969; Sickinger, 1969a, b; Hofmann, 1972).

Most recent investigations have shown that in extensive ileal resection and severe enteric bile acid loss the bile acid concentration in the large intestine is not above normal. Nevertheless such patients suffer from considerable diarrhoea accompanied by steatorrhoea (Hofmann, 1972). It is obvious that the free fatty acids, hydroxy fatty acids in particular, are the cause of this diarrhoea. The bacterial hydroxylation of oleic acid produces 10-hydroxystearic acid which has a similar structure to ricinoleic acid (d-12-hydroxyoleic acid, familiar as the main ingredient of castor oil) (Meyer, 1890; Thomas 1972). Clinical investigations and perfusion studies on the colon have shown that it is not only the hydroxy fatty acids but also the non-hydroxylated fatty acids which inhibit sodium absorption and thus water absorption in the colon. One of the most important factors would appear to be the physical state of the fatty acids. It is possible that hydroxy fatty acids have a higher water solubility and are thus the main cause of the so-called "fatty acid diarrhoea" (Hofmann *et al.*, 1970a, b; Ammon and Phillips, 1972; Soong *et al.*, 1972; Hofmann, 1972; Bright-Asare and Binder, 1973).

Therapy with large doses of cholestyramine is generally without effect after extensive ileal resection. A fat-free diet or a replacement of long-chain triglycerides by medium-chain triglycerides is needed. Hofmann (1972) recommends in addition only small 4 g-doses of cholestyramine in the morning and evening. The hydroxylation of the fatty acids can be reduced at the same time by disinfecting the small intestine, e.g. with tetracyclines or lincomyzin, at intervals.

## C. Bacterial Deconjugation of Bile Acids (Blind Loop Syndrome; Diverticula, etc.)

### *1. Pathogenesis*

Many examinations of the normal intestinal flora have led to the conclusion that the proximal section of the small intestine is comparatively sterile and only the distal sections harbour a great number of bacteria (e.g. Kalser *et al.*, 1966).

However, Gorbach *et al.* (1967) established consistently and reproducibly that there is a grampositive flora comprising streptococci, staphylococci, lactobacilli and moulds in the entire small intestine of adults. The number of bacteria in the upper small intestine seldom exceeds $10^3$ to $10^4$/ml but there is a tendency for the bacterial count to increase in the lower section. Anaerobic bacteria predominate here. The mechanisms which prevent these bacteria from uncontrolled proliferation are not known. One essential factor would appear to be the acidity of the gastric juice which controls or prevents the entry of various bacteria and another the normal peristalsis which prevents bacteria rising from the colon or the caecum into the small intestine (Tabaqchali and Booth, 1970).

An increase in the bacterial population can occur under various pathological conditions. These changes are known as the "blind loop syndrome" or "stagnant loop syndrome". One point all these changes have in common is not necessarily motility disturbance, i.e. the localized stagnation of the intestinal content but a localized or generalized proliferation of the small intestinal flora. There are three different basic gastro-intestinal disturbances as shown in Table 12.

Using strictly anaerobic methods Drasar *et al.* (1966) demonstrated that in the conditions listed in Table 12 bacteroids and anaerobic lactobacilli predominated in the flora of the small intestine. Changes in the flora are general or localized depending on the basic disturbance. For example, in the case of duodenal diverticula bacteroids occur in greater numbers only in the upper jejunum, in multiple jejunal diverticula in the entire small intestine and finally in distal resection of the small intestine only in the lower sections (Tabaqchali and Booth, 1970).

Direct bacterial action on the intestinal mucosa and disturbed lipolysis have long been discussed as causes of steatorrhoea in conditions where the intestinal flora is disturbed. Dawson and Isselbacher (1960) were the first to assume impaired bile acid metabolism because conjugated bile acids are normally hydrolysed to unconjugated bile acids by bacterial action in the colon. Hydrolysis gives rise to free bile acids,

Table 12

Causes of pathological flora in the small intestine
(according to Tabaqchali and Booth 1970, modified)

| | | |
|---|---|---|
| A. Impairment of stomach function<br>Billroth II operation, syndrome of the afferent loop, malfunctioning gastrojejunostomy, atrophy of the gastric membrane. | | |
| B. Stasis of the contents of the small intestine | | |
| | (a) postoperative: | blind loops,<br>enteroanastomosis. |
| | (b) strictures: | congenital strictures,<br>regional enteritis (M. Crohn),<br>tuberculosis of the small intestine. |
| | (c) adhesions: | postoperative,<br>radiotherapy. |
| | (d) diverticulosis of the small intestine | |
| | (e) motility disturbances: | sclerodermia,<br>diabetic neuropathy,<br>vagotomy,<br>ganglionic blocking agents. |
| | (f) incomplete obstruction of the bile ducts with cholangitis. | |
| C. Free communication between the large and small intestine | | gastrocolic fistulae,<br>enterocolic fistulae,<br>extensive resection of the small intestine. |

dehydroxylation at $C_7$ to the secondary bile acids (deoxycholic acid from cholic acid and lithocholic acid from chenodeoxycholic acid). Midtvedt and Norman (1967) as well as Hill and Drasar (1968) then demonstrated that not all the bacteria in the small intestine are able to affect this deconjugation and dehydroxylation but that only anaerobic, e.g. bacteroids, Veilonella, Clostridia and anaerobic lactobacilli can do so.

The deconjugation of bile acids takes place *in vivo* only in those sections of the intestine where stasis is present, where the local conditions encourage the growth of anaerobic organisms. Bacteroids play the main part in the deconjugation (Gorbach and Tabaqchali, 1969). The free bile acids in the small intestine had increased in ten patients with the blind loop syndrome (cholic acid 0·3–3·9 mM/l, desoxycholic acid 0·15–1·5 mM/l and chenodeoxycholic acid 0·05–1·1 mM/l); after broad spectrum antibiotics had been given orally the bacterial count in the small intestine was reduced to normal and, at the same time, the free bile acids were no longer present in the intestinal content. The steatorrhoea dropped to a normal level (Tabaqchali and Booth, 1966; Rosenberg *et al.*, 1967).

Two causes of steatorrhoea have been discussed: firstly, damage of intestinal mucosa by free bile acids, and secondly, conjugated bile acid deficiency and thus impaired micelle formation.

Although morphological damage of the mucosa of the small intestine by free bile acids is possible (Dawson and Isselbacher, 1960; Donaldson, 1965), *in vivo* the epithelial cells of the small intestine do not suffer morphological or functional damage even when bile acid deconjugation is increased (Tabaqchali and Booth, 1967, quoted in Tabaqchali and Booth, 1970). Most recent investigations by Ament *et al.* (1972) again indicate however that morphological damage of the epithelial cells, i.e. defective fat absorption, may be the cause of steatorrhoea in cases of enteric stasis.

In six patients with steatorrhoea resulting from enteric stasis Tabaqchali *et al.* (1968) determined the concentration of conjugated bile acids in the upper jejunum. The total concentration had dropped to less than 5 mM/l (normal 5–10 mM/l). The greatest reduction was seen in the case of taurine conjugates. This bile acid concentration is no longer sufficient for normal micelle formation (Hofmann, 1963a). In a slightly acid environment free bile acids are unfortunately less soluble than their conjugates and are therefore no longer active in micelle formation (Hofmann and Small, 1967; Holt, 1967). Moreover some of the bile acid in the small intestine is in a non-ionized form and is passively absorbed in the entire small intestine (Dietschy *et al.*, 1966; Hislop *et al.*, 1967). This reduces the enteric bile acid concentration even further. The increased passive absorption of free, i.e. deconjugated, bile acids in the upper and middle small intestine causes the serum level of free bile acids to rise in patients with the blind loop syndrome (Lewis *et al.*, 1969).

The blind loop syndrome may also be accompanied by macrocythaemia irrespective of steatorrhoea. This is a consequence of vitamin $B_{12}$ deficiency. All experiments indicate that vitamin $B_{12}$ is competitively taken up by bacteria, in particular those of the *Escherichia coli* group (Donaldson *et al.*, 1962; Tabaqchali and Booth, 1967; Schjönsby *et al.*, 1973). The serum folic acid level is higher than normal, probably as a result of increased folic acid synthesis by the intestinal bacteria (Donaldson, 1964). Iron deficiency may be a result of the primary disease. Bile acids are necessary to the absorption of vitamin D. $H^3$-labelled vitamin D is therefore less completely absorbed in blind loop patients than in normal persons. This lack of vitamin D may lead to osteomalacia (Badenoch *et al.*, 1965; Cooke *et al.*, 1963).

*1. Diagnosis*

The symptomatology of the blind loop syndrome is determined by the basic morphological or functionally detectable defect. The specific symptoms of individual diseases will not be examined here (see Table 12). Steatorrhoea and possibly diarrhoea may be sub-symptoms of the disturbance in each case. There may, for example, be no symptoms in the case of duodenal or jejunal diverticula. There are no characteristic symptoms in less than 50% cases of duodenal diverticula and in the majority of cases of small intestinal diverticula.

Steatorrhoea in cases of regional enteritis may be a side-symptom to which little attention is paid. There may be additional enteric bile acid loss in regional ileitis or after ileal resection. In diabetic neuropathy with steatorrhoea, diarrhoea is usually the most prominent symptom (so-called diabetic diarrhoea or steatorrhoea). The state of the small intestinal flora is not pathological in all cases of diabetic steatorrhoea (Corsini *et al.*, 1967; Malins and Mayne, 1969; Goldstein *et al.*, 1970) (see p. 185). Detection of pathological flora and bile acid analyses of the intestinal contents and serum are too complex for practical purposes. So in many cases the diagnosis of steatorrhoea in the blind loop syndrome is a diagnosis by elimination. The quantitative faecal fat determination method is used for this purpose.

It has lately become possible to determine the increased deconjugation of bile acids by means of the breath test (Fromm and Hofmann, 1971) (see p. 160). $C^{14}$-glycocholic acid (cholyl glycine-1-$C^{14}$) is given after a test meal. An increase in the $CO_2{}^{14}$ exhaled indicates increased deconjugation of the labelled glycocholic acid. If $C^{14}$-excretion in the faeces is determined at the same time or cholic acid labelled with $H^3$ (tritium), this method can be used to differentiate between bile acid malabsorption, e.g. in the case of enteric bile acid loss and increased bacterial deconjugation. The blind loop syndrome may also be accompanied by a secondary hyperoxaluria (see p. 160).

In the blind loop syndrome the daily faecal fat excretion rarely exceeds 40 g. This means that the stool weight is usually normal or only slightly raised as there is generally a selective malabsorption of triglycerides and fat-soluble vitamins; unless of course there is diarrhoea caused by increased excretion of hydroxy fatty acids. The biopsy of the small intestine is histologically normal and when examined by microscope or stereomicroscope. The D-xylose test may produce pathological results. However, the exact mechanism of D-xylose malabsorption is not yet known (Tabaqchali and Booth, 1970). The Schilling test gives pathological results. If intrinsic factor is given at the same time absorption does not improve. A megaloblastic anaemia does not usually develop for several years. Sternal puncture material does not necessarily show any characteristic changes because there may also be anaemia due to iron deficiency or infection arising from the primary disease (Tabaqchali and Booth, 1970).

*2. Therapy*

Oral doses of antibiotics, usually tetracycline or chlortetracycline, reduce the steatorrhoea to a normal level in a few days. The dose is 1–2 g/day. Treatment is continued for 7–10 days.

It has not yet been ascertained whether prolonged therapy with small doses is appropriate (Tabaqchali and Booth, 1970). Neomycin is not usually of any use as it has comparatively little effect on anaerobic organisms. This antibiotic itself causes triglyceride malabsorption when given in large doses (see p. 180). The positive reaction to antibiotic therapy again confirms the aetiological significance of the pathological intestinal flora. As the anaerobic flora declines, the conjugated bile acids in the small intestine rise to a normal level and the pathologically high proportion of free bile acids in the intestinal content and in the serum returns to normal. If there are signs of a megaloblastic anaemia parenteral substitution with vitamin $B_{12}$ is indicated. If osteomalacia is present vitamin D or a combination of the fat-soluble vitamins A, D, E and K (e.g. Adek-Falk$^{R}$) should be given parenterally. The blind loop syndrome can often be remedied surgically, e.g. by the resection of blind sacks in the small intestine or the removal of strictures and fistulae.

## D. Disturbances in Intestinal Mucosa Transport (Malabsorption)

*1. Primary Malabsorption (Primary Sprue)*

The term primary malabsorption syndrome covers three diseases, some of whose causes are unknown:

gluten-induced sprue,
tropical sprue,
unclassifiable sprue (idiopathic sprue).

This concise account of the malassimilation syndrome will only deal with gluten-induced sprue. Tropical sprue is of no importance in our latitudes although there have been patients with tropical sprue who have never been in the tropics, the cause of which has not yet been fully explained (Klipstein, 1968, 1970; Baker and Mathan, 1968, 1970). Primary, non-tropical malabsorption syndromes which show no or only an incomplete reaction to a gluten-free diet are termed unclassifiable sprue. The diagnosis of unclassifiable sprue is thus a diagnosis by elimination (Rubin *et al.*, 1970).

*2. Gluten-induced Sprue (Coeliac Disease or Adult Coeliac Disease; Non-tropical Sprue)*

*a. Pathogenesis.* Gee (1888) was the first to describe this disease involving diarrhoea and chronic nutritional disturbance, under the heading of "coeliac affectation" in infants. Even at that time it was Gee's opinion that this disease also occurs in adults.

In 1932 Thaysen provided the first detailed description of adult coeliac disease. Then in 1950 Dicke recognized the connection between cereal products and this disease. Further investigations showed that the toxic factor is the water-soluble gliadin fraction of gluten (Krainick and Debatin, 1953). In both infants and adults coeliac disease is caused by a genetic disturbance in the peptide splitting in the epithelial cells of the small intestine. The disease is therefore inheritable Even today it is not known exactly which peptide or peptides, i.e. split products of the water-soluble gliadin fraction, causes the morphological changes in the mucosa. It is possible that a peptidase deficiency results in incomplete peptide splitting and that unsplit peptide acts either as a toxin or antigen (Kowlessar *et al.*, 1970; Reed, 1970). The mucosa would then be destroyed by specific antibodies (Reed, 1970).

However, Douglas and Peters (1970) have since shown that although the peptic-tryptic digestion is disturbed in untreated gluten-induced sprue, when therapy with gluten-free diet had brought about a remission there was no difference in the peptic-tryptic digestion compared with normal persons. The impaired gluten-breakdown in untreated sprue could therefore also be a consequence of lesions in the small intestinal mucosa. Contact with gliadin-containing products or extracts causes a typical mucosal lesion (Paulley, 1954; Sakula and Shiner, 1957). It is typical that the most severe mucosal changes are to be found in the upper small intestine. If, however, gluten is introduced directly into the normal ileum of patients with gluten-induced sprue the typical mucosal lesion develops there too (Rubin *et al.*, 1960).

Under the microscope or stereomicroscope a distinction may be made between "sub-total" and "partial" villous atrophy (Fig. 8a, 9a). In sub-total villous atrophy a further distinction can be made between "flat mucosa" and "flat mucosa with mosaic patterns" (Booth *et al.*, 1962). Other authors distinguish between "severe", "moderate" and "slight" mucosal changes (Benson *et al.*, 1964; Rubin *et al.*, 1960).

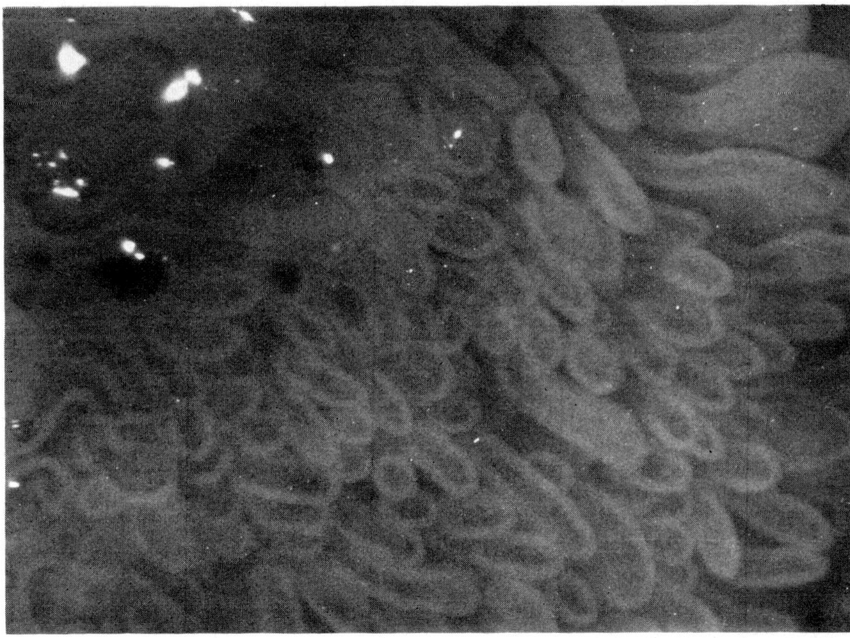

(a)

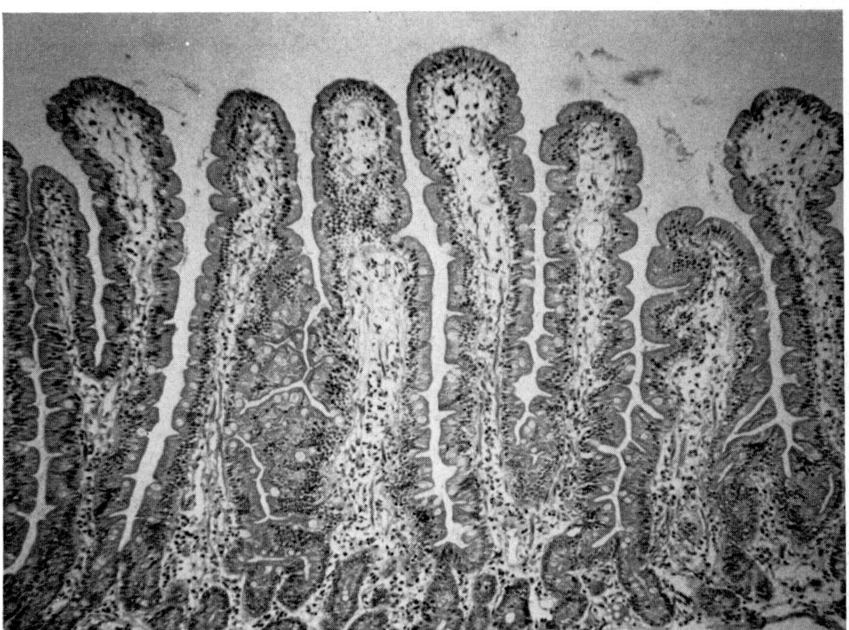

(b)

Fig. 8. Normal small intestine: (a) stereomicroscopic aspect; (b) histology.

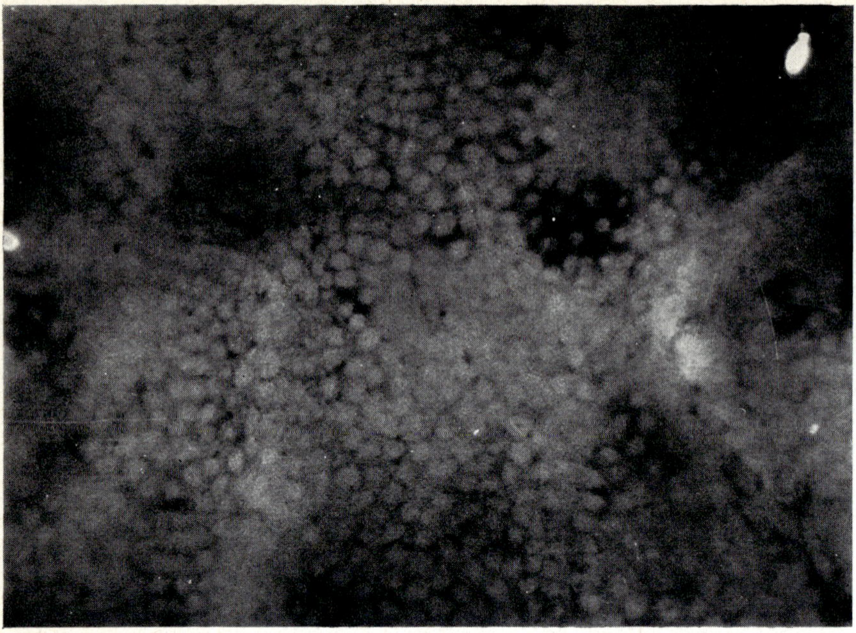

(a)

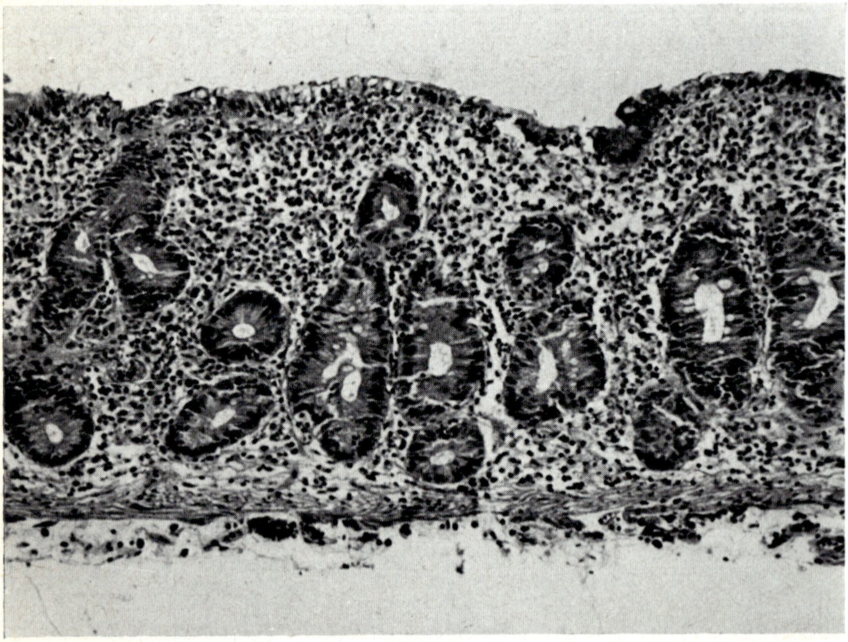

(b)

Fig. 9. Subtotal villous atrophy: (a) stereomicroscopic aspect; (b) histology.

The epithelium is flattened, irregular and sometimes stratified (Fig. 8b, 9b). The cell nuclei are irregular in size. Microscopically the subtotal villous atrophy shows a completely flat mucosa. The furrows are often enlarged and always deeper. In partial villous atrophy broad, blunt residual villi are still to be observed (Shiner and Doniach, 1960). Cell regeneration in the lengthened crypts is increased but the number of mature epithelial cells is reduced owing to increased cytolysis. The shape of the villi is however determined by the number of mature epithelial cells. So gluten-induced sprue differs from other diseases in that villous atrophy is accompanied by a rise in cell turnover. An increase in synthesis of the membranaceous, lysosomal, microsomal and mitochondrial enzymes can be demonstrated histochemically although the total enzyme content of the epithelial cells is reduced. The dynamic process can be compared with a haemolytic anaemia (Creamer, 1964; Riecken *et al.*, 1966a; Riecken, 1970). The lamina propria is usually infiltrated to a greater or lesser extent by lymphoid cells, plasma cells and granulocytes or eosinophiles. The lymph cavities are often distended. Because of the extended furrows the mucosa is of normal thickness (Shiner and Doniach, 1960). All clinical symptoms and all changes determined in the laboratory are the consequence of this mucosal lesion and the resulting functional disturbances. Most prominent are disturbances in the active mucosa transport and the passive diffusion from the lumen of the small intestine into the blood stream or the lymphatic system. On the other hand, the transfer of numerous substances from the blood stream and the lymphatic system into the lumen is increased. As the severity of the histological changes diminishes in the distal section of the small intestine, there is an intestinal absorption reserve for certain substances (Booth, 1966). If this is exceeded, or as in the case of some substances such as calcium or iron which can only be absorbed in certain sections of the intestine, the result is impaired absorption and, in time, deficiency symptoms.

The triglyceride absorption is reduced chiefly through the destruction of the epithelium and a reduction in the surface of the small intestine. Hydrolysis of triglycerides in the lumen is normal but the triglyceride content of the lymph in the thoracic duct is lowered (Blomstrand, 1955). The proportion of saturated fatty acids in the faeces increases for three reasons:

i. increased endogenous fatty acid secretion;
ii. bacterial conversion of unsaturated fatty acids to saturated fatty acids; and
iii. selectively better absorption of unsaturated fatty acids compared to saturated fatty acids.

James *et al.* (1961) held the view that diarrhoea in gluten-induced sprue is caused by an increase of hydroxy fatty acids, in particular hydroxy-stearic acid. This was not confirmed by other authors to begin with (Cooke, 1968) but more recent investigations performed by Soong *et al.* (1972) clearly indicated that abnormal fatty acids, hydroxy fatty acids in particular, were responsible for diarrhoea in gluten-induced sprue.

The water and electrolyte transport in the small intestine is also impaired. The total potassium pool is clearly reduced although the serum potassium level may still be normal. The sodium pool is not reduced unless the sprue is severe (Cooke, 1957; Reitemeier *et al.*, 1956). Calcium on the other hand is actively absorbed chiefly in the duodenum. As the mucosal damage is at its most severe here, calcium absorption is disturbed at an early stage. Transport is dependent on vitamin D. In cases of severe sprue only 18% of the calcium is absorbed by the small intestine. Calcium also passes into the intestine with the pancreatic and intestinal secretions and is only incompletely reabsorbed. Finally it is bound by the unabsorbed nutritional fatty acids and excreted in the faeces in the form of calcium soap (Fink and Laszlo, 1957). The absorption of magnesium is also impeded in a similar way; there is in particular a rise in magnesium loss through the faeces (Balint and Hirschowitz, 1961; McIntyre *et al.*, 1960). Iron absorption is also substantially disturbed (Badenoch and Callender, 1954, 1960).

Damage to the intestinal mucosa causes loss of protein from the mucosa and increased protein excretion in faeces (secondary exudative enteropathy). There is however not always a significant relationship between this secondary exudative enteropathy and the hypoproteinaemia which is often present. The pathogenesis of hypoproteinaemia is complex. The main causes are increased protein loss in faeces and impaired amino acid absorption (Parkins, 1960).

*b. Clinical aspects.* The onset of the disease in adults is often caused by particular stresses such as physical trauma, infection, other intercurrent diseases or pregnancy. Coeliac disease has frequently not been manifest in childhood but it must be assumed that an asymptomatic sprue had existed in childhood and remained latent. The disease usually becomes clinically manifest between the ages of 30 and 40 but can occur in patients over 60.

The classic symptoms are chronic diarrhoea, weakness and loss of weight. Stools are excessively large, the stool weight being at least 400 g/day. Stools have a rancid odour but the typical whitish colour is not due to the fat content but to bacterial decomposition of the bile pigments. There is diarrhoea in 80–95% of the patients, general debility in 88–95% and loss of weight in about the same proportion. This loss of weight, however, does not only depend on the extent of the steatorrhoea but also on anorexia and nausea to be observed in about 30–40%.

Other symptoms, generally to be found in less than half the patients, are abdominal discomfort, flatulence, glossitis, haemorrhagic tendency, tetany, ostalgia, paraesthesia, mental disturbances, nocturnal polyuria and hypothermia, sometimes fever. These are symptoms which are not provoked by the intestinal lesion itself. Glossitis, haemorrhagic tendency, tetany and ostalgia are the consequences of vitamin K deficiency, vitamin D deficiency and calcium deficiency. Hypothermia is obviously caused by malnutrition and secondary pituitary insufficiency (Dent *et al.*, 1961).

Loss of weight is the most frequent objective finding, occurring in 55%. Flatulence and oedema occur in more than half the cases. Individual intestinal loops are often palpable through the abdominal wall. There is never any pain caused by pressure. In 10–13% of the cases the liver is enlarged. There is seldom a fatty degeneration of the liver. The spleen is seldom enlarged, generally of normal size and frequently even comparatively small. Relative hypotonia, watchglass nails and drumstick fingers and finally hyperpigmentation as in Addison's disease occur in 20–40%. In addition to paraesthesia signs of peripheral neuropathy are to be found (Cooke *et al.*, 1953, 1966; Bossak and Wang, 1957).

*c. Laboratory findings.* Anaemia is present in about half the cases. This is generally hypochromic. The serum iron level is lowered in practically all cases and the oral iron absorption test produces pathological findings. The iron-binding capacity is raised. Iron deficiency can occasionally be the main symptom of adult coeliac disease (Kilpatrik and Katz, 1969). Megaloblastic bone marrow is also to be found in some cases. Leucopenia and thrombocytopenia occur in less than half the patients.

In about one-third of the patients the total serum protein is diminished. There is occasionally a marked drop in globulin as far as severe hypo- or dysglobulinaemia (Green and Wollaeger, 1960). There is a drop in the number of IgA-producing cells in the interstice of the intestinal mucosa (Pittingale, 1971). There is however an incidence of malabsorption syndromes in primary, in particular primary acquired immunoglobulin deficiency (Crabbe and Heremans, 1966; Bull and Tomasi, 1967).

The serum calcium, the ionized calcium and the protein-bound calcium is reduced in two-thirds of the patients. Reduced serum phosphate also occurs but much more rarely. The alkaline serum phosphatase is increased in over 60% (Gossmann, 1966). As a consequence of vitamin K deficiency the Quick value falls to a pathological level in about 70%.

In about half the patients there is evidence of a low total serum lipid level caused by a drop in all lipid fractions.

*d. Specific diagnosis.*

*i. Triglyceride malabsorption.* Here the determination of stool weight, which is frequently over 400 g/day is recommended The most reliable evidence of disturbed triglyceride absorption is to be obtained by the method of van de Kamer *et al.* (1949) or the gravimetric method Faecal fat excretion is generally over 50 g/day. The $J^{131}$-triolein test produces pathological results.

*ii. Carbohydrate absorption.* The D-xylose test shows pathological results. The D-xylose urinary excretion is pathologically low (below 20% of the dose given) and the D-xylose serum level is under 25 mg% after 60 min.

*iii. Folic acid absorption.* The determination of folic acid in the serum gives rise to technical difficulties. Absorption studies produce shallow curves in a small proportion of patients. The excretion of formamino-glutamic acid after administration of histidine is increased yet there is no clear correlation to the reduced serum folic acid to be established (Knowles, 1962).

*iv. Vitamin $B_{12}$ absorption.* The Schilling test in gluten-induced sprue rarely shows pathological results—in contrast to tropical sprue—as the ileal mucosa is usually unchanged (Cooke, 1968).

*v. Faecal nitrogen excretion.* The nitrogen content of the faeces is determined by Kjeldahl's method or as indophenol blue after chloramine-T oxidation (Stegemann and Loeschke, 1962). With a protein intake of 100–120 g/day the faecal nitrogen content is under 2·5 g/day. In cases of gluten-induced sprue an increased faecal nitrogen content is to be observed in about 60% (Badenoch and Callender, 1960). Faecal nitrogen was 5·0 ± 1·2 g/day in a series of 74 cases of adult coeliac disease (Wilson and Dietschy, 1971).

*vi. Radiography of small intestine.* Eighty-five per cent of patients with gluten-induced sprue show characteristic, but only relatively specific signs of malabsorption. The most important are dilatation of the intestinal loops, segmentation, dilution of the barium contrast medium. The coarsening of the mucosal folds gives rise to a "pile of plates" appearance. The so-called "moulage" appearance, resulting from complete loss of the mucosal structure, is less common. In only 73% of cases with bioptically and histologically determined sprue is there radiological evidence of malabsorption (Adlersberg *et al.*, 1954; Laws *et al.*, 1963; Prevot, 1966; Isbell *et al.*, 1969). But radiological examination is of prime importance in eliminating other inflammatory or neoplastic diseases of the small intestine, e.g. regional enteritis or malignant lymphoma.

*vii. Aspiration biopsy.* Aspiration biopsy is essential to confirm diagnosis. The typical location for the biopsy is the upper jejunum, directly below the flexura duodenojejunalis or, if this point cannot be reached, the lower duodenum. The extent of villous atrophy can be assessed comparatively well microscopically or stereomicroscopically. In order that the structure and height of the villi and the depth of the crypts may be correctly assessed, the tissue must be embedded and cut with great care, and axially aligned (Rubin and Dobbins, 1965; Riecken *et al.*, 1966b).

*e. Therapy.* An attempt must be made with a gluten-free diet for all forms of primary malabsorption. It is not easy to administer this diet in practice because all products which contain even traces of wheat, rye or barley are forbidden. The diet must be completely free of gluten. Gluten-free bread and bakery goods are being produced today, however. All foods, especially commercially produced foods, must be tested for complete lack of gluten. The children's hospital of the University of Zurich will supply a list of the proven gluten-free foods obtainable in Germany and Switzerland, including bread and other bakery goods (Schmerling, 1967).

When starting the diet care must be taken that the fat content is reduced to about 50 g in order to eliminate quickly symptoms such as flatulence and diarrhoea. A low-fat diet is not very palatable, however, and often a high calorie content is desirable. For this reason it is advisable to attempt to replace the nutritional triglycerides by medium-chain triglycerides. Because of their smaller molecular diameter and the simple cellular transport, medium-chain triglycerides with a fatty acid chain of $C_8$–$C_{12}$ are better absorbed than the long-chain nutritional triglycerides even in cases of sub-total villous atrophy and damage to the epithelium of the small intestine (Holt, 1967; Sickinger, 1968a, b, 1969a, b) (see p. 128).

Improvement is usually not so rapid in adults suffering from coeliac disease as in infants and it often takes six weeks to obtain results (Haemmerli, 1970). For this reason fat-soluble vitamins (A, D, E and K) (e.g. Adek-Falk[R]) should be given parenterally at least in the early stages of treatment. The therapy also requires parenteral administration of iron and often of calcium and possibly vitamin $B_{12}$ and folic acid. In adults the condition of the intestinal mucosa including the depth of crypts does not generally return to normal until three months on a gluten-free diet (Fig. 10a, b).

The diet must often be continued indefinitely. Spontaneous remissions

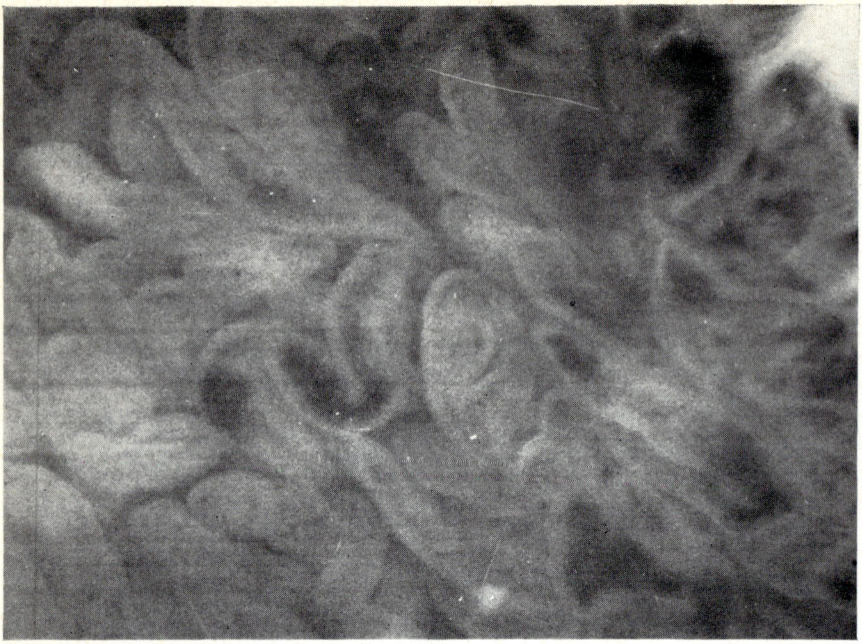

(a)

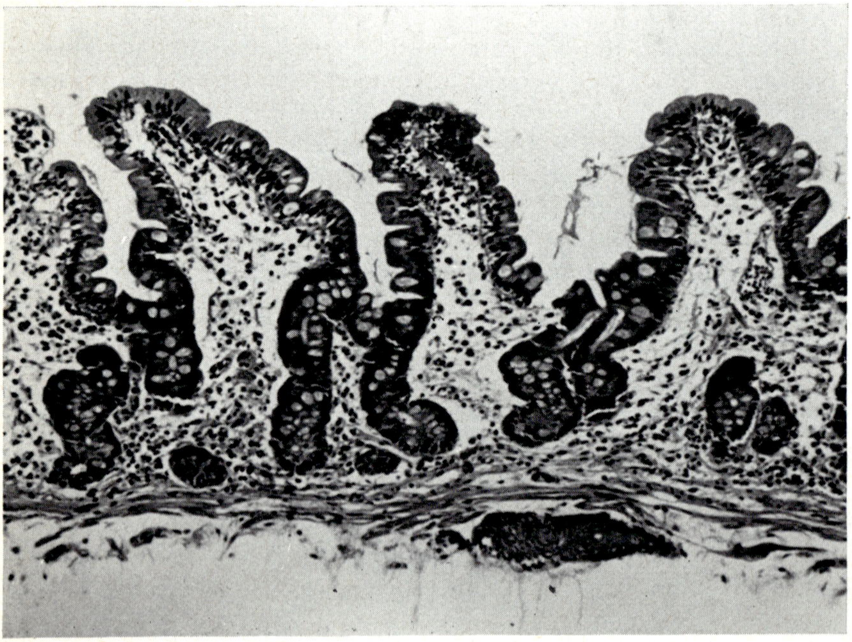

(b)

Fig. 10. Small intestine in Coeliac disease after three months of therapy with gluten-free diet: (a) stereomicroscopic aspect; (b) histology.

often occur in adults and there is often a temptation to introduce gluten into the diet again after one to two years free from symptoms. The result is almost always a recurrence of the pathological changes in the intestinal mucosa although the clinical signs of malabsorption only occur in some patients after a time. For 20 years therapy with glucocorticoids with a normal diet has repeatedly been found to effect an improvement in the intestinal mucosal damage and malabsorption. But treatment with glucocorticoids can only be regarded as an additional treatment (Wall *et al.*, 1970). Another manifestation of gluten-induced sprue is, for example, the enteric osteopathy already mentioned—a combination of osteomalacia and osteoporosis. Osteomalacia has even been found in cases of gluten-induced sprue without steatorrhoea (Moss *et al.*, 1965; Hunstein *et al.*, 1968).

Enteric osteopathy is diagnosed via the increased alkaline serum phosphatase, an iliac crest biopsy providing histological confirmation. Secondary (or primary) immunoglobulin deficiency has also been mentioned (see p. 188). A further consequence of damage to the epithelium of the small intestine is a secondary disaccharidase deficiency and, in particular, a secondary lactase deficiency (McGill and Newcomer, 1970). There appears to be a close correlation between gluten-induced sprue and dermatitis herpetiformis (Friedman and Hare, 1965; Fraser *et al.*, 1967; Fry *et al.*, 1967; Marks and Shuster, 1970; Marks *et al.*, 1970; Brow *et al.*, 1971; Weinstein *et al.*, 1971). A marked incidence of malignant gastro-intestinal lymphoma and carcinoma has also been observed in cases of gluten-induced sprue. The interrelationship is not yet completely clear (Joske, 1960; Creamer, 1964; Harris *et al.*, 1967; Ross and Garabedian, 1970). Recently Lancaster-Smith *et al.* (1971) reported diffuse interstitial lung processes in coeliac disease. Neuropathy has also been observed frequently (Cooke and Smith, 1966). This has nothing to do with vitamin $B_{12}$ or folic acid deficiency (Cooke *et al.*, 1966). It may be that pyridoxin deficiency plays some part (Morris *et al.*, 1970). Psychiatric disorders are more frequent in patients with coeliac disease but there is no statistically significant incidence of specific diseases (Goldberg, 1970).

### 3. *Secondary Malabsorption* (*Secondary Sprue*)

It is in particular dermatitis herpetiformis (Johnson and Alpert, 1971; Trier, 1971), intestinal lymphoma and hypo- or agammaglobulinaemia (Bull and Tomasi, 1968) which give rise to difficulties in distinguishing secondary from primary malabsorption. All three diseases are regarded as complications of gluten-induced sprue and as the cause of malabsorption (literature quoted by Ross and Garabedian, 1970).

*4. Regional Enteritis*

This disorder causes general malabsorption, depending on extent and localization, by reducing the absorbing surface of the mucous membrane. In numerous cases, especially in inflammatory stenoses, increased bacterial growth in a section of the small intestine may be the cause of triglyceride malabsorption (blind loop syndrome) (Tabaqchali and Booth, 1970).

*5. Radiation Injury to Small Intestine*

In X-ray treatment impaired cell generation in the crypts leads to a decrease in the height of the villi and to megaloblastosis and megalocytosis in the epithelium of the small intestine. Abscesses may also develop occasionally in the crypts. After discontinuation of radiation recovery is generally rapid. Clinical symptoms are generally slight (Reeves *et al.*, 1965; Sickinger *et al.*, 1965; Trier and Browning, 1966; Wiernik, 1966; Tankel *et al.*, 1965; Read, 1970; Hagemann and Lesher, 1971).

*6. Allergic (Eosinophilic) Enteritis*

This rare polyaetiological disease may give rise to the typical morphological and functional picture of a generalized malabsorption (Burhenne and Carbone, 1966; Waldmann *et al.*, 1967; Fahrländer, 1967; Dalinka and Masters, 1970; Jacobson, 1970; Kaplan *et al.*, 1970; Klein *et al.*, 1970; Leinbach and Rubin, 1970).

*7. Intestinal Lambliasis*

Lambliasis is often a result of another disease with more marked symptoms (Yardley *et al.*, 1964). The parasites are to be found in the lumen of the small intestine and on the microvilli of the epithelium but also penetrate into the epithelial cells and as far as the lamina propria (Brandborg *et al.*, 1967). There is no close relationship between the extent of infestation and gastro-intestinal symptoms. The lambliae can be eliminated by means of a parasiticide, e.g. quinacrin. Steatorrhoea is reduced or completely cured (Jeffries *et al.*, 1969).

*8. Coccidiosis*

A coccidial infection of the small intestine can lead to villous atrophy and to lesions of the microvilli of the epithelium (Brandborg *et al.*, 1970).

*9. General Mastocytosis (Urticaria Pigmentosa)*

Diarrhoea is rare in this disease and steatorrhoea even more uncommon. The cause of triglyceride malabsorption is a clumping of the villi, there being a diffuse infiltration of the submucosa with eosinophilic granulocytes and a small number of mast cells. It is also possible however that metabolic products of the mast cells cause motility disturbances of the small intestine (Bank and Marks, 1963; Ammann and Spycher, 1972).

*10. Amyloid Degeneration*

The extent and cause of the malabsorption in amyloidosis depends on the location and extent of the amyloid deposits. The following are thought to be the main causes: damage to intestinal mucosa by amyloidosis, vascular insufficiency, pancreatic insufficiency and a blind loop syndrome resulting from motility disturbances (Beddow and Tildon, 1960; Schein, 1947; Herskovic *et al.*, 1964; Casad and Bocian, 1965).

*11. Sclerodermia*

There is no correlation between the extent of intestinal affectation and the extent of malabsorption in this case either. Hardening of the submucosa where absorption is normal can lead to impaired lymph drainage and triglyceride transport (Greenberger *et al.*, 1968b). Occasionally, however, there is also marked malabsorption where fibrosis occurs only in patches and muscular atrophy is present (Kahn *et al.*, 1966; Alpert and Warner, 1968). The general opinion at present is therefore that the motility disturbance leads to stasis and bacterial overgrowth, i.e. to the blind loop syndrome (Levinson and Kirsner, 1970).

The treatment of steatorrhoea in these inflammatory, infiltrative and sclerotic processes is therefore disinfection of the small intestine with tetracycline or chlorotetracycline as, in certain circumstances, for regional enteritis and amyloid degeneration (Kahn *et al.*, 1966; Alpert and Warner, 1968; Tabaqchali and Booth, 1970) (see p. 167).

As sclerodermia may lead to a peri- or panarteritis affecting the pancreas, pancreatic insufficiency must also be considered as a cause of steatorrhoea in sclerodermia. Acute recurrent pancreatitis results in a secretory pancreatic insufficiency which requires replacement therapy (Toth and Alpert, 1971).

*12. Malabsorption Resulting from Medication*

It is known today that a number of medicaments cause various absorption disturbances under certain conditions (Dobbins, 1968). The most thorough examinations have been made of neomycin which can cause temporary malabsorption. According to most recent investigations the primary cause is its direct effect on the epithelial cells of the small intestine which results in shortening of the villi. Lymphocytes and pigment-containing macrophages are to be found in the lamina propria (Dobbins *et al.*, 1968). This leads to a disturbance in the absorption of fat, amino acids, cholesterol, monosaccharides and disaccharides, sodium, calcium, carotene, vitamin $B_{12}$, iron and bile acids. The loss of bile acids is, however, not the cause of steatorrhoea as the bile acid pool is reduced to only a small extent and the intraluminal bile acid concentration does not drop below the critical micellar concentration (Hardison and Rosenberg, 1969). Yet most recent findings show that neomycin precipitates lipids from the micellar phase (Thompson *et al.*, 1971). The disaccharidase activity in the epithelial cells also drops, one of the results being lactose malabsorption (Cain *et al.*, 1968). Other antibiotics such as tetracycline have similar effects (Greenberger *et al.*, 1966). Alcohol impairs the absorption of folic acid in the jejunum (Halsted *et al.*, 1967). Diphenylhydantoin, biguanidine, colchicine, *p*-aminosalicylic acid, methotrexate and clofibrate are other substances which can cause various disturbances in the absorption in the small intestine (Dobbins 1968; Caspary, 1971; Race *et al.*, 1970). Cholestyramine causes steatorrhoea by binding the bile acids in the small intestine (Hashim *et al.*, 1961). Details of pathogenesis will not be discussed here.

*13. Disturbed Arterial Circulation in the Small Intestine*

Arteriosclerotic stenoses of the arteria mesenterica cranialis seldom lead to malabsorption (Marston, 1968). Ischaemia affecting function only occurs where there is occlusion of two of the three vascular trunks supplying the small intestine (arteria coeliaca, arteria mesenterica cranialis and arteria mesenterica caudalis). Of five patients with ischaemia, detected by angiography and confirmed by surgery, in the arteria mesenterica cranialis only three had steatorrhoea. Neither was any lesion found in the mucosa of the small intestine as the cause of steatorrhoea. Motility disturbances, leading to increased bacterial overgrowth in the small intestine, have also been discussed with regard to the pathogenesis of steatorrhoea. In two patients steatorrhoea was eliminated by means of revascularization (Watt *et al.*, 1967).

*14. Proximal Resection of Small Intestine*

In contrast to distal resection enteric bile acid loss only occurs here where resection is extensive. Malabsorption symptoms do not therefore generally occur after proximal resection unless one-half to two-thirds of the small intestine has been removed. The occurrence of a malabsorption syndrome depends on three factors:

a. the remaining intestinal surface;
b. the passage time; and
c. the mixing with pancreatic ferments.

(Booth, 1965, 1966; Kistler, 1967.)

Steatorrhoea is the most prominent symptom but nitrogen excretion may also be increased. Depending on the extent of resection the absorption of disaccharides, monosaccharides and fat- and water-soluble vitamins is also disturbed. In contrast to distal resection only extensive proximal resection effects vitamin $B_{12}$ absorption. The large volume of faeces contains an increased amount of water and electrolytes. The residual intestine undergoes a functional and structural adaptation process after resection.

Influenced by the larger quantity of food the number of epithelial cells per unit of length of the villi increases and the small intestine expands (Porus, 1965; Dowling, 1967; Weser, 1971). According to Beck *et al.* (1968) we may therefore distinguish between three postoperative phases:

a. immediate postoperative phase;
b. convalescence and adaptation;
c. permanent state.

This functional and structural adaptation plus the use of the substitution and dietary therapy possible today, means that patients with only 25 cm of small intestine can survive (Beck *et al.*, 1968).

*Therapy.* In the immediate postoperative phase priority is given to infusion to replace electrolytes and protein. It must be remembered that one litre of watery stools can mean a loss of up to 120 mEq potassium, 200 mEq sodium and 150 mEq chlorine. A larger quantity of magnesium is also excreted in the faeces. Fifteen hundred calories should be given daily in the form of parenteral infusions containing glucose, fructose, amino acids and triglycerides. A gradual change to solid food will be possible in the course of several months. Tinctura opii (approximately $3 \times 10$ drops/day), codeinum phosphoricum ($3 \times 25$ mg/day) or diphenoxylate (Reasec[R]) for long-term treatment may be given to inhibit the peristaltic action of the small intestine and to treat the diarrhoea. Doses of silica (Entero Teknosal[R]) can be given to improve the consistency of unpleasant watery stools causing severe anal irritation.

During the adaptation phase and even later in cases of extensive resection it is advisable to replace nutritional triglycerides by medium-chain triglycerides. If steatorrhoea of over 25 g/day continues, substitution of electrolytes, potassium, calcium and possibly magnesium should be continued as a prophylactic measure. Similarly parenteral substitution of fat-soluble vitamins A, D, E and K (e.g. Adek-Falk[R]) will be necessary. The parenteral administration of vitamin $B_{12}$ and folic acid is also to be recommended (Kistler, 1967; Beck *et al.*, 1968; Winawer, 1966). Additional antibiotic therapy, e.g. with tetracyclines or chlorotetracyclines may be necessary in cases of increasing bacterial growth in the residual intestine.

Surgical measures to reduce the rate of passage—vagotomy or the insertion of an antiperistaltic segment—have been attempted with varying success. The residual intestine is often too short for the second operation; it is then simpler to perform a resection of the longitudinal muscles in the remaining terminal segment of the small intestine, extending it by about 1 cm. This creates a sphincter mechanism which delays passage (Schiller *et al.*, 1967; Shepard, 1966). One occasional result of extensive resection of the small intestine is hypersecretion with hyperchlorhydria of the stomach because of reduced formation of one inhibitor, probably enterogastrone. This may necessitate vagotomy and pyloroplasty (Windsor *et al.*, 1969).

## E. Specific or Selective Absorption Disturbances

### *1. Disaccharidase Deficiency; Secondary Disaccharidase Deficiency*

Secondary disaccharidase deficiency is the result of damage to the epithelium of the small intestine. As in primary disaccharidase deficiency, lactase deficiency is the main factor here as there is less lactase activity than the other disaccharides and it is therefore particularly susceptible to damage. Little is known of the factors which cause this. It is assumed that virus infections, nutritional diseases, e.g. Kwashiorkor, chemical substances, e.g. drugs, are the causes. Of the last named group particular mention should be made of substances which impair protein synthesis such as colchicine, neomycin and puromycin. These drugs can also lead to steatorrhoea in a similar way to X-ray treatment. All diseases of the small intestine which cause damage of the brush border or the epithelium, chiefly all forms of sprue (gluten-induced, tropical and unclassified sprue) also lead to a reduction or a loss of disaccharidase activity.

In contrast to patients with tropical sprue, those with gluten-induced sprue normally show no intolerance to milk as the lactase activity is normal in the usually intact lower small intestine, thus compensating lactase deficiency in the upper small intestine.

The possibility of secondary lactase deficiency is the subject of discussion in the case of mesenteric circulation disorders with ischaemia of the small intestine, cystic fibrosis of the pancreas, lambliasis, ulcerative colitis, regional enteritis and finally infectious hepatitis and Whipple's disease (McGill and Newcomer, 1970).

### *2. Primary Glucose–Galactose Malabsorption*

This is a congenital defect in the glucose–galactose transport system of the small intestine and the renal tubular system (Lindquist and

Meeuwisse, 1962; Laplane *et al.*, 1962). The patients, usually infants, have diarrhoea and glucosuria. Steatorrhoea does not occur. Diarrhoea ceases only when glucose and galactose are eliminated from the diet. This disease has also been observed in adults (Rommel and Grimmel, 1967). Glucose and galactose in the diet must be replaced by fructose which is absorbed normally.

### 3. *a-β-Lipoproteinaemia*

In *a-β*-lipoproteinaemia, also known as acanthocytosis or Bassen–Kornzweig syndrome, a disturbance in chylomicron synthesis leads to an accumulation of triglycerides in the intestinal epithelium. Fat absorption is thus impaired and steatorrhoea develops (Isselbacher *et al.*, 1964; Dobbins, 1966; Levy *et al.*, 1966; Ways *et al.*, 1967; Gotto *et al.*, 1971).

By way of symptomatic therapy of fat malabsorption nutritional fat is replaced by medium-chain triglycerides which are transported direct in the blood of the portal vein. The formation of chylomicrons is not necessary (Isselbacher, 1965).

### 4. *Cystinuria*

Cystinuria is caused by a disturbance in the transport of dibasic amino acids in the small intestine and often also in the renal tubular system (Milne, 1964). In the course of time the patients develop cystine calculae in the efferent urinary tract. Growth may be affected, depending on the extent of the disease and patients with cystinuria often show retarded growth. Steatorrhoea does not occur (Milne, 1967).

### 5. *Hartnup Syndrome*

The intestinal transport of numerous monoamino–monocarboxylic amino acids is disturbed here (Baron *et al.*, 1956). The clinical symptoms, pellagra-type skin changes, cerebellar ataxia and other neurological symptoms result from the malabsorption of essential amino acids. The absorption of tryptophane is also disturbed. Steatorrhoea is not known in such cases (Milne, 1964, 1967).

### 6. *Malabsorption of Vitamin $B_{12}$*

In 1959 Herbert described cases of possible selective vitamin $B_{12}$ malabsorption. Imerslund (1960) also Gräsbeck *et al.* (1960) observed a familial syndrome in children with isolated vitamin $B_{12}$ malabsorption and normal secretion of intrinsic factor, usually accompanying proteinuria and pathological renal changes. More recent investigations have shown however that this may also have been a sub-symptom of an undeveloped primary or secondary malabsorption (Ben-Bassat *et al.*, 1969; Eidelmann *et al.*, 1966; Corcino *et al.*, 1970).

*7. Impaired Intestinal Lymph Drainage*

*a. Lymphatic disorders.* Lymph drainage disturbances in the small intestine lead primarily to a protein loss, i.e. exudative enteropathy. As the long-chain triglyceride absorbed by the epithelial cells of the small intestine is transported in the form of chylomicrons via the lymphatic channels, disturbances of the enteric lymph drainage can also result in triglyceride malabsorption. Steatorrhoea may be a symptom of a lymph drainage disorder in the small intestine. As a result of this disturbance, which may be caused by hypoplasia of the enteric lymphatic system or by a stenosis of the lymphatic channels, the lymphatic channels in the villi and the submucosa are distended as far as the serous membrane. This condition is known as intestinal lymphangiectasia or intestinal lymphatic oedema. A distinction is made between primary intestinal lymphatic oedema (primary exudative enteropathy) and secondary intestinal lymphatic oedema, depending on the cause.

In the case of primary intestinal lymphatic oedema there is a congenital hypoplasia of the lymphatic channels in the intestines or in other parts of the body or there is retarded development of the lymphatic system. Primary intestinal lymphatic oedema, which may be part of a general lymphatic oedema, becomes manifest mainly between the ages of 11 and 28. It is therefore also known as "primary lymphatic oedema praecox" (Allen, 1934).

In secondary intestinal lymphatic oedema lymph drainage disorders and intestinal lymphangiectasia are caused by another primary disease, e.g. retroperitoneal fibrosis, Whipple's disease (intestinal lipodystrophy), lymphoma of the mesenteric lymphatic nodes (lymphosarcoma, Hodgkin's disease, fungoid mycosis), vascular congestion in the general cardiovascular system (insufficiency of right heart, constrictive pericarditis, tricuspid insufficiency). There are numerous other diseases of the gastro-intestinal tract, including inflammatory processes, which may also cause secondary exudative enteropathy but which are not accompanied by intestinal lymphatic oedema.

The clinical aspects, diagnosis and therapy of intestinal lymphatic oedema will now be outlined. Reference is also made to literature: Martini *et al.*, 1963; Pomerantz and Waldmann, 1963; Waldmann, 1966, 1970).

*b. Clinical aspects and diagnosis.* Gastro-intestinal symptoms are generally slight or absent altogether. Diarrhoea occurs occasionally. There may be vomiting after drinking milk. Lymphatic oedema of the extremities may draw attention to the disease. Lymphography will then show that it is a hypoplastic form of lymphatic oedema. Hypoproteinaemia is present when the enteric protein loss is greater than synthesis. The serum levels of not only albumin, but also immunoglobulin, in particular IgG globulin, and transferrin and coeruloplasmin are reduced. The enteric protein loss can be determined by means of $Cr^{51}$-albumin, $Cu^{67}$-coeruloplasmin, $Fe^{51}$-dextran or $J^{131}$-polyvinyl–pyrrolidon (literature in Waldmann, 1966, 1970). Lymphopenia is also characteristic. The daily faecal fat loss is frequently still normal and seldom exceeds 30 g. The D-xylose test and other absorption tests show normal results. There may be no changes in the small intestine to be detected by radiography. Some patients show a moderate coarsening of the mucosal contours; there may be also hypotonia of the intestinal loops and accumulation of contrast (Marshak *et al.*, 1961; Waldmann *et al.*, 1961; Wagner *et al.*, 1968). A biopsy of the small intestine is the decisive diagnostic factor: it shows dilatation and telangiectasia of the lymphatic channels in the villi and sub-mucosa (Figs. 11a, b).

*c. Therapy.* The intestinal lymph flow partly depends on the quantity of absorbed triglyceride which must be transported via the lymphatic channels. The lymph flow is but slight when the diet contains no fat. If only 10% long-chain triglyceride is added to the diet, the lymph flow increases by 40% (Hashim, 1968). As the enteric protein loss (exudative enteropathy) and impaired fat transport (cause of steatorrhoea) are caused by a strain on the enteric lymphatic system, the diet must be practically free of fat (Jeffries *et al.*, 1964) or the nutritional fat must be more or less completely replaced by medium-chain triglycerides. These triglycerides, with a chain-length of $C_8$–$C_{12}$ are not resynthesized intracellularly to triglycerides and are not transported in chylomicrons via the lymphatic channels but pass direct into the portal blood as free fatty acids (Holt, 1967; Sickinger, 1968a, b). A fat-free diet or substitution with medium-chain triglycerides leads immediately to a normalization of the faecal fat excretion, the enteric protein loss is reduced or becomes completely normal (Holt, 1964; Sickinger, 1968a, b). The intestinal lymphangiectasia also improves under this treatment (Creutzfeldt *et al.*, 1969). Secondary lymphatic oedema also improves but priority must be given to treatment of the primary disease, e.g. with tetracyclines in the case of Whipple's disease.

## F. Non-classifiable Disorders

### *1. Diabetic Enteropathy (Diabetic Diarrhoea and Steatorrhoea)*

Steatorrhoea and diarrhoea are facultative symptoms of diabetic enteropathy. These are quite rare complications of insulin deficiency diabetes.

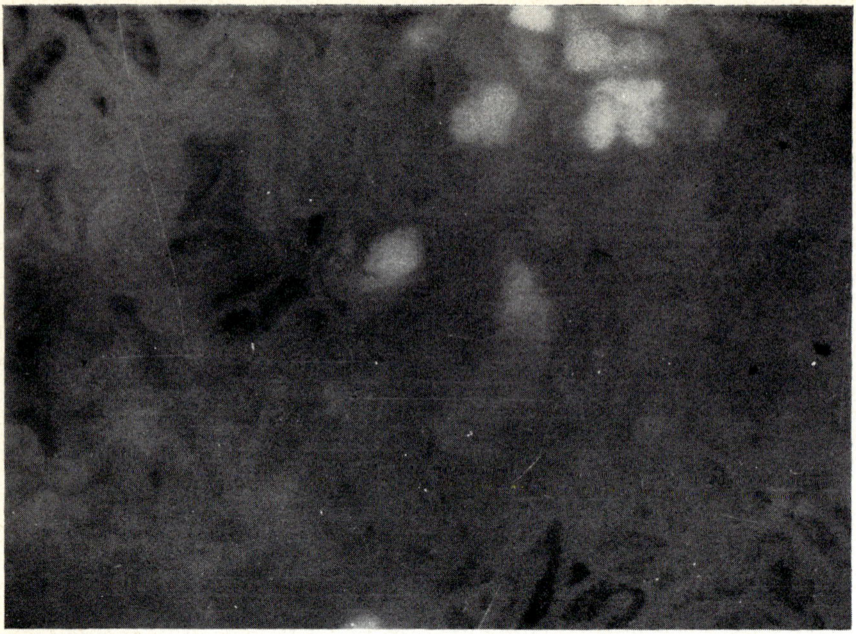

(a)

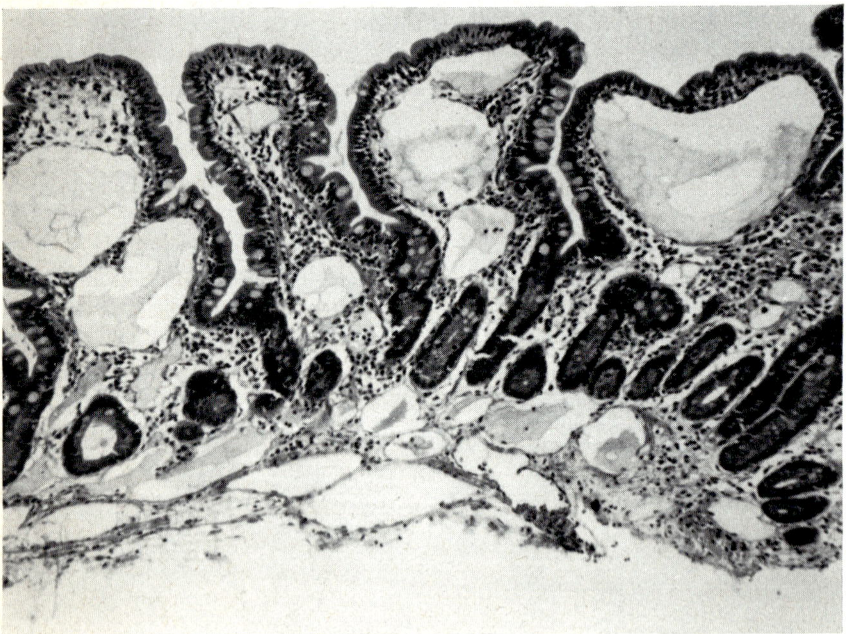

(b)

Fig. 11. Primary intestinal lymphatic oedema ("primary lymphanicctasia"): (a) stereomicroscopic aspect; (b) histology.

The steatorrhoea may have various causes. Because of a frequently observed coincidence of diabetic neuropathy and steatorrhoea a disorder of the autonomic nervous system has also been assumed (Aktan and Klotz, 1958). Pathological anatomical examinations however produced neither evidence of a neurogenic cause nor of any other causative factors (Berge *et al.*, 1956). More recent investigations have shown that in some patients there is a pathological increase in the flora of the small intestine as in the blind loop syndrome (Tabaqchali and Booth, 1967; Goldstein *et al.*, 1970).

Thin, watery stools and very frequent motions, chiefly at night or only at night, are typical of the clinical picture. In some cases motions are more frequent after meals. The male sex predominates and steatorrhoea develops generally between the ages of 30 and 50, diabetes mellitus having been present for two to ten years. The diabetes mellitus is often unstable. Orthostatic disturbances in circulatory regulation, irregular sweat production, particularly a localized reduction, are other characteristic symptoms. Faecal fat and nitrogen excretion are increased. Radiography often shows atonia of the stomach with functional emptying disturbances. The small intestinal passage time is shortened; individual loops may be hypotonic; the mucosal contours are then coarsened. A biopsy of the small intestinal mucosa shows no changes (Malins and French, 1957). Diabetic diarrhoea would appear to involve the same disorder as diabetic enteropathy, yet in a less marked form. It occurs much more frequently, often alternating with obstipation. Recent investigations have shown a close relationship between diabetic diarrhoea and diabetic neuropathy (Malins and Mayne, 1969).

There is no specific therapy for diabetic steatorrhoea or diarrhoea. The basic step is an improved stabilization of the diabetes. If increased bacterial growth in the small intestine is suspected treatment with tetracycline, chlorotetracycline or lincomycin may be tried.

### *2. Hypoparathyroidism*

Hypoparathyroidism may be accompanied by steatorrhoea—sometimes only intermittently. Nothing is known as yet about the cause of this steatorrhoea. One theory is that it may be pancreatogenic (Morse *et al.*, 1961).

### *3. Hyperthyroidosis*

Hyperthyroidosis may occasionally be the cause of slight steatorrhoea. Diarrhoea is more frequent. Both diarrhoea and steatorrhoea cease after treatment of the primary endocrinopathy (Bernstein and Riding, 1970; Middleton, 1971).

*4. Agammaglobulinaemia*

Immunoglobulin A (IgA) is formed in the plasma cells of the lamina propria of the small intestinal mucosa. It is secreted together with a carrier protein which originates from the epithelial cells. Various investigations have shown that IgA has a protective function (Bull and Tomasi, 1968). IgA deficiency sometimes occurs with malabsorption but the causal relationships have not yet been explained. Crabbe and Heremans (1966) describe a female patient with selective IgA deficiency, atrophy of the small intestinal mucosa and malabsorption. There was a distinct improvement in malabsorption when a gluten-free diet was given. However, the histologically evident improvement in the small intestinal mucosa was not accompanied by an increase in the serum IgA level. An IgA deficiency also sometimes occurs in gluten-induced sprue (Eidelmann *et al.*, 1966; Hobbs and Hepner, 1968). Other patients with IgA deficiency and malabsorption did not however react to therapy with a gluten-free diet (Waldmann and Laster, 1964; Collins and Ellis, 1965). Hobbs and Hepner (1968) also report a low level of immunoglobulin M (IgM) in patients with untreated gluten-induced sprue and a return of the IgM plasma level to normal with a gluten-free diet.

IgA or IgM deficiency alone would not appear to be the cause of malabsorption because patients with primary congenital IgA deficiency, ataxia and telangiectasia do not suffer from malabsorption (Eidelmann and Davis, 1968). The present view is that malabsorption occurs only in the case of primary acquired IgA deficiency and not in the case of a primary congenital deficiency. A strict classification is not yet possible. Neither are the causal relationships known as yet (Bull and Tomasi, 1968).

## REFERENCES


Adlersberg, D. A., Marshak, R. H., Colcher, H., Drachman, S. R. and Friedman, A. I. (1954). The roentgen appearances of the small intestine in sprue. *Gastroenterology* **2,** 548–556.

Admirand, W. H. (1972). Hyperoxaluria and bowel disease. *New Engl. J. Med.* **286,** 1412–1413.

Admirand, W. H., Earnest, D. and Williams, H. (1971). Hyperoxaluria and bowel disease. *Trans. Ass. Am. Physiol.* **84,** 307–312.

Aktan, H. S. and Klotz, A. P. (1958). Fat absorption and pancreatic function in diabetes mellitus. *Ann. Int. Med.* **49,** 820–828.

Allen, E. V. (1934). Lymphedema of extremities: classification, etiology and differential diagnosis: A study of 300 cases. *Arch. Int. Med.* **54,** 606–624.

Alpert, L. I. and Warner, R. R. P. (1968). Systemic sclerosis: case presenting with tetracycline-responsive malabsorption syndrome. *Am. J. Med.* **45,** 468–473.

Ament, M. E., Shimoda, S. S., Saunders, D. R. and Rubin, C. E. (1972). Pathogenesis of steatorrhea in three cases of small intestinal stasis syndrome. *Gastroenterology* **63,** 728–747.

Ammann, R. (1970). Die chronische pankreatitis. *Deut. Med. Wschr.* **95,** 1.

Ammann, R. (1971). 10 Jahre perorale dünndarmbiopsie bei ambulanten patienten. *Schw. Med. Wschr.* **101,** 1004–1008.

Ammann, R. und Filipini, L. (1967). Zur funktions-diagnostik des pankreaskarzinoms. *Deut. Med. Wschr.* **92,** 1636–1637.

Ammann, R. und Spycker, C. (1972). Malabsorption syndrom bei generalisierter Mastozytose (Urticaria pigmentosa). *Schw. Med. Wschr.* **102,** 213–220.

Ammann, R., Haemmesli, U. P., Leuthold, E., Von Fetten, A., Weidmann, P. und Hafter, E. (1968). Nützliches und überflüssiges in der dünndarmdiagnostik. *Schw. Med. Wschr.* **98,** 1044–1047.

Ammon, H. V. and Phillips, S. F. (1972). Fatty acids inhibit intestinal water absorption in man: fatty acid diarrhea? *Gastroenterology* **62,** 717.

Artom, C. and Reale, L. (1935). The formation of intermediate products in the pancreatic digestion of neutral fat. *Arch. Sci. Biol. Bologna* **21,** 368–380.

Astaldi, G. and Stroselli, E. (1960). Peroral biopsy of the intestinal mucosa in hepatic cirrhosis. *Am. J. Dig. Dis.* **5,** 603–612.

Austad, W. I., Lack, L. and Tyor, M. P. (1967). Importance of bile acids of an intact distal small bowel for fat absorption. *Gastroenterology* **52,** 638–646.

Ayulo, J. A. (1970). Rapid duodenal intubation employing a wire guide. *Amer. J. Dig. Dis.* **15,** 1099–1104.

Badenoch, J. and Callender, S. T. (1954). Iron metabolism in steatorrhea: the use of radioactive iron in studies of absorption and utilization. *Blood* **9,** 123–133.

Badenoch, J. and Callender, S. T. (1960). Effect of corticosteroids and gluten-free diet on absorption of iron in idiopathic steatorrhoea and coeliac disease. *Lancet* **1,** 192–194.

Badenoch, J., Bedford, P. D. and Evans, J. R. (1965). Massive diverticulose of the small intestine with steatorrhea and megaloblastic anemia. *Quart. J. Med.* **24,** 321–330.

Badley, B. W., Murphy, I. M., Bouchier, I. H. and Sherlock, S. (1969). The role of bile salts in steatorrhea of chronic liver disease. *Gastroenterology* **56,** 1136.

Bahls, G. (1970). Chologene Diarrhoen nach Ileumresektion und ihre Behandlung mit Cholestyramin. *Z. Gastroenterol.* **8,** 41–43.

Baker, S. J. and Mathan, V. I. (1968). Syndrome of tropical sprue in South India. *Am. J. Clin. Nutr.* **21,** 984–993.

Baker, S. J. and Mathan, V. I. (1970). Tropical sprue. *In* "Modern Trends in Gastroenterology" (W. I. Card and B. Creamer eds.), Vol. 4, pp. 198–228. Butterworths, London.

Balint, J. A. and Hirschowitz, B. I. (1961). Hypomagnesemia with tetany in non-tropical sprue. *New Engl. J. Med.* **265,** 631–633.

Bank, S. and Marks, I. N. (1963). Malabsorption in systemic mast cell disease. *Gastroenterology* **45,** 535–549.

Baroana, E., Orrego, O., Fernandez, E., Amenbar, E., Maldonado, E., Tag, F. and Salinas, A. (1962). Absorption function of small intestine in liver cirrhosis. *Am. J. Dig Dis.* **7,** 318–330.

Baron, D. N., Dent, C. E., Harris, H., Hart, E. W. and Jepson, J. B. (1956). Hereditary pellagra-like skin rash with temporary cerebellar ataxia. Constant renal amino-aciduria, and other bizarre biochemical features. *Lancet* **2,** 421–428.

Beck, K. und Gnauck, R. (1962). Uber die Steatorrhoe bei Leberzirrhose. *Gastroenterologia* (Suppl.) **97,** 144–147.

Beck, K., Helms, M. und Augustin, R. (1968). Die Behandlung von Nahrungsausnutzungsstörungen unter Verwendung von Fetten mit mittelkettigen Fettsäuren. *Med. Ernaehrung* **9,** 201–204.

Beddow, R. M. and Tilden, I. L. (1960). Malabsorption syndrome due to amyloidosis of the intestine secondary to lepromatous leproxy: report of a case. *Ann. Int. Med.* **53,** 1017–1027.

Ben-Bassat, I., Feinstein, A. and Ramot, B. (1969). Selective vitamin $B_{12}$ malabsorption with proteinuria in Israel. *Israel J. Med. Sci.* **5,** 62–68.

Benson, J. A., Culver, P. J., Ragland, S., Jones, C. M., Drummey, G. D. and Bougas, E. (1957). The D-xylose absorption test in malabsorption syndromes. *New Engl. J. Med.* **256,** 335–339.

Benson, G. D., Kowlessar, O. D. and Sleisenger, W. A. (1964). Adult celiac disease with emphasis upon response to the gluten-free diet. *Medicine* **43,** 1–40.

Benzonana, G., Entressangles, B., Marchir-Mouren, S., Pasero, L., Sarda, L. and Desnuelle, P. (1964). Further studies on pig pancreatic lipase. *In* "Metabolism and Physiological Significance of Lipids" (R. M. C. Dawson and D. N. Rhodes eds.) pp. 141–154. Wiley, New York.

Berge, K. G., Spraque, R. G. and Bennett, W. A. (1956). The intestinal tract in diabetic diarrhea: a pathologic study. *Diabetes* **5,** 289–294.

Bergmann, M. (1952). Uber die peristaltische Wirksamkeit der Gallensäuren und ihre klinische Anwendung. *Wien. Klin. Wschr.* **64,** 704–707.

Berk, R. N. and Scay, D. G. (1972). Cholerheic enteropathy as a cause of diarrhea and death in radiation enteritis and its prevention with cholestyramine. *Gastroenterology* **62,** 722.

Berndt, W. und Müller-Wieland, K. (1969). Vergleichende Bewertung der Wirksamkeit von Pankreasfermentpräparaten. II. Verfahren zur Beurteilung und abschlieszenden Bewertung. *Z. Gastroenterol.* **7,** 314–322.

Bernstein, A. and Riding, W. D. (1970). Hyperthyroidism and stearrhoea. *Postgrad. Med. J.* **46,** 318–320.

Binder, H. S. (1970). Celiac sprue "Unmasking" after vagotomy and hiatal hernia repair. *New Engl. J. Med.* **283,** 520–521.

Bircher, J. und Haemmerli, U. P. (1967). Diättherapie bei gastroenterologischen Erkrankungen. Versuch einer kritischen Stellungnahme. *Schweiz. Med. Wschr.* **97,** 1687–1696.

Bishop, R. F. (1965). Bacterial flora of stomach and small intestine after gastric surgery. *Ernaehrungsforsch.* **10,** 417–422.

Blomstrand, R. (1955). A study on the intestinal absorption of fat in normal adults and in nontropical sprue with carbon-labelled oleic acid and palmitic acid. *Acta Med. Scand.* **152,** 129–138.

Bloom, B., Chaikoff, I. L., Reinhardt, W. O., Entenman, C. and Dauben, W. G. (1950). The quantitative significance of the lymphatic pathway in transport of absorbed fatty acids. *J. Biol. Chem.* **184,** 1–8.

Bloom, B., Chaikoff, I. L. and Reinhardt, W. O. (1951). Intestinal lymph as pathway for transport of absorbed fatty acids of different chain lengths. *Am. J. Physiol.* **166,** 451–455.

Bloomstrand, R. and Ahrens, E. H., Jr. (1958). The absorption of fats studied in a patient with chyluria: III Cholesterol. *J. Biol. Chem.* **233,** 327–330.

Blum, M. and Spritz, N. (1966). The metabolism of intravenously injected isotopic cholic acid in Laennec's cirrhosis. *J. Clin. Invest.* **45,** 187–193.

Booth, C. C. and Mollin, D. L. (1957). Importance of the ileum in the absorption of vitamin $B_{12}$. *Lancet,* **2,** 1007.

Booth, C. C., Stewart, J. S., Holmes, R. and Brackenbury, W. (1962). "Intestinal Biopsy". Ciba Foundation Study Group N 14. Churchill, London.

Booth, C. C. (1965). Treatment of malabsorption syndrome after intestinal resection. *Gastroenterologia* **104,** 49–58.

Booth, C. C. (1966). Pathophysiologie der Dünndarmresorption. *Internist* **7,** 197–208.

Borgström, B. (1954). On the mechanism of pancreatic lipolysis of glycerides. *Biochem. Biophys. Acta* **13,** 491–504.

Borgström, B. (1955). Transport of $^{14}C$-decanoic acid in porta and inferior vena cava blood during absorption in the rat. *Acta Physiol. Scand.* **34,** 71–74.

Borgström, B. (1960). Studies on intestinal cholesterol absorption. *J. Clin. Invest.* **39,** 809–815.

Borgström, B. (1964). Lipid absorption-physicochemical considerations. *In* "Metabolism and Physiological Significance of Lipids" (R. M. C. Dawson and D. N. Rhodes, eds.), pp. 221–228. Wiley, New York.

Borgström, B. (1965). The dimensions of the bile salt micelle. Measurement by gel filtration. *Biochim. Biophys. Acta* **106,** 171–183.

Borgström, B., Lundh, G. and Hofmann, A. (1963). The site of absorption of conjugated bile salts in man. *Gastroenterology* **45,** 229–238.

Bossak, E. T. and Wang, C. I. (1957). Clinical aspects of the malabsorption syndrome (idiopathic sprue). *In* "The Malabsorption Syndrome" (D. Adlersberg, ed.), pp. 112–134. Grune and Stratton, New York.

Braddock, L. R. I., Fleisher, D. R. and Barbero, G. J. (1968). A physical chemical study of the Van De Kamer method for fecal fat analysis. *Gastroenterology* **55,** 165–172.

Brandborg, L. L., Rubin, C. E. and Quinton, W. E. (1959). A multipurpose instrument for suction biopsy of the esophagus, stomach, small bowel and colon. *Gastroenterology* **37,** 1–16.

Brandborg, L. L., Tankersley, C. B., Gottlieb, S., Barancik, M. and Sartor, V. E. (1967). Histological demonstration of mucosal invasion by Giardia Lamblia on man. *Gastroenterology* **52,** 143–150.

Brandborg, L. L., Goldberg, St. B. and Breidenbach, W. C. (1970). Human coccidiosis: a possible cause of malabsorption. *New Engl. J. Med.* **283,** 1306–1313.

Bright-Asare, P. and Binder, H. J. (1973). Stimulation of colonic secretion of water and electrolytes by hydroxy fatty acids. *Gastroenterology* **64,** 81–88.

Brooks, F. P. (1972). Testing pancreatic function. *New Engl. J. Med.* **286,** 300–302.

Brow, J. R., Parker, F., Weinstein, W. M. and Rubin, C. E. (1971). The small intestinal mucosa in dermatitis herpetiformis: I Severity and distribution of the small intestinal lesion and associated malabsorption. *Gastroenterology* **60,** 355–361.

Bruusgaard, A. (1972). Schilling test versus changes in bile acid pattern in testing terminal: ileal function. *In* "Bile Acids in Human Diseases" (P. Back and W. Gerok, eds.), pp. 238–241. Schattauer Verlag, Stuttgart, New York.

Bull, D. M. and Tomasi, T. B. (1968). Deficiency of immunoglobulin in intestinal disease. *Gastroenterology* **54,** 313–320.

Burhenne, H. J. and Carbone, J. V. (1966). Eosinophilic (allergic) gastroenteritis. *Am. J. Roentgenol.* **96,** 332–338.

Cain, G. D., Reiner, E. B. and Patterson, M. (1968). Effects of neomycin on disaccharidase activity of the small bowel (human). *Arch. Int. Med.* **122,** 311–314.

Carey, M. C. and Small, J. M. (1972). Micelle formation by bile salts. *Arch. Int. Med.* **130,** 506–527.

Casad, B. E. and Bocian, J. J. (1965). Primary systemic amyloidosis simulating acute idiopathic ulcerative colitis. *Am. J. Dig. Dis.* **10,** 63–74.

Caspary, W. F. (1971). Effect of biguanides on intestinal transport of sugars, amino acids and calcium. *Arch. Exp. Pathol. Pharmakol.* **269,** 421–422.

Chalfin, D. and Holt, P. R. (1966). Metabolism of octanoic acid by rat intestinal slices and homogenates. *Fedn. Proc. Fedn. Am. Socs. Exp. Biol.* **25,** 639.

Choudhoury, D. C. R., Nickolson, G. I. and Cooke, W. T. (1964). Simple capsule for multiple intestinal biopsy specimens. *Lancet* **2,** 185–186.

Clark, B. and Hübscher, G. (1960). Biosynthesis of glycerides in mucosa of the small intestine. *Nature* **185,** 35–37.

Clark, B. and Hübscher, G. (1962). Glycerokinase in mucosa of the small intestine of the cat. *Nature* **195,** 599–600.

Clark, S. B. and Holt, P. R. (1968). Rate-limiting steps in steady-state intestinal absorption of trioctanvin-1-14C. Effect of biliary and pancreatic flow diversion. *J. Clin. Invest.* **47,** 612–623.

Clark, S. B. and Holt, P. R. (1969). Inhibition of steady-state intestinal absorption of long-chain triglyceride by medium-chain triglyceride in the unanesthetized rat. *J. Clin. Invest.* **48,** 2235–2243.

Clark, S. B., Brause, B. and Holt, P. R. (1969). Lipolysis and absorption of fat in the rat stomach. *Gastroenterology* **56,** 214–222.

Classen, M. und Koch, H. (1968). Perorale Dünndarmbiopsie. *Deut. Med. Wschr.* **93,** 2203–2204.

Cohen, M., Morgan, R. G. H. and Hofmann, A. F. (1969). One-step quantitative extraction of medium-chain and long-chain fatty acids from aqueous samples. *Lipid Res.* **10,** 614–616.

Cohen, M., Morgan, R. G. H. and Hofmann, A. F. (1971). Lipolytic activity of human gastric and duodenal juice against medium and long chain triglycerides. *Gastroenterology* **60,** 1–15.

Collins, J. R. and Ellis, D. S. (1965). Agammaglobulinemic malabsorption and rheumatoid-like arthritis. *Am. J. Med.* **39,** 476–482.

Cooke, W. T. (1957). Water and electrolyte upsets in the steatorrhea syndrome. *In* "The Malabsorption Syndrom" (D. Adlersberg, ed.), pp. 47–62. Grune and Stratton, New York.

Cooke, W. T. (1968). Adult celiac disease. *In* "Progress in Gastroenterology" (G. B. J. Glass, ed.), Vol. 1, pp. 299–338. Grune and Stratton, New York.

Cooke, W. T. and Smith, W. T. (1966). Neurological disorders associated with adult coeliac disease. *Brain* **89,** 683–722.

Cooke, W. T., Penney, A. L. P. and Hawkins, C. F. (1953). Symptoms, signs and diagnostic features of idiopathic steatorrhea. *Quart. J. Med.* **22,** 59–65.

Cooke, W. T., Cox, E. V., Fone, D. J., Meynell, M. J. and Gaddie, R. (1963). The clinical and metabolic significance of jejunal diverticula. *Gut* **4,** 115–131.

Cooke, W. T., Johnson, A. G. and Woolf, A. L. (1966). Vital staining and electron microscopy of the intramuscular nerve endings in the neuropathy of adult coeliac disease. *Brain* **89,** 663–682.

Corcino, J. J., Waxman, S. and Herbert, V. (1970). Absorption and malabsorption of vitamin $B_{12}$. *Am. J. Med.* **48,** 562–569.

Corsini, G., Gandolfi, E. Bonechi, I. and Curri, B. (1966). Postgastrectomy malabsorption. *Gastroenterology* **50,** 358–365.

Corsini, G., Gandolfi, E., Bonechi, I. and Curri, B. (1967). Fat absorption in diabetes mellitus. *Diabetes* **16,** 455–461.

Crabbe, P. A. and Heremans, J. F. (1966). Lack of gamma A-immunoglobin in serum of patients with steatorrhea. *Gut* **7,** 119–127.

Creamer, B. (1964). Malignancy and the small intestine mucosa. *Brit. Med. J.* **2,** 1435–1436.

Creutzfeldt, W. (1964). Funktionsdiagnostik bei Erkrankungen des Pankreas. *Verh. Deut. Ges. Inn. Med.* **70,** 781–801.

Creutzfeldt, W. (1969). Das Zollinger-Ellison-Syndrom. *Verh. Deut. Ges. Inn. Med.* **75,** 242–264.

Creutzfeldt, W., Kern, E., Kümmerle, F. und Schumacher, J. (1961). Die Ausfallerscheinungen nach totale Pankreatiktomie und ihre Behandlung. *Ergeb. Inn. Med. Kinderheilk.* **16,** 79–124.

Creutzfeldt, W. und Widmann, R. (1956). Untersuchungen über die Funktion des Exokrinen Pankreas bei Leber- und Gallewegserkrankungen mit Hilfe des Mecholyl-Athertestes. *Klin. Wschr.* **34,** 968–974.

Creutzfeldt, W., Sickinger, K., Emrich, D. und Gregl, A. (1969). Der Einfluss der mittelkettigen Triglyceride auf die exzudative Enteropathie bei den verschiedenen Formen des primären Lymphoedema praecox. *In* "Aktuelle Gastroenterologie" (H. Bartelheimer and N. Heisig, eds.), pp. 141–195. Thieme, Stuttgart.

Creutzfeldt, W., Fehr, H. und Schmidt, H. (1970). Verlaufsbeobachtungen und diagnostische Verfahren bei der chronisch-rezidivierenden und chronischen Pankreatitis. *Schweiz. Med. Wschr.* **100,** 1180–1189.

Crosby, W. H. and Kugler, H. W. (1962). Intraluminal biopsy in the small intestine. *Am. J. Dig. Dis.* **2,** 236–242.

Dalinka, M. K. and Masters, C. J. (1970). Eosinophilic enteritis. Report of a case without gastric involvement. *Radiology* **96,** 543–544.

Dasher, G. F. (1952). Surface activity of naturally occurring emulsifiers. *Science* **116,** 660–663.

Dawson, A. M. and Isselbacher, K. J. (1960). Studies on lipid metabolism in the small intestine with observations on the role of bile salts. *J. Clin. Invest.* **39,** 730–740.

Dent, C. E., Stokes, J. F. and Carpenter, M. E. (1961). Death from hypothermia in steatorrhoea. *Lancet* **1,** 748–749.

Desnuelle, P. and Savary, P. (1963). Specifities of lipases. *J. Lipid Res.* **4,** 368–384.

Dicke, W. K. (1950). *In* "Een onderzoek naar de nadelige invloed van sommige graansoorten op de lijder aan coeliakie". Thesis, Univ. Utrecht.

Dietschy, J. M., Salomon, H. S. and Siperstein, M. D. (1966). Bile acid metabolism: I. Studies on the mechanisms of intestinal transport. *J. Clin. Invest.* **45,** 832–846.

Dobbins, W. O. (1966). An ultrastructural study of the intestinal mucosa in congenital $\beta$-lipoprotein deficiency with particular emphasis upon the intestinal absorption cell. *Gastroenterology* **50,** 195–210.

Dobbins, W. O. (1968). Drug-induced steatorrhea. *Gastroenterology* **54,** 1193–1195.

Dobbins, W. O., Herrero, B. A. and Mansbach, C. M. (1968). Morphologic alterations associated with neomycin induced malabsorption. *Am. J. Med. Sci.* **255,** 63–77.

Donaldson, R. M., Jr. (1964). Normal bacterial populations of the intestine and their relation to intestinal function. *New Engl. J. Med.* **270,** 994–1001.

Donaldson, R. M. (1965). Studies on the pathogenesis of steatorrhea in the blind loop syndrome. *J. Clin. Invest.* **44,** 1815–1825.

Donaldson, R. M., Jr., Corrigan, H. and Natsios, G. (1962). Malabsorption of $^{60}$Co-labelled cyanocobalamin in rats with intestinal diverticula: II. Studies on contents of the diverticula. *Gastroenterology* **43,** 282–290.

Dornberger, G. R., Comfert, M. W. and Wollaegen, E. E. (1948). Pancreatic function as measured by analysis of duodenal contents before and after stimulation with secretion. *Gastroenterology* **11,** 701–713.

Douglas, A. P. and Peters, T. J. (1970). Peptide hydrolase activity of human intestinal mucosa in adult coeliac disease. *Gut* **11,** 15–17.

Dowling, R. H. (1967). Compensatory changes in intestinal absorption. *Brit. Med. Bull.* **23,** 275–278.

Dowling, R. H. (1972). The enterohepatic circulation. *Gastroenterology* **62,** 122–140.

Dowling, R. H., Rose, G. A. and Sutor, D. J. (1971). Hyperoxaluria and renal calculi in ileal disease. *Lancet* **1,** 1103–1106.

Drasar, B. S., Hill, M. J. and Shiner, M. (1966). The deconjugation of bile salts by human intestinal bacteria. *Lancet* **1,** 1237–1238.

Dreher, K. D., Schulman, J. H. and Hofmann, A. F. (1967). Surface chemistry of the monoglyceride-bile salt system: its relationship to the function of bile salts in fat absorption. *J. Colloid Interface Sci.* **25,** 71–83.

Dreiling, D. A. and Janowitz, H. D. (1957). Laboratory diagnosis of pancreatic disease: secretion test. *Am. J. Gastroenterol.* **28,** 268–279.

Drube, H. C. (1963). Untersuchungen zur medikementösen Verdauungs insuffizienz. *Z. Gastroenterol.* **1,** 358–366.

Drummey, G. D., Benson, J. A. and Jones, C. M. (1961). Microscopical examination of the stool for steatorrhea. *New Engl. J. Med.* **264,** 85–87.

Eidelmann, S. S. and Davis, D. S. (1968). Immunoglobulin content of intestinal mucosal plasma-cells in ataxia telangiectasia. *Lancet* **1,** 884–886.

Eidelmann, S. S., Parkins, R. A. and Rubin, C. E. (1966). Abdominal lymphoma presenting as malabsorption. *Medicine* **45,** 111–137.

Eisenburg, J., Schwandt, P., Christoforis, A., Koczorek, K. H., Forrell, M. M., Kiefhaber, P. und Frey, K. W. (1969). Untersuchungen zur Fettresorption bei Kranken mit Leberzirrhose. *Fortschr. Med.* **87,** 185–188.

Engstrom, J. F., Rybak, J. J. and Duber, M. (1968). Evidence for a lipase system in canine gastric juice. *Am. J. Med. Sci.* **256,** 346–351.

Entressangles, B. L., Paséro, L., Savary, P., Sarda, L. et Desnuelle, P. (1961. Influence de la nature des chaines sur la vitesse de leur lipase pancréatique. *Bull. Soc. Chim. Biol.* **43,** 581–591.

Entressangles, B. L., Savary, P., Constantin, M. J. et Desnuelle, P. (1964). Comportement *in vitro* et *in vivo* des chaînes countes situées en position interne dans les triglycerides. *Biochim. Biophys. Acta* **84,** 140–148.

Fahrländer, H. (1967). Uber allergische Ernährungen des Dünndarms. *Wien. Klin. Wschr.* **79,** 644–650.

Fink, S. and Laszlo, D. (1957). A metabolic study following oral calcium$^{45}$ administration in a patient with non-tropical sprue. *Gastroenterology* **32,** 689–703.

Fisher, H. and Kaunitz, H. (1964). Effects of medium- and long-chain saturated triglycerides on blood and liver cholesterol of chicken and rats. *Proc. Soc. Exp. Biol. Med.* **116,** 278–280.

Földes, J., Magyar, I., Szücs, J. und Gyertyanffy, S. (1966). Bauchspeicheldrüsextrakt auf die Steatorrhoe bei Leberzirrhose und nach subtotale Gastroectomie. *Z. Gastroenterol.* **4,** 284–288.

Forth, W., Rummel, W. und Glasner, H. (1966). Zur resorptions hemmende Wirkung von Gallensäuren. *Arch. Exp. Pathol. Pharmakol.* **254,** 364–380.

Frazer, A. C. (1952). Studies on the aetiology of the sprue syndrome. *Gastroenterologia* **78,** 357–364.

Frazer, A. C. and Sammons, H. G. (1945). The formation of mono- and di-glycerides during the hydrolysis of triglyceride by pancreatic lipase. *Biochem. J.* **39,** 122–128.

Fraser, N. G., Murray, D. and Alexander, J. O. (1967). Structure and function of the small intestine in dermatitis herpetiformis. *Brit. J. Dermatol.* **79,** 509–518.

Fredrickson, D. S., Levy, R. I. and Lees, R. S. (1967). Fat transport in lipoproteins—integrated approach to mechanisms and disorders. *New Engl. J. Med.* **276,** 273–281.

Freund, G. and Weinsier, R. L. (1966). Standarized ketosis in man following medium chain triglyceride ingestion. *Metabolism* **15,** 980–991.

Friedmann, A. I. and McEwan, G. (1963). Small bower absorption in portal cirrhosis with ascites. *Am. J. Gastroenterol.* **39,** 114–119.

Friedman, M. and Hare, P. J. (1965). Gluten-sensitive enteropathy and eczema. *Lancet* **1,** 521–524.

Friedner, S. and Moberg, S. (1967). Determination of total faecal lipids including medium-chain triglycerides. *Clin. Chim. Acta* **18,** 345–349.

Fröhlicher, E. (1936). Die Resportion von Gallensäuren aus verschiedenen Dünndarmabschnitten. *Biochem. Z.* **283,** 273–279.

Fromm, H. (1972). A prospective comparison of different tests of ileal function. *In* "Bile Acids in Human Diseases" (P. Back and W. Gerok, eds.), pp. 223–237. Schattauer Verlag, Stuttgart, New York.

Fromm, H. and Hofmann, A. F. (1971). Breath test for altered bile-acid metabolism. *Lancet* **2,** 621–625.

Fry, L., Keir, P., McMinn, R. M. H., Cowan, J. D. and Hoffbrand, A. V. (1967). Small-intestinal structure and function and haematological changes in dermatitis herpetiformis. *Lancet* **2,** 729–733.

Furman, R. H. (1968). Effects of medium chain length triglycerides on serum lipids. *In* "Medium-Chain Triglycerides" (J. R. Senior, ed.), pp. 51–61. University of Pennsylvania Press, Philadelphia, U.S.A.

Furman, R. H., Howard, R. P., Brusco, O. J. and Alaupovic, P. (1965). Effects of medium chain length triglyceride (MCT) on serum lipids and lipoproteins in familial hyperchylomicronemia (dietary fat-induced lipemia) and dietary carbohydrate-accentuated lipemia. *J. Lab. Clin. Med.* **66,** 912–926.

Galapaux, E. A., Templeton, R. D. and Borken, E. L. (1938). The influence of bile on the motility of the dog's colon. *Am. J. Physiol.* **121,** 130–136.

Gee, S. (1888). On celiac affectation. *St. Barth. Hosp. Rep.* **24,** 17–32.

Goldberg, D. (1970). A psychiatric study of patients with diseases of the small intestine. *Gut* **11,** 459–465.

Goldstein, F., Wirts, C. W. and Kowlessar, O. D. (1970). Diabetic diarrhea and steatorrhea: microbiologic and clinical observations. *Ann. Int. Med.* **72,** 215–218.

Goodman, W. S. (1965). Cholesterol ester metabolism. *Physiol. Rev.* **45,** 747–839.

Gorbach, S. L. and Tabaqchali, S. (1969). Bacteria, bile and the small bowel. *Gut* **10,** 963–972.

Gorbach, S. L., Plant, A. G., Nahas, L. and Weinstein, L. (1967). Studies of intestinal microflora: II. Micro-organisms of the small intestine and their relations to oral and fecal flora. *Gastroenterology* **53,** 856–867.

Gossmann, H. (1966). Calziumstoffwechsel bei Erkrankungen des Dünndarms. *Internist* **7,** 236–242.

Gotto, A. M., Levy, R. I., John, K. and Fredrickson, D. S. (1971). On the protein defect in abetalipoproteinemia. *New Engl. J. Med.* **284,** 813–818.

Gracey, M., Burke, V. and Anderson, C. M. (1969). Assessment of medium-chain triglyceride feeding in infants with cystic fibrosis. *Arch. Dis. Childhood* **44,** 401–403.

Grande, F. (1962). Dog serum lipid responses to dietary fats differening in chain length of saturated fatty acids. *J. Nutr.* **76,** 255–264.

Gräsbeck, R., Gordin, R., Kantero, I. and Kuhlbäck, B. (1960). Selective vitamin $B_{12}$ malabsorption and proteinuria in young people. A syndrome. *Acta Med. Scand.* **167,** 289–296.

Green, P. A. and Wollaeger, E. E. (1960). The clinical behaviour of sprue in the United States. *Gastroenterology* **38,** 399–418.

Greenberger, N. J., Franks, J. J. and Isselbacher, K. S. (1965). Metabolism of 1-$C^{14}$ octanoic and 1-$C^{14}$ palmitic acid by rat intestinal slices. *Proc. Soc. Exp. Biol. Med.* **120,** 468–472.

Greenberger, N. J., Rodgess, J. B. and Isselbacher, K. J. (1966). Absorption of medium and long chain triglycerides: factors influencing their hydrolysis and transport. *J. Clin. Invest.* **45,** 217–227.

Greenberger, N. J., Tzagournis, M. and Graves, T. M. (1968a). Stimulation of insulin secretion in man by medium chain triglycerides. *Metabolism* **17,** 796–781.

Greenberger, N. J., Dobbins, W. O., Ruppert, R. D. and Jesseph, J. E. (1968b). Intestinal atony in progressive systemic sclerosis (Scleroderma). *Am. J. Med.* **45,** 301–308.

Grözinger, K. H., Vollwein, A. and Böhler, R. (1972). Untersuchungen zur Verdaurungswirkung von Enzymsubstitutions präraraten. *Med. Klin.* **67,** 458–461.

Haemmerli, U. P. (1970). Klinik des Malabsorptionssyndroms. *Therapiewoche* **20,** 3195–3198.

Haemmerli, U. P. und Ammann, R. (1963). Malabsorptionssyndrom. Moderne Untersuchungsmethoden und Differentialdiagnose. *Schweiz. Med. Wschr.* **93,** 1517–1527.

Haessler, H. A. and Isselbacher, K. J. (1963). The metabolism of glycerol by intestinal mucosa. *Biochim. Biophys. Acta* **73,** 427–436.

Hagemann, R. F. and Lesher, S. (1971). Irradiation of the g.i. tract: compensatory response of stomach, jejunum and colon. *Brit. J. Radiol.* **44,** 599–602.

Halsted, C. H., Griggs, R. C. and Harris, J. W. (1967). The effect of alcoholism on the absorption of folic acid ($H^3$-PGA) evaluated by plasma levels and urine excretion. *J. Lab. Clin. Med.* **69,** 116–131.

Hardison, W. G. M. and Rosenberg, I. H. (1966). Malabsorption of bile salts as a cause of steatorrhea after ileal resection. *Am. J. Clin. Nutr.* **18,** 312.

Hardison, W. G. M. and Rosenberg, I. H. (1967). Bile-salt deficiency in the steatorrhea following resection of the ileum and proximal colon. *New Engl. J. Med.* **277,** 337–342.

Hardison, W. G. M. and Rosenberg, I. H. (1968). The relation of bile salt wasting to steatorrhea during neomycin administration. *Gastroenterology* **54,** 1243.

Hardison, W. G. M. and Rosenberg, I. H. (1969). The effect of neomycin on bile salt metabolism and fat digestion in man. *J. Lab. Clin. Med.* **74,** 564–573.

Harris, O. D., Cooke, W. T., Thompson, H. and Waterhouse, J. A. H. (1967). Malignancy in adult coeliac disease and idiopathic steatorrhea. *Am. J. Med.* **42,** 899–912.

Hashim, S. A. (1968). Studies of medium chain fatty acid transport in portal blood. *In* "Medium-Chain Triglycerides" (J. R. Senior, ed.), pp. 81–90. University of Pennsylvania Press, Philadelphia, U.S.A.

Hashim, S. A., Bergen, S. S. and Van Itallie, T. B. (1961). Experimental steatorrhea induced in man by bile acid sequestrant. *Proc. Soc. Exp. Biol. Med.* **106,** 173–175.

Hashim, S. A., Bergen, S. S., Jr., Krell, K. and Van Itallie, T. B. (1964). Intestinal absorption and mode of transport in portal vein of medium chain fatty acids. *J. Clin. Invest.* **43,** 1238.

Haslewood, G. A. D. (1964). The biological significance of chemical differences in bile salts. *Biol. Rev. Cambridge Phil. Soc.* **39,** 537–574.

Haverback, B. J., Dycc, B. J., Gutentag, P. J. and Montgomery, D. W. (1963). Measurement of trypsin and chymotrypsin in stool. A diagnostic test for pancreatic exocrine insufficiency. *Gastroenterology* **44,** 588–597.

Hedberg, C. A., Melnyk, C. S. and Johnson, C. F. (1966). Gluten enteropathy appearing after gastric surgery. *Gastroenterology* **50,** 796–804.

Herbert, V. (1959). "The Megaloblastic Anemias". Grune and Stratton, New York, London.

Herskovic, T., Bartholomew, L. G. and Green, P. A. (1964). Amyloidosis and malabsorption syndrome. *Arch. Int. Med.* **114,** 629–633.

Hill, M. J. and Drasar, B. S. (1968). Degradation of bile salts by human intestinal bacteria. *Gut* **9,** 22–27.

Hillman, H. S. (1968). Postgastrectomy malnutrition. *Gut* **9,** 576–584.

Hislop, I. G., Hofmann, A. F. and Schoenfield, L. J. (1967). Determinants of the rate and site of bile acid absorption in man. *J. Clin. Invest.* **46,** 1070–1071.

Hobbs, J. R. and Hepner, G. W. (1968). Deficiency of $\gamma$M-globulin in coeliac disease. *Lancet* **1,** 217–220.

Hofmann, A. F. (1963a). The function of bile salts in fat absorption: the solvent properties of dilute micellar solutions of conjugated bile salts. *Biochem. J.* **89,** 57–68.

Hofmann, A. F. (1963b). The behaviour and solubility of monoglycerides in diluted micellar bile salt solution. *Biochim. Biophys. Acta* **70,** 308–316.

Hofman, A. F. (1965). Clinical implications of physico-chemical studies on bile salts. *Gastroenterology* **48,** 484–494.

Hofmann, A. F. (1966). A physicochemical approach to the intraluminal phase of fat absorption. *Gastroenterology* **50,** 56–64.

Hofmann, A. F. (1967). The syndrome of ileal disease and the broken enterohepatic circulation: cholerheic enteropathy. *Gastroenterology* **52,** 752–757.

Hofmann, A. F. (1968). Functions of bile in the alimentary canal. *In* "Handbook of Physiology" (C. F. Code, ed.), Section 6, Vol. V, pp. 2507–2533. Williams and Wilkins, Baltimore, U.S.A.

Hofmann, A. F. (1971). Bile acid metabolism in liver disease. *In* "Alkohol und Leber" (W. Gerok, K. Sickinger and H. H. Hemikeuser, eds.), pp. 421–433. Schattauer Verlag, Stuttgart.

Hofmann, A. F. (1972). Bile acid malabsorption caused by ileal resection. *Arch. Int. Med.* **130,** 597–605.

Hofmann, A. F. and Borgström, B. (1962). Physico-chemical state of lipids in intestinal content during their digestion and absorption. *Fedn. Proc. Fedn. Am. Socs. Exp. Biol.* **21,** 43–50.

Hofmann, A. F. and Borgström, B. (1964). The intraluminal phase of fat digestion in man: The lipid content of the micellar and oil phases of intestinal content obtained during fat digestion and absorption. *J. Clin. Invest.* **43,** 247–257.

Hofmann, A. F. and Grundy, S. M. (1965). Abnormal bile salt metabolism in a patient with extensive lower intestinal resection. *Clin. Res.* **13,** 254.

Hofmann, A. F. and Poley, J. R. (1969). Cholestyramine treatment of diarrhea associated with ileal resection. *New Engl. J. Med.* **281,** 397–402.

Hofmann, A. F. and Small, D. M. (1967). Detergent properties of bile salts: correlation with physiological function. *Ann. Rev. Med.* **18,** 333–376.

Hofmann, A. F., Poley, J. R., Mekhjian, H. S. and Phillips, S. F. (1970a). Hydroxy fatty acids: An apparent cause of diarrhea in patients with ileal resection and steatorrhea. *J. Clin. Invest.* **49,** 44a–45a.

Hofmann, A. F., Thomas, P. J., Smith, L. H. and McCall, J. T. (1970b). Pathogenesis of secondary hyperoxaluria in patients with ileal resection and diarrhea. *Gastroenterology* **58,** 960.

Hogben, C. A. M. (1969). The alimentary tract. *Ann. Rev. Physiol.* **22,** 381–406.

Holt, P. R. (1964). Dietary treatment of protein loss in intestinal lymphangiectasia. The effect of eliminating dietary long-chain triglycerides on albumin metabolism in this condition. *Pediatrics* **34,** 629–633.

Holt, P. R. (1967). Medium-chain triglycerides. A useful adjunct in nutritional therapy. *Gastroenterology* **53,** 961–966.

Holt, P. R., Hashim, S. A. and Van Itallie, T. B. (1965). Treatment of malabsorption syndrome and exudative enteropathy with synthetic medium chain triglycerides. *Am. J. Gastroenterol.* **43,** 549–559.

Horino, M., Machlin, L. J., Hertelendy, F. and Kipnis, D. M. (1968). Effect of short-chain fatty acids on plasma insulin in ruminant and nonruminant species. *Endocrinology* **83,** 118–128.

Hunstein, W., Sickinger, K. und Creutzfeldt, W. (1969). Uber das Auftreten von Osteomalazien bei Sprue ohne Steatorrhea. *In* "Aktuelle Gastroenterologie" (H. Bartheimer, N. Heising, eds.), pp. 200–203. Thieme, Stuttgart.

Iber, F. L. (1968). Treatment of pancreatic insufficiency. *John's Hopkins Bull.* **122,** 172–179.

Imerslund, O. (1960). Idiopathic chronic megaloblastic anemia in children. *Acta Paediat.* **49,** suppl. **120,** 115.

Isbell, R. G., Carlson, H. C. and Hoffmann, H. N. (1969). Roentgenologic-pathologic correlation in malabsorption syndromes. *Am. J. Roentgenol.* **107,** 158–169.

Isselbacher, K. J. (1965). Factors influencing the absorption of medium chain triglycerides. *Gastroenterology* **49,** 337–338.

Isselbacher, K. J. and Budy, D. (1963). Synthesis of lipoproteins by rat intestinal mucosa. *Nature* **200,** 364–365.

Isselbacher, K. J., Scheig, R., Plotkin, G. R. and Caulfield, J. B. (1964). Congenital $\beta$-lipoprotein deficiency: an hereditary disorder involving a defect in the absorption and transport of lipids. *Medicine* **43,** 347–361.

Jacobson, L. B. (1970). Diffuse eosinophilic gastroenteritis: An adult form of gastroenteropathy. *Am. J. Gastroenterol.* **54,** 580–588.

James, A. T., Webb, J. P. W. and Kellock, T. D. (1961). The occurrence of unusual fatty acids in faecal lipids from human beings with normal and abnormal fat absorption. *Biochem. J.* **78,** 333–339.

Jeejeebhoy, S. A. and Kozak, G. (1970). Determination of fecal fats containing both medium and long chain triglycerides and fatty acids. *Clin. Biochem.* **3,** 157–163.

Jeffries, G. H., Weser, E. and Sleisinger, M. H. (1964). Malabsorption. *Gastroenterology* **46,** 434–466.

Jeffries, G. H., Weser, E. and Sleisinger, M. H. (1969). Malabsorption. *Gastroenterology* **56,** 777–797.

Johnson, D. P. and Alpert, M. E. (1971). Dermatitis herpetiformis: a disease associated with intestinal malabsorption. *Am. J. Gastroenterol.* **55,** 21–32.

Johnston, J. M. (1968). Mechanism of fat absorption. *In* "Handbook of Physiology" (C. F. Code, ed.), Section 6, Vol. III, pp. 1353–1375. Williams and Wilkins, Baltimore, U.S.A.

Jordan, P. H., Jr. and Grossman, M. I. (1959). Effect of dosage schedule on the efficacy of substitution therapy in pancreatic insufficiency. *Gastroenterology* **36,** 447–451.

Joske, R. A. (1960). Primary carcinoma of the jejunum with atrophic jejunitis and intestinal malabsorption. *Gastroenterology* **38,** 810–816.

Kahn, I. J., Jeffries, G. H. and Sleisinger, M. H. (1966). Malabsorption in intestinal scleroderma: correction by antibiotics. *New Engl. J. Med.* **274,** 1339–1344.

Kalser, M. H. (1964). Malabsorption syndromes. *In* "Gastroenterology" (H. L. Bockus, ed.), Vol. 2, pp. 423–502. Saunders, Philadelphia, London.

Kalser, M. H., Cohen, R., Arteaga, I., Yawn, E., Mayoral, L., Hoffert, W. R. and Frazier, D. (1966). Normal viral and bacterial flora of the human small and large intestine. *New Engl. J. Med.* **274,** 500–505.

Kalser, M. H., Leite, C. A. and Warren, W. D. (1968). Fat assimilation after massive distal pancreatectomy. *New Engl. J. Med.* **279,** 570–576.

Kaplan, S. M., Goldstein, F. and Kowlessar, O. D. (1970). Eosinophilic gastroenteritis. Report of a case with malabsorption and protein-losing enteropathy. *Gastroenterology* **58,** 540–545.

Kelleher, J., Walker, B. E. and Losowsky, M. S. (1970). An assessment of the Van De Kamer method for estimation of fecal fat. *Clin. Chim. Acta* **30,** 267–271.

Kern, F. and Borgström, B. (1965). Quantitative study of the pathways of triglyceride synthesis by hamster intestinal mucosa. *Biochim. Biophys. Acta* **98,** 520–531.

Kilpatrick, Z. M. and Katz, J. (1969). Occult celiac disease as a cause of iron deficiency anemia. *J. Am. Med. Ass.* **208,** 999–1001.

Kistler, H. J. (1967). Die Nachbehandlung von Patienten mit ausgedehnten Dünndarmresektionen. *Schweiz. Med. Wschr.* **97,** 457–463.

Kiyasu, J. Y., Bloom, B. and Chaickoff, I. L. (1952). The portal transport of absorbed fatty acids. *J. Biol. Chem.* **199,** 415–419.

Klein, N. C., Hargrove, R. L., Sleisinger, M. H. and Jeffries, G. H. (1970). Eosinophilic gastroenteritis. *Medicine* **49,** 299–319.

Klipstein, F. A. (1968). Progress in gastroenterology: tropical sprue. *Gastroenterology* **54,** 275–293.

Klipstein, F. A. (1970). Recent advances in tropical malabsorption. *Scand. J. Gastroenterol.* **5,** Suppl. 6 (Quadr. Rev.) 93–114.

Knowles, J. P. (1962). Excretion of formimino-glutamic acid in steatorrhea. *Gut* **3,** 42–48.

Kowlessar, O. D., Warren, R. E. and Bronstein, H. D. (1970). Celiac disease: enzyme defect on immune mechanism? *In* "Progress in Gastroenterology" (G. B. J. Glass, ed.), pp. 409–429. Grune and Stratton, New York.

Krainick, H. G. and Debatin, F. (1953). Der schädliche Mehleffekt bei der Kindlichen Cöliakie. *Klin. Wschr.* **31,** 958–959.

Kramer, P., Kearney, M. M. and Ingelfinger, F. J. (1962). The effect of specific foods and water loading on the ileal excreta of ileostomized human subjects. *Gastroenterology* **42,** 535–546.

Kritchevsky, D. and Tepper, S. A. (1965). Influence of medium-chain triglyceride (MCT) on cholesterol metabolism in rats. *J. Nutr.* **86,** 67–72.

Kritchevsky, D. and Rabinowitz, J. L. (1966). Influence of dietary fat on fatty acid biosynthesis in rat. *Biochim. Biophys. Acta* **116,** 185–188.

Kümmerle, F., Beck, K. und Tenner, R. (1969). Leben ohne Pankreas. *Deut. Med. Wschr.* **94,** 691–694.

Kuo, P. T. and Huang, N. N. (1965). Effect of medium-chain triglyceride upon fat absorption and plasma lipid and depot fat of children with cystic fibrosis of pancreas. *J. Clin. Invest.* **44,** 1924–1933.

Lack, L. and Weiner, I. M. (1967). Role of intestine during the enterohepatic circulation of bile salts (Editorial). *Gastroenterology* **52,** 282–287.

Lagerlöf, H. O. (1972). Pancreatic function and pancreatic disease studied by means of resection. *Acta Med. Scand.* Suppl. **128.**

Lancaster-Smith, M. J., Benson, M. K. and Strickland, I. D. (1971). Coeliac disease and diffuse interstitial lung disease. *Lancet* **1,** 473–475.

Laplane, R., Polonovski, C., Etienne, M., Debray, P., Lods, J. C. et Pissarro, B. (1962). L'intolerance aux sucres a transport intestinal actif. Ses rapports avec l'intolerance au lactose et le syndrome coeliaque. *Arch. Fr. Pédiat.* **19,** 895–944.

Laws, J. W., Booth, C. C., Shawdon, H. and Stewart, J. S. (1963). Correlation of radiological and histological findings in idiopathic steatorrhoea. *Brit. Med. J.* **1,** 1311–1314.

Lee, D. S., Hashim, S. A. and Van Itallie, T. B. (1968). Effect of long chain triglyceride on chylous transport of medium chain fatty acids. *Am. J. Physiol.* **214,** 294–297.

Leinbach, G. E. and Rubin, C. E. (1970). Eosinophilic gastroenteritis: A simple reaction to food allergens. *Gastroenterology* **59,** 874–889.

Levinson, J. D. and Kirsner, J. B. (1970). Infiltrative disease of the small bowel and malabsorption. *Am. J. Dig. Dis.* **15,** 741–766.

Levy, R. I., Fredrickson, D. S. and Laster, L. (1966). The lipoproteins and lipid transport in abetalipoproteinemia. *J. Clin. Invest.* **45,** 531–541.

Lewis, B., Panveliwalla, D., Tabaqchali, S. and Wootton, I. D. P. (1969). Serum-bile-acids in the stagnant-loop syndrome. *Lancet* **1,** 219–220.

Lindquist, B. and Meeuwisse, G. W. (1962). Chronic diarrhea caused by monosaccharide malabsorption. *Acta Paediat.* **51,** 674–685.

Lindstedt, S. (1957). The turnover of cholic acid in man. *Acta Physiol. Scand.* **40,** 1–9.

Lindstedt, S. and Norman, A. (1956). The turnover of bile acids in the rat: bile acids and steroids. *Acta Physiol. Scand.* **38,** 121–128.

Linscheer, W. G. (1970). Malabsorption in cirrhosis. *Am. J. Clin. Nutr.* **23,** 488–492.

Lindscheer, W. G., Patterson, J. F., Moore, E. W., Clermont, R. J., Robins, S. J. and Chalmers, T. C. (1966). Medium and long chain fat absorption in patients with cirrhosis. *J. Clin. Invest.* **45,** 1317–1325.

Lindscheer, W. G., Slone, D. and Chalmers, T. C. (1967). Effects of octanoic acid on serum-levels of free fatty acids, insulin, and glucose in patients with cirrhosis and in healthy volunteers. *Lancet* **1,** 593–597.

Linscheer, W. G., Platt, R. R. and Blum, A. L. (1968). Elevated levels of a medium chain fatty acid in cerebrospinal fluid of patients with cirrhosis. *Gastroenterology* **54,** 1296.

Loder, R. M., Mueller, V. C., Trier, J. S., Dobbins, W. O., Barrett, B. and Rubin, C. E. (1964). An improved design for a hydraulic biopsy tube. *Gastroenterology* **46,** 418–420.

Losowsky, M. S. and Walker, B. E. (1969). Liver disease and malabsorption. *Gastroenterology* **56,** 589–600.

Lundh, G. (1958). Intestinal digestion and absorption after gastrectomy. *Acta Chir. Scand.* **231,** *Suppl.* pp. 1–83.

Lundh, G. (1962). Pancreatic exocrine function in neoplastic and inflammatory disease: a simple and reliable new test. *Gastroenterology* **42,** 275–280.

Lundh, S. and Nordenstam, H. (1970). Pancreas calcification and pancreas cancer. *Acta Chir. Scand.* **136,** 493–496.

McGill, D. B. and Newcomer, A. D. (1970). Primary and secondary disacharidase deficiencies. *In* "Progress in Gastroenterology" (G. B. J. Glas, ed.), Vol. II, pp. 392–408. Grune and Stratton, New York.

McIntyre, I., Hanna, S. and Booth, C. C. (1960). Intracellular magnesium deficiency in man. *Clin. Sci.* **20,** 297–305.

McKay, C. (1970). Postgastrectomy steatorrhea. *Am. J. Surg.* **120,** 324–328.

McKay, D. G., Kaunitz, H., Csavossy, I. and Johnson, R. E. (1967). Electron microscope studies of the absorption of lipids. II. Medium chain saturated triglycerides. *Metabolism* **63,** 127–136.

McPherson, J. R. (1970). Jejunal biopsy. *Med. Clin. N. Amer.* **54,** 851–862.

Malins, J. M. and French, J. M. (1957). Diabetic diarrhea. *Quart. J. Med.* **26,** 467–472.

Malins, J. M. and Mayne, N. (1969). Diabetic diarrhea. A study of thirteen patients with jejunal biopsy. *Diabetes* **18,** 858–866.

Mansbach, C. M., Wilkins, R. M., Dobbins, W. O. and Tyor, M. P. (1968). Intestinal mucosal function and structure in the steatorrhea of Zollinger-Ellison syndrome. *Arch. Int. Med.* **121,** 487–494.

Maratka, Z. und Sedka, J. (1964). Eine einfache Methode zur Magen- und Darmbiopsie. *Gastroenterologia* **102,** 369–372.

Marin, S. A., Clark, M. L. and Senior, J. R. (1968). Distribution of D-xylon in sequestered fluid resulting in false-positive tests of malabsorption. *Ann. Int. Med.* **69,** 1155–1162.

Marin, G. A., Clark, M. L. and Senior, J. R. (1969). Studies of malabsorption occurring in patients with Laennec's cirrhosis. *Gastroenterology* **56,** 727–736.

Marks, J. and Shuster, S. (1970). Dermatitis Herpetiformis. The role of gluten. *Arch. Dermatol.* **101,** 452–457.

Marks, J., Birkett, D., Shuster, S. and Roberts, A. F. (1970). Small intestine mucosal abnormalities in relatives of patients with dermatitis herpetiformis. *Gut* **11,** 493–497.

Marshak, R. H., Wolf, B. S., Cohen, N. and Janowitz, D. N. (1961). Protein-losing disorders of the gastrointestinal tract: Roentgen features. *Radiology* **77,** 893–905.

Marston, A. (1964). Patterns of intestinal ischaemia. *Ann. Roy. Coll. Surg.* **35,** 151–181.

Martini, G. A., Dölle, A. W., Petersen, F., Triske, H. und Strohmeyer, G. (1963). Die exsudative Gastroenteropathie, ein polyaetiologisches Syndrom. *Internist* **4,** 197–209.

Mattson, F. H. and Volpenheim, R. A. (1964). The digestion and absorption of triglycerides. *J. Biol. Chem.* **239,** 2772–2777.

Meihoff, W. W. and Kern, F., Jr. (1968). Bile salt malabsorption in regional ileitis, ileal resection, and mannitol-induced diarrhea. *J. Clin. Invest.* **47,** 261–267.

Mekhjian, H. S., Philips, S. F. and Hofmann, A. F. (1968). Conjugated bile salts block water and electrolyte transport by the human colon. *Gastroenterology* **54,** 1256.

Mekhjian, H. S., Philips, S. F. and Hofmann, A. F. (1971). Colonic secretion of water and electrolytes induced by bile acids: Perfusion studies in man. *J. Clin. Invest.* **50,** 1569–1577.

Meyer, H. (1890). Uber den wirksamen Bestandteil der Rizinusöls. *Arch. Exp. Pathol. Pharmakol.* **28,** 145–154.

Middleton, W. R. J. (1971). Thyroid hormones and the gut. *Gut* **12,** 172–177.

Midtvedt, T. and Norman, A. (1967). Bile acid transformations by microbial stains belonging to genera found in intestinal contents. *Acta Pathol. Microbiol. Scand.* **71,** 629–638.

Milne, M. D. (1964). Disorders of amino acid transport. *Brit. Med. J.* **1,** 327–336.

Milne, M. D. (1967). Hereditary abnormalities of intestinal absorption. *Brit. Med. Bull.* **23,** 279–284.

Moldow, W. E. and Connelly, R. R. (1968). Epidemiology of pancreatic cancer in Connecticut. *Gastroenterology* **55,** 677–686.

Moore, J. G., Englert, E., Jr., Bigler, A. H. and Clark, R. W. (1971). Simple fecal tests of absorption. A prospective study and critique. *Amer. J. Dig. Dis.* **16,** 97–105.

Morris, J. S., Ajdukiewicz, A. B. and Read, A. E. (1970). Neurological disorders and adult coeliac disease. *Gut* **11,** 549–554.

Morse, W. I., Cochrane, W. A. and Landrigan, P. L. (1961). Familial hypoparathyroidism with pernicious anemia, steatorrhea and adrenocortical insufficiency, a variant of mucoviscidosis. *New Engl. J. Med.* **264,** 1021–1026.

Moss, A. J., Waterhouse, C. and Terry, R. (1965). Gluten-sensitive enderopathy with osteomalacia but without steatorrhea. *New Engl. J. Med.* **272,** 825–830.

Müller-Wieland, K. (1962). Folgen einen exokrinen Pankreasinsuffizienz. *Deut. Arch. Klin. Med.* **208,** 361–370.

Müller-Wieland, K. und Berndt, W. (1969). Vergleich der enzymatischen Aktivität verscheidener Pankreasfermentpräparate *in vitro. Deut. Med. Wschr.* **94,** 1870–1872.

Munk, I. (1884). Zur kenntnis von der resorption: bildung und ablagerung der fette im tier körper. *Arch. Pathol. Anat.* **95,** 407–467.

Nestel, P. J., Carroll, K. F. and Silverstein, M. S. (1964). Influence of free fatty acid metabolism on glucon tolerance. *Lancet* **2,** 115–117.

Nygaard, K., Helsingen, N. und Rootwelt, K. (1970). Adaption of vitamin $B_{12}$ absorption after ileal bypass. *Scand. J. Gastroenterol.* **5,** 349–351.

Oberhauser, E., Orrego-Matte, H., Salinas, A. and Baraona, E. (1962). Further studies on intestinal absorption in liver cirrhosis, using an intraintestinal reference substance (polyethylene glycol). *Am. J. Dig. Dis.* **7,** 669–711.

Palay, S. L. and Karlin, L. J. (1959). An electron microscope study of the intestinal villus. 2. The pathway of fat absorption. *J. Biophys. Biochem. Cytol.* **5,** 373–394.

Paris, R. and Clement, G. (1968). Biosynthesis of triglycerides from double-labeled 2-monopalmitin on the intestinal mucosa. *Biochim. Biophys. Acta* **152,** 63–74.

Parkins, R. A. (1960). Protein-losing interopathy in the sprue syndrome. *Lancet* **2,** 1366–1368.

Paulino-Netto, A., Dreiling, D. A. and Baronophy, I. D. (1960). The relationship between pancreatic calcification and cancer of the pancreas. *Ann. Surg.* **151,** 530–537.

Paulley, J. W. (1954). Observations in the aetiology of idiopathic steatorrhoea. Jejunal and lymph-node biopsies. *Brit. Med. J.* **2,** 1318–1321.

Pihl, B. G., Glotzer, D. J. and Patterson, J. F. (1966). Absorption of medium chain fatty acids by dog colon. *J. Appl. Physiol.* **21,** 1059–1062.

Pimparkar, B. J., Tulsby, E. G., Kalser, M. H. and Bockus, H. L. (1961). Correlation of radioactive and chemical fat determinations in the malabsorption syndrome. I. Studies in normal and functional disorders of the gastrointestinal tract. *Am. J. Med.* **30,** 910–926.

Pinter, K. G., McCracken, B. H., Lamar, C., Jr. and Goldsmith, G. A. (1964).

Fat absorption studies in various forms of steatorrhea. *Am. J. Clin. Nutr.* **15,** 293–298.

Pittingale, K. W. (1971). Immunoglobulin-containing cells in the coeliac syndrome. *Gut* **12,** 291–296.

Playoust, M. C. and Isselbacher, K. J. (1964). Studies in the intestinal absorption and intramucosal lipolysis of a medium chain triglyceride. *J. Clin. Invest.* **43,** 878–885.

Playoust, M. R., Lack, L. and Weiner, I. M. (1965). Effect of intestinal resection on bile salt absorption in dogs. *Am. J. Physiol.* **208,** 363–369.

Pomerantz, M. and Waldmann, T. A. (1963). Systemic lymphatic abnormalities associated with gastrointestinal protein loss secondary to intestinal lymphangiectasia. *Gastroenterology* **45,** 703–711.

Porus, R. L. (1965). Epithelial hyperplasia following massive small bowel resection in man. *Gastroenterology* **48,** 753–757.

Prevot, R. (1966). Neue Erkantnisse auf dem Gebiet der röntgenologischen Dünndarmdiagnostik. *Internist* **7,** 223 231.

Race, T. R., Paes, I. C. and Faloon, W. W. (1970). Intestinal malabsorption induced by oral colchicine. Comparison with neomycin and cathartic agents. *Am. J. Med. Sci.* **259,** 32–41.

Ralston, A. W. and Hoerr, C. W. (1942). The solubilities of the normal saturated fatty acids. *J. Org. Chem.* **7,** 546–555.

Randle, P. J., Garland, P. B., Hales, C. N. and Newsholme, E. D. (1963). Glucose fatty acid cycle: its role in insulin sensitivity and metabolic disturbances of diabetis mellitus. *Lancet* **1,** 785–789.

Raper, H. S. (1913). Experiments bearing on the functions of the liver in the metabolism of fats. *J. Biol. Chem.* **14,** 111–134.

Read, A. E. (1970). Malignant disease and steatorrhea. *In* "Modern Trends in Gastroenterology" (W. I. Card and B. Creamer, eds.), Vol. 4, pp. 180–197. Butterworths, London.

Reed, L. S. (1970). Pathogenesis of celiac disease in adults. *N.Y. State J. Med.* **70,** 2095–2102.

Reeve, J. and Franks, J. J. (1968). Fatty acid synthesis by jejunal slices from rats fed medium and long chain triglycerides. *Am. J. Physiol.* **214,** 1425–1428.

Reeves, R. J., Cavanaugh, P. J., Sharpe, K. W., Thorne, W. A., Winkler, C. and Sanders, A. P. (1968). Fat absorption studies and small bowel X-ray studies in patients undergoing $Co^{60}$ teletherapy and/or radium application. *Am. J. Roentgenol.* (*Rad. Ther. Nuclear Med.*) **94,** 848–851.

Reissell, P. K., Mandella, P. A., Poon-King, T. M. W. and Hatch, F. T. (1966). Treatment of hypertriglyceridemia: I. Total caloric restriction followed by refeeding a low carbohydrate, high fat diet in the carbohydrate-induced type (Eight cases); II. Low fat diet plus medium-chain triglycerides in the fat-induced type (two cases). *Am. J. Clin. Nutr.* **19,** 84–98.

Reitemeier, R. J., Higgins, J. H., Lee, P. R. and Scholer, J. F. (1956). The absorption of water and sodium from the small bowel of patients with non-tropical sprue. *J. Clin. Invest.* **35,** 730.

Rick, W. (1971). Laboratoriumsdiagnostik der Verdauungs- und Resorptionsstörungen. *In* "Wissenschaftliche Berichte" (E. Merck, ed.), Nr. 6, pp. 60–130. Darmstadt.

Riecken, E. O. (1970). Vergleigende bioptische Untersuchungen zur formalen pathogenese der Dünndarmschleimhautveränderungen bei der heimischen Sprue. *Klin. Wschr.* **48,** 1216–1225.

Riecken, E. O., Stewart, J. S., Booth, C. C. and Pearse, A. G. E. (1966a). A histochemical study on the role of lysosomal enzymes in idiopathic steatorrhea before and during the gluten free diet. *Gut* **7,** 317–332.

Riecken, E. O., Stewart, J. S. and Dowling, R. H. (1966b). Neuere Methoden in der Diagnostik intestinaler Störungen. *Internist* **7,** 209–217.

Rommel, K. and Grimmel, K. (1967). Galaktosemalabsorption im Erwachsenenalter. *Klin. Wschr.* **45,** 559–564.

Rosenberg, I. H., Hardison, W. G. and Bull, D. M. (1967). Abnormal bile-salt patterns and intestinal bacterial overgrowth associated with malabsorption. *New Engl. J. Med.* **276,** 1391–1397.

Ross, J. R. (1971). Postgastrectomy syndromes and their management. *Surg. Clin. N. Amer.* **51,** 615–632.

Ross, J. R. and Garabedian, M. (1970). Systemic manifestations of gluten enteropathies and gluten sensitivity in some other diseases. *In* "Progress in Gastroenterology" (G. B. J. Glass, ed.), Vol. II, pp. 430–442. Grune and Stratton, New York.

Rothmann, M. M. and Katz, A. B. (1964). Analyses of feces. *In* "Gastroenterology" (H. L. Bochus, ed.), Vol. II, 2nd edn, pp. 694–722. Saunders, Philadelphia, London.

Rowe, G. G. (1967). Control of tenermus and diarrhea by cholestyramine administration. *Gastroenterology* **53,** 1006.

Rubin, C. E. (1966). Electron microscopic studies of triglyceride absorption in man. *Gastroenterology* **50,** 65–77.

Rubin, C. E. and Dobbins, W. O. (1965). Peroral biopsy of the small intestine. A review of its diagnostic usefulness. *Gastroenterology* **49,** 676–697.

Rubin, C. E., Brandborg, L. L., Phelps, P. C. and Taylor, H. C. (1960). Studies of celiac disease: I. The apparent identical and specific nature of the duodenal and proximal jejunal lesion in celiac disease and idiopathic sprue. *Gastroenterology* **38,** 28–49.

Rubin, C. E., Eidelmann, S. and Weinstein, W. M. (1970). Sprue by any other name. *Gastroenterology* **58,** 409–413.

Sabesin, S. M. and Isselbacher, K. J. (1965). Protein synthesis inhibition: mechanism for the production of impaired fat absorption. *Science* **147,** 1149–1151.

Sakula, J. and Shiner, M. (1957). Coeliac disease with atrophy of the small intestine mucosa. *Lancet* **2,** 876–877.

Sanbar, S. S. and Martin, J. M. (1967). Stimulation by octanoate of insulin release from isolated rat pancreas. *Metabolism* **16,** 482–484.

Sanbar, S. S., Hetenyi, G., Forbath, N. and Evans, J. R. (1965). Effects of infusion of octanoate on glucose concentration in plasma and the rates of glucose production and utilization in dogs. *Metabolism* **14,** 1311–1323.

Sarda, L. et Desnuelle, P. (1958). Action de la lipase pancreatique sur les esters en emulsion. *Biochim. Biophys. Acta* **30,** 513–521.

Sarles, H. (1971). Alcoholism and pancreatitis. *Scand. J. Gastroenterol.* **6,** 193–198.

Sarles, H., Sarles, J. C., Camatte, R., Muratore, R., Gaini, M., Guien, C. L., Pastor, J. and Le Roy, F. (1965). Observations on 205 confirmed cases of acute pancreatitis and chronic pancreatitis. *Gut* **6,** 545–559.

Saunders, D. R. (1967). Medium chain triglycerides and the Van De Kamer method. *Gastroenterology* **52,** 135–136.

Scheig, R. (1968). Hepatic metabolism of medium chain fatty acids. *In* "Medium

Chain Triglycerides" (J. R. Senior, ed.), pp. 39–47. University of Pennsylvania Press, Philadelphia, U.S.A.

Schein, J. (1947). Syndrome of non tropical sprue with hitherto undescribed lesions of the intestine. *Gastroenterology* **8,** 438–460.

Schiller, W. R., DiDis, L. J. A. and Anderson, M. C. (1967). Production of artificial Sphincters "Ablation of the longitudinal layer of the intestine". *Arch. Surg.* **95,** 436–441.

Schjönsby, H., Drasar, B. S., Tabaqchali, S. and Booth, C. C. (1973). Uptake of vitamin $B_{12}$ by intestinal bacteria in the stagnant loop syndrome. *Scand. J. Gastroenterol.* **8,** 41–47.

Schmidt, U. (1971). Klinik und Therapie der exokrinen Pankreasinsuffizienz. *In* "Wissenschaftliche Berichte" (E. Merck, ed.), nr. 6, pp. 160–195. Darmstadt.

Schonheyder, F. and Volgvartz, K. (1946). The gastric lipase in man. *Acta Physiol. Scand.* **11,** 349–360.

Schultis, K. und Wagner, E. (1968). Zur Enzymsubstitution nach Pankreatektomie und bei Insuffizienz des exokrinen Pankreas. *Deut. Med. Wschr.* **93,** 1685–1691.

Schwabe, A. D., Bennett, L. R. and Bowman, L. P. (1964). Octanoic acid absorption and oxydation in humans. *J. Appl. Physiol.* **19,** 335–337.

Seliger, G., Krassner, R. L., Beranbaum, E. R. and Miller, F. (1971). The spectrum of roentgen appearance in amyloidosis of the small and large bowel; Radiologic-pathologic correlation. *Radiology* **100,** 63–70.

Senior, J. R. (1965). A simple and reliable method for distinguishing steatorrhea of pancreatic or intestinal origin. *Clin. Res.* **13,** 261.

Senior, J. R. (1968). Steatorrhea and the measurement of fecal fat. *Gastroenterology* **55,** 310–311.

Senior, J. R. and Isselbacher, K. J. (1960). Activation of long-chain fatty acids by rat-gut mucosa. *Biochim. Biophys. Acta* **44,** 399–400.

Senior, J. R. and Isselbacher, K. J. (1963). Demonstration of intestinal monoglyceride lipase: An enzyme with a possible role in intracellular completion of fat digestion. *J. Clin. Invest.* **42,** 187–195.

Sheehy, T. W. and Flock, M. H. (1964). "The Small Intestine". Hoeber Medical Edition, New York.

Shepard, D. (1964). Antiperistaltic bowel segment in the treatment of the short bowel syndrome. *Ann. Surg.* **163,** 850–855.

Shimoda, S. S. and Rubin, C. E. (1968). The Zollinger-Ellison syndrome with steatorrhea. I. Anticholinergic treatment followed by total gastrectomy and colonic interposition. *Gastroenterology* **55,** 695–704.

Shiner, M. and Doniach, I. (1960). Histopathologic studies in steatorrhea. *Gastroenterology* **38,** 419–440.

Shmerling, D. H. (1967). Die glutenfreie Ernährung bei Cöliakie. *Schweiz. Med. Wschr.* **97,** 706–713.

Sickinger, R. (1964). Uber die Steatorrhea bei Leberzirrhose und den Versuch ihrer Substitution mit Pankreasfermenten. Inaug. Dis. Freiburg.

Sickinger, K. (1965). Oraler und intravenöser D-Xylose-Test bei Leberzirrhose und Hepatitis. *Z. Gastroenterol.* **13,** 193–202.

Sickinger, K. (1968a). Therapie der Steatorrhea durch Substitution des Nahrungsfettes mit mittelkettigen Triglyceriden. *Deut. Med. Wschr.* **93,** 1600–1603.

Sickinger, K. (1968b). Bilanzuntersuchungen bei Patienten mit Maldigestion, Malabsorption und primärer exsudativer Enteropathie unter mittelkettigen Triglyceriden. *Med. Ernaehrung* **9,** 145–148.

Sickinger, K. (1969a). Die Behandlung der chologenen. Diarhoe und Steatorrhoe der enteralen Gallensäureverlustsyndroms mit Cholestyramin und mittelkettigen Triglyceriden. *Deut. Med. Wschr.* **94,** 1151–1157.

Sickinger, K. (1969b). Behandlung der Steatorrhoe mit Pankreasfermenten und mittelkettigen Triglyceriden. *Artzl. Fortbild* **17,** 289–295.

Sickinger, K. (1973). Quantitative Stuhlanalyse. *Med. Klin.* **68,** 1243–1247.

Sickinger, K. und Hannemann, H. (1968). Die titrimetrische Stuhlfettbestimmung nach Van De Kamer bei Gabe von mittelkettigen Triglyzeriden. *Klin. Wschr.* **46,** 1005–1007.

Sickinger, K., Musshoff, K., Stephan, F. und Appels, A. (1965). Resportionsstudien nach Röntgenbestrahlung des Abdomens bei maligner Lymphogranulomatose unter Verwendung der D-Xylong Resorptionstests und des $J^{131}$-Trioleintests. *Strahlentherapie* **138,** 340–346.

Simmonds, W. J. (1955). Some observations on increase in thoracic lymph flow during intestinal absorption of fat in unanesthetized rats. *Aust. J. Exp. Biol. Med. Sci.* **33,** 305–313.

Sjövall, J. (1960). Bile acids in man under normal and pathological conditions: bile acids and steroids. *Clin. Chim. Acta* **5,** 33–41.

Sleisinger, M. H. (1969). Malabsorption syndrome. *New Engl. J. Med.* **281,** 1111–1117.

Small, D. M., Dowling, R. H. and Redinger, R. N. (1972). The intero-hepatic circulation in bile salts. *Arch. Int. Med.* **130,** 552–573.

Smith, L. H., Fromm, H. and Hofmann, A. F. (1972). Acquired hyperoxaluria, nephrolithiasis and intestinal disease. *New Engl. J. Med.* **286,** 1371–1375.

Smits, B. J., Wilding, P. and Cooke, W. J. (1968). Ready absorption of medium chain triglycerides in the steatorrhea syndrome. *Gut* **9,** 28–33.

Soergel, K. H. (1969). Mechanism of diarrhea in the Zollinger-Ellison syndrome. *In* "Non-Insulin Producing Tumors of the Pancreas" (L. Demling and R. Ottenjan, eds), pp. 152–161. Thième, Stuttgart.

Soong, C. S., Thompson, J. B., Poley, J. R. and Hess, D. R. (1972). Hydroxy fatty acids in human diarrhea. *Gastroenterology* **63,** 748–757.

Stalder, G. A. and Kayasseh, L. (1972). Die diagnotische Bedeutung der Lundh-Tests bei der Pankreasinsuffizienz. *Deut. Med. Wschr.* **97,** 432–433.

Stanley, M. and Nemchausky, B. (1966). Estimation of bile salt turnover in rats in normal subjects and in patients with steroid wasting syndromes. *J. Lab. Clin. Med.* **68,** 1019–1020.

Stanley, M. and Nemchausky, B. (1967). Fecal $C^{14}$-bile acid excretion in normal subjects and patients with steroid-wasting syndromes secondary to ileal dysfunction. *J. Lab. Clin. Med.* **70,** 627–639.

Stegemann, H. und Loeschke, V. (1962). Mikrobestimmung von Stickstoff als Indopherrolblau nach Chloramin-T-oxydation. *Z. Physiol. Chem.* **329,** 241–248.

Strauss, E. W. (1966). Electron microscopic study of intestinal fat absorption *in vitro* from mixed micelles containing linolenic acid, monoolein, and bile salt. *J. Lipid Res.* **7,** 307–323.

Strauss, E. W. (1968). Morphological aspects of triglyceride absorption. *In* "Handbook of Physiology" (C. F. Code, ed.), Section 6, Vol. III, pp. 1377–1406. Williams and Wilkins, Baltimore, U.S.A.

Summerskill, W. H. J. (1959). Malabsorption and jejunal ulceration due to gastric hypersecretion with pancreatic islet-cell hyperplasia. *Lancet* **1,** 120–123.

Sun, D. C. H., Albacete, R. A. and Chen, J. K. (1967). Malabsorption studies in cirrhosis of the liver. *Arch. Int. Med.* **119,** 567–572.

Tabaqchali, S. and Booth, C. C. (1966). Jejunal bacteriology and bile-salt metabolism in patients with intestinal malabsorption. *Lancet* **2,** 12–15.
Tabaqchali, S. and Booth, C. C. (1967). Relationship of the intestinal bacterial flora to absorption. *Brit. Med. Bull.* **23,** 285–290.
Tabaqchali, S. and Booth, C. C. (1970). Bacteria and the small intestine. *In* "Modern Trends in Gastroenterology" (W. I. Card and B. Creamer, eds), Vol. 4, pp. 143–179. Butterworths, London.
Tabaqchali, S., Hatzioanou, J. and Booth, C. C. (1968). Bile salt deconjugation and steatorrhoea in patients with the stagnant-loop syndrome. *Lancet* **2,** 12–16.
Tamio, I., Grant, D. B., Fosbrooke, A. S., Segall, M. M. and Lloyd, J. K. (1968). Effects of single oral load of medium-chain triglyceride on serum lipid and insulin levels in man. *J. Lipid Res.* **9,** 661–666.
Tankel, H. I., Clark, D. H. and Lee, F. D. (1965). Radiation enteritis with malabsorption. *Gut* **6,** 560–569.
Tantibhedhyangkul, P., Hashim, S. A. and Van Itallie, T. B. (1967). Effects of ingestion of long-chain and medium-chain triglycerides on glucose tolerance in man. *Diabetes* **16,** 796–799.
Tattrie, N. H., Bailey, R. H. and Kates, M. (1958). The action of pancreatic lipase on stereoisomeric triglycerides. *Arch. Biochem. Biophys.* **78,** 319–327.
Thaysen, T. E. H. (1932). "Non-tropical Sprue". Levin and Mursgaard, Kopenhagen.
Thomas, P. J. (1972). Identification of some enteric bacteria which convert oleic acid to hydroxystearic acid *in vitro. Gastroenterology* **62,** 430–435.
Thompson, G. R., Barrowman, J., Gutierrez, L. and Dowling, R. H. (1971). Action of neomycin on the intraluminalphase of lipid absorption. *J. Clin. Invest.* **50,** 319–323.
Toth, A. and Alpert, L. I. (1971). Progressive systemic sclerosis terminating as periarteritis nodosa. *Arch. Pathol.* **92,** 31–36.
Treadwell, C. R. and Vahouny, S. V. (1968). Cholesterol absorption. *In* "Handbook of Physiology" (C. F. Code, ed.), Section 6, Vol. 3, pp. 1407–1438. Williams and Wilkins, Baltimore, U.S.A.
Trier, J. S. (1971). Dermatitis herpetiformis and celiac sprue. *Gastroenterology* **60,** 468–469.
Trier, J. S. and Browning, T. H. (1966). Morphologic response of the mucosa of human small intestine to X-ray exposure. *J. Clin. Invest.* **45,** 194–204.
Valdivieso, V. D. and Schwabe, A. D. (1966). Absorption of medium-chain lipids from the rat cecum. *Am. J. Dig. Dis.* **11,** 474–479.
Van De Kamer, J. H., Huinnick, B. and Weijers, H. A. (1949). Rapid method for the determination of fat in feces. *J. Biol. Chem.* **177,** 347–355.
Van Deest, B. W., Fordtran, J. S., Morawski, S. G. and Wilson, J. D. (1968). Bile salt and micellar fat concentration in proximal small bowel contents of ileectomy patients. *J. Clin. Invest.* **47,** 1314–1324.
Van Goidsenhoven, G. E., Henke, W. J., Vacca, J. B. and Knight, W. A., Jr. (1963). Pancreatic function in cirrhosis of the liver. *Am. J. Dig. Dis.* **8,** 160–173.
Vlahcevic, Z. R., Buhac, I., Bell, C. C. and Swell, L. (1970). Abdominal metabolism of secondary bile acids in patients with cirrhosis. *Gut* **11,** 420–422.
Vlahcevic, Z. R., Miller, J. R., Farrar, J. T. and Swell, L. (1971). Bile acid metabolism in patients with cirrhosis: I. Kinetic aspects of cholic acid metabolism. *Gastroenterology* **60,** 491–498.
Vlahcevic, Z. R., Juttijudata, P., Bell, C. C., Jr. and Swell, L. (1972). Bile acid metabolism in patients with cirrhosis: II. Cholic and chenodeoxycholic acid metabolism. *Gastroenterology* **62,** 1174–1181.

Vogel, R. M., Weinstein, L. D., Herskovic, T. and Spiro, H. M. (1967). Mechanisms of steatorrhea in the Zollinger-Ellison Syndrome. *Ann. Int. Med.* **67,** 816–822.

Von Erdmann, G. (1968). Die Verwendung mittelkettiger Triglyceride in der Pädiatrie. *Med. Ernaehrung* **9,** 244–246.

Von Tappeiner, H. E. (1878). Uber die Aufsaugung von Gallensäuren Alkoholien im Dünndarm. *Wien. Sitzungsbericht* **77,** 281–286.

Wagner, A., Schneider, V. und Georgi, M. (1968). Zur Röntgendiagnostik beim enteralen Proteinverlustsyndrom. *Fortschr. Roentgenstr.* **109,** 280–291.

Wagner, E. (1967). Exocrine pancreatic function before and after Billroth: II. Gastrectomy. *German Med. Monthly* **12,** 527–532.

Waldmann, T. A. (1966). Protein-losing enteropathy. *Gastroenterology* **50,** 422–443.

Waldmann, T. A. (1970). Protein losing enteropathy. *In* "Modern Trends in Gastroenterology" (W. I. Card and B. Creamer, eds), Vol. 4, pp. 125–142. Butterworths, London.

Waldmann, T. A. and Laster, L. (1964). Abnormalities of albumin metabolism in patients with hypogammaglobulinemia. *J. Clin. Invest.* **43,** 1025–1035.

Waldmann, T. A., Steinfeld, J. L., Dutcher, T. F., Davidson, J. D. and Gordon, R. S. (1961). The role of the gastrointestinal system in "idiopathic hypoproteinemia". *Gastroenterology* **41,** 197–207.

Waldmann, T. A., Wochner, R. D., Laster, L. and Gordon, R. S. (1967). Allergic gastroenteropathy. A cause of excessive gastrointestinal protein loss. *New Engl. J. Med.* **276,** 761–769.

Wall, A. J., Ungar, B., Baird, C. W., Langford, I. M. and MacKay, I. R. (1967). Malnutrition after partial gastrectomy. *Am. J. Dig. Dis.* **12,** 1077–1086.

Wall, A. J., Douglas, A. P., Booth, C. C. and Pearce, A. G. E. (1970). Response of the jejunal mucosa in adult coeliac disease to oral prednisolone. *Gut* **11,** 7–14.

Watt, J. K., Watson, W. C. and Haase, S. (1967). Chronic intestinal ischaemia. *Brit. Med J.* **3,** 199–202.

Ways, P. O., Parmentier, C. M., Kayden, H. J., Jones, J. W., Saunders, D. R. and Rubin, C. E. (1967). Studies on the absorptive defect for triglyceride in abetalipoproteinemia. *J. Clin. Invest.* **46,** 35–46.

Weiner, I. M. and Lack, L. (1968). Bile salt absorption: enterohepatic circulation. *In* "Handbook of Physiology" (C. F. Code, ed.), Section 6, Vol. III, pp. 1439–1455. Williams and Wilkins, Baltimore, U.S.A.

Weinstein, W. M., Brow, J. R., Parker, F. and Rubin, C. E. (1971). The small intestinal mucosa in dermatitis herpetiformis: II. Relationship of the small intestinal lesion to gluten. *Gastroenterology* **60,** 362–369.

Welbourn, R. B. (1967). Nutritional aspects of gastric surgery. *Rev. Surg.* **24,** 233–239.

Weser, E. (1971). Intestinal adaption to small bowel resection. *Am. J. Clin. Nutr.* **24,** 133–135.

Whitfield, A. G. W., Crane, C. W., French, J. M. and Bayley, T. J. (1965). Life without a pancreas. *Lancet* **1,** 675–677.

Wiernik, G. (1966). Changes in the villous pattern of the human jejunum associated with heavy radiation damage. *Gut* **7,** 149–153.

Willig, F., Körber, W. und Cornelius, H. (1970). Zur messung der Stuhlfetts nach dem Prinzip der Kapazitätsanderung eines Kondensators. *Z. Gastroenterol.* **8,** 304–311.

Wilson, F. A. and Dietschy, J. M. (1971). Differential diagnostic approach to clinical problem of malabsorption. *Gastroenterology* **61,** 911–931.

Wilson, F. A. and Dietschy, J. M. (1972). Approach to the malabsorption syndromes associated with disordered bile acid metabolism. *Arch. Int. Med.* **130,** 584–594.

Winawer, S. J., Broitman, S. A., Wolochow, D. A., Osborne, M. P. and Zamcheck, N. (1966). Successful management of massive small-bowel resection based on assessment of absorption defects and nutritional needs. *New Engl. J. Med.* **274,** 72–78.

Windsor, C. W. O., Fejfar, J. and Woodward, D. A. K. (1969). Gastric secretion after massive small bowel resection. *Gut* **10,** 779–786.

Wirts, C. W. (1963). Studies of the mechanism of postgastrectomy steatorrhoea. *Ann. Int. Med.* **58,** 25–36.

Wollaeger, E. E., Comfort, M. W. and Caqitt, O. T. (1948). Efficiency of gastro-intestinal tract after resection of head of pancreas. *J. Am. Med. Ass.* **137,** 838–845.

Wolochow, D. A., Broitman, S. A., Williams, L. A. and Zamcheck, N. (1965). A rapid method for quantitative determination of fecal fat based on the principle of electrical capacitance. *J. Lab. Clin. Med.* **65,** 334–341.

Yardley, J. H., Takano, J. and Hendrix, T. R. (1964). Epithelial and other mucosal lesions of the jejunum in giardiasis. Jejunal biopsy studies. *Bull. John's Hopkins Hosp.* **115,** 389–406.

Zieve, L. and Mulford, B. (1967). Secretion of pancreatic enzymes: 3. Response of patients with cirrhosis to secretion and pancreozymia. *Am. J. Dig. Dis.* **12,** 303–309.

Zurier, R. B., Hashim, S. A. and Van Itallie, T. B. (1965). Effect of medium chain triglyceride on cholestyramine-induced steatorrhea in man. *Gastroenterology* **49,** 490–495.

4

# Quantitative Effects of Dietary Fat and Cholesterol on Serum Cholesterol in Man

R. B. McGANDY and D. M. HEGSTED

*Department of Nutrition,*
*Harvard School of Public Health,*
*Boston, Massachusetts, U.S.A.*



## I. INTRODUCTION

Over the past 15 years or so, a number of well-controlled studies have done much to advance our understanding of the dietary regulation of levels of circulating lipids (total cholesterol, for the most part) in adult males. Although a number of both macro- and micro-constituents of the diet, as well as the dynamical state of energy balance, have been shown to influence blood lipids significantly, by far the greatest regulatory power can be ascribed to dietary lipids. The amount and type (in terms of chain length and saturation) of the fatty acids in dietary triglycerides and the amount of dietary cholesterol can induce very large changes in blood lipids; and these dietary components can account for the great bulk of the variability in mean blood cholesterol levels found among adult male population groups in the world.

On the other hand, all studies correlating intakes of dietary fats or other materials with levels of blood lipids among individual members or relatively homogeneous population groups have repeatedly shown that intrinsic factors, presumably genetic, play a role in determining the level maintained by any particular individual. In metabolic ward studies in which diet and energy balance can be maintained constant, differences in individuals receiving the same diet persist. Failure to appreciate the interdependent role of diet and heredity has led to unfortunate conclusions.

Among middle-aged American males, the mean serum cholesterol level is in the range of 220–240 mg/100 ml with reported standard deviations of 30–40 mg/100 ml. Thus, 90 % of adult American men have serum cholesterol levels between about 160 and 300 mg/100 ml. Reported dietary intakes of American males (National Diet–Heart Study Research Group, 1968; Kannel and Gordon, 1970) indicate that only 5 % of the population takes in on the average day less than 300 mg of dietary cholesterol, less than 10 % of the calories as saturated fatty acids, or less than 32 % of the calories as fat. Thus, in terms of what is known about the dietary changes needed to reduce the serum cholesterol level, American diets are almost uniformly "hypercholesterolgenic".

The difficulties in determining the exact composition of the average diet of an individual should be appreciated, however. In groups of individuals in which diets have been examined a few months apart, whether by dietary history (Reshef and Epstein, 1972) or by weighing the actual food consumed (Marr *et al.*, 1959), correlation coefficients of the order of 0·8 for the total fat consumed were obtained. Although this degree of correlation is reasonably high and suggests some confidence in the history, it is not known whether the variation observed in individual diets represents actual change between the two histories or the collection of atypical data during one or the other period. There is, in fact, no way to determine with accuracy the *average* diet of an individual nor to identify those dietary histories which are unsatisfactory. Thus, in surveys such as those mentioned in the previous paragraph the individuals recorded as having atypical diets may represent those in which the history is least satisfactory.

Given the errors or uncertainties of dietary data, the large variation in the levels of serum cholesterol in individuals eating the same diet, and the variation in diets from time to time, it is not surprising that within populations such as those which have been studied there is no significant correlation between the nature of the diet and the serum cholesterol level in individuals examined. This has been misinterpreted to mean that diet has no effect or is not responsible for the generally elevated levels of serum cholesterol in such populations. Rather, the data indicate that dietary patterns are so similar that they are overshadowed by the genetic effects. This is clear since it has been repeatedly shown that the level of serum cholesterol will be reduced in the great majority of such individuals by a modification of the dietary and, furthermore, that the individuals with the highest levels of serum cholesterol are generally those who are most responsive to changes in the composition of the dietary fat. Abundant evidence is now available to demonstrate this both in highly restricted groups, such as those in a metabolic ward, or in free-living populations.

The large inherent differences in the cholesterol levels of individuals consuming similar diets do impose difficulties in attempting to quantitate the effects of such diets upon the serum cholesterol level. In addition, the serum cholesterol in an individual is subject to variation at different sampling times. In most people's experience, the standard deviation of an individual subject is of the order of 10–12 mg/100 ml when under strict dietary control and of the order of 15 mg/100 ml or so in free-living populations. Variability will ordinarily be larger in those individuals with the higher lipid levels. This kind of variability limits to a great degree the conclusions that can be drawn from groups composed of few subjects.

It is now also recognized that the pattern of lipoproteins in blood varies in individuals and Fredrickson *et al.* (1967) have identified at least five different types. The prevalence of these various types within population groups is not known and indeed there are, as yet, no criteria for classifying the majority of people even though their serum lipid levels may be well above desirable limits. So far, the classification has been limited to only those with very high lipid levels, i.e. above the 95th percentile. Although some information is available upon the response of such individuals to various kinds of dietary modification, and different types of diets are recommended for different types of hyperlipoproteinaemias, the quantitative aspects of the relationship between diet and the various classes of serum lipids and lipoprotein in different types are completely unexplored. Such differences undoubtedly contribute to some of the differences observed by different authors but the extent of this is unknown.

It should also be apparent that differences in the response of patients with severe degrees of hyperlipidaemia might be expected and that generalizations from the response of selected patients are rarely warranted.

In spite of these difficulties, consistent, quantifiable, and predictable changes in the level of serum cholesterol are obtained by modifications of the dietary fat if the groups are sufficiently large to overcome the inter- and intra-individual variability. Serum triglycerides vary widely during the day and are immediately dependent upon the preceding meal pattern. Thus, they are not usually interpretable unless fasting samples are examined and even in fasting samples the variance will usually be substantially larger than with serum cholesterol. Much less data are available upon the effects of variations in dietary fat upon serum triglycerides/phospholipids than upon serum cholesterol.

The relationship between diet and blood lipids in free-living populations is more difficult to ascertain since as already discussed one does not have ways for accurate dietary assessment of fat intakes, energy balance, or other factors which may have effects. When dietary changes are instituted in such population groups, the magnitude of the change is more variable and on the whole dampened compared to metabolic ward studies. No doubt this reflects varying degrees of adherence to the dietary programme.

We do not intend to deal in any detail with the many and varied papers which demonstrate that the level of serum cholesterol can be modified by modifying the composition of the dietary fat or the general epidemiologic data relating dietary fat, serum cholesterol level, and atherosclerotic heart disease. It is our position that these relationships have been shown and that dietary or other measures which lower serum cholesterol are called for as public health measures in populations with elevated serum cholesterol levels and atherosclerotic heart disease. Rather, we intend to focus on some of the unresolved questions related to the effects of different kinds or amounts of specific fats or fatty acids.

Undoubtedly, the most important paper in the general area of dietary fat and serum cholesterol level was the paper of Keys *et al.* (1957). Groups of "stabilized" schizophrenics were fed a series of diets in which the amount and kind of fat was varied. Multiple regression equations were developed to relate the change in the serum cholesterol to change in the dietary content of saturated (S), monounsaturated (M), and polyunsaturated (P) fatty acids. From some 40 different diets available for comparison, the equation of best fit was

$$\Delta \text{ Chol} = -1{\cdot}68 + 2{\cdot}76 \, \Delta \text{S} + 0{\cdot}05 \, \Delta \text{M} - 1{\cdot}35 \, \Delta \text{P}$$

where $\Delta$ Chol is expressed as mg/100 ml and $\Delta$ S, $\Delta$ M, and $\Delta$ P are the change in the calories contributed by each class of fatty acids. The constant, $-$ 1·68, and the coefficient for $\Delta$ M of 0·05 did not contribute significantly to the equation. Thus, these were eliminated which yielded the final equation

$$\Delta \text{ Chol} = 2{\cdot}74 \; \Delta \text{ S} - 1{\cdot}31 \; \Delta \text{ P}.$$

This equation was later simplified to

$$\Delta \text{ Chol} = 1{\cdot}2 \; (2 \text{ S-P}).$$

The major conclusions of Keys *et al.* were, therefore, that the mono-unsaturated fatty acids are essentially neutral and that the addition or subtraction of these from the diet have no effect upon serum cholesterol; that increasing the saturated fatty acids raises serum cholesterol and raising polyunsaturated fatty acids decreases the serum cholesterol—the ratio of activity being approximately 2:1 and in opposite directions. Only those saturated fatty acids with carbon chains greater than ten were considered to act as saturated fatty acids.

In a subsequent paper Keys *et al.* (1958) fed diets in which the ratio of S:P was held constant but the content of M varied substantially. These gave essentially the same serum cholesterol levels and apparently confirmed the prediction that the content of M was not a significant factor in the regulation of the level of serum cholesterol.

The Harvard studies (Hegsted *et al.*, 1965) were similar in design to those of Keys *et al.* They were based upon a diet consisting of low fat foods which provided (on composite analysis) 16·3 g of fat, 16 % of the calories from protein, and a relatively constant daily level of dietary cholesterol (306 mg). To this low-fat diet the oils to be tested were added at the appropriate level and additional calories as needed were furnished by carbohydrate sources—starch, sugars, cereals and breads, and potatoes. Dietary plans allowed for appropriate individualized calorie intakes ranging from 2200–3000 kcal. per day as needed to maintain constant body weight. In the first series of experiments, the test oils were used to provide diets of 22 and 38 % of fat calories; in the second series only the higher level was utilized. The test oils were used mainly by incorporating them into recipes for baked and dessert products, salad dressings, ice cream and milk, and so forth. Dietary cholesterol was included at three levels (116, 306, and 686 mg/day) by removing or adding eggs to the diet. In all the studies, a control or base line diet was designed to simulate the usual American diet in regard to dietary fats. Basically, it was the same as the test diets except that ordinary whole milk and ice cream were used, as well as mixed commercial fats and oils. By analysis, this diet yielded 38 % of the calories from fat and contained 331 mg of cholesterol.

All feeding studies were of 4 weeks' duration with fasting (morning) blood samples being obtained on the 24th and 28th day of each test period, a period sufficient for adaptation to a new diet. Values of specified lipid classes were averaged for purposes of statistical analysis of responsiveness. The control diet was fed during various periods throughout the entire series of studies and served as the reference for measuring change. Each subject, then, served as his own control. Changes in the intake of dietary fatty acids and dietary cholesterol were managed in the same way, the point of reference always being the control diet.

The subjects were a group of chronic schizophrenics, white males in their 40s and 50s who were psychiatrically stable and free of physical illness and who were cooperative and available for long-term studies. They were selected after screening a larger group in the hospital and individuals with markedly elevated or very low serum cholesterol levels while consuming the house diet were deliberately excluded. None were obese and the average serum cholesterol level while consuming the control diet was approximately 225 mg/100 ml.

In the first study, 36 different diets were studied, each being fed to a group of 9 or 10 men for a period of 28 days. These included a variety of fats and mixtures of fat selected primarily to evaluate the effects of the entire range of intakes of saturates (S), monounsaturates (M) and polyunsaturates (P) that can be achieved with ordinarily available oils. The extremes of S, M, and P intakes were achieved with coconut oil, olive oil, and safflower oil, respectively. The composition of the total dietary fat was, of course, influenced by the fat present in the basal diet. Thus, in the diets supplying 38 % of the fat calories, the coconut oil diet supplied 85 % of the total as S, in the olive oil diet there were 69 % of the total as M, and in the safflower oil diet 65 % of the total as P. These represent about the extremes that can be achieved in these kinds of studies.

The overall multiple regression equation, similar to that developed by Keys *et al.*, from these data was

$$\Delta \text{ Chol} = 2{\cdot}32\text{ S} + 0{\cdot}32\text{ M} - 1{\cdot}46\text{ P} + 6{\cdot}51\text{ C} + 0{\cdot}83$$

in which Δ Chol is the change in serum cholesterol in mg/100 ml, S, M, and P are the change in the saturated, monounsaturated, and polyunsaturated fatty acids in the diet expressed as percentage of calories, and C is the change in cholesterol intake in 100 mg/day. This equation has a multiple correlation coefficient, R, of 0·94 and $R^2$, the percentage of the variance explained by the equation, is 0·88. The standard deviation from regression is 12·98 mg/100 ml.

As in the data of Keys *et al.* (1957), the coefficient of M makes no significant contribution to the equation. When this variable was omitted from the equation, the equation based upon S, P, and C alone was

$$\Delta \text{ Chol} = 2{\cdot}16 \text{ S} - 1{\cdot}65 \text{ P} + 6{\cdot}77 \text{ C} - 0{\cdot}53. \quad (1)$$

The multiple correlation coefficient is 0·936 (Fig. 1).

The equation of this kind developed by Keys *et al.* (1965a, 1965b)

$$\Delta \text{ Chol} = 1{\cdot}3 \text{ (2S-P)} + 1{\cdot}5 \text{ Z}\dagger \quad (2)$$

has a coefficient of S which is somewhat larger relative to P than equation (1). In comparing the two equations, Keys and Parlin (1966) conclude that the Keys *et al.* equation applied to the data of Hegsted *et al.* gives an R of 0·92, not significantly less than the value of 0·936. However, the data of Keys *et al.* were somewhat less well explained by equation (1) than by equation (2). In particular, equation (1) appeared to over-predict the change in serum cholesterol compared to those found by Keys *et al.* when diets relatively high in polyunsaturated oils and which lowered the serum cholesterol were fed.

In the studies reported by Thomasson *et al.* (1967) ten different combinations of trilaurin (completely saturated), olive oil (68% mono-unsaturated) and safflower oil (72% polyunsaturated) were fed in a formula diet which contained 50% of the calories as the experimental fat. The ten fat mixtures gave a wide variety of ratios of S, M, and P. As all dietary groups had the same initial level of 145 mg cholesterol per 100 ml serum the common regression equations can be expressed as follows

$$\Delta \text{ Chol} = 0{\cdot}435 \text{ S} - 0{\cdot}290 \text{ P} + \text{K},$$

in which K = 139 mg/100 ml (men) or 120 mg/100 ml (women).

It may be noted that the ratio of activity of S:P in the equation for men is approximately 1·4 and this approximates the ratio obtained by Hegsted *et al.* which was 1·6. Both are substantially lower than the ratio of 2 found by Keys *et al.*

It should be noted, of course, that it is not certain whether one would expect the same results under the conditions of Thomasson *et al.*, Keys *et al.*, and Hegsted *et al.* The background of the subjects used was obviously different. Formula feeding often results in a fall in serum cholesterol (Hashim *et al.*, 1959; McCann *et al.*, 1959) which may reflect the fact that the diets are free of cholesterol but other dietary factors may have an effect as well. As discussed later, it is not known whether lauric acid has the same quantitative effect upon serum cholesterol as other saturated

† Z is the square root of the cholesterol intake (see discussion of dietary cholesterol on p. 225).

fatty acids. Finally, a number of the subjects in Thomasson's study lost some weight, especially those which received the highest level of trilaurin, and this may have influenced to some degree the serum cholesterol levels achieved.

## II. TOTAL FAT IN THE DIET

Hegsted *et al.* (1965) also analysed the same data by examining only the composition of the dietary fat, i.e. ignoring the amount of fat in the diet. It should be noted that in this type of analysis the sum of S, M, and P is inevitably 100 % and a third variable can be predicted from any two variables alone. Also, the study was not particularly well designed for this analysis since most of the groups studied were consuming diets with 38 % of the calories from fat and only 7 groups of the total of 36 groups available received the diets with 22 % of the calories as fat. Nevertheless, in this analysis, the equation based upon fatty acid content of the total

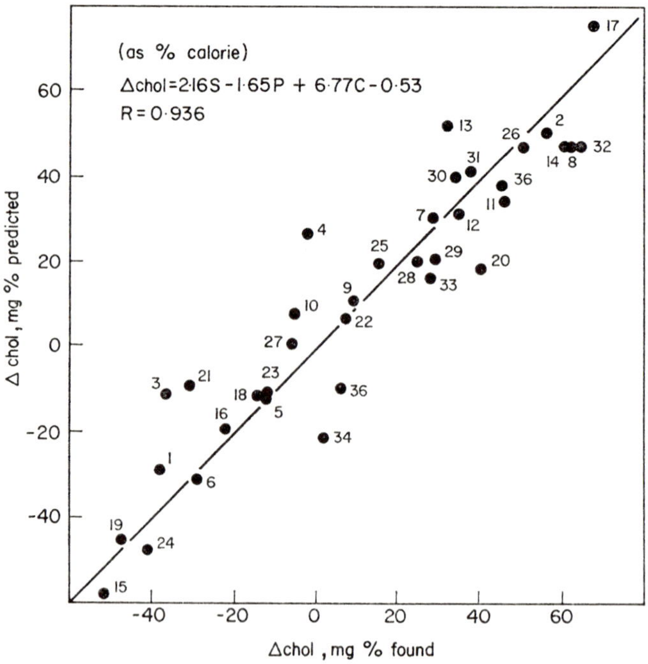


Fig. 1. A scatter diagram indicating the correlation between the change in serum cholesterol (Δ Chol) actually found and those predicted by the regression equation indicated. S and P are the change in the percentage of total calories provided by saturated and polyunsaturated fatty acids. C is the change in dietary cholesterol expressed as 100 mg units. Taken from Hegsted *et al.* (1965).

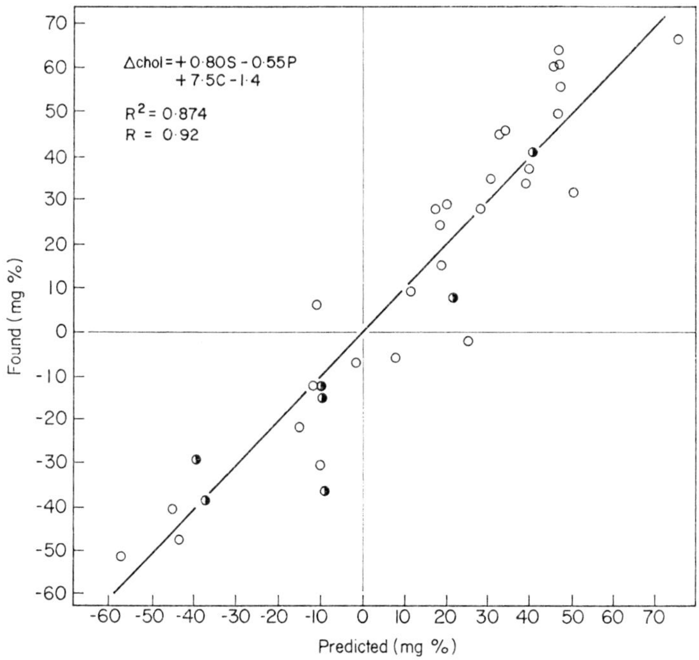


Fig. 2. The same data shown in Fig. 1 but S and P are the change in the percentage of the dietary fat which was supplied as saturated and polyunsaturated fatty acids. Half-filled circles indicate diets in which the total fat supplied 22% of the total caloric intake; open circles are diets in which the total fat supplied 38% of the calories.

dietary fat (Fig. 2) was equally efficient in predicting change in serum cholesterol as the equation in which the fatty acid content was expressed as a percentage of the calories shown in Fig. 1.

This conclusion is similar to that reached by Grande *et al.* (1972). Their equation predicts that when the composition of the dietary fat is such that 2 S-P = 0 varying the amount of fat should have no effect upon the serum cholesterol. They, therefore, compared four different diets which varied in the amount and composition of fat but in which the S and P contents were such that 2 S-P = 0. The essential details of this comparison are shown in Table 1. Note that Diet 1 had only about 5% of the calories as fat. The serum cholesterol levels were unaffected by the change in fat content of the diet. As expected, the triglyceride levels were elevated upon the lower levels of fat and tended to be inversely related to the fat content of the diet.

These conclusions may not be entirely in accord with the data presented by Vergroesen and de Boer (1971). Using formula diets these investigators fed 90% trilaurin + 10% safflower oil, olive oil, and safflower oil as the source of fat in diets which provided 20, 35, and 50% of the calories as fat. With the 90% trilaurin + 10% safflower oil or olive oil diets the serum cholesterol level rose modestly as the intake went from 20 to 35 to 50% of the calories. These increases were not statistically significant. Increasing the safflower oil content of the diet lowered significantly the serum phospholipid levels while serum cholesterol levels showed the same tendency. However, the differences in the composition of the fat influenced serum cholesterol much more than did the changes in the amount of fat in the diet.

Table 1

Diets of varying fat content which produced similar levels of serum cholesterol (from Grande *et al.*, 1972)

| | DIETS | | | |
|---|---|---|---|---|
| | 1 | 2 | 3 | 4 |
| Fat calories, % of total | 5·4 | 13·7 | 29·9 | 29·9 |
| Total dietary glycerides, g | 12·6 | 35·5 | 80·0 | 80·7 |
| Saturated acids ($C_{12}$–$C_{16}$), g | 4·3 | 6·6 | 11·1 | 20·1 |
| Monounsaturated acids, g | 4·5 | 18·9 | 47·0 | 19·6 |
| Polyunsaturated acids, g | 1·7 | 7·4 | 18·4 | 36·9 |
| Serum cholesterol, mg/100 ml | 221 | 228 | 225 | 227 |
| Triglycerides, mg/100 ml | 222 | 180 | 149 | 145 |

Whether one accepts the conclusion of Grande *et al.* (1972) that one can substitute fat of the appropriate composition for carbohydrate in the diet and have no effect upon the serum cholesterol level or not, it is quite clear that at all levels of fat intake which are of practical significance in developed countries the primary factors determining serum cholesterol level is the composition of the fat and not the amount of fat in the diet. Undoubtedly, the reason that lowering of serum cholesterol is usually observed when the fat content of a diet is lowered is that the dietary recommendation usually consists of the removal of various sources of saturated fatty acids. Thus, the fat remaining in the diet is relatively less saturated as well as lower in amount. It should be recognized, however, that the recommendation to lower the fat content of a diet imposes limitation upon one's ability to manipulate the composition of the fat in the diet. Furthermore, lowering the fat content of the diet will normally result in an increase of the carbohydrate content. This may result in an elevation of the level of serum triglycerides in a significant fraction of the population. The most effective practical diets for lowering the level of cholesterol are those in which saturated fats are replaced by polyunsaturated fat, maintaining the total fat intake at a reasonable level.

It should also be noted that when the fat content of the diet is held constant or when only the composition of the dietary fat is considered, additional restraints are placed upon the data. Since $S + M + P = 100$, a combination of two of these variables provides a complete description of the data and the other can be calculated by difference. Thus, in the experiments of Thomasson *et al.* (1967) referred to previously, the equation

$$\Delta \text{Chol} = 0{\cdot}7\ S + 0{\cdot}3\ M + K$$

in which K = 100 mg/100 ml or 99 mg/100 ml for men and women respectively, described the results as well as the equation involving S and P. One could conclude from this equation that S was $2\frac{1}{2}$ times as hypercholesterolaemic as M.

The studies of Keys *et al.* (1958) in which M was varied while holding the ratio of S:P constant supports the conclusion that M *per se* has no effect upon the serum cholesterol level. Yet it should be recognized that the terms *raised*, *lowered*, or *has no effect* are only meaningful relative to something else. One might ask, for example, what would the serum cholesterol be in a diet containing only M if this fatty acid has no effect on serum cholesterol. Clearly, it would have to be determined by something. The problem is largely a semantic one. The equations are descriptive. Only when the mechanisms are known by which the various classes of fatty acids affect circulating cholesterol will it be possible to describe how the regulation of serum cholesterol is accomplished.

## III. EFFECTS OF SPECIFIC SATURATED FATTY ACIDS

The great bulk of monounsaturated fatty acids in practical diets consists of oleic, elaidic- and erucic acid, and most of the polyunsaturated fatty acids consists of linoleic acid. Relatively little quantitative work is available to indicate whether other mono- or polyunsaturated acids have the same influence as oleic and linoleic acids but this is of little practical significance. The exception to this might be in populations in which a considerable intake of dietary fat is derived from fish.

On the other hand, the saturated fatty acids vary substantially. Both butterfat and coconut oil which are known to be very hypercholestero-laemic contain substantial amounts of fatty acids with chain lengths of 14 or less and the possibility exists that their peculiar effects might be explained by the combination of saturated fatty acids they contain. The palmitic and stearic acid content of various dietary fats also varies substantially. Thus, if the several saturated fatty acids vary greatly in their effect upon serum cholesterol, this would be of substantial practical importance.

Cocoa butter is relatively unique. It contains approximately 65% saturated fatty acids of which over half is stearic acid and the remainder mostly palmitic acid and about 35% oleic acid. Various authors (Hegsted *et al.*, 1965; Keys *et al.*, 1965b) have noted that this fat was less hypercholesterolaemic than would be expected from its composition, suggesting that stearic acid might be less hypercholesterolaemic than palmitic acid or other saturated fatty acids.

The data available from the first study of Hegsted *et al.* (1965) were analysed by multiple regression equations in an attempt to determine the relative influence of the various fatty acids. Included in the analysis were $S_{10}$ (saturated fatty acids of 10 carbons or less), $S_{12}$ (lauric acid), $S_{14}$ (myristic acid), $S_{16}$ (palmitic acid), $S_{18}$ (stearic acid), M (monounsaturated acids, practically oleic acid), P (polyunsaturated acids, practically linoleic acid) and dietary cholesterol. This regression analysis indicated that most of the variance could be explained by four variables—$S_{14}$, $S_{16}$, P, and dietary cholesterol.

However, it was pointed out that these regression coefficients are not unique and that the various independent variables were not randomly or independently distributed in the various diets fed. Thus, while it seemed likely that myristic, palmitic, and linoleic acid and dietary cholesterol were the primary independent variables influencing the serum cholesterol and that lauric acid ($S_{12}$), stearic acid ($S_{18}$), and monounsaturates (M) which were also important constituents of the diets had little effect, this was not proven by the analysis.

Additional studies (McGandy *et al.*, 1970) were designed in an attempt to better elucidate the specific influences of saturated fatty acids independently of one another and independently of accompanying mono- and polyunsaturated. Since tripalmitin and tristearin are poorly absorbed, it is not possible to approach this problem through addition of pure triglycerides of these specific fatty acids to the diet. We instead utilized semi-synthetic, mixed triglycerides made by randomly trans-esterifying natural fats with triglycerides of specific fatty acids. Of course, even with this technique there are limitations to the kinds of end products one can achieve. One reaches a point where substantial amounts of trisaturates are produced even when using natural oils low in saturates as starting points—safflower and olive oils were utilized in these studies. In order to test the effect of higher levels of myristic, palmitic, and stearic acids, we utilized some preparations based on medium-chain triglycerides (MCT) as the oil with which the specific long-chain acids were transesterified.

These materials were fed under conditions similar to those previously described, all with diets supplying 38% of the calories as fat. Data from thirty different diets were available for comparison.

These studies were somewhat less instructive than was hoped probably because of the limitations in one's ability to substitute specific fatty acids at a sufficiently high level. The most striking feature was that when myristic, palmitic, and stearic acids were transesterified with MCT in order to yield triglycerides containing approximately 50% of the specific fatty acids, myristic and palmitic were markedly hypercholesterolaemic whereas stearic acid was only slightly so compared to MCT alone. This appeared to confirm the conclusion of Keys *et al.*

However, when the semi-synthetic fats prepared with safflower oil and olive oil were compared, only modest differences between the effects of the saturated fatty acids could be detected although they were hypercholesterolaemic compared to the base oils alone. Lauric acid appeared to be slightly less hypercholesterolaemic than the remaining three saturated fatty acids.

Grande *et al.* (1970) compared the effects of cocoa butter and palm kernel oil and what they called an "imitation cocoa butter" and "imitation palm kernel oil". Cocoa butter and palm kernel oil both contain 54–59% saturated fatty acids but over half of these are stearic acid in cocoa butter whereas nearly all of the saturated fatty acids are composed of $C_{12}$–$C_{16}$ acids in palm kernel oil. The imitation cocoa butter was a mixture of palm oil, hydrogenated soyabean oil (mostly stearic acid), olive oil and safflower oil in the proportions which yielded essentially the same fatty acid composition as cocoa butter itself. The imitation palm kernel oil was made of hydrogenated soyabean oil, olive oil and safflower oil in the proportions which yielded the same ratios of total S, M, and P as the palm kernel oil but the S was largely stearic acid rather than $C_{12}$–$C_{16}$ acids. The two "imitation fats" were transesterified.

The four fats were compared in a Latin Square design with four groups of subjects receiving each fat for 18 days. The experimental diets contained 83 g of the experimental fats and a total of 105 g fat/day (approximately 27% of the calories).

The overall mean serum cholesterol levels were 203 $\pm$ 29, 199 $\pm$ 29, 217 $\pm$ 34, and 193 $\pm$ 31 mg/100 ml for cocoa butter, imitation cocoa butter, palm kernel oil, and imitation palm kernel oil, respectively.

The conclusions were as follows: Since the cocoa butter and the imitation cocoa butter gave similar results the effects on serum cholesterol were due to the fatty acid composition and not to some peculiar property of cocoa butter.

The palm kernel oil gave a significantly higher serum cholesterol value than the other three which were not different. This is consistent with the greater hypercholesterolaemic effect of lauric-, myristic- and palmitic acid compared to stearic acid.

It was concluded that the results are consistent with the hypothesis that "stearic acid, like oleic acid or mixed carbohydrate, has no effect upon the serum cholesterol concentration in man".

This study does, however, provide a good example of the extreme difficulties in sorting out the finer details in this area. The imitation palm kernel oil contained 15% of $C_{12}$–$C_{16}$ saturated fatty acids whereas the imitation cocoa butter contained 27%, the difference being made up by stearic acid. The polyene content was 11% compared to 8% in the latter product. Nevertheless, the mean cholesterol value based upon a total of 30 men was 193 mg/100 ml in the former and 199 mg/100 ml in the latter group, an insignificant difference. The difference in cholesterol values, comparing the values obtained on each man when receiving the two diets, was also insignificant. The intra- and inter-individual variability poses great limitations even with groups as large as 30 men per experimental group.

The relative effects of lauric, myristic, palmitic, and stearic acids have also been studied by Vergroesen and de Boer (1971). Triglycerides of these fatty acids were transesterified in approximately 1:2 ratios with both safflower and olive oil in order to produce products containing approximately 30% of the appropriate fatty acid. These preparations were fed as a source of 50% of the total calories in formula diets.

As would be expected, the diets based upon safflower oil produce lower cholesterol values than those based upon olive oil. However, within each group of oils, those containing lauric and myristic acids produced higher cholesterol levels than those containing palmitic or stearic acids, and lauric and myristic acids did not appear to be different nor did palmitic acid relative to stearic acid. Thus, in these studies the short-chain acids appeared to be relatively more hypercholesterolaemic than the long-chain acids.

In summary, therefore, there is considerable evidence that the saturated fatty acids may vary substantially in their hypercholesterolaemic effects. Most of the data support the thesis that stearic acid has less effect upon serum cholesterol than lauric, myristic, or palmitic acids, but do not support the contention that it is completely without effect under most conditions.

Similarly, the data so far available suggest that lauric and myristic acids may be somewhat more hypercholesterolaemic than palmitic acid but the data are not sufficient to quantitate this difference under all conditions.

It is unfortunate that this problem is not better defined since the principal source of stearic acid in most modern diets will come from meat. If stearic acid is indeed substantially less hypercholesterolaemic than the other saturated fatty acids under usual dietary conditions, it will be of practical importance in the design of diets aimed at lowering the level of serum cholesterol. Fats such as butterfat and coconut oil are clearly among the most hypercholesterolaemic in the usual diet. It is perhaps of less practical importance to know whether this is due to the high content of total saturated fatty acids or partially due to the combination of fatty acids they happen to contain.

## IV. EFFECTS OF DIETARY CHOLESTEROL

In the first study of Hegsted *et al.* (1965) the effects of the addition of dietary cholesterol as egg were studied in the presence of three different fats—coconut oil, olive oil, and safflower oil. Removal of all egg from the low-fat diet resulted in an intake of 116 mg of dietary cholesterol/day. The data (Fig. 3) indicated that the response in serum cholesterol was

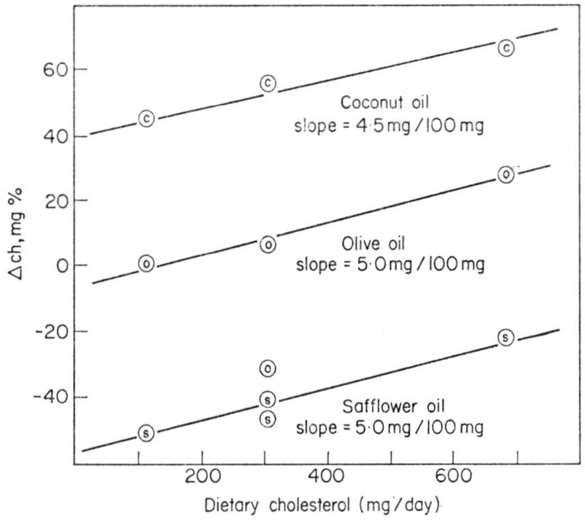


Fig. 3. Change in serum cholesterol at different levels of cholesterol intake supplied by egg. The diets contained 38% of the calories as fat supplied principally by coconut oil, olive oil, or safflower oil. The response to dietary cholesterol appears to be approximately linear and similar in the three diets. Taken from Hegsted *et al.* (1965).

approximately 5 mg/100 ml of serum for each 100 mg of cholesterol added. Insofar as the data available were concerned, there appeared to be a linear response to the addition of cholesterol and since the slopes of the lines were similar regardless of the oil in the diet, there appeared to be no interaction with the kind of fat in the diet. That is, the kind of fat did not appear to accentuate or modify the response to the dietary cholesterol.

It should be noted that in these specific experiments in which the cholesterol intake was deliberately varied, the slope of the dose-response lines—4·5 to 5 mg/100 ml/100 mg—was somewhat less than that calculated from the multiple regression equations (pp. 217 and 218) which was between 5 and 7 depending upon the other variables included in the equation.

Keys *et al.* (1965a) have concluded that the response of the serum cholesterol to changes in the dietary intake is not linearly related to the intake. Rather, they believe that the change in serum cholesterol is approximately proportional to the square root of the cholesterol intake. Keys and Parlin (1966) draw upon some 19 studies in the literature to support the proposition that the change in serum cholesterol is approximately predicted by their equation.

More recently, Mattson *et al.* (1972) examined the effects of three different cholesterol intakes between 106 and 317 mg cholesterol/1000 kcal. The cholesterol was supplied as egg yolk and formula diets were used. These contained approximately 40% of the calories as fat; the fat being a mixture of olive oil, palm oil, and cocoa butter designed to approximate the fatty acid composition of an average American diet. In these studies the change in serum cholesterol was essentially linearly related to intake and was approximately 12 mg for each 100 mg of cholesterol in 1000 kcal. This value would be equivalent to 4·8 mg/100 mg cholesterol/day assuming an average calorie intake of 2500 kcal. This is no different from the value obtained by Hegsted *et al.*

Both Connor *et al.* (1964) and Beveridge *et al.* (1960) found that the serum cholesterol concentration was not markedly affected by dietary cholesterol once substantial intakes were achieved. Metabolic studies (Taylor *et al.*, 1960; Wilson and Lindsey, 1965; Taylor *et al.*, 1966) indicate that cholesterol absorption is limited at high intakes and there is presumably feedback control over hepatic cholesterol synthesis. The failure of very high intakes of cholesterol to modify serum cholesterol levels substantially when added to diets that already contain considerable amounts of cholesterol presumably accounts for the general feeling some years ago that dietary cholesterol had very little to do with the level in the serum.

Since the response at very high levels of intake is of little practical significance, it appears fair to conclude that at this time it should be accepted that the response of serum cholesterol is about 4 to 5 mg/100 ml for each 100 mg of dietary cholesterol consumed. One might suspect that this would be better defined if the effects of body size or caloric intake were considered but this is as yet uncertain.

Mattson *et al.* calculate that in the National Diet–Heart Study (1968) approximately 50% of the lowering of the serum cholesterol that was obtained could be accounted for by the change in cholesterol intake. They thus suggest that changes in the intake of cholesterol may be more important than changes in the dietary fat. We do not agree with this conclusion. It is true that at the present time restriction of the intake of cholesterol, primarily by restricting the consumption of eggs and dairy products, may be the most easily achieved means of lowering the serum cholesterol level. However, the potential for lowering cholesterol is greater by the modification of dietary fat. The practical application of this will require the development of more acceptable kinds of foods containing modified fats.

## V. PRACTICAL EXPERIENCE

It would only be logical in a chronic disease, such as atherosclerotic heart disease, to assume that modification of the various risk factors at an early age would be more effective than their modification after atherosclerosis is already far advanced. The limited data available support this logic. In Leren's study (1970), for example, a reduction in the re-occurrence of heart attacks after dietary modification was only apparent in the younger men in the study. Pathological data on young American men demonstrate that atherosclerosis is already far advanced in many young men in their 20s (Enos *et al.*, 1955; Strong and McGill, 1962). Thus, attention should be directed toward the modification of serum cholesterol during adolescence, the period in which serum cholesterol levels begin to rise to those levels which typify those of adults in industrial societies.

Recently, several groups of investigators have shown that total cholesterol can be profoundly influenced by alterations in dietary lipids in adolescence. Working in boys' boarding schools, our group (McGandy *et al.*, 1972; Ford *et al.*, 1972) has shown that reducing saturated fatty acids and total cholesterol and increasing polyunsaturated fatty acids in the ordinary school diet led to prompt reduction in mean serum cholesterol levels of 10% in one school and 15% in another. Complete adherence in these studies, as with the free-living adult studies already cited, could not be assured. In the school where better dietary adherence was possible, the mean serum cholesterol level of teenage boys eating the school diet was about 180 mg/100 ml and this was lowered to about 152 mg/100 ml on a diet providing 10% of the calories from saturated fatty acids (instead of 15%), 10% from polyunsaturated fatty acids (instead of 3%), and 300 mg of cholesterol/day (instead of 540).

In similar studies done in Holland (Vergroesen and de Boer, 1971), a reduction in blood cholesterol of from 192 mg/100 ml to 149 mg/100 ml in the first part of the trial and from 198 mg/100 ml to 160 mg/100 ml in the second part of the experiment, has been reported in a group of institutionalized teenage boys and girls after substituting ordinary institution dietary fats with products containing large quantities of linoleic acid. Here, too, complete dietary adherence was not assured so that these responses probably do not represent maximal ones.

Although there is still some disagreement as to the quantitative roles that various lipid components of the diet play in defining the serum cholesterol, there is already extensive experience in the development of diets which are practical for the lowering of serum cholesterol in population groups. These follow the generalities that are clear from the previous discussion and involve reducing the intake of saturated fatty acids, increasing the intake of polyunsaturated fatty acids, and lowering the intake of dietary cholesterol. Numerous studies (Christakis *et al.*, 1966; National Diet–Heart Study, 1968; Research Committee to the Medical Research Council, 1968; Turpeinen *et al.*, 1968; Dayton *et al.*, 1969; Leren, 1970) have shown that mean reductions of blood cholesterol from 10 to 15% can be achieved in middle-aged men and can be maintained for years. The magnitude of this effect is about one-half to two-thirds of what could be achieved under metabolic ward conditions. This difference almost certainly represents the degree of non-adherence which is always a fact in life in dealing with free-living population groups. The degree of non-adherence is certainly affected by the availability and acceptability of foods with a modified fat composition. More satisfactory adherence will depend largely upon the development of satisfactory foods of wide variety which permits the consumption of a modified fat diet with relative ease. Many modified foods are now available which could be put on the market but many improvements are also required.

Whether the modification of the serum cholesterol by such diets will, in fact, lead to a reduction in the prevalence of coronary artery disease is not yet proven. However, the preliminary results are encouraging and it is only logical to attempt to remove those risk factors which have so far been identified.

## REFERENCES

Beveridge, J. M. R., Connell, W. F., Mayer, A. G. and Haust, H. L. (1960). The response of man to dietary cholesterol. *J. Nutr.* **71,** 61–65.

Christakis, G., Rinzler, S. H., Archer, M., Winslow, G., Jampel, S., Stephenson, J., Friedman, G., Fein, H., Kraus, A. and James, G. (1966). The anti-coronary club. A dietary approach to the prevention of coronary heart disease—a seven year report. *Am. J. Publ. Hlth* **56,** 299–314.

Connor, W. E., Hodges, R. E. and Bleiler, R. A. (1961). The serum lipids in men receiving high cholesterol and cholesterol-free diets. *J. Clin. Invest.* **40,** 894–901.

Dayton, S., Pearce, M. L., Hashimoto, S., Dixon, W. J. and Tomiyasu, U. (1969). A controlled clinical trial of a diet high in unsaturated fat in preventing complications of atherosclerosis. *Circulation* **40,** Suppl. II, 1–63.

Enos, W. F., Jr., Beyer, J. C. and Holmes, R. H. (1955). Pathogenesis of coronary disease in American soldiers killed in Korea. *J. Am. Med. Ass.* **158,** 912–914.

Ford, C. H., McGandy, R. B. and Stare, F. J. (1972). An institutional approach to the dietary regulation of blood cholesterol in adolescent males. *Preventive Med.* **1,** 426–445.

Fredrickson, D. S., Levy, R. I. and Lees, R. S. (1967). Fat transport in lipoproteins—integrated approach to mechanisms and disorders. *New Engl. J. Med.* **276,** 34–44, 94–103, 148–156, 215–225, 273–281.

Grande, F., Anderson, J. T. and Keys, A. (1970). Comparison of effects of palmitic and stearic acids in the diet on serum cholesterol in man. *Am. J. Clin. Nutr.* **23,** 1184–1193.

Grande, F., Anderson, J. T. and Keys, A. (1972). Diets of different fatty acid composition producing identical serum cholesterol levels in man. *Am. J. Clin. Nutr.* **25,** 53–60.

Hashim, S. A., Clancy, R. E., Hegsted, D. H. and Stare, F. J. (1959). Effect of mixed-fat formula feeding on serum cholesterol in man. *Am. J. Clin. Nutr.* **7,** 35–42.

Hegsted, D. M., McGandy, R. B., Myers, M. L. and Stare, F. J. (1965). Quantitative effects of dietary fat on serum cholesterol in man. *Am. J. Clin. Nutr.* **17,** 281–295.

Kannel, W. B. and Gordon, T. (1970). The Framingham Study: Diet and the Regulation of Serum Cholesterol. Department of Health, Education and Welfare, National Institutes of Health, Bethesda, Maryland.

Keys, A. and Parlin, R. W. (1966). Serum cholesterol response to changes in dietary lipids. *Am. J. Clin. Nutr.* **19,** 175–181.

Keys, A., Anderson, J. T. and Grande, F. (1957). Prediction of serum–cholesterol responses of man to changes in fats in the diet. *Lancet* **2,** 959–966.

Keys, A., Anderson, J. T. and Grande, F. (1958). Effect of serum cholesterol in man of mono-ene fatty acid (oleic acid) in the diet. *Proc. Soc. Exp. Biol. Med.* **98,** 387–391.

Keys, A., Anderson, J. T. and Grande, F. (1965a). Serum cholesterol response to changes in the diet: II. The effect of cholesterol in the diet. *Metabolism* **14,** 759–765.

Keys, A., Anderson, J. T. and Grande, F. (1965b). Serum cholesterol response to changes in the diet: IV. Particular saturated fatty acids in the diet. *Metabolism* **14,** 776–787.

Leren, P. (1970). The Oslo diet-heart study. Eleven year report. *Circulation* **42,** 935–942.

Marr, J. W., Heady, J. A. and Morris, J. N. (1959). Repeat individual weighed dietary surveys. *Proc. Nutr. Soc.* **18,** xii.

Mattson, F. H., Erickson, B. A. and Kligman, A. M. (1972). Effect of dietary cholesterol on serum cholesterol in man. *Am. J. Clin. Nutr.* **25**, 589–594.

McCann, M. B., Trulson, M. F., Waddell, W. R., Dalryimple, W. and Stare, F. J. (1959). The effects of various vegetable oils on the serum lipids of adult American males. *Am. J. Clin. Nutr.* **7**, 35–42.

McGandy, R. B., Hegsted, D. M. and Myers, M. L. (1970). Use of semi-synthetic fats in determining effects of specific dietary fatty acids on serum lipids in man. *Am. J. Clin. Nutr.* **23**, 1288–1298.

McGandy, R. B., Hall, B., Ford, C. and Stare, F. J. (1972). Dietary regulation of blood cholesterol in adolescent males: A pilot study. *Am. J. Clin. Nutr.* **25**, 61–66.

National Diet–Heart Study Research Group (1968). The national diet-heart study: final report. *Circulation* **37**, Suppl. I, 1–203.

Research Committee to the Medical Research Council (1968). Controlled trial of soya bean oil in myocardial infarction. *Lancet* **2**, 693–699.

Reshef, A. and Epstein, L. M. (1972). Reliability of a dietary questionnaire. *Am. J. Clin. Nutr.* **25**, 91–95.

Strong, J. P. and McGill, H. C. (1962). The natural history of coronary atherosclerosis. *Am. J. Pathol.* **40**, 37–49.

Taylor, C. B., Patton, D., Yogi, N. and Cox, G. E. (1960). Diet as source of serum cholesterol in man. *Proc. Soc. Exp. Biol. Med.* **103**, 768–772.

Taylor, C. B., Mikkelson, B., Anderson, J. A. and Forman, D. T. (1966). Human serum cholesterol synthesis measured with the deuterium label. *Arch. Pathol.* **81**, 213–231.

Thomasson, H. J., de Boer, J. and de Iongh, H. (1967). Influence of dietary fats on plasma lipids. *Path. Microbiol.* **30**, 629–647.

Turpeinen, O., Miettinen, M., Karvonen, M. J., Roine, P., Pekkarinen, M., Lehtosuo, E. J. and Alivirta, P. (1968). Dietary prevention of coronary heart disease: Long-term experiment: I. Observations on male subjects. *Am. J. Clin. Nutr.* **21**, 255–276.

Vergroesen, A. J. and de Boer, J. (1971). Quantitative und qualitative Effekte mehrfach ungesättigter und anderer Fettsäuren in der menschlichen Diat. *In* "Polyenfettsäuren", Vol. 22, pp. 76–89. Scientific Publications of the German Nutrition Society, Steinkopff Verlag, Darmstadt.

Wilson, J. D. and Lindsey, C. A., Jr. (1965). Studies on the influence of dietary cholesterol on cholesterol metabolism in the isotopic steady state in man. *J. Clin. Invest.* **44**, 1805–1814.

# 5 The Role of Fat in the Treatment of Diabetes Mellitus

A. J. HOUTSMULLER

*Erasmus University, Rotterdam, The Netherlands*



## I. INTRODUCTION

The incidence of diabetes mellitus is increasing all over the world. This increase seems to be clearly associated with two factors, notably the higher average life expectancy and improved standard of living, plus the improved survival rate of young diabetic patients who can now reach reproductive age and produce genetically predisposed offspring.

This disorder, syndrome or disease (see Editorial, *Lancet*, 1971) is, as generally assumed, hereditary based and becomes manifest due to predisposing factors of which obesity, multiple pregnancies and infections are accepted with a reasonable degree of certainty. In particular, diet plays an important role—which is strikingly demonstrated during long periods of starvation when 80 % of manifest diabetes can disappear, for example, during World War II (Schöfling and Graeve, 1956a,b).

## II. DESCRIPTION OF THE SYNDROME

Since the pathophysiological basis of diabetes mellitus has not yet been completely elucidated, it is usually defined as a disorder characterized by an absolute or relative deficiency of normally-functioning insulin (Levine, 1970). An insulin deficiency, by whatever cause, results immediately in three serious biochemical disturbances, notably:

1. an increased release of glucose from the liver;
2. a decreased uptake of glucose by insulin-sensitive tissues such as muscular and adipose tissue, resulting in increased blood sugar level;
3. an increased lipolysis from the adipose tissues and liver.

These disturbances may develop acutely or be of a chronic nature. Clinically, a distinction can be made between the juvenile diabetes syndrome, insulin-dependent, often beginning at an early age with emaciation, polyuria and keto-acidosis and the maturity-onset diabetes syndrome, primarily insulin-independent, occurring at a later age, particularly in women and characterized by adiposity, hyperglycaemia and hyperlipaemia.

Vascular disorders, macro- as well as micro-angiopathy, occur frequently at an early stage with either syndrome. The cause of these abnormalities is as yet largely unknown. However, the disturbed insulin metabolism seems to be the main reason.

## III. CARBOHYDRATE- AND FAT METABOLISM IN DIABETES MELLITUS

Fat metabolism in diabetes cannot be considered separately from carbohydrate metabolism. Carbohydrates and fats are supplied to the bloodstream via the intestine. During the passage through the intestine they are adapted for absorption by the intestinal mucosa. The processes involved will not be discussed here (see Ch. 3). After a short survey of carbohydrate- and fat metabolism the abnormalities caused by insulin deficiency will be discussed in more detail.

### A. Normal Carbohydrate Metabolism

After the necessary conversion to monosaccharides the carbohydrates pass through the intestinal wall exclusively as glucose, fructose and galactose and reach the liver via the vena portae (after which only glucose appears in the bloodstream). The rate of absorption in the intestine is not the same for the various monosaccharides; the fructose absorption is much slower than that of glucose (Soskin and Levine, 1952). On the other hand the uptake of fructose by the liver proceeds more quickly than that of glucose (Levine and Haft, 1970) which even increases in the case of insulin deficiency. This leads to a different degree of fat formation from glucose or fructose; fructose being the more efficiently converted to fat. Kipnis (1967) estimated that the glucose conversion in man, in the liver, after an oral glucose loading, was 2/3 of the glucose supplied. For injected $^{14}C$-fructose Atwell and Waterhouse (1971) found 31% conversion to glucose. Both sugars can, to a considerable degree, be converted into fats, in which process mainly two organs are involved—the liver and the adipose tissue. The glucose (fructose) is converted into acetyl-CoA, after which via various routes mainly palmitic and oleic acid are formed. The first possibility is the formation of malonyl-CoA from acetyl-CoA for which ATP is necessary. Subsequently from 7-malonyl-CoA molecules and acetyl-CoA the $C_{16}$ fatty acid palmitic acid is formed. In addition to this *de novo* synthesis fatty acids can be formed in mitochondria by chain elongation.

To a lesser degree oleic acid and also some other saturated or mono-unsaturated fatty acids (C14-O, C16-1, C18-0 and C18-1) are formed. These fatty acids are subsequently coupled to α-glycerophosphate, which is also formed from glucose, leading to the formation of fats. These fats which mainly originate from the liver are called endogenous triglycerides, as opposed to the exogenous triglycerides which are derived from dietary fats.

The endogenous triglycerides are subsequently coupled in the liver to a protein carrier which leads to the formation of lipoproteins. The lipoproteins appear in the bloodstream where they can be recognized on account of their physico-chemical properties. At ultracentrifugal analysis they form the group of very low density lipoproteins (VLDL), using one of the various electrophoretic methods of analysis they constitute the so-called pre-β-lipoproteins. (For a recent review see Houtsmuller, 1969.)

The chemical composition of VLDL is approximately 10% protein, 55% triglycerides, 13% cholesterol and 22% phospholipids; their flotation rate in the ultracentrifuge ($S_f$) is 20–400. The pre-β-lipoproteins reach the various tissues via the bloodstream where, by means of lipoprotein lipase they are gradually split (see Figs 1, 2 and 3). The fatty acids liberated in this process can be used by the tissues for the

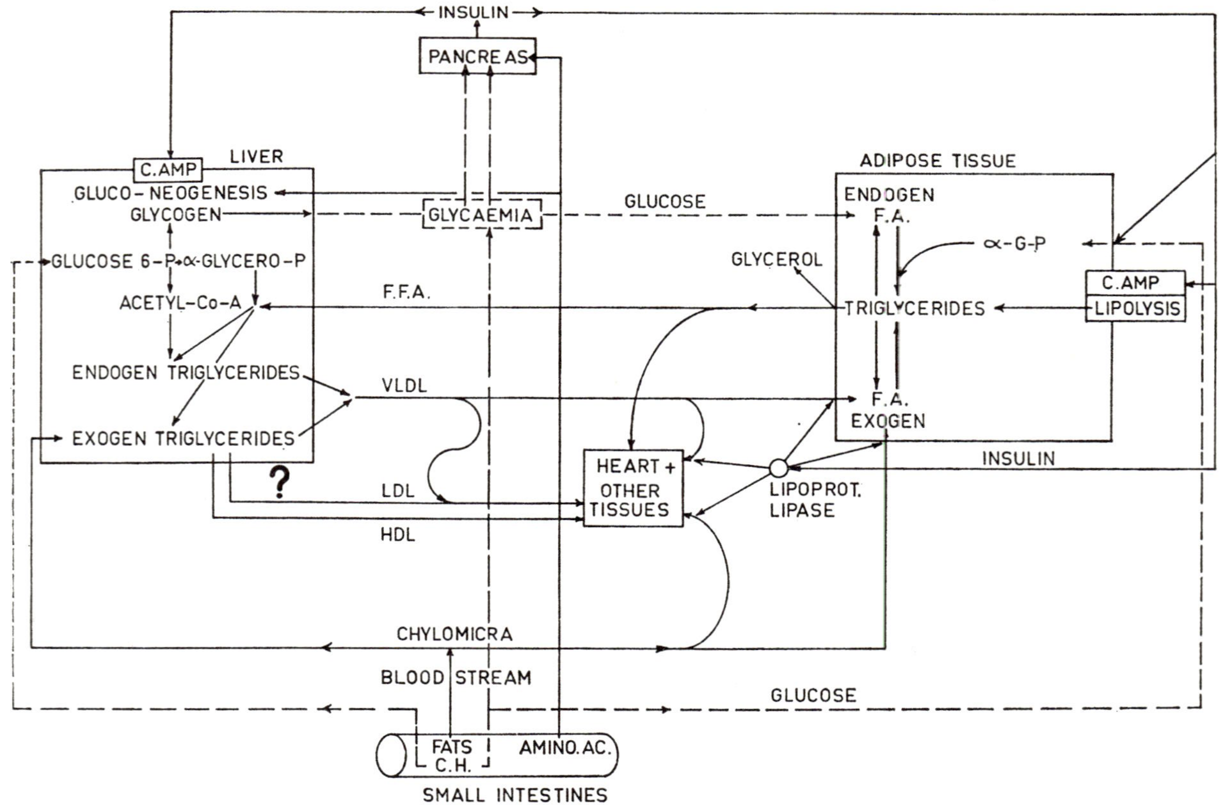


Fig. 1. Survey of the metabolism of dietary carbohydrates and fats in the liver and fatty tissue under the control of insulin. The dietary fats are offered to the tissues as chylomicrons and split by the insulin–sensitive lipoprotein–lipase system. Via re-esterification in the liver these so-called exogenous triglycerides (VLDL) are brought into the blood stream. They are stored in the fatty tissues and—when necessary—the triglycerides are split and the free fatty acids and glycerol released into the blood stream. The dietary carbohydrates are partly converted in the liver into endogenous triglycerides and are transported also as VLDL in the blood stream. In the fat tissue mainly α-glycerophosphate, necessary for the synthesis of triglycerides, is formed from these

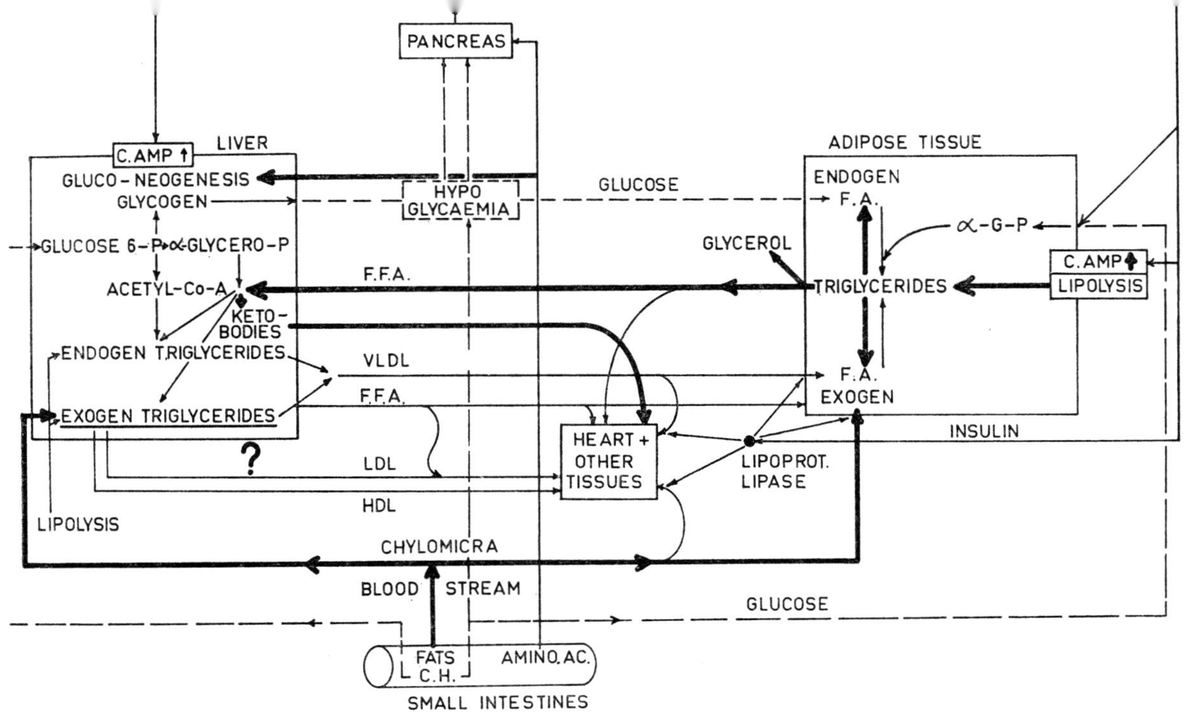


Fig. 2. Under extreme dietary conditions such as an almost carbohydrate-free diet, the required carbohydrates are formed from proteins, glycerol (gluconeogenesis). The chylomicrons which are offered on a large scale to the liver are converted maximally into exogenous triglycerides. They will appear in the blood stream partly as VLDL and partly as free fatty acids because of insufficient supply of α-glycerophosphate. An appreciable fraction of these free fatty acids are converted to ketone bodies, which serve as substrate in various organs (e.g. kidneys, brain, muscle tissues—including heart). The insulin level falls because of the weaker glucose stimulus. In fat tissue the chylomicrons are hydrolysed by the now less active lipoprotein–lipase system; the fatty acids are taken up and re-esterified with α-glycerophosphate into triglycerides. The lipolysis has been stimulated by decreased insulin concentration. Glycerol and FFA are released into the blood at an increased rate. From part of the FFA triglycerides are formed in the liver. The degree of α-glycerophosphate formation determines the concentration of VLDL in the plasma. Fatty tissue depletion is probable.

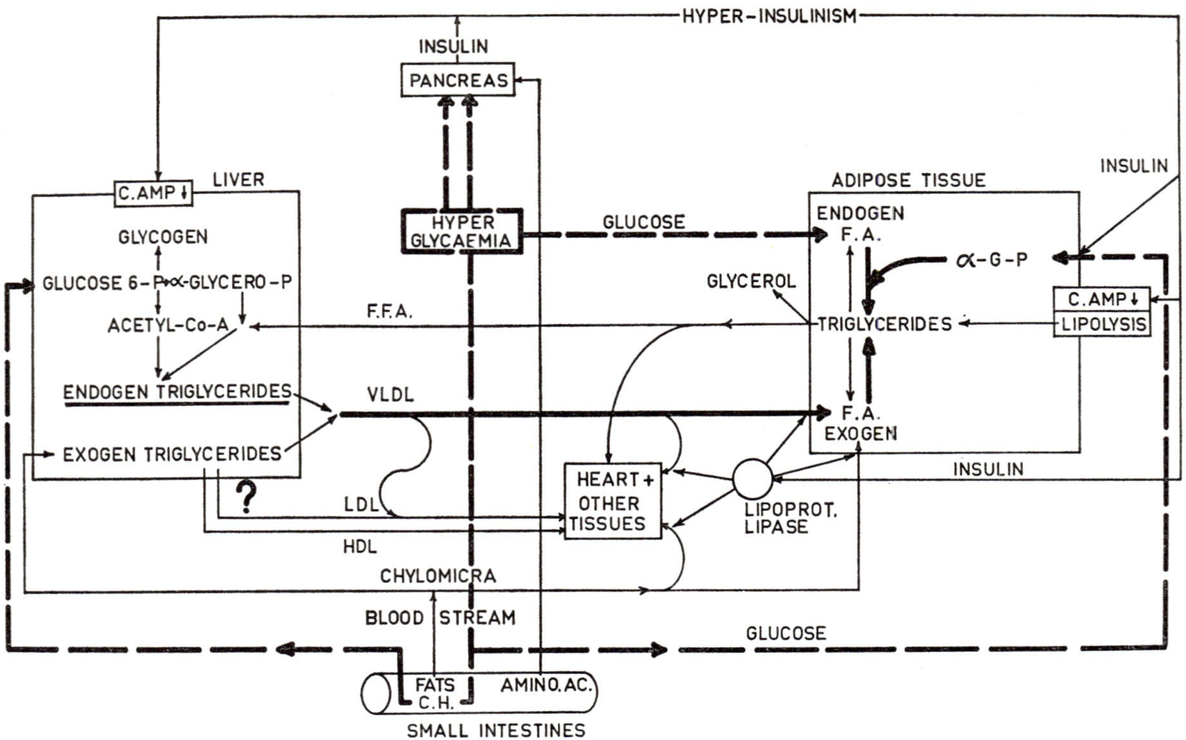


Fig. 3. Under extreme dietary conditions such as an almost fat-free diet the endogenous triglyceride formation is stimulated maximally in the liver, resulting in considerably increased VLDL levels. Because of hyperglycaemia the insulin level rises, as a result of which the lipoprotein–lipase system is activated and cyclic AMP formation blocked. The VLDL are now metabolized at maximal rate and FFA is taken up in the various tissues. Tissue lipolysis is minimal just as the glycerol and free fatty acid levels in the plasma. Fat tissue deposits increase.

production of energy (ATP synthesis) or can be stored as fat. The latter process takes place mainly in the adipose tissue.

The adipose tissue is one of the most active organs in fat metabolism. Its function is the synthesis and storage of fats or release of fatty acids, dependent on the conditions. Glucose offered to the adipose tissue is taken up with the help of insulin and is, to a considerable degree, converted into α-glycerophosphate, which is necessary for triglyceride

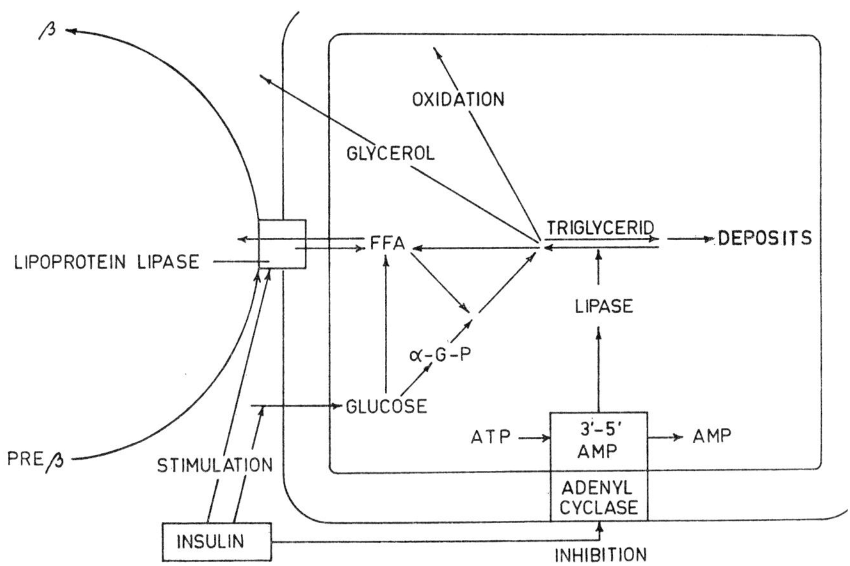


Fig. 4. Uptake and storage of triglycerides derived from plasma or synthesized *de novo* by cells of adipose or vascular tissue in relation to the stimulating or inhibiting effects of insulin.

synthesis with fatty acids derived from lipoproteins. In adipose tissues fatty acids are also synthesized as in the liver, although to a lesser degree (Goldrick, 1967). However, this differs considerably in man and various animal species. These endogenous adipose tissue triglycerides are supplemented with fats from the diet. The dietary fats which are transported as chylomicrons, are split at the capillary walls of the adipose tissues by lipoprotein lipases likewise the VLDL. The fatty acids are taken up and by coupling to α-glycerophosphate transformed into triglycerides (see Fig. 4). It is interesting to note that the triglycerides formed in this way are a reflection of the fatty acid pattern of the dietary fats. The deposits formed from endogenous and exogenous fat are in turn subject to lipolysis by the action of intracellular lipases so that there is a dynamic equilibrium between triglyceride synthesis and lipolysis.

The work of Sutherland and Robinson (1969) revealed that at least one of the above fat-cell lipases, which splits the triglycerides, can cause lipolysis in an activated form only. This activation is dependent on the concentration of cyclic AMP which is also called a "second messenger" since in a way it represents the specific stimulus of many hormones and

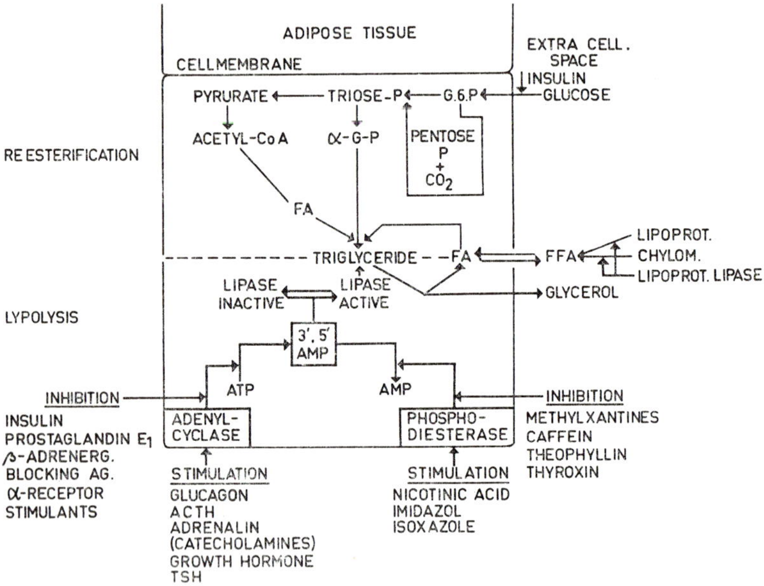


Fig. 5. Scheme of fatty acid synthesis and lipolysis in the fat cell. Insulin stimulates uptake of glucose, which is converted into α-glycerophosphate and to saturated or monounsaturated acids from which triglycerides are formed. The latter are split by the intracellular lipase after which glycerol and free fatty acids are released into the blood stream. This lipase is activated by cyclic AMP which, in turn, is inhibited by insulin and stimulated by other hormones.

pharmaceuticals. The cyclic AMP is formed by the enzyme adenylatecyclase from ATP and broken down by phosphodiesterase. Both enzyme systems are in turn influenced by a series of hormones and pharmaceuticals. The adenylatecyclase for instance is inhibited by insulin and prostaglandin $E_1$ and $E_2$ and further by β-adrenergic blocking agents, whereas it is stimulated by glucagon, ACTH, growth hormone, catecholamines (adrenalin!), TSH and β-adrenergic stimulating agents. The phosphodiesterase is inhibited by methylxanthines (caffeine, theophylline) and probably thyroxine, whereas it is stimulated by nicotinic acid, imidazole and isoxazole (see Fig. 5).

By regarding the cyclic AMP centrally in the process of lipolysis, there appears to be a logical relationship between the action of the many hormones acting on the lipolysis. Probably one of the main regulating hormones is insulin, which affects adipose tissue in the following way:

1. glucose uptake in the adipose tissue increases—resulting in an increased fatty acid synthesis;
2. glucose conversion into α-glycerophosphate increases;
3. insulin has an inhibiting effect on the adenylatecyclase as a result of which less cyclic AMP is formed and lipolysis decreases;
4. it increases the lipoprotein–lipase activity of fat cells, so that more fatty acid uptake may occur from the various circulating lipoproteins, particularly from the chylomicrons and very low density lipoproteins.

Figure 5 shows the process of the lipolysis in the fat cell.

## B. Normal Fat Metabolism

Dietary fats are split in the intestinal lumen, after emulsification, by the pancreatic lipase during which process free fatty acids and glycerol are formed via di- and monoglycerides. After uptake in the intestinal wall these components are re-esterified to form triglycerides, from which chylomicrons are formed after addition of cholesterol, phospholipoids and proteins. These are transported via the lymph spaces and enter the venous bloodstream via the ductus thoracicus. For further details the reader is referred to one of the many surveys. Probably triglycerides are also formed in the wall of the small intestine from endogenous fatty acids which can be compared with endogenous triglyceride synthesis in the liver (Havel, 1970). The chylomicrons reach the various tissues via the bloodstream, from where they normally disappear very quickly with a half-life of 5–15 minutes (Fredrickson *et al.*, 1967). Boberg and Halberg (1969) calculated that fat emulsions can be taken up from the bloodstream by the tissues as chylomicrons in amounts up to 10 g triglycerides/h.

Part of the chylomicrons is taken up by the liver and an important part goes directly to the tissues (Havel, 1969). It is not certain whether for uptake in the liver lipoprotein–lipases are necessary. However, these are engaged in the uptake of fatty acids from the chylomicrons by most other tissues notably by the adipose tissue, for which a hydrolytic lipolysis is essential. The lipoprotein–lipases necessary for this process can normally be found in the capillary endothelium and other tissues and can easily be demonstrated in the plasma after intravenous administration of very small amounts of heparin. In most organs the fatty acids thus taken up are oxidized but liver- and adipose tissue deal differently with the liberated fatty acids. In the liver they are oxidized, and converted into phospholipoids or synthesized to form triglycerides. They reappear as pre-$\beta$-lipoproteins in the bloodstream. The pre-$\beta$-lipoproteins originating from the liver are subject to the same metabolic fate as those which have been formed from carbohydrates, as has already been described.

Thus, in adipose tissue fatty acids from dietary fats are taken up both directly from chylomicrons and indirectly via the triglycerides formed in the liver.

Adipose-tissue fat can be split into glycerol and free fatty acids via the process of lipolysis described earlier. The glycerol, which can no longer be used for the resynthesis into triglycerides, and the free fatty acids may serve as energy sources for most organs. By far the greater part of the fatty acids is transported as so-called free fatty acids which, however, are complex bound to albumin. According to Fredrickson *et al.* (1967) more than 25 g/hr of free fatty acids can be transported via the plasma, in spite of their low concentrations—0·3 to 0·7 mmol/plasma in the fasting state. They are partly taken up in the tissues at a rate of up to 360 $\mu$mol/min (Eaton *et al.*, 1969), partly converted in the liver again into very low density lipoproteins, especially in the fasting state. The triglycerides found in the plasma can therefore originate

1. from free fatty acids originating from adipose tissue after lipolysis;
2. in a carbohydrate-rich diet by direct synthesis in the liver;
3. in a fat-rich diet from chylomicrons.

See also Figs 1, 2 and 3.

## C. Diabetes Mellitus

Disturbances of insulin metabolism are the main factors in the diabetes mellitus syndrome. It is generally assumed that in the juvenile diabetes syndrome there is an almost complete absence of normally functioning insulin. Insulin suppletion is therefore essential in the treatment of this form. The problem is quite different in maturity-onset diabetes, where apart from hyperglycaemia and hyperlipaemia, obesity is almost invariably observed. Characteristic of this syndrome are the regularly observed simultaneous increase of insulin and blood sugar levels in the plasma; apparently the body, even with a high insulin concentration, is not able to bring about a normoglycaemia.

The level of the fasting plasma insulin concentration seems to be connected with the degree of obesity (Bagdade *et al.*, 1967a, b) or rather with fat cell size (Sjöström, 1972; Sjöström *et al.*, 1972). The insulin secretion after glucose uptake is delayed in obese diabetics but continues for a longer period than in normal test subjects. Because of this abnormally slow onset of insulin secretion the increase in the blood sugar content cannot be regulated rapidly enough by uptake in liver and other tissues. The resulting hyperglycaemia often evokes a very high insulin level which is often followed by a reactive, although mild, hypoglycaemia.

In order to compare the abnormal insulin secretion of obese diabetic patients with healthy people, Kipnis and Perley (1966) introduced an insulin/glucose ratio. Seltzer and Smith (1959) and Seltzer *et al.* (1967) suggested the use of the insulinogenic index, based on the difference between the fasting values of glucose and insulin and their increased levels after glucose administration measured at the same time.

Bagdade *et al.* (1967) tried to relativate the insulin response at different body weights by expressing it as a change in percentage with respect to the fasting insulin concentration. With this method he found that invariably the fasting insulin concentration correlated directly with the ideal body weight. Most investigators concluded in this way the existence of a reduced insulin secretion in obese diabetic patients.

These observations and the methods elaborated to compare different groups of patients are all characterized by their non-physiological maximal stimulation of the $\beta$-cells by a single 100-g glucose load instead of comparing the groups in a more physiological way as for instance the reaction to daily food uptake. We did not find any correlation at all between the insulin responses to a maximal glucose load and the reactions after repeated meal distributions during 24 hr in obese diabetics and obese controls in carbohydrate-rich and fat-rich periods (to be published). Also Salans (1973) found in obese patients during high carbohydrate intake compared to low carbohydrate intake an apparently improved glucose and insulin response in oral glucose tolerance tests. There was however, in contrast a worsening of plasma glucose and insulin responses after normal meals.

Cerasi and Luft (1967) considered the basal abnormality in diabetes to be a retardation in the initial insulin response to glucose in the first few minutes. However, not all investigators agreed upon a decreased insulin response to glucose in obese diabetics. Notably Reaven *et al.*

(1971) deny this categorically. Neither did Stephan *et al.* (1972) find any difference in insulin secretion between obese patients with or without diabetes, nor did they find a relationship between basal plasma insulin concentration and body weight or basal plasma insulin and corresponding plasma glucose. The last word with regard to this matter has definitely not yet been said. Another problem which is still unsolved is the difference in insulin reaction after weight loss between obese patients with or without diabetes. Whereas after weight reduction the otherwise normal obese patients show a reduced insulin secretion (Stephan *et al.*, 1972), the reverse seems to be the case in obese diabetics who seem to display a normalization of the insulin secretion (Karam *et al.*, 1965). Be that as it may, most patients with maturity-onset diabetes appear to have so much circulating plasma insulin that this explains why no acidotic phenomena occur. Insulin is in fact a main regulator of storage and preservation of nutritious substances. Normally the islets of Langerhans produce 22–44 units of insulin/day, 40% of which is used immediately in the liver to stimulate several intrahepatic enzyme systems. Insulin is broken down very rapidly and has a half-life of 5–10 min; it circulates at levels of about 10–20 μunits/ml plasma which after glucose uptake rise to 100–150 μunits/ml (Levine, 1970). Acute blocking of the insulin function, for instance by injection of insulin antibodies, will result within a few minutes in the development of the diabetic syndrome with increased blood sugar content and fatty acid concentration in the blood. This means that the β-cells must produce continuously a basal amount of insulin, which in man is estimated at 0·94 μg/hr (Catt, 1970).

What are the stimuli of insulin production and control? Since most of them originate in the diet it is necessary to investigate further this phenomenon. *In vivo*, glucose appears to be the most important substance influencing insulin secretion. Other stimuli (metabolites, hormones, etc.) also appear to be effective but only in the presence of glucose. Apart from glucose the potassium and calcium cations must be present in a certain minimal concentration to enable insulin stimulation, furthermore it seems that the glucose metabolism in the β-cell itself must be intact. The insulin secretion after glucose appears to proceed in two phases; the first rapid phase occurs within one minute after stimulation, reaches its maximum after about two minutes and is exhaustible; the second slower phase is connected with the insulin synthesis and reaches its maximum after 30–60 minutes. This phase is stimulated by growth hormone (Catt, 1970). The β-cells are fully permeable to glucose, which is metabolized to form, e.g. ATP. The rate of glucose oxidation is most likely controlled by the intracellular concentration of cyclic AMP as the $\beta$-cells contain the intact adenylatecyclase and phosphodiesterase system (Kipnis, 1970).

Apart from glucose some metabolites of proteins and fats are also insulin-release stimulants. Particularly the amino acids arginine and leucine are potential although weaker stimulants (Floyd *et al.*, 1970) and to a smaller degree also the fatty acids and $\beta$-keto-acids. Crespin *et al.* (1969) found a large increase of insulin in the plasma during infusion of sodium oleate and glycerol, consistently followed by hypoglycaemia. This has previously been observed in dogs by Seyffert and Maddison (1967). Also triglycerides (Pelkonen *et al.*, 1968) and short-chain fatty acids (Montagne and Taylor, 1968) show an insulin-stimulating effect. Furthermore several nutritious substances also appear to stimulate insulin secretion via gastro-intestinal hormones as secretin, pancreozymin, glucagon, etc. Their mechanisms are only partly known. For further details the reader is referred to, e.g. the review article by Kahil *et al.* (1970).

*1. Insulin Deficiency and Liver Metabolism*

Insulin acts in the liver by decreasing the concentration of cyclic AMP. In insulin deficiency an elevated cyclic AMP concentration, resulting from a lack of inhibition of adrenalin, glucagon, glycocorticoids, etc., gives an increased glycogenolysis, an increased gluconeogenesis from pyruvate and amino acids, a decreased glycogen formation, a decreased potassium uptake and an accelerated metabolism of fats (and fatty acids).

The glucose uptake in the liver as such is not influenced by insulin deficiency (Catt, 1970) owing to the high rate of transport by the cell membrane–glucose carrier system. Glucose breakdown, however, is insulin sensitive. In this process various enzymes play a role as: glucokinase, phosphofructokinase and pyruvatekinase, which are active unidirectional and four other enzymes which can reverse these reactions to the process of gluconeogenesis, notably: pyruvate-carboxylase, phospho-enol pyruvate-carboxykinase, fructose-1, 6-diphosphatase and glucose-6-phosphatase (Atwell and Waterhouse, 1971). Glucokinase is decreased in insulin deficiency, glucose-6-phosphatase, on the other hand, is increased. Phosphofructokinase in the liver probably is stimulated by insulin, this is definitely the case in striated muscles (Beitner and Kalant, 1971).

Figure 6 shows the glycolysis scheme in the liver. Another enzyme, fructokinase, which rapidly converts fructose in the liver into fructose-1-phosphate is not insulin sensitive, so that in diabetes fructose is metabolized and converted into fatty acids much more rapidly than glucose.

Normally about 10–30% of the fructose supplied is converted into glucose (Atwell and Waterhouse, 1971). On the basis of studies with human liver tissue (obtained during operations) Herman *et al.* (1970) found that the phosphorylation reaction for fructose proceeds much more rapidly than that for glucose; in particular the fructokinase

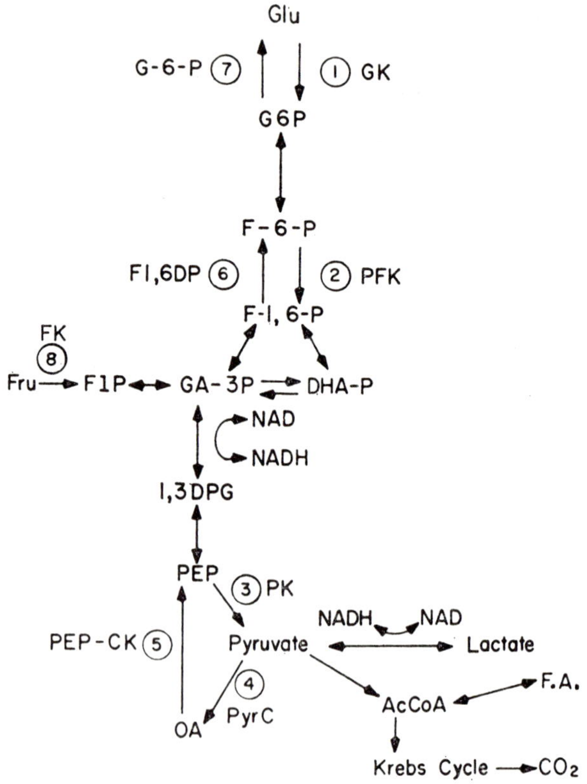


Fig. 6. Glycolysis in liver (after Atwell). The enzymes glucokinase (1), phosphofructokinase (2) and pyruvate kinase (3) give irreversible reactions. See text for explanation of the abbreviations.

activity was much higher than that of glucokinase and hexokinase. These data also show that the rate of glycolysis eventually determines the amount of fatty acids synthesized from it. This is of practical significance since it is common practice in the dietary treatment of patients with diabetes not to restrict fructose as a carbohydrate source, because it has hardly any insulin-stimulating activity. However, then the fact is completely overlooked that the synthesis of saturated triglycerides (especially palmitic acid) from fructose is strongly promoted, whereas by the simultaneous reduction of insulin secretion the insulin-sensitive lipoprotein–lipase system is less stimulated, which in turn may cause a decreased splitting of the triglycerides formed. The above data also explain why sucrose and fructose cause higher triglyceridaemia than glucose (Nestel *et al.*, 1970; Macdonald, 1965, 1966). In insulin deficiency the four above-mentioned enzyme systems which stimulate gluconeogenesis are increased. By the raised cyclic AMP concentration several metabolic steps are stimulated, also promoting gluconeogenesis:

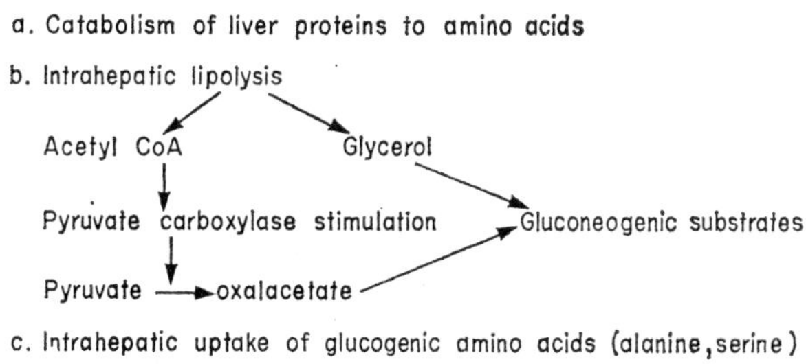


The glucose thus formed can be considered useful in diabetes, especially for the central nervous system, which does not need insulin for its glucose uptake. The increased circulating free fatty acids probably hamper the glucose uptake in other tissues, especially in heart and skeletal muscles, as was postulated by Randle *et al.* (1963). They described a distinct biochemical syndrome, the so-called glucose–fatty acid cycle, which assumes for plasma glucose and free fatty acids a competition concerning the uptake in muscles. Normally the FFA are taken up into the muscle cells more rapidly than glucose which is even accentuated in insulin deficiency. The cycle thus provides a primitive mechanism, which tends to maintain sufficient glucose for glucose-dependent tissues such as the central nervous system.

The triglyceride formation in the liver does not only depend on the fatty acid synthesis, but possibly to an even stronger degree on the availability of sufficient α-glycerophosphate. Jackson *et al.* (1971) are of the opinion that during insulin deficiency, which causes the liver to utilize glucose less easily, other precursors which are all easily available can be used for oxidation instead, for example fructose, amino acids, lactate, pyruvate and glycerol. Therefore Jackson *et al.* conclude that the hypertriglyceridaemia often found in diabetes is caused mainly by increased gluconeogenesis. In more severe insulin deficiency large amounts of free fatty acids are rapidly supplied from the fatty tissues to the liver, as their uptake in the liver is not impeded (Heimberg, 1971); although the normal breakdown is impeded. If this condition is sufficiently prolonged it will lead to fatty infiltration of the liver. Production is now intensified and will result in, for example, synthesis of β-hydroxy-β-methyl-glutaryl-CoA, which is split into aceto–acetic acid and acetyl-CoA.

The water-soluble aceto–acetate and its reduced form, β-hydroxy-butyric acid, are now formed in excess and released into the bloodstream, where these rather strong acids may give rise to acidosis. In the lungs and urinary bladder, for example, the aceto–acetic acid will be decarboxylated to acetone, which explains the origin of the three keto-bodies formed during diabetic acidosis. In the formation of fatty acids from glucose in the liver two rate-limiting steps are recognized: firstly, oxidative decarboxylation of pyruvate to acetyl-CoA which means an irreversible utilization of glucose and secondly, carboxylation of acetyl-CoA to malonyl-CoA, the first specific step in lipogenesis. In insulin deficiency the acetyl-CoA carboxylase is inhibited by the rise of intra-cellular free fatty acids and fatty-acyl-CoA (Numan *et al.*, 1965), which explains the decreased lipogenesis from glucose. So another of the possible pathways to reduce blood glucose concentrations is blocked in this way.

The supply of fatty acids to the liver plays an important role in the hepatic synthesis of triglycerides. Heimberg *et al.* (1969) and Heimberg (1971) found in the isolated rat liver a direct relation between the output of triglycerides and free fatty acids taken up by the liver, however, only to a certain (high) maximum as the output capacity of triglycerides is limited. This acts as a rate-limiting process and causes an accumulation of triglycerides in the liver after too high a supply of free fatty acids.

The output of triglycerides is lowered during insulin deficiency, both with regard to the relative and to the maximal output. An important fact therefore is that although during a relative insulin deficiency the triglycerides output from the liver became higher on increased supply of free fatty acids to the liver, it was still lower than normal. Moreover this output of triglycerides appeared to be directly proportional to the chain length of the fatty acids, but inversely proportional to their number of double bonds. This observation might have important consequences for the diet of diabetic patients, e.g. an increased linoleic acid content of the diet should result in a decreased triglyceride output from the liver; this might explain partly the observed lowering effect on serum triglyceride of diets rich in linoleic acid. How far these processes also play a role in man remains yet to be seen. To summarize: insulin deficiency is responsible for four changes in liver metabolism:

a. the synthesis of triglycerides from carbohydrates decreases;
b. the synthesis of triglycerides from free fatty acids supplied both from the diet and from adipose tissue decreases;
c. the lipolysis of triglycerides stored in the liver increases;
d. in case of rapid fatty acid uptake by strong lipolysis from adipose tissue a fatty infiltration of the liver is risked.

### 2. *Insulin Deficiency and Fat Cell Metabolism*

As already described (p. 238) cyclic AMP appears to play a central role in the metabolism of fat cells (adipocytes) and the effects of insulin can be explained largely by its influence on the cyclic AMP concentration. Metabolism of adipose tissue in man, however, is not the same everywhere. Omental fat for instance is more active in triglyceride synthesis than subcutaneous adipose tissue (Björntorp *et al.*, 1969a) and vice versa—the basal lipolysis is twice as high in subcutaneous fat cells as in omental fat cells (Goldrick and McLoughlin, 1970), probably as a result of the larger size of the subcutaneous adipocytes. Several lipases have been demonstrated in the adipose tissue. Schwartz and Jurigas (1971) isolated from rat epididymal-adipose tissue a series of lipases, e.g. a triglyceride lipase, di- and monoglyceride lipase and short-chain triglyceride lipase (tributyrinase). Only the first one, the triglyceride lipase which is also called hormone-sensitive lipase, is influenced by the cyclic AMP level.

Adipose tissues also contain varying amounts of $\alpha$- and $\beta$-adrenergic receptors, and therefore react differently to noradrenalin (Burns and Langley, 1970). According to Kjellberg and Östman (1971) noradrenalin intensifies via the $\beta$-adrenergic receptors lipolysis and inhibits this via the $\alpha$-adrenergic receptors, whereas the final effect is dependent also on the feeding condition. Insulin is active on various levels of the carbohydrate- and fat-metabolism of the fat cells. Insulin deficiency causes a decrease in the production of $\alpha$-glycerophosphate, necessary for the resynthesis of triglycerides from fatty acids and promotes lipolysis also by the raised cyclic AMP level which activates the intracellular triglyceride-splitting lipase. In serious insulin deficiency this process rapidly leads to depletion of the fat deposits. Fat cell metabolism in maturity-onset diabetes is completely different with its high absolute insulin levels, which although insufficient in normalization of the blood sugar level, are largely sufficient for the fat cell metabolism.

Intact adipose tissue of maturity-onset diabetics metabolizes less glucose than adipose tissue from non-diabetics (Grodsky *et al.*, 1963). According to Kahlenberg and Kaland (1964) this is caused by a defect in the membrane transport of glucose in the diabetic fat cell, so that the glucose metabolism of the fatty tissue is inhibited at various places. The fat cells (adipocytes) in maturity-onset adipose diabetics appear in general to be much larger than in control persons, whereas their number does not increase (Björntorp and Sjöström, 1971). This is also observed in adipose patients without diabetes (Björntorp and Karlsson, 1971). Sometimes also an increased number of adipocytes is found, caused by overfeeding in the very first years of life. The explanation will have to be found in the function of the adipocytes, which must store the excess supply of nutritious substances in the form of fat. To this end insulin is necessary, leading to increased insulin release and increased plasma insulin levels. The latter, however, appears to occur mainly during carbohydrate feeding (Grey and Kipnis, 1971). These investigators found that in obese patients the height of the insulin level was dependent on the carbohydrate supply in the diet. If this was replaced isocalorically by fat, the insulin level decreased. This was confirmed by our group (Houtsmuller *et al.*, 1973). If carbohydrates were again supplied in the diet, the insulin level rose, even during loss of weight by calorie restriction. The fact that the composition of the diet is indeed determinative of the basal insulin level was recently confirmed by Muller *et al.* (1971), who, observing control persons on carbohydrate restriction, noted a rapid decrease of the basal insulin level coupled to a rise in glucagon. Also, the insulin stimulation to protein was distinctly decreased whereas that of glucagon rose. Glucagon increases adipose cell cyclic-AMP level, so causing lipolysis and offering fuel to the body in the form of released fatty acids, sparing at the same time plasma glucose. This increased lipolysis could be promoted in diabetes by an often strongly increased glucagon level (Muller, 1970). The same applies to growth hormone levels, which in diabetes also regularly appear to be raised (Lundbaeck *et al.*, 1971). However, there is also the influence of a diet- and day-rhythm; after food uptake endogenous liver triglycerides are transported to the (fat) tissues whereas in the fasting state more fatty acids shift from the fat deposits to the liver by lipolysis. This rhythm has been demonstrated by Schlierf (1971) and Barter *et al.* (1971) who found the highest levels of insulin during the daytime. The hypertrophic fat cells which are formed during an excessive uptake of calories seem to become less insulin-sensitive (Rabinowitz and Zurker, 1962), which means an increasing stress to the $\beta$-cells of the pancreas. In patients with a diabetic predisposition on a genetic basis, this may lead to exhaustion of insulin production, after which a diabetic condition due to relative insulin deficiency will become manifest. It is interesting to note that on subsequent loss of body weight the sensitivity to insulin of the now smaller fat cells may increase again.

The *de novo* synthesis of fatty acids from glucose is generally low in the human adipocytes (Melatti *et al.*, 1970), but varies widely in individuals. Subcutaneous fat cells with a low basal-fat synthesis activity without insulin in the incubation medium are also the least insulin sensitive. On the basis of his *in vitro* experiments Mellati *et al.* (1970) calculated that a normal average person with a total body adipose-tissue mass of 15 kg of which less than 10% is omental fat can convert only about 3 g glucose/24 hr into fatty acids in the fat tissues. As these findings have been confirmed (Ditschuneit, 1971) this means that it is the liver which is mainly responsible for *de novo* fat synthesis from glucose.

Considerable progress in the study of adipose-tissue metabolism was made after it became possible to determine number and size (Hirsch and Gallian, 1968) of the fat cells, as a result of which the fat cell activity could be calculated on the basis of cell number instead of on basis of weight (diameter) and fatty acid production respectively. Björntorp and Karlsson (1971) found no difference in activity in fat cells of various sizes if calculated on the basis of the number of cells. They found a significant positive correlation between fat cell size and glucose conversion into triglycerides of the adipocytes in adipositas. The larger fat cells had a higher lipoid-to-protein ratio than the small cells. Salans *et al.* (1968) found with a somewhat different technique no difference in basal glucose uptake by adipocytes of obese patients or control persons; he found however, significant differences if calculated on a basis per unit of tissue lipid. The sensitivity of the adipocytes to insulin, was distinctly inversely correlated to cell size. The small fat cells of children are the most sensitive to insulin, whereas the larger fat cells in adipositas have a reduced insulin sensitivity, which is normalized after losing weight.

These results correspond well with clinical observations which indicated a disturbed glucose metabolism in obese patients without clinical diabetes caused by a relative insulin resistance, accompanied by an increased plasma insulin content (hyperinsulinaemia) (Karan *et al.*, 1963; Bagdade *et al.*, 1967a). This insulin resistance is caused by a decreased insulin sensitivity of the fatty tissue of unknown origin. In a recent literature survey Nikkilä and Taskinen (1970) placed more emphasis on this relative inefficiency of the circulating insulin in relation to hyperglycaemia in obese patients. They assume a normal $\beta$-cell response to an exaggerated hyperglycaemic stimulus. Most authors cited by him found, in patients with hypertriglyceridaemia, an increased insulin response to a standard glucose-loading and a positive correlation between the plasma triglycerides and the insulin levels. In obese patients as a rule hyperinsulinaemia and hypertriglyceridaemia were observed. On the basis of his own investigations and those of others Nikkilä supposed the real cause of adiposity to be a primary disturbance in the peripheral glucose uptake with a secondary hyperinsulinaemia. An important fact in this connection is the observation by Farquhar *et al.* (1966) that the plasma triglyceride response to a carbohydrate-rich diet is strongly correlated to the observed glucose tolerance before this diet is instituted.

Nikkilä could divide his obese patients into a group with hypertriglyceridaemia and a group without this abnormality. He could not demonstrate any difference between basal plasma insulin level and insulin secretion in both groups (determined with a method in which a constant-rate of 131J-labelled bovine insulin was infused with a subsequent assay of the specific activity of plasma immunoreactive insulin and calculation of the insulin secretion rate as the ratio of insulin infusion rate and the immunoreactive insulin specific activity). Both groups though had significantly higher insulin parameters (plasma insulin, basal insulin secretion rate and insulin secretion responses to stimuli) that non-obese control persons. Patients with manifest insulin-independent diabetes, however, invariably showed too low an insulin response to a glucose load but could display very high serum triglycerides. Finally the patients with hypertriglyceridaemia displayed a delayed glucose removal after intravenous glucose-loading in relation to the observed plasma insulin levels.

According to Salans and Dougherty (1971) it is possible that the enlarged adipocytes develop altered cellular properties and Smith (1971) and Jahnke *et al.* (1970) indeed demonstrated a decreased ability of insulin to promote glucose oxidation and lipogenesis in enlarged human adipocytes. Of great importance seems the observation by Salans *et al.* (1970) that the kind of the diet followed can influence decisively insulin sensitivity of isolated fat tissue, e.g. a high carbohydrate diet will increase the insulin sensitivity. This corresponds with the observations of Grey and Kipnis (1971), that the insulin level in obese patients is dependent on the amount of carbohydrates in the diet. They assume that the insulin resistance in the obese patients demonstrates an adaptive mechanism, which protects the body against the danger of serious hypoglycaemia, caused by strong insulin stimulation after excessive carbohydrate uptake. According to Hartman *et al.* (1971)

the lipolytic mechanisms of the enlarged adipocytes have not been diminished. According to Nestel *et al.* (1969) the large adipocytes have an even greater lipolysis. Moreover, the turnover of free fatty acids in adipositas seems enhanced (Björntorp *et al.*, 1969b).

To keep the metabolism of the adipocytes in equilibrium, either the activity of the adenylatecyclase–cyclic AMP system should be reduced, or the glucose oxidation increased; for both situations more insulin is necessary. This is possibly one of the causes of insulin resistance of adipose tissues in obesity. The observation that large adipocytes need more insulin than small fat cells seems to be of great significance especially in diabetes complicated by obesity, since adiposity apparently causes a vicious circle—more and more insulin and nutrients being claimed by the adipose tissues at the expense of other organs.

The fat composition of subcutaneous adipose tissue is not different for control persons and adult diabetics having the same dietary composition (Dayton *et al.*, 1967; Hirsch *et al.*, 1960). Albutt and Chance (1969) found the same in normal and diabetic children on a standard diet. They also found a correlation between the content of linoleic acid in fasting plasma and fatty tissue in diabetic children who had been on a diet rich in linoleic acid for some years. The half-life of linoleic acid in human subcutaneous fatty tissue was calculated by Dayton *et al.* (1967) to be between 350 and 680 days. Hirsch *et al.* (1960) found in subcutaneous fat a 30% increase in linoleic acid after feeding corn oil (with about 50% linoleic acid) for 10 weeks, which in children could be achieved after 6–8 weeks (Hashim and Asfour, 1968). During rapid weight increase a fairly fast increase of the linoleic acid concentration of the subcutaneous fat occurred (Dayton *et al.*, 1967). It is clear, however, that it can be negatively influenced by the endogenous triglyceride production from carbohydrates in the diet.

Summarizing: the influence of an increased amount of adipose tissue will result in the necessary increase of plasma insulin to keep fat cell metabolism in equilibrium. The so-called insulin "resistance" should be considered a consequence of obesity instead of being the primary cause (Gordon, 1962). The increased lipolysis in adipose tissue of obese patients enhances the level of the free fatty acids in the plasma, which are taken up by the muscles in preference to glucose, so decreasing glucose consumption resulting in a further insulin stimulation (Lassers *et al.*, 1971). Another consequence is that because of the increased supply of glucose and fatty acids to the liver an increased synthesis of triglycerides is induced, which is reflected in a higher plasma level of pre-$\beta$-lipoproteins.

## IV. CLINICAL CONSEQUENCES OF DISTURBED FAT METABOLISM IN DIABETES MELLITUS

As has already been stated, insulin deficiency does not only cause hyperglycaemia by increasing glucose release from the liver and decreasing uptake in peripheral tissues but also increases plasma free fatty acids by lipolysis from fatty tissue and liver. This lipolysis causes not only a higher content of glycerol and free fatty acids in the plasma but also an increased triglyceride content of Fredrickson's type IV-hyperlipaemia, the so-called carbohydrate-induced lipaemia. During acute absolute insulin deficiency this type of hyperlipaemia will change to type V, since the chylomicrons are no longer sufficiently split.

There is no agreement whether hyperlipaemia in diabetes mellitus is a normal phenomenon. Neither is it clear to what degree this lipaemia is decisively influenced by the composition of the diet. The question whether there is a correlation between the severity of the disturbances in the carbohydrate metabolism and the degree of hyperlipaemia has not been answered adequately. There seems to be a greater correlation between the obesity of diabetic patients and the plasma lipid level. From older data it has already become clear that in assessing the presence or absence of hyperlipaemia, differences exist between plasma lipoids in patients with and without keto acidosis. In uncontrolled diabetes the free fatty acids and triglycerides are increased most and earliest, serum cholesterol the least, whereas the phospholipoids pursue a middle course (Adlersberg, 1958). The hyperlipaemia can reach an extreme degree (Albutt and Chance, 1969).

Adlersberg and Wang (1955) described total lipoid values up to 16 g/100 ml and cholesterol concentrations up to 1480 mg/100 ml. Adlersberg (1958) compared diabetic patients in different states of the disease with control persons. The diabetic patients with a normal blood sugar level had only a slight increase in total fatty acids, triglycerides and total lipoids compared to the control persons. As soon as the blood sugar values became higher the hyperlipaemia rapidly became more severe. The cholesterol, however, remained normal longest. The most abnormal blood lipid compositions were observed in patients with increased blood sugar values and vascular complications. In the pre-insulin area blood cholesterol content in diabetes was also distinctly increased (Joslin *et al.*, 1952), which can be explained by diets rich in saturated fat and cholesterol.

Most investigators found no strict correlation between blood cholesterol and other lipid parameters as, e.g. triglycerides, FFA, etc. Generally an increase in triglycerides or pre-$\beta$-lipoproteins has been found, even in well-regulated diabetes. Also, a rising level of blood lipids is noticed connected to increasing age (Jackson *et al.*, 1971; Pomerance and Kunkel, 1950; Baker *et al.*, 1955; Ejarque *et al.*, 1959; Albrink and Man, 1958; New, 1963; Schrade *et al.*, 1963; Braunsteiner, 1966). In a few studies gaschromatographic methods were used (Schrade *et al.*, 1963; Tuna *et al.*, 1968). Tuna *et al.* (1968) compared 61 diabetics and 21 normal control persons matched for age and sex. The diabetic diet consisted of 35% of calories derived from fats, no supplements rich in polyunsaturated fats were used. The normal control group was on the usual American diet. The only difference between the two diets was a moderate reduction in the fat consumption of the diabetic groups compared to the normals. Total serum fatty acids were clearly increased in diabetic patients with retinopathy and nephropathy or poor control (blood glucose repeatedly higher than 200 mg/100 ml). Regarding their total fatty acid composition in the control group the major fatty acids were found to be palmitic, oleic and linoleic, each represented more than 20% of the total fatty acids measured. Myristic, palmitoleic, stearic, eicosatrienoic and arachidonic acids each formed 1–7% of the total fatty acids. In uncomplicated diabetes only the percentage of palmitoleic acid was significantly lower than normal, stearic acid being increased. In absolute concentrations there was a moderate-to-striking increase in palmitic, oleic and stearic acids.

In diabetic retinopathy and nephropathy an increase in the percentages of myristic and oleic acids of the total fatty acids and definite decreases in the percentages of linoleic, eicosatrienoic and arachidonic acids were found. In absolute terms however, there was an increase in all fractions. These disturbances were seen most strikingly in diabetes with poor control, and probably reflect mobilized fat deposits. The most striking fact seems to be the increased relative deficiency of essential fatty acids in diabetes, with complications. Whether or not this deficiency reflects a need of increased linoleic acid or is a symptom of a diet high in carbohydrates with an increased endogenous production of saturated fatty acids needs to be elucidated. Our own investigations point to the latter possibility which, however, does not exclude the first one. After isocaloric substitution for carbohydrates of polyunsaturated fatty acids in the diet of diabetics, a marked decrease of plasma triglycerides and even cholesterol is seen within ten days. After some months the exudates of diabetic retinopathy—an expression of the plasma lipid level—disappear (Houtsmuller, 1968, 1972).

We have to remember that plasma fatty acids are normally determined in a fasting state and probably reflect the fat deposit composition. It is too often forgotten that they are not representative of the normal, non-fasting blood lipid composition (Schlierf *et al.*, 1971) and, for example, fasting fatty acid values are often the highest of the 24-hr values. It is not only patients with manifest diabetes who show a deviating lipoid spectrum; deviations in the serum lipoids can also be observed in latent diabetes.*

One can see, from the WHO definition of latent diabetes given below, how difficult it is to distinguish between latent diabetes and obesity. Braunsteiner *et al.* (1965) found, in a systematic investigation, latent diabetes in 16 out of 20 patients with hypertriglyceridaemia. The plasma free-fatty-acid concentration in their patients was also increased. They are of the opinion that the increase of triglycerides might be one of the first symptoms of diabetes. These data are even more important now there is increasing evidence that a greatly increased change on myocardial infarction can be expected in patients with a latent or even chemical diabetes.

Righetti *et al.* (1973) compared, on a basis of hyperlipaemia, 48 overt diabetics and 40 latent ones against a group of 47 patients with hyperlipaemia only. Hypertriglyceridaemia and vascular disease (coronary sclerosis and peripheral sclerosis) were more frequent among diabetics than among non-diabetics, and more common among latent diabetics than among overt treated diabetics. These unexpected data were explained by the effect of treatment.

Albrink *et al.* (1962) was one of the first to find abnormalities in the plasma lipid composition of relatives of patients with a known diabetes —confirming the already suspected hereditary basis of this disease (see also Jakobson *et al.*, 1965). Of late, serum lipid abnormalities have also been found in patients with peripheral vascular diseases. Greenhalgh *et al.* (1971) reported hyperlipaemia in 51 out of 166 patients with peripheral vascular diseases, as opposed to 3 out of 50 control persons, the upper limit of normal plasma cholesterol was 262 mg/100 ml, and of triglycerides, 161 mg/100 ml. The most frequently occurring abnormality was an increased content of triglycerides. Ghilchik and Morris (1971) made the interesting observation that the insulin secretion in this type of patient was strongly reduced and could be compared with the pattern of juvenile diabetes.

* *Definition of latent diabetes:*

1. a person in whom the GTT has produced a normal result but who is known to have been diabetic according to a GTT at some time during pregnancy, during infection, when under some other stress, or when obese;
2. a person who has abnormal blood glucose responses (similar to those found in diabetes mellitus) to provocative tests, such as the cortisone-augmented GTT.

From "Diabetes Mellitus", report of a World Health Organization expert committee. World Health Organization technical report series (1965), 310.

There is general agreement about the fact that the dietary carbohydrates in obese diabetic patients cause a prolonged increased plasma–glucose level and increased insulin concentration (Reaven *et al.*, 1967). Bierman *et al.* (1972) however, are not of this opinion. According to most authors this increased supply of glucose and insulin will result in an increased production of triglycerides in the liver, visible in the plasma as an increase in pre-$\beta$-lipoproteins (Salans and Reaven, 1966). In hereditary diabetes with adiposity (and self-production of insulin) and in adiposity with disturbed carbohydrate metabolism, both hyperglycaemia and hyperinsulinaemia are increased, which intensifies the production of triglycerides. Also the basal insulin level is increased (Bagdade *et al.*, 1967) and perhaps most important, the absolute insulin levels in the obese diabetics after glucose stimulation are very strongly increased for a prolonged period, which means an intense stimulation of the liver functions* (see also Jackson *et al.*, 1971).

A possible explanation for the hyperinsulinaemia in mild, adult-onset diabetes is suggested by Estrick *et al.* (1967) who observed an exaggerated insulin secretion by dietary protein in obese diabetes, compared to normals. After a protein load, plasma insulin levels were higher in diabetics than in controls; the inverse was found after a glucose load.

Some indications are available to explain the disturbances in the removal, "clearance", of the hypertriglyceridaemia in diabetes mellitus. Most of them originate from the studies of Bierman *et al.* (1970), Bagdade *et al.* (1968) and Bierman (1971). The pre-$\beta$-lipoproteins from the plasma must be split by lipoprotein lipase before they can be incorporated into the various tissues. There is a distinct disturbance in these mechanisms in types I and V of Fredrickson, where the level of one of the lipoprotein lipases was found to be lowered, just as in myxoedemia (Porte *et al.*, 1965), whereas the lipoprotein lipase in diabetic hyperlipaemia (secundary type IV) seems to be lowered also. This triglyceride lipase is present in postheparin plasma, is insulin sensitive and is decreased in type I, contrary to the diglyceride lipase which splits diglycerides and is probably identical to a monoglyceride lipase (Greten *et al.*, 1970). Both lipases are activated by heparin just like phospholipases (Bierman *et al.*, 1940). Bagdade *et al.* (1968) demonstrated that acute insulin deprivation in insulin-dependent diabetic patients caused a sharp increase in triglycerides by a retarded removal, for which the now decreased lipoprotein lipase was responsible.

* The fact that on comparison of obese patients with and without diabetes the former display less insulin increase after glucose loading than the latter and that the rise per cent of the insulin values with respect to the basal levels are even lower than those of non-adipose normal persons, sometimes make the enormous absolute insulin values look of less importance.

Most patients with diabetes, however, are not in as distinct an insulin-deficient condition as those reported by Bagdade. More interesting is therefore the statement of Bierman (1971) that there appears to be a relative lipoprotein–lipase deficiency in diabetes which can not be detected with normal heparin stimulation, but can be found after exhaustion of it by a continuous heparin infusion. In this process a difference is found between adiposity with and without diabetes. In the latter disease lipoprotein lipase is not exhaustible by continuous heparin infusion, while in obese diabetes it is. The lipoprotein–lipase activity has so far never been assessed at different times for 24 hours. Regarding the rhythm in the insulin level which is high in the daytime and much lower at night, it is very likely that the triglyceride production as well as clearance in the daytime (after meals) is high and falls at night. The fact that the triglyceride level rises during the night points to an increased lipolysis, probably combined with a decreased removal. In our own diurnal studies however, distinct lipolysis at night was seen only in obese patients (Houtsmuller *et al.*, 1973).

## V. HYPERLIPAEMIA AND DIABETIC ANGIOPATHY

There are many indications that the prevalence of vascular degenerative diseases is higher in diabetics than in the general population (Kinsell, 1955). Joslin (1937) concluded that in the pre-insulin period 50% of the causes of death in diabetic patients was diabetic coma, against only 1% in 1950. Fatal vascular lesions in 1930 amounted to 20% against 76% in 1950. Scherf and Boyd (1955) found that 90% of the diabetics showed signs of artherosclerosis after 10 years of diabetes. Schettler and Wahl (1969) made an instructive survey of many statistical data. In particular, the combination of diabetes with hypertension and gallstones appeared to be fatal. Recently it has become clear that nowadays more than 75% of all causes of death in diabetes are caused by chronic vascular disorders (Entmacher and Marks, 1965). Although macro-angiopathy is not specific for diabetes it is present in this disease very frequently and in a severe degree. Notably the frequency of coronary atherosclerosis is twice as high in male diabetics as in non-diabetic patients, whereas this figure for females is even three times as high (Clawson and Bell, 1949), which is particularly important as coronary heart disease in pre-menopausal non-diabetic females is rare. The question now arises whether the degree of the abnormality of the various metabolic aspects of diabetes may account for these serious vascular disorders. The literature on this subject is certainly not unanimous; yet most investigators tend to correlate the degree of diabetic abnormalities directly with the degree of macro-angiopathy; for the micro-angiopathy this seems to be less easy. Root *et al.* (1950) are very positive on this subject as they found a distinct correlation between poorly controlled diabetes, with blood sugars above 200 mg% and with a tendency to acidosis, and an increased incidence of macro-angiopathy.

Ricketts (1955) is of a somewhat different opinion on the relation of atherosclerosis, and degree of control in diabetes. He clearly stated that the "levels of blood lipids . . ., are directly related . . ., to the degree of diabetic control". Thus according to him the problem of diabetic macro-angiopathy can be simplified and related to the degree of accompanying hyperlipaemia, which is also one of the fundamental factors in non-diabetic atherosclerosis.

Adlersberg and Wang (1955) found severe vascular abnormalities even in mild cases of diabetes with "essential" extreme hyperlipaemia. In a prospective study Lowy and Barach (1958) found a higher incidence of lipid abnormalities in those diabetic patients who later showed manifest vascular abnormalities; again blood cholesterol level appeared to be the main predictive factor. Adlersberg and Risler (1959) found however, that triglycerides in diabetic vascular abnormalities were often more increased than cholesterol, which previously had not been investigated systematically. Albrink *et al.* (1963) likewise found a distinct correlation between increased triglyceride concentrations in blood and vascular complications in diabetes. Brausteiner *et al.* (1966) stated as an essential point in the treatment of diabetic vascular complications that neither sulphonylurea nor insulin therapy appeared to be able to prevent hypertriglyceridaemia, not even when the blood sugars were normalized. However, they did not pay attention to the diets of the patients. In this respect the recent publications by Lundbaeck *et al.* (1971) drawing attention to the increased growth-hormone levels in almost all stages of diabetes, seem to be of great importance.

Constam (1965) published the remarkable observation that the late prognosis of the macro- and micro-angiopathic complications of his diabetic patients was dependent on the quality of the therapy in the first five to ten years. This was fully confirmed later on by Caird *et al.*, 1969. Although neither of these two authors investigated serum lipids systematically, the supposition seems to be justified that by the sharp regulation of diabetes the serum lipids hardly deviated from normal or not at all. Constam did not describe the diets of his patients, but judged therapy as very good if the repeated blood sugars were lower than 180 mg/100 ml in more than half of the controls and keto-acidose was nearly always absent. His insulin-dependent patients had a better prognosis than those with so-called mild adult-onset diabetes. Constams' explanation points to a difference in age, the patients with mild adult-onset diabetes being much older than his insulin dependent patients. More likely, in our opinion, is the fact that those with adult-onset diabetics still have self-production of insulin, which can be assumed to be very high, promoting the already mentioned hypertriglyceridaemia. The insulin-dependent patients however, have no possibility for hyper-insulinaemia, pending between hypo- and hyperglycaemic coma. In fact, insulin-dependent diabetics very rarely have exudative diabetic retinopathy, which is, as we have shown, an expression of hypertriglyceridaemia (Houtsmuller, 1968, 1972). This hypertriglyceridaemia in patients with adult-onset diabetes could very well be one of the important reasons for the early and severe atherosclerosis in these patients. Regarding the question whether hyperlipaemia can be the cause of diabetic angiopathy, the results of Fanconi (1955) are alarming. He treated diabetic children from 1932–46 with a diet very rich in saturated fats, and fructose, and low in proteins. Within 16 years all of his diabetic children had a nephropathy, and after 21 years all had died! Prospective investigations in this direction have hardly been carried out. One of the few is that of Ryan *et al.* (1970), who followed a group of juvenile insulin-dependent diabetics who, after 25 years of diabetes still did not show vascular complications. In the following 1–20 years (with an average of 12 years) a third of these patients started to display minimal macro- or micro-vasculopathy. The authors claim that by good control of the carbohydrate metabolism it should be possible to prevent angiopathy or at least postpone it for a prolonged period. Elkeles *et al.* (1971) found in a group of insulin-independent diabetics most of the micro-vascular abnormalities (retinopathy, peripheral neuropathy) in the group with the lowest insulin response to glucose. As expected he also found that this group showed the lowest fasting triglyceride values and the lower body weight. The patients with the higher insulin response also showed a higher degree of excessive weight and more severe triglyceridaemia. The suggestion of Elkeles *et al.* (1971) that the insulin response to glucose is more important in the pathogenesis of diabetic (micro-) vascular complications than the blood sugar level meanwhile seems of great importance.

From Elkeles' studies it is clear that we have to distinguish more sharply between micro- and macro-angiopathy in connection with diabetes. As for the micro-vascular complications, a lack of insulin, perhaps accentuated by a high growth-hormone level, results in a high blood-glucose level. This elevated blood sugar forces intracellularly alternative glucose pathways—of which the polyol and glucuronic acid cycle are the most important. Growth hormone is known to have a counterbalancing effect upon insulin, resulting in high blood glucose levels. This may stimulate the polyol pathway, an alternative pathway of glucose metabolism in which no phosphorylation of glucose is required. When glucose enters into the cells in increased concentration, the hexokinase enzyme which is saturated at normal physiological glucose concentrations is now unable to phosphorylate all intracellular glucose, so that the rather simple insulin-independent polyol pathway is now stimulated, involving the reduction of free glucose to sorbitol. Also the rate-limiting enzyme for this pathway, aldose reductase, is quite active and not so readily saturated even at very high glucose concentrations. At the same time the means of disposing of this polyol, its oxidation to fructose, is limited in many tissues. As a consequence the intracellular production of sorbitol, in insulin-independent cells systems such as brain, retina and endothelial tissue, is increased which can result in intracellular oedema by the osmotic activity of the sorbitol molecule (Morrison *et al.*, 1972). This oedema seems to be one of the serious dangers in micro-angiopathy and neuropathy. Besides the increase of sorbitol in insulin-independent cells sorbitol may accumulate also in insulin-dependent cell systems. Beaumont *et al.* (1971) is of the opinion that growth hormone interacts into the interrelationship of glucose and fatty acid metabolism. By counterbalancing the insulin effects in diabetes fatty acid oxidation is now increased, the levels of acetyl CoA in tissues are raised, which simultaneously increases levels of citrate. The accumulated citrate inhibits phosphofructokinase, so that fructose-6-phosphate accumulates in turn, forming excess glucose-6-phosphate and glucose intracellularly. This intracellular glucose is now converted easily to sorbitol. As the growth hormone mobilizes fatty acids from fat deposits and so raises the FFA level of the plasma, the intracellular fatty acid concentration is increased, resulting in further fatty acid oxidation.

Also in insulin-dependent cell systems the sorbitol increase may be a main cause of their deterioration—thus lack of insulin may be the chief cause of diabetic micro-angiopathy.*

The glucuronic acid cycle, which is also insulin independent, converts phosphorylated glucose to glucose-1-phosphate and uridine diphosphoglucose, in which form it enters the glucuronic acid cycle, from which excess glycoproteins and mucopolysaccharides can be formed, resulting in basal membrane thickening (Spiro, 1959; Kent, 1971).

Contrary to the opinion that a shortage of insulin is the main cause of

* N.B. the sorbitol introduced into the diabetic diet cannot enter into cells with the exception of liver cells, where it is metabolized.

diabetic vascular complications the concept that an excess of insulin is responsible for these phenomena is supported by several investigations. These, however, considered mainly the causes of macro-angiopathy. Mahler (1967) is a convinced promoter of this concept, which is supported by the following biochemical data:

1. insulin stimulates the incorporation of $C^{14}$-labelled precursors of fats into the lipids of the arterial wall;
2. patients with adult-onset diabetes often have a strongly increased plasma insulin content;
3. insulin injected in animals produces an increase in atherosclerosis.

The plasma lipoproteins are split by lipoprotein lipase after which the liberated fatty acids are taken up in the arterial wall where they are coupled to the $\alpha$-glycerophosphate which is produced there. These phenomena are stimulated by insulin as is the uptake of glucose; on the other hand an intracellular triglyceride-splitting enzyme exists (Mahler, 1967) in the arterial wall, whose function is to split the accumulated intracellular lipids so promoting their removal (see Fig. 4). This lipase, which according to Mahler shows some resemblance to intracellular fat cell lipase, is inhibited by insulin, so that by increased insulin concentrations an accumulation of lipids in the arterial wall is stimulated and removal suppressed. A low plasma insulin content would then have a favourable effect, e.g. by increasing lipolysis from the arterial wall. Many supporters of this hypothesis were present at the Fifth Capri Conference April 7–8 1971 (Lundbaek and Keen, 1971), where, e.g. Keen explained the relation between glucose intolerance and arterial diseases in patients without overt diabetes via hyperglycaemia leading to hyperinsulinaemia, as a result of which the increased lipogenesis and retarded lipolysis in the arterial wall as suggested by Mahler could occur. Woolf and Nikkilä appeared to be of the same opinion. Supporting clinical evidence was published by Tzagournis *et al.* (1967) who found increased insulin secretion according to a standard GTT in 22 out of 25 patients under 50 years with myocardial infarction.

Sloan *et al.* (1970) had similar results in a group of patients with peripheral atherosclerotic vascular diseases. They compared carefully 51 patients with this disease with a control group matched for weight and height. In the atherosclerotic group a significantly increased and prolonged insulin reaction after glucose stimulation was observed.

Malherbe *et al.* (1971) likewise found a prolonged and increased insulin response in patients with myocardial infarction without excessive weight and without family history of diabetes compared with matched control persons—although only after an oral glucose stimulus, whereas an intravenous glucose stimulus displayed no difference in insulin reaction. This points to the different $\beta$-cell stimulation of the two methods.

Animal experiments also point to the harmful effect of excess insulin. Stout (1970) administered long-acting insulin to chickens over a period of five months and found definitely more intimal lipid infiltration in the aortas of these chickens than in the control group. In another experiment (Stout, 1971) rats were injected with sodium (1-$^{14}$C)-acetate with and without insulin. The animals were killed one hour later. The results showed that insulin stimulated significantly the incorporation of sodium (1-$^{14}$C)-acetate into intracellular aorta lipids.

Duff *et al.* (1949, 1950, 1954) in a long series of experiments with rabbits found even as early as 1949–54 that alloxan-diabetic rabbits fed a cholesterol-rich diet showed much less aortic atherosclerosis than the control animals. Indeed, a large proportion of the diabetic animals presented no atherosclerosis whatever, although the plasma cholesterol levels were of the same degree in the two groups. When substituting insulin into the alloxan-diabetic rabbits, the inhibition of aortic atherosclerosis was thus obviated.

Cruz *et al.* (1961) injected insulin into one femoral artery of 19 alloxan-diabetic dogs and saline in the other. He reported a significant increase of artery tissue cholesterol and fatty acids in the insulin-injected leg on comparing this leg with the saline-administered one. One has to remember with regard to these results that the fact that in Fredrickson's type I hyperlipaemia with a very elevated level of blood lipids no increased atherosclerosis occurs, probably due to the inefficiency of the lipoprotein lipase in this disease to split the plasma lipids. An identical process plays an important role in experimental animal diabetes, e.g. the now insufficient insulin-dependent lipoprotein–lipase system.

Even more difficult than finding a correlation between the possible causes of increased macro-angiopathy in diabetes is to discover the causes of micro-angiopathy. The only well known factor is the time elapsing between the first manifestation of diabetes and the manifestation of micro-angiopathy, which appears to be 10–15 years (Constam, 1965; Mehnert, 1969). A good recent survey is given by Mehnert (1969) who discusses the pros and cons of the two opposing standpoints:

1. good control of carbohydrate metabolism will inhibit micro-angiopathy;
2. micro-angiopathy seems to be independent of any therapeutic approach to regulate CHO metabolism.

An argument used by the advocates of the latter point of view is based on thickening of the basal membrane of the capillaries which seems to exist already before the biochemical abnormalities of carbohydrate- and fat metabolism become manifest. However, Mehnert rightly points out that this thickening is not necessarily synonymous with clinical micro-angiopathia. Moreover, the data on this subject are scarce and controversial, thus, for example, Williamson *et al.* (1970) and Kilo *et al.* (1972) found an increase in thickening of the basal membrane with age whereas 43 % of the diabetics examined showed basal membranes no thicker than those of control persons. Also Osterby Hansen *et al.* (1966) and Amherdt *et al.* (1971) were not able to demonstrate a thickening of the basal membrane, compared with matched controls. An important argument, in favour of the other hypothesis, that the diabetically-changed metabolism itself has a deteriorating influence on the micro-angiopathy, is the fact that only after diabetes has been manifest for a number of years does micro-angiopathy occur, or at least become clinically manifest. If heredity does play a role in the development of the diabetic micro-angiopathy it is impossible to explain why most patients do not develop this abnormality until 30–50 years after birth, i.e. usually 5–15 years after the disease becomes manifest. Moreover it was observed by Mehnert (1969) that in the periods of starvation, as during World War II, micro-angiopathy seemed to be inhibited to the same extent as the diabetic condition.

Finally, experimental investigations with rats made diabetic by streptozotocin such as those of Renold (1971) and Lenenberger *et al.* (1971) who demonstrated retinal microangiopathy occurring after six months also support the concept that disturbances in the diabetic metabolism are to be held responsible for clinical retinal micro-angiopathy. The failure of common therapeutic measures to prevent micro-angiopathy therefore should probably be explained by their inadequacy and/or lack of adherence of the treated patients to the therapy.

## VI. THE ROLE OF FAT IN THE TREATMENT OF DIABETES MELLITUS

From the previous sections it should be clear that diabetic patients, even if their disease is well regulated, have a tendency to develop hyperlipaemia which is known to promote atherosclerosis. For this reason a fat-rich diet seems at first sight to be illogical. On the other hand it has been demonstrated that in most of the insulin-independent diabetics a hyperinsulinaemia occurs which might promote hypertriglyceridaemia.

This combination of hypertriglyceridaemia and hyperinsulinaemia promotes atherosclerosis in particular. As a carbohydrate-rich diet will aggravate hyperinsulinaemia in these patients this would also seem to be the wrong therapeutic approach. To find what the optimal dietary pattern in diabetes should be in order to prevent the development of the main cause of death of diabetic patients, namely angiopathy, two groups of data may provide important information, notably:

geographical differences in dietary treatment of diabetes mellitus, including war conditions;
results of experimental diets, taking a strict or non-strict diabetes treatment into consideration.

## A. Geographical Differences in Diets

Although much research has been carried out on the relation of dietary compositions and different health aspects in various countries, those concerning dietary influences on diabetes are few. Even scarcer are data which could throw light on the question whether differences in composition of the diets prescribed to diabetics influence the development of macro- or micro-angiopathy. One of the problems is the low average life expectancy of the population in the developing countries, which therefore does not reach the age for the detection of maturity-onset diabetes. Ahuja (1969) for instance, reported that the average age in India in 1969 was 44 years so that most diabetics examined belonged to the group of the juvenile diabetics. A low atherosclerosis and myocardial infarction prevalence was found in Jamaicans, Japanese, Bantu negroes and Yemenite Jews with diabetes who, however, as a rule have a diet deficient in calories.

West and Kalbfleisch (1971) described the difficulties as follows:

> "Among the problems which have made it difficult to evaluate the associations between prevalence of diabetes and nutritional factors have been the paucity of systematically collected data on nutrition in populations where prevalence of diabetes has been established (and vice versa), the lack of uniformity in methods and definitions, and difficulties in obtaining representative samples of age-matched populations."

Early in diabetes research a variety of this disease, which was hardly encountered in Western Europe, was recognized in the tropics and was called the J-type by Hugh-Jones (1955). This type is characterized by a start at early age, thinness, the need for a large amount of insulin but usually no development of ketonuria. This abnormality was also reported from Ceylon and India. According to Tripathy and Kar (1965) this type was caused by undernutrition, and feeding CHO (rice) in large amounts, often only once every 24 hours. Tripathy assumes the presence of a constant high concentration of growth hormone in the long periods between meals during which the fat deposits are completely mobilized resulting in high free fatty acid values in the plasma. This may explain the great insulin need. In addition to the growth hormone also a raised glucagon level can explain the "insulin resistance" in these thin young diabetics (Unger, 1971). It is important that in this type serious vascular abnormalities are observed both of the macro- and micro-angiopathic type in the absence of frequent acidosis.

Contrary to the undernourished diabetics without ketoacidosis of the tropics, diabetes appears to be extremely rare in groups of people in the arctics such as the Eskimoes. So Sageld *et al.* (1966) reported the extremely low incidence of diabetes of only 0·06% among Eskimoes. The diet of these people consists mainly of fish, and although Sagild suggested that racial characteristics were responsible, the possibility of the combination of a low CHO diet with large amounts of polyunsaturated fat in the diet should, however, seriously be considered as a cause of this low frequency. Supporting this concept is the observation of Mouratoff *et al.* (1969) who compared another group of Eskimoes from Alaska with Indians from the same area and likewise found in both groups a very low diabetes frequency. Both groups had a diet rich in protein, low in carbohydrates and moderate in fat and were physically very active. Further details were not given.

A detailed comparative study on diabetes prevention and nutrition in various countries was carried out by West and Kalbfleisch (1966), who in four countries, namely Uruguay, Venezuela, Malaya and East-Pakistan, ascertained the possible relation between diabetes frequency and nutritional habits. Only persons of over 30 years were examined. The existence of possible diabetes was investigated with the aid of an oral glucose load. In Uruguay 6·9% appeared to have "diabetes", in Venezuela 7·3%, in Malaya 3·5% and in East-Pakistan 1·5%.

The diet in Uruguay was typically Western, i.e. rich in calories, animal protein and animal fat. The diet in Pakistan and Malaya was typically Eastern, i.e. low in calories, protein and animal fat. The greater part of the calories originated from rice. The Venezuela diet lay in between these two extremes. Another important aspect was that in Uruguay 34·4% of the persons examined were obese, in Venezuela 14·8%; in Pakistan and Malaya no obesity was found. The only correlation which could be found was that of obesity and diabetes, irrespective of the composition of the diet which had led to this obesity. West and Kalbfleisch (1971) also reported in 1971 an extension of their investigation to ten countries. Groups of people in Uruguay, Venezuela, Malaysia, East-Pakistan, Costa Rica, El Salvador, Guatemala, Honduras, Nicaragua and Panama were examined.

In general a positive association was observed between the prevalence of diabetes and fat- and sugar-uptake, in addition to a negative association between the prevalence of diabetes and the total carbohydrate consumption. However, it should be noted that the total caloric uptake was lowest in the groups which received a carbohydrate-rich diet. The incidence of diabetes was further correlated with increased serum cholesterol levels. Although in general a correlation was suspected between sugar uptake and diabetes, there appeared to be impressive differences between the groups examined. For example the sugar uptake in Malaysia and Venezuela was the same, the frequency of diabetes, however, was twice as high in Venezuela. In Malaysia much more sugar was used than in El Salvador, yet the diabetes frequency was the same. However, the main conclusion of West and Kalbfleisch, was undoubtedly that when the diabetics in the various countries were matched for adiposity possible inter-racial differences were no longer demonstrable. So probably the incidence of diabetes is better correlated with an excess of (carbohydrate) caloric intake rather than the quantity of sugar actually consumed.

From the few geographical investigations on the possible correlation between nutrition and diabetic vascular diseases, the only conclusion that can be drawn for the time being is that obesity invariably plays an important role in induction of diabetes and diabetic angiopathy. Interesting in this connection is the study by Schöffling and Graeve (1956b) of the starvation period in Germany 1943–47, which was accompanied by a drastic drop in both macro- and micro-angiopathy. However, one should realize that apart from the change to a low-caloric diet (mainly carbohydrates) during the starvation period, there was also less smoking and more physical exercise. Yet the investigation by Schöffling indicates that some (drastic!) measures are able to have a favourable influence on the prevention of diabetic angiopathy.

## B. Dietary Experiments

Contrary to the relative lack of usable epidemiological facts regarding nutrition and diabetes, many nutrition experiments concerning this relationship have been published. These can be divided in two main groups:

those in which the level of blood and urine glucose concentration were assessed (sharp diabetes control versus free diabetes treatment);

those where the difference in composition of the diet was assessed (fat versus carbohydrates).

In the last few years some investigations have been carried out to see whether saturated fats behave differently from unsaturated ones, whereas the question whether short-chain or long-chain carbohydrates have different effects in the treatment of the varying forms of diabetes appears hardly to be under discussion, certainly not in more prolonged investigations. Finally it is striking that there are almost no prospective investigations in progress studying the influence of dietary changes on the prognosis of an already existing diabetes.

It has taken a long time for us to become aware of the interrelation between carbohydrate and fat metabolism; even in 1952 Joslin wrote that carbohydrates in the normal individual are almost totally stored as liver- and muscle glycogen, lying in the order of magnitude of 200–500 g, and that the fat in the livei originated from the dietary fats.

In the first 20 years of this century fat was the main source of calories for the diabetic: the development of obesity was encouraged. Around 1918 the reduced-calorie diet of Allen found acceptance. After the introduction of insulin the allowed amount of carbohydrate could be steadily increased. Joslin and White (1965) advised a "normal" ratio of 50% cal. carbohydrate, protein 15% and fat 35%, whereas at that time the American Diabetes Association (ADA) recommended 40% carbohydrate in addition to 15% protein and 45% fat. In 1971 a committee of the ADA (Bierman *et al.*, 1971) suggested a diet with 45% or even more carbohydrates. This report was extremely carefully worded, which is probably a demonstration of the sharp division of contradictory opinions existing at the moment concerning the way diabetics should be nourished. Even with regard to the problem of whether diabetes patients should be well-controlled or only superficially regulated there appears to be no unanimous opinion. As almost all investigations suffer from the restriction of the criteria used: namely, only some criteria of carbohydrate metabolism were studied, mainly blood sugars and urine reduction, the existence of this uncertainty is not astonishing. The complexity of the problem is also increased by the fact that often no sharp separation is made between macro- and micro-angiopathy; the macro-angiopathy as a phenomenon is non-specific for diabetes and cannot be differentiated from atherosclerosis without diabetes; the micro-angiopathy however, appears to be almost specific for diabetes. Keiding *et al.* (1952b) were the first to observe a distinct higher frequency of macro- and micro-angiopathy in poorly controlled diabetes while Fanconi (1955) was one of the first to set out the dangers of various dietary possibilities sharply against each other. He described the late effects of various diets in diabetic children: notably the "Fruchte-Gemüse-Dauerkost" propagated by him from 1934–48 which was poor in protein and very rich in saturated fat appeared to be fatal. As already mentioned, 21 years after the beginning of this treatment none of the children were alive. Fanconi suspected that the high (saturated) fat content of the diet in addition to the protein restriction particularly promoted the fatal nephropathy. The Joslin school which is accepted by most clinicians, has always held the view that a rigid diabetes control can retard micro-angiopathy. Preferably, conclusive results should be based on prospective studies which, however, in Marble's opinion (Marble, 1965) could not be achieved because they were impractical and unjustifiable especially with insulin-dependent diabetics.

The follow-up period should be sufficiently long and preferably one should start with patients between 20 and 30 years. Furthermore the beginning of the diabetes must be sufficiently characterizable, which especially for maturity-onset diabetes is often impossible since it can remain asymptomatic for a long time. One of the most assessible retrospective studies is that by Johnsson (1960) from Sweden who followed two groups of young patients, the first from 1922–35 on a strictly regulated diet and the second one from 1936–45 on a free diet. The micro-angiopathy in the latter group was significantly more serious than that in the first. A remarkable detail was that patients with frequent hypoglycaemic comas showed a very low micro-angiopathy frequency. As stated previously (see p. 257), Rickets (1965) adopted a more careful attitude in assessing the influence of diabetic control on angiopathy. In vascular abnormalities the concentration of plasma mucopolysaccharides as well as of lipoproteins appeared to have increased. Ricketts found that in most cases of distinct hyperlipaemia the diabetes control was insufficient. Mucopolysaccharides, however, were also increased in well controlled diabetes. Ricketts also cited a critical assessment by Knowles of 300 publications on diabetes control, from which it appears that almost all studies which had appeared up till then were more or less insufficient, as here also the criteria used were only glycosuria and blood sugars. Regarding the micro-angiopathy there seemed to be little difference in results between free diet and strict control according to Knowles. However, as already said it remains essential to keep the assessment of macro- and micro-angiopathy separate. Although micro-angiopathy in the form of blindness caused by diabetic retinopathy is dramatic, a much greater hazard is of course the occurrence of the myocardial infarction, a macro-angiopathic complication.

In our opinion chronic renal insufficiency complicating diabetes is a combination process of both abnormalities. In 1968 Knowles considered diabetes control as "a return to normal of the abnormalities caused by insulin insufficiency", leaving undecided the question whether prevention of the thickening of the basal membrane of the muscle capillaries, which can also be found in blood relatives of diabetes patients (Siperstein *et al.*, 1968) should be included. Knowles still hesitated to decide whether a close control of the patients would have a favourable influence on the prevention of diabetic retinopathy on account of the commonly accepted argument that the real cause of diabetic retinopathy is unknown and probably mainly genetically determined.

Since then a number of facts have been published demonstrating the dominating influence of the biochemical disturbances in insulin deficiency as a cause of diabetic retinopathy. (See for instance the already mentioned results of Renold (1971) with rats diabetic due to streptozotocin treatment and the results of Bloodworth in dogs made diabetic with growth hormone.) Griffiths *et al.* (1971) observed in patients with haemochromatosis who were kept alive the occurrence of diabetic retinopathy, the degree of which was dependent on the length of period of haemochromatosis. On account of these experiments it seems that the supporters of the heredity theory who see the development of diabetic micro-angiopathy independent of the control will have to reconsider their—rather negative—therapeutic approach. Caird (1968) and Constam (1965) adopted a more positive attitude. The results of Joplin *et al.* (1971) are even more positive than those of Caird. These authors found a favourable effect of the adherence to a strict diet even in patients with manifest diabetic retinopathy.

Whereas the main attention in the controversy of the merits of a strictly controlled diet versus a free one is gradually shifting from blood sugar levels to plasma lipids as the more important criterion, the problem really should be settled using criteria such as insulin, growth hormone and glucagon, etc., concentrations in the blood. Some important conclusions can be drawn from nutritional experiments in normals and diabetics. In general the more carbohydrate in the diet the larger the synthesis of triglycerides. These facts are more pronounced in older people or patients with carbohydrate intolerance (Glueck *et al.*, 1969). Also the conversion of short-chain carbohydrates into saturated triglycerides is greater than that of starch (Kaufmann *et al.*, 1966; Macdonald, 1965; Nestel *et al.*, 1970). We ourselves investigated, during a study on triglyceride formation in diabetes in some control persons, the effects of isocaloric conversion of glucose, fructose and starch into triglycerides, some effect being observed of fructose in the case of 40 cal % carbohydrate. Nestel *et al.* (1970) found that for diets with about 70–80 % carbohydrates invariably higher plasma triglyceride levels of sucrose instead of starch whereas the insulin response in the sucrose periods was invariably the highest. This insulin response was obtained by measuring insulin reactions after intravenous glucose administrations. If the percentage of fats was increased, the triglyceride formation was mainly controlled by the type of fat, polyunsaturated fats giving the lowest values. The observation by Nestel *et al.* that the removal of triglycerides was stimulated mostly by polyunsaturated fatty acids was particularly interesting. On the basis of the above data it can be assumed that the lipogenic effect of sucrose with respect to starch is neutralized by a sufficient concentration of polyunsaturated fatty acids. This is particularly essential in the case of carbohydrate-sensitive patients as was demonstrated by Little *et al.* (1970).

This means that a diet high in polyunsaturated fatty acids is most recommendable even for normal persons, as the lower the lipid content of the plasma the lower will be the risk of atherosclerosis. Furthermore, it appears that the basal insulin level and the insulin secretion after carbohydrates increase gradually with the percentage of dietary carbohydrates. The type of carbohydrates also plays an important role. Rosen and Shafrir (1972) found for equal glucose and fructose loads four times as much insulin stimulation after glucose. Yet in both cases the free fatty acid level dropped in the same order of magnitude which reflects an increased triglyceride formation in fat tissue. The glycerol release, however, was not equal, being much higher after fructose load, which means less antilipolytic action of fructose. From these facts it seems that the insulin-independent uptake of fructose supplies sufficient energy to form α-glycerophosphate for FFA esterification, with at the same time an insufficient insulin level to block lipolysis. Grey and Kipnis (1971) observed, when testing obese persons, a rise of 50 % in basal plasma insulin when a low carbohydrate diet was isocalorically replaced by high carbohydrate diet. Even when a hypocaloric diet was given the insulin level appeared to rise considerably after replacing the diet poor in carbohydrates by one rich in carbohydrates which may mean a fundamental change in the concept of hyperinsulinaemia in adipose patients—in which case in general a peripheral insulin antagonism is assumed.

Rabinowitch described as early as 1935 a decreased atherosclerosis development in patients with diabetes mellitus, whom he treated with a low-calorie and carbohydrate-rich diet. He held the diet-induced fall in serum cholesterol level responsible for this.

Singh (1955) made a survey of the experimental data concerning the effects of carbohydrate-rich nutrition in diabetes in addition to his own experiences with 80 mild insulin-dependent diabetics, who because of the carbohydrate-rich diet gradually seemed to need less insulin. On GTT investigation 74 of the patients demonstrated a decreasing two-hour glucose value which points to a sufficient endogenous insulin secretion. He however, put his patients on not only a high-carbohydrate diet, but also on a caloric restriction of 1600–2200 calories, so that his results are not easy to evaluate. Kempner *et al.* (1958) published the results of their 15 years' experience with rice diets (more than 90% of the calories originating from carbohydrates) in 100 diabetics with micro-vascular complications, particularly diabetic retinopathy. The mean period of treatment was 22 months, a rather short period. The mean blood sugar values and insulin requirement decreased; acidosis was hardly observed. The most likely factor was again the weight decrease of the obese patients which *per se* may be responsible for the decrease of the cholesterol levels observed and the improvement of the clinical symptomatology. At the beginning of the treatment a distinct diabetic retinopathy was observed in 48 patients. In 13 of this group the aspect of the fundus retinae improved, in 15 there was no progression. The assessment of a possible improvement of the retinopathy by the rice diet itself is further hampered by the fact that hypertension and the obesity were also favourably influenced. No mention is made of the effect on the 28 patients from his series who did not require insulin therapy and so had a good chance of developing hypertriglyceridaemia. After reading of such results, one is inclined to prescribe a carbohydrate-rich diet to diabetic patients forgetting that the results are mainly caused by the loss of body weight. As will be seen later, the results with a high-fat diet are the same or, in case of a linoleic-rich diet, even much better. The effect of a low-fat diet in diabetic retinopathy was described more accurately by Van Eck (1959) who observed 12 patients who had been on this diet for some months up to three years. The daily diet consisted of maximally 20 g fat and 80 g protein, the other calories were obtained from *ca* 400 g carbohydrates. It was striking that on replacement of the fat present in the previous diet *ca* 100 g/day, by *ca* 400 g carbohydrates the patients did not require an increased amount of insulin, provided this replacement took place gradually. Only in a few cases the body weight changed. A striking feature was the decrease of the serum cholesterol and total triglyceride content in most patients; also the hard retinal exudates, mainly composed by and originating from plasma lipoproteins (especially very low density lipoproteins), decreased after a few months or disappeared in five out of ten patients which suggests a correlation between plasma lipids and these exudates. Bierman and Hamlin (1961) were amongst the first to recognize the hyperlipaemic effect of a high-carbohydrate diet in diabetes. For five insulin-dependent patients two liquid-formula diets were compared with (a) a 40% corn oil, 45% carbohydrate and 15 cal% protein composition and (b) an 85% carbohydrate, 15% protein composition without fat. On the second high-carbohydrate diet the fasting plasma triglycerides rose two- to four-fold. The insulin requirement did not increase in his investigation. There was no decrease in the cholesterol content as described by Van Eck, probably as this was already lowered by the previous corn oil–carbohydrate diet. Ernest *et al.* (1965) described the effect of a 70% carbohydrate, 20% protein, 10% fat diet in nine insulin-dependent patients with diabetic retinopathy. Most of the patients showed a distinct weight decrease at the beginning, after which constant weight was maintained. The mean insulin requirement likewise decreased, so that it is not surprising that the plasma lipids decreased even in the first few weeks after the beginning of the diet. The main detail was the uniform regression in the hard retinal exudates which became visible after about six months. The proliferative abnormalities, consisting of newly formed inferior capillaries, were not influenced favourably.

The same result, however, was reported by King *et al.* (1963) who with a 70 cal% corn-oil diet also observed a decrease in cholesterol and total lipids, followed by a decrease of retinal exudates. Patel *et al.* (1969) described a group of 25 diabetics in India, who on account of their vegetarian principles followed a diet with an average of 67% carbohydrates. The mean age of the patients was 50 years, all were adult-onset, non-insulin dependent diabetics. During this treatment the blood sugar level could be regulated easily by changing the dose of oral antidiabetic drugs; some patients gained weight. Blood lipids were not assessed, possible vascular complications were not reported. Brunsell *et al.* (1971) examined the glucose and insulin reactions of nine non-diabetics and thirteen non-insulin dependent borderline or mild diabetics with two diets, which each were administered for ten days. One diet contained 40% fat, 45% carbohydrates and 15% protein, the other diet 85% carbohydrate and 15% protein. The carbohydrates consisted of dextrose and dextromaltose. On comparing the two groups the GTT appeared to have decreased during the carbohydrate-rich diet, however, the insulin secretion had not changed. The fasting glucose levels were lower for all patients during the carbohydrate-rich diet; the basal insulin levels were likewise decreased. The incremental insulin area or the percentage insulin area however, did not. At the first sight these data are remarkable. The differences in basal insulin levels, however, do not give a good picture of the total group investigated. The insulin concentrations were not lower for the seven non-diabetic patients, this effect was achieved by great differences in levels in two of the diabetic patients examined, of which in total only five out of thirteen were examined.

It seems very unlikely that on account of this irregular insulin distribution it may be postulated that the mean fasting insulin levels of the diabetics decreased during the carbohydrate-rich period. Unfortunately it was not indicated clearly which of the two diets was given first since an exchange from 40 % fat in short-chain carbohydrates may have a different effect on the insulin levels, than a change from carbohydrate to fat. It is also regrettable that the composition of the fat was not given. Finally it is remarkable that the basal insulin levels of the five diabetic patients were not higher than those of the control persons, 18·1 versus 20·8 $\mu$units/ml, whereas their body weight differed, 127·6% against 116·4%. However, the correlation between excess of weight and increased basal insulin levels of the persons examined individually was clear. Brunsell *et al.* (1971) reported an increase in triglyceride levels during the carbohydrate-rich period although details were not given.

Bierman (1972) added that the acute insulin response after intravenous glucose loading increased significantly on high-carbohydrate diets. This fact easily explains the decrease in fasting glucose levels and weakens the suggestion of Bierman that by a high-carbohydrate diet in diabetes the peripheral sensitivity for insulin is enhanced. His conclusions regarding diet for diabetics are rather dangerous. In spite of his own findings that an increase in carbohydrate content of the food increases triglycerides-production also (Bierman and Hamlin, 1961; Brunsell *et a.*, 1971) he stated:

> "The implications with regard to the carbohydrate content of the diabetic diet may be simply stated: there is no evidence to support disproportionate restriction of dietary carbohydrate in the diabetic diet when fasting hyperglycaemia is otherwise treated by insulin or by oral agents. In the subject with mild glucose intolerance and normal fasting plasma glucose concentration, restriction of calories, since such individuals tend to be obese, usually suffices to normalize glucose tolerance. In that case as well, there is no rationale for disproportionate restriction of carbohydrate while calories are being reduced. The empirical improvement with 'carbohydrate restriction' that is noted in clinical practice in such patients could

> easily be attributable to the well-established effect of simultaneous caloric restriction . . .. Higher carbohydrate diets may have some long term benefits since such diets are associated with lower proportions of dietary fat and cholesterol. Whether or not over the long term this will improve the outlook for the diabetic patient so prone to develop severe atherosclerosis prematurily remains to be determined."

The facts Bierman overlooks are firstly that people will not easily reduce their weight in the western countries, and secondly that in taking a diet rich in polyunsaturated fatty acids, the cholesterol content is cut down at least to the same ratio.

Summarizing the scarce publications on extreme carbohydrate-rich diets in diabetes it appears that the insulin requirement does not increase, provided the carbohydrate conversion proceeds gradually. From some publications it appears that the weight may decrease (Kempner) and probably connected with this is a decrease of cholesterol and total triglyceride (Van Eck), probably also caused by weight decrease since Bierman *et al.* observed a rise in triglycerides. The most positive result seems to come from the retinopathy improvement. Notably the hard exudates disappeared in most patients of Kempner, Van Eck, Ernest and King which invariably seem to have been preceded by a decrease in plasma lipids. These investigations, however, are partly controversial regarding the triglyceride behaviour, so that far-reaching conclusions cannot for the time being be drawn.

## VII. RESULTS OF A FAT-RICH DIET ON DIABETES

Only a few publications exist on this subject contrary to the many investigations into the prevention of cardiovascular diseases in non-diabetic persons. I shall restrict myself only to the investigations with polyunsaturated fatty acids since the poor experiences with diets high in saturated fat from the pre-insulin period should not be repeated.

Since the observation by Kinsell *et al.* (1952) that administration of linoleic acid causes a strong decrease in plasma lipids, some investigations have been carried out on diabetes patients. In a discussion on diet and diabetes Kinsell (1967) reported:

> "The arguments in support of such a diet are, paradoxically enough, essentially the same as those advanced in support of the high-carbohydrate–low-fat diet, namely, that for the average patient a better diabetic control is achieved and, conceivably some beneficial effect upon vascular complications results."

Thus Kinsell confirmed less emphatically that the effect on the diabetes control as such is the same for carbohydrate- and fat-rich diets, i.e.

dependent on the intensity of the treatment rather than on the composition of the diet. In the case of strict diabetes control, it is not illogical that the blood lipids are hardly increased or not at all as long as there is no excessive weight and the blood sugars do not deviate too much from the normal values.

Unfortunately with our level of prosperity this strict control is an exception, so that it is indeed important to know how blood lipids are influenced by dietary measures under practical conditions. In general, diet experiments have established that a high concentration of linoleic acid has a greater lipid-decreasing effect than a diet low in fat and rich in carbohydrates.

Kinsell *et al.* (1959a) named three conditions as essential for every diabetes diet: 1. acceptability; 2. optimal balance between diet and long-acting insulin to avoid hyper- and hypoglycaemia and 3. maintaining the plasma lipids at the lowest possible level. Bearing in mind the "ideal" diabetes control as formulated by Knowless (1968)—"return to normal of the abnormalities caused by insulin insufficiency"—a fourth condition might be added namely: normalization of insulin, growth hormone and probably also glucagon levels should be tried.

Kinsell (1959a) also reported that, when during balance experiments in diabetes patients, linoleic acid was replaced isocalorically by saturated fat not only the blood lipids increased considerably, but also the blood sugars rose and more insulin was necessary to control the diabetes. Kinsell *et al.* (1959b) reported an improvement of some patients with severe diabetic retinopathy after a linoleic-acid diet was given. However, details were not given, so that it is impossible to evaluate the type of this improvement. In 1960 the AMA committee on food and nutrition took up a prudent stand upon the fat in the diabetes diet (Pollack, 1960). Reference was made to the possible favourable effect of a diet rich in polyunsaturated fatty acids; however, percentages were not given. King *et al.* (1963) describe favourable experiences mentioned earlier with a diet rich in corn oil. For a period of three years they compared 28 patients on a normal fat-rich diet with 17 patients for whom this diet had been replaced by a diet rich in corn oil. The two groups did not differ with regard to age, sex, duration of diabetes or treatment. The plasma lipids decreased in these periods during the corn-oil diet but no distinct influence was observed on diabetic control, insulin requirement and weight. There was, however, a marked reduction in the extent of the retinal exudates; 80% improved against 29·7% spontaneous improvement in the eyes of the control persons. However, the visual acuity did not improve. Kinsell and Schlierf (1965) stressed again that atherosclerosis is aggravated by a prolonged increased concentration of plasma lipids, but can be inhibited by unsaturated fatty acids. It is obvious that these data can be of great importance for diabetes treatment. It is to be regretted that Kinsell and Schlierf did not give more quantitative data which would have made them more meaningful. Nevertheless on account of the much more extensive experience with the treatment of macro-angiopathic disorders on basis of atherosclerosis in non-diabetics with high linoleic-acid diets it seems rather logical to expect to some extent the same effects in the treatment of diabetic vascular disease, especially as there is increasing evidence for a direct relation between the hard exudates characteristic of diabetic retinopathy and the degree of hyperlipaemia (TG + TC). The following points support this concept.

1. Hard exudates are hardly ever found in young insulin-dependent diabetics, at least if sufficient exogenous insulin is given. In these cases severe triglyceridaemia will not occur. If juvenile diabetes is uncontrolled, severe hyperlipaemia (which apparently is a necessary condition) exists and hard retinal exudates will develop rapidly.
2. Reduction of hyperlipaemia in patients with hard retinal exudates with any effective dietary measure or drug treatment will result in a gradual disappearance of the ocular lesion. Kempner *et al.* (1958), Van Eck (1959) and Ernest *et al.* (1965) succeeded with low-fat diets, King *et al.* (1963) with a high corn-oil diet, Esmann *et al.* (1963) with PAS and Duncan *et al.* (1968), Harrold *et al.* (1969) and Houtsmuller (1968) with clofibrate (Atromid$^{R}$). Moreau and Pichon (1970) even go as far as stating that there can be no exudative retinopathy without hyperlipaemia.

Houtsmuller (1972) found that with a diet rich in polyunsaturated fatty acids, the exudates in diabetic retinopathy disappeared within three to six months in most cases, independently of weight-changes, only the reduction of plasma lipids being of importance. The fact should not be overlooked that a low-carbohydrate diet, with a high proportion of polyunsaturated fat (up to 50 cal%) more effectively lowers blood lipids than the standard American Heart Association fat-controlled diet (Hulley *et al.*, 1972).

Hulley reported that the chief effect of the standard AHA diet appeared to be a reduction of the level of $\beta$-lipoproteins and that of carbohydrate restriction a lowering of pre-$\beta$-lipoproteins also.

Although less effective than polyunsaturated fatty acids as linoleic acid, triglycerides made with medium-chain fatty acids (10 or less carbon atoms) (MCT) can induce lower plasma lipids than the long-chain saturated fatty acids. Van Itallie *et al.* (1969) studied the effects of MCT in great detail not only in normal people but also in patients with maturity-onset diabetes. MCT caused a short-lasting ketonaemia unlike corn oil which was used as a control fat. Both MCT and corn oil improved the tolerance to orally-ingested glucose, according to the authors probably due to stimulation of a $\beta$-cytotropic enteric hormone (secretin), whereas the ketonaemia as such already stimulates insulin secretion, at least in normal people (Pi-Sunyer *et al.*, 1969). Both MCT and corn oil temporarily decreased the plasma glucose level. As could be expected, on account of the similarity between MCT and carbohydrate metabolism, the insulin response was higher after MCT uptake.

Some German groups have advocated for a few years an extremely fat-rich diet—the so-called "Punkt Diät" (20% protein, 10% carbohydrates, 9% alcohol and 60% fat). Although consumption of this diet is not limited, normally insufficient calories are taken up to maintain body weight. According to Wessels *et al.* (1970) this diet causes ketonaemia, reduces blood glucose and insulin concentrations as well as plasma triglycerides. Whether this type of diet will be useful in the treatment of diabetes still remains to be proven. The positive aspect is the decreased insulin release and the greater feeling of satiety, which is especially advantageous in reducing obesity, the most common and most difficult to treat abnormality in the adult diabetic syndrome. A definite disadvantage of this extreme dietary composition will be the high risk of developing in the long run, certain nutritional deficiencies due to the low carbohydrate content. These can be prevented of course by supplementing the water soluble vitamins and minerals such as calcium, iron, etc., but this will require more insight into nutritional requirements than is present normally.

We studied the long-term effects of dietary fats on plasma lipids and diabetic retinopathy in 21 hospitalized patients of which 12 were insulin-dependent. They received eucalorically liquid-formula diets (LFD) with 50 cal% safflower oil, 15% casein and 35% maltodextrose. After discharge from the hospital they followed diets with mainly the same composition but instead of safflower oil a margarine with 50–55% linoleic acid was given while the maltodextrose was replaced by bread (and potatoes). The average results of this treatment on plasma triglycerides and cholesterol concentrations are given in Fig. 7. Furthermore, fasting blood glucose levels fell gradually during the first weeks and remained constant afterwards. Insulin requirement in the insulin-dependent patients decreased to 13%. Four of the 21 patients did not respond to this dietary change, all with moderate-to-severe renal impairment, which probably could be an explanation for this failure. In

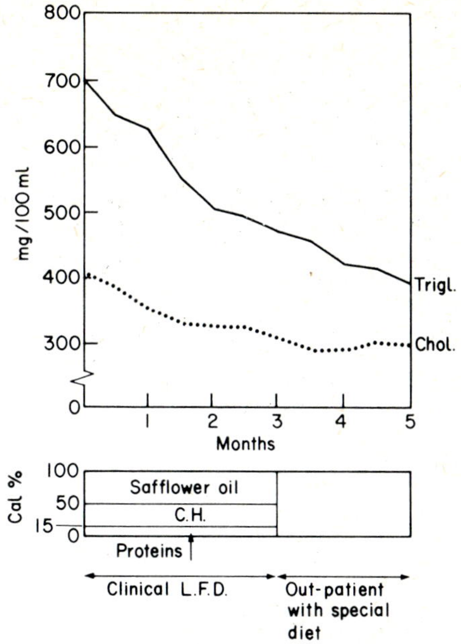


Fig. 7. Influence of 50 cal% safflower oil given eucalorically in the form of a liquid-formula diet with 15 cal% casein and 35 cal% maltodextrose on blood lipid concentrations of 21 patients with diabetic retinopathy and serious hyperlipaemia. After three months the liquid-formula diet was replaced calorically by normal meals prepared with a margarine with 50–55% linoleic acid, the maltodextrose by starch.

one female patient even an increasing lipaemia (triglycerides) was observed, due to insufficient lipoprotein–lipase activity.

The retinal abnormalities improved as could be expected by the decreased blood lipid values (for example, see Fig. 8) although the visual aquity did not improve. This disappointing result corresponds well with the experiences of King (1959), van Eck (1959) and others. The following clinical case studies are given to illustrate the possibilities of dietary manipulation with liquid-formula diets.

*Patient 1*: male, 36-years-old, insulin-dependent diabetic with retinopathy. After stabilization of the plasma lipids he received isocalorically an LFD with 50 cal% safflower oil, 35 cal% lactose and 15 cal% protein. As shown in Fig. 9 plasma lipids fell dramatically. Changing the LFD composition to 35 cal% safflower oil and 50 cal% sucrose induced a rapid increase of plasma triglycerides but thus decreased when starch was given instead of sucrose. During the high safflower-oil period insulin requirement was again definitely lower.

Another example of this type of patient is the following.

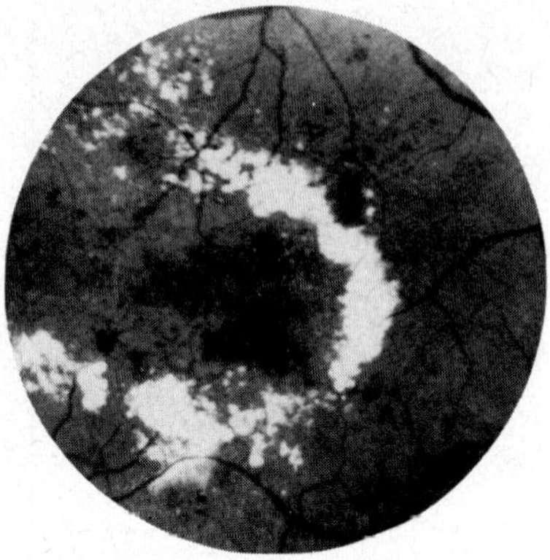

(a)

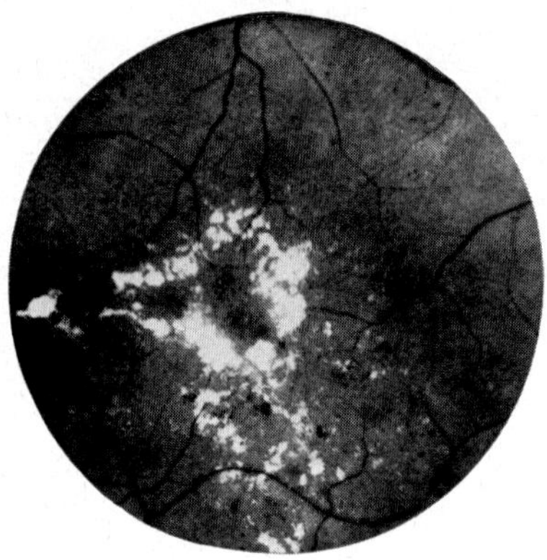

(b)

Fig. 8. Examples of decrease of retinal exudates in diabetic retinopathy under the influence of safflower oil: (a) before therapy; (b) during therapy.

*Patient 2*: female, 57-years-old, insulin dependent diabetic with retinopathy. As Fig. 10 shows blood-lipid concentrations decreased very significantly on the 50 cal% safflower oil LFD accompanied by a clear fall in insulin requirement. Again there was a strong increase in blood lipids during the period in which sucrose was given. On substituting starch for sucrose they decreased but not to the same level as during the period rich in safflower oil.

Typical in both patients is the extreme sensitivity for sucrose, suggesting that severe reduction of sucrose in the diet of this type of patient is necessary; while a high concentration of oils rich in linoleic acid are needed to induce minimal blood-lipid concentrations. In a previously

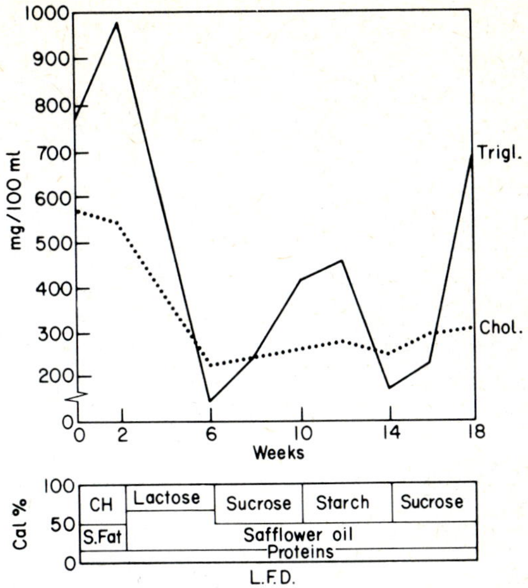


Fig. 9. Serum cholesterol and triglyceride concentrations of patient 1.

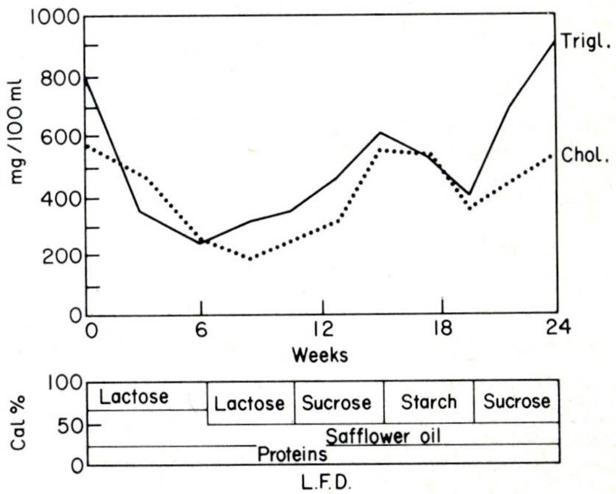


Fig. 10. Serum cholesterol and triglyceride concentrations of patient 2.

published experiment (Houtsmuller, 1967, 1968) the effects of 2 g clofibrate/day, given for two years, on plasma lipids and retinal exudates of 40 patients with diabetic retinopathy were described. Again a significant decrease of plasma cholesterol and triglyceride concentrations resulted in an improvement of the retinal aspect. Blood glucose and insulin levels were not influenced. However, it should also be noted

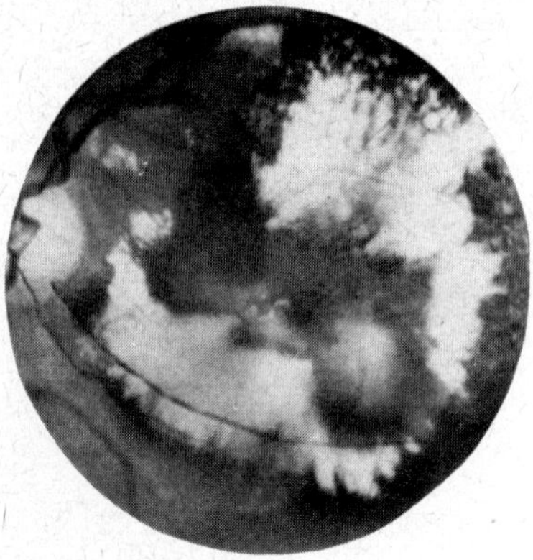

(A)

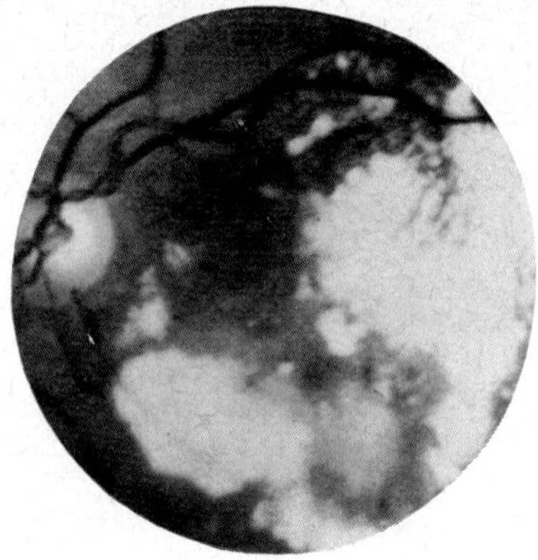

(B)

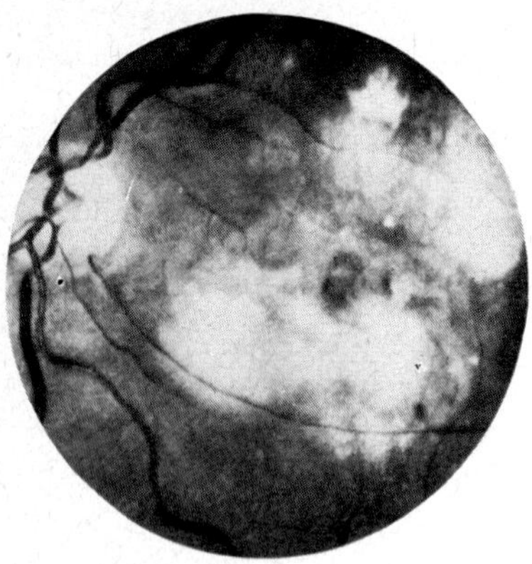

(C)

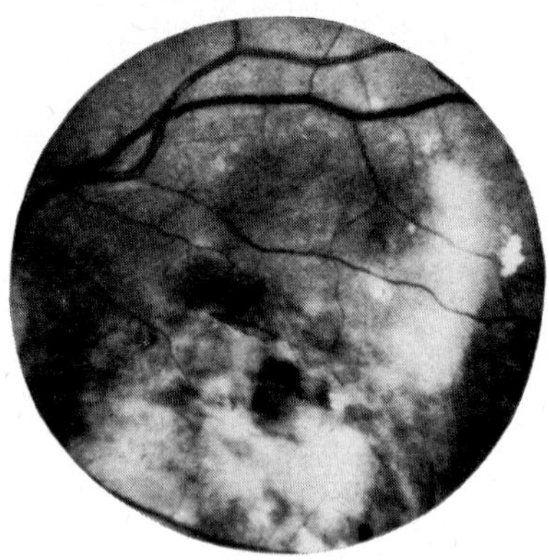

(D)

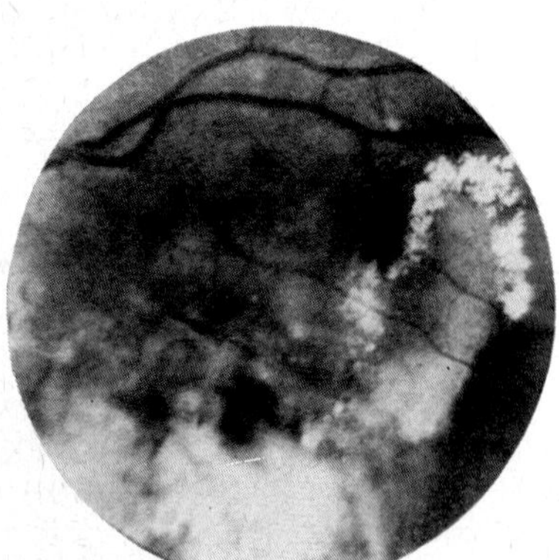

(E)

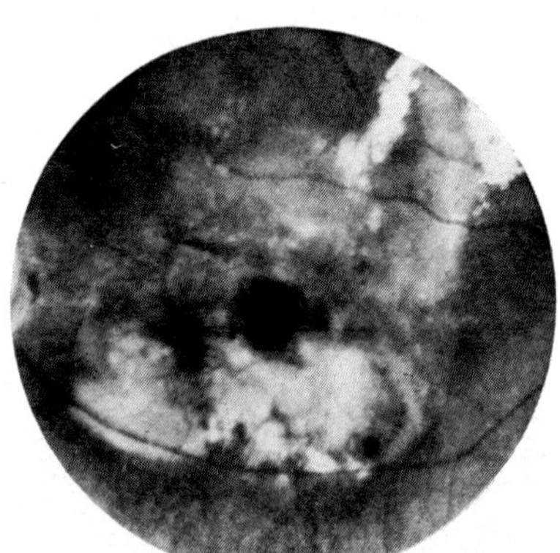

(F)

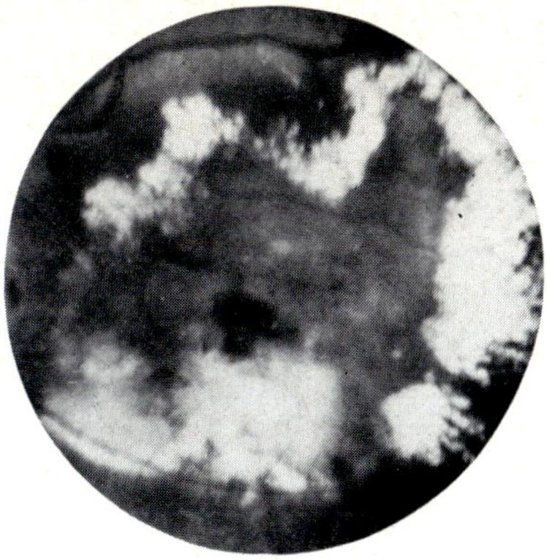

(G)

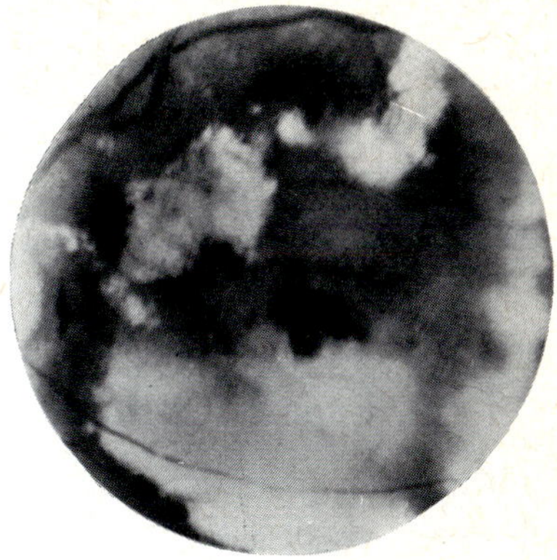

(H)

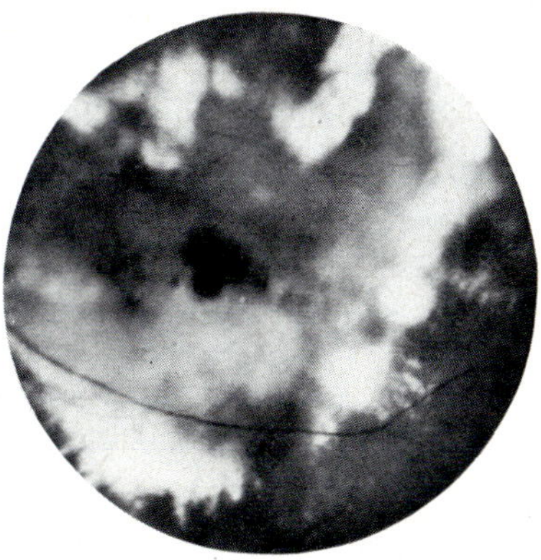

(I)

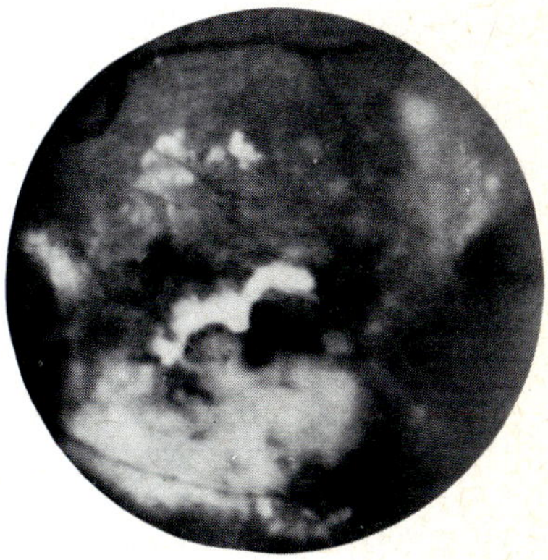

(J)

Fig. 11 A–J. Female patient with diabetic retinopathy, 63-years-old, insulin-independent with gross hyperlipaemia at first examination. Blood cholesterol 423 mg%, blood triglycerides 640 mg%.

A and B represent observation period of six months, with rapid increase of retinal exudates; C and D show the effect of clofibrate, the decrease of blood lipids and the corresponding decrease of hard exudates; E, F and G show the effect of a saturated-fat diet, causing a rise in blood lipids and increase in hard exudates; H, I and J show the effect of 15 cal% linoleic acid, effecting a decrease of blood lipids, followed by a gradual decrease of hard exudates.

that 20% of the controls in this double blind study showed a "spontaneous" improvement of the retinal exudates apparently not related to their blood lipid levels. At the end of this study (in 1964) the same 40 patients and another 50 more were put on a *ca* 15 cal% linoleic-acid containing diet and the course of their lipaemia and retinopathy was followed prospectively for seven years. Every three months a complete blood lipid analysis was obtained, whereas every three to six months a colour photograph was taken of the retinal fundus which were assessed in accordance with the criteria of T. R. Fraser (Oakley *et al.*, 1967). Of the original 93 patients 28 dropped out of the study because of other diseases or death.

Hyperlipaemia improved significantly in 52% of the patients while 15% did not react to the dietary change and in 33% the condition even worsened probably due to insufficient adherence to the prescribed diet. The retinal exudates improved in 54%, did not change in 18% and progressed in 28%. The correlation between the dietary influences on lipaemia and retinopathy was again striking—in 87% a synchronous change was observed supporting the hypothesis that the retinal exudates in diabetes are directly related to the level of the plasma lipids (see for an example Fig. 11 A–J).

These data demonstrate convincingly that to continue a diet rich in linoleic acid can be useful in the treatment of exudative diabetic retinopathy. Even more important is the observation that the life expectancy of these patients (death rate 32% in five years) was higher than of a previously observed group wherein a death rate of *ca* 60% during five years was recorded (Houtsmuller and Henkes, 1964), although both groups were comparable regarding age and sex, severity of the diabetic retinopathy and nephropathy.

Finally, we carried out a clinical investigation to find the best diet for patients with diabetes mellitus. Theoretically this should be a diet which keeps the blood sugars and plasma lipids as low as possible with as few fluctuations as possible in the day and night rhythm and with the smallest possible fluctuations in insulin level. Regarding the carbohydrates it is clear that starch should be preferred to short-chain carbohydrates. As for the fats, on the basis of the foregoing it is to be expected that the linoleic-acid rich fats have a more favourable result than the saturated fats. To avoid great fluctuations during the day as caused by the normal three-meals rhythm, the technique of Schlierf *et al.* (1971) was followed according to which an equal amount of food was administered from 8 a.m. every two hours, six times in total. Altogether, 14 clinical patients were studied—seven obese and three lean insulin-independent diabetics and four non-diabetic obese patients (see Table 1). The patients received for three periods of ten days isocaloric amounts of three different diets in a randomized sequence. The basic compositions of the three diets were:

1. 20 cal% protein, 50 cal% butter and 30 cal% starch.
2. 20 cal% protein, 50 cal% sunflower oil (*ca* 65% linoleic acid), 30 cal% starch.

3. 20 cal % protein, 30 cal % fat mixture of equal parts of butter and sunflower oil, 50 % starch.

Table 1

| | Sex | Age | Length (cm) | Weight (kg) | Geigy index |
|---|---|---|---|---|---|
| Obese diabetes | | | | | |
| | ♀ | 52 | 160 | 110 | +46 |
| | ♀ | 65 | 160 | 89 | +25 |
| | ♀ | 72 | 165 | 94 | +26 |
| | ♀ | 75 | 154 | 105 | +45 |
| | ♀ | 60 | 155 | 89 | +28 |
| | ♀ | 60 | 152 | 76 | +17 |
| | ♀ | 58 | 175 | 96 | +22 |
| Lean diabetes | | | | | |
| | ♂ | 62 | 180 | 69 | −12 |
| | ♀ | 45 | 160 | 53 | − 9 |
| | ♂ | 66 | 169 | 65 | − 6 |
| Non-diabetic obese patients | | | | | |
| | ♀ | 69 | 158 | 96 | +34 |
| | ♀ | 44 | 170 | 97 | +29 |
| | ♀ | 69 | 163 | 93 | +28 |
| | ♀ | 55 | 170 | 103 | +32 |

The participants were kept in bed for most of the day for the full 30 days, kept at body weight (+ 0·5 kg) which was daily controlled. The change from one diet to the other did not cause distinct changes in weight in any of them. On the last day of each ten-day period venous blood samples were taken with a syringe at two-hour intervals from 8 a.m. until midnight, after which for practical reasons the two latest samples were taken at four-hour intervals. They were analysed on glucose-, insulin-, triglycerides-, free fatty acids-, cholesterol concentrations. For the results see Figs 12a,b,c, 13a,b,c, 14a,b, 15a,b,c and 16a,b,c respectively. At the end of each experimental period also lipoprotein lipase activities were measured.

Although the relatively small number of patients in each group did

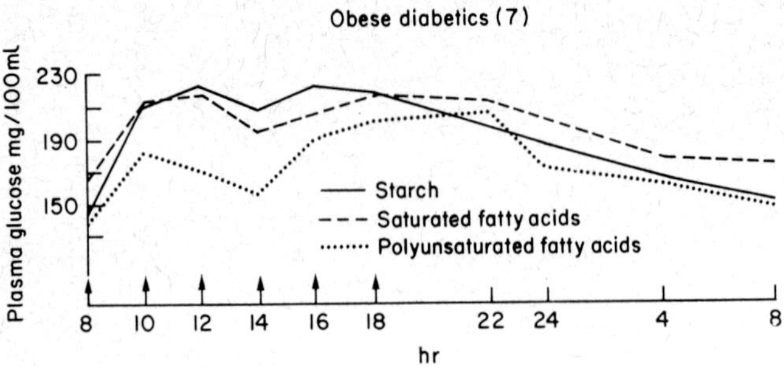


(A)

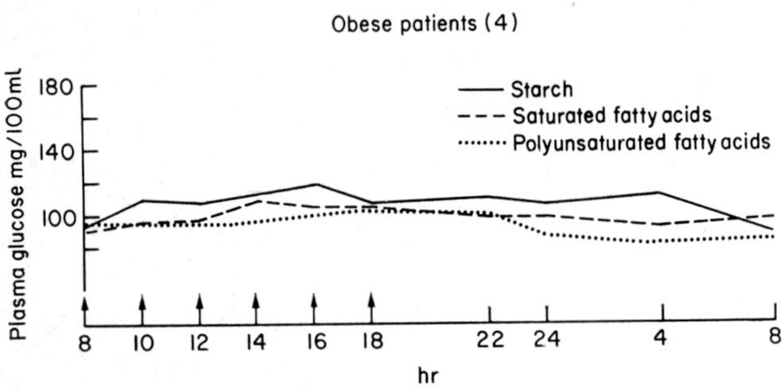


(B)

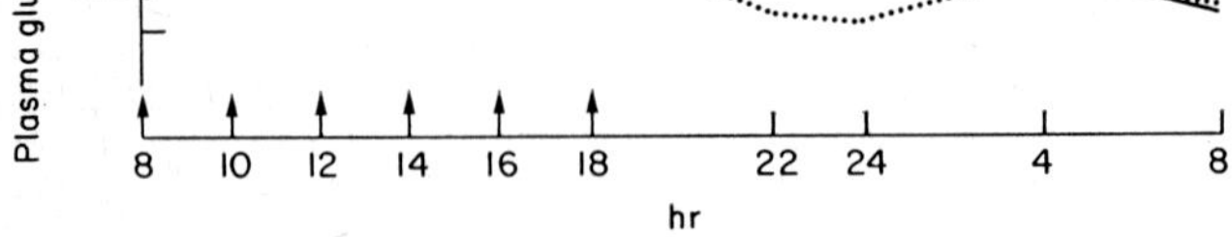


(C)

Fig. 12 A–C. 24-hr Plasma glucose levels of obese patients and diabetic patients with or without obesity. The glucose levels of obese diabetics are the highest of the three groups. Comparing the three feeding periods, only in the obese diabetics a significant lower glucose level was found during the polyunsaturated fatty acid period. Isocaloric meals were given at the times indicated with arrows.

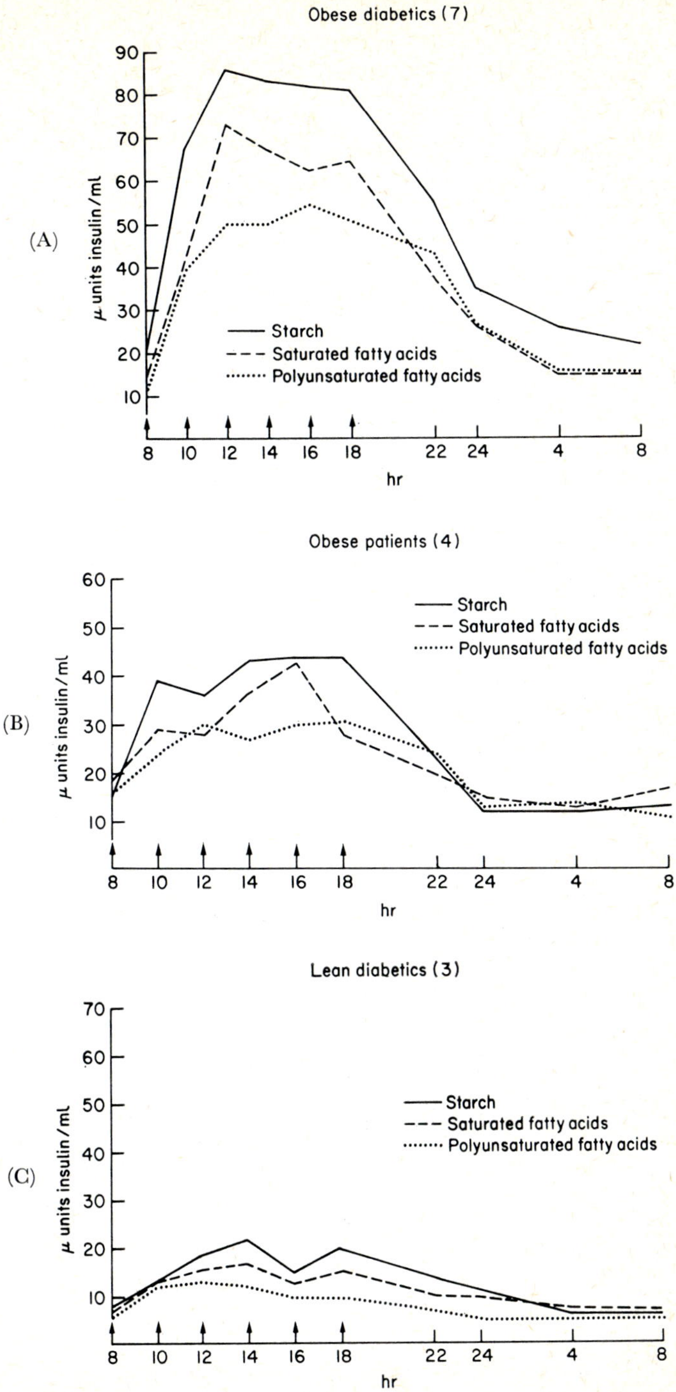


Fig. 13 A–C. 24-hr Plasma insulin levels of obese patients and diabetic patients with or without obesity. These obese diabetic demonstrated highly significant increased insulin levels, the lean diabetics had a very small insulin secretion. It is to be noticed that the insulin levels reached the fasting level at midnight except for the obese diabetic group. For the three groups the 24-hr insulin area was lowest during the polyunsaturated fatty acid period. Isocaloric meals were given at the times indicated with arrows.

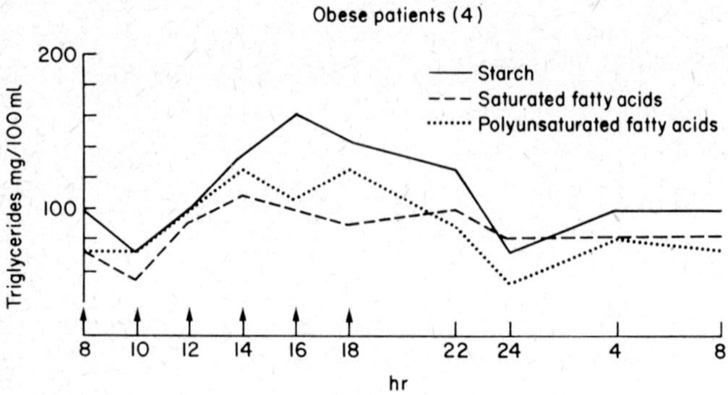


(A)

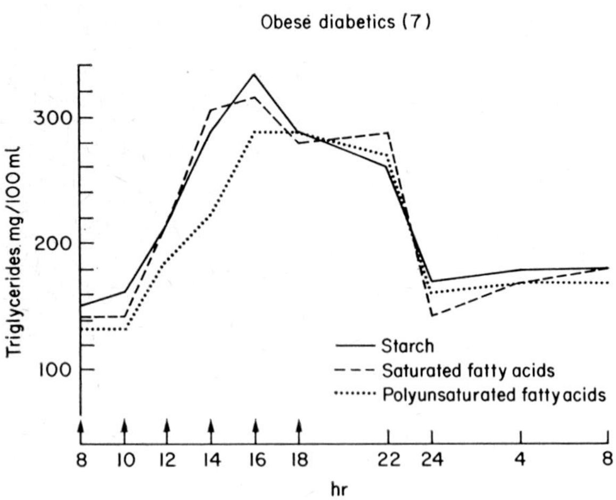


(B)

Fig. 14 A–B. 24-hr Plasma-triglycerides levels of obese non-diabetic patients and obese diabetics. Differences in the three feeding periods were not significant. Isocaloric meals were given at the times indicated by arrows. No data is available on the lean diabetic patients.

not allow definitive conclusions for all parameters, the following interesting trends can be recognized.

1. *Blood glucose* levels in the diabetic groups were higher than of the non-diabetic obese patients for the full 24 hours. Lower 24-hr values were induced by the diet rich in linoleic acid only in the obese diabetics. The other two groups did not show a statistically significant response of this criterion on the three different diets.

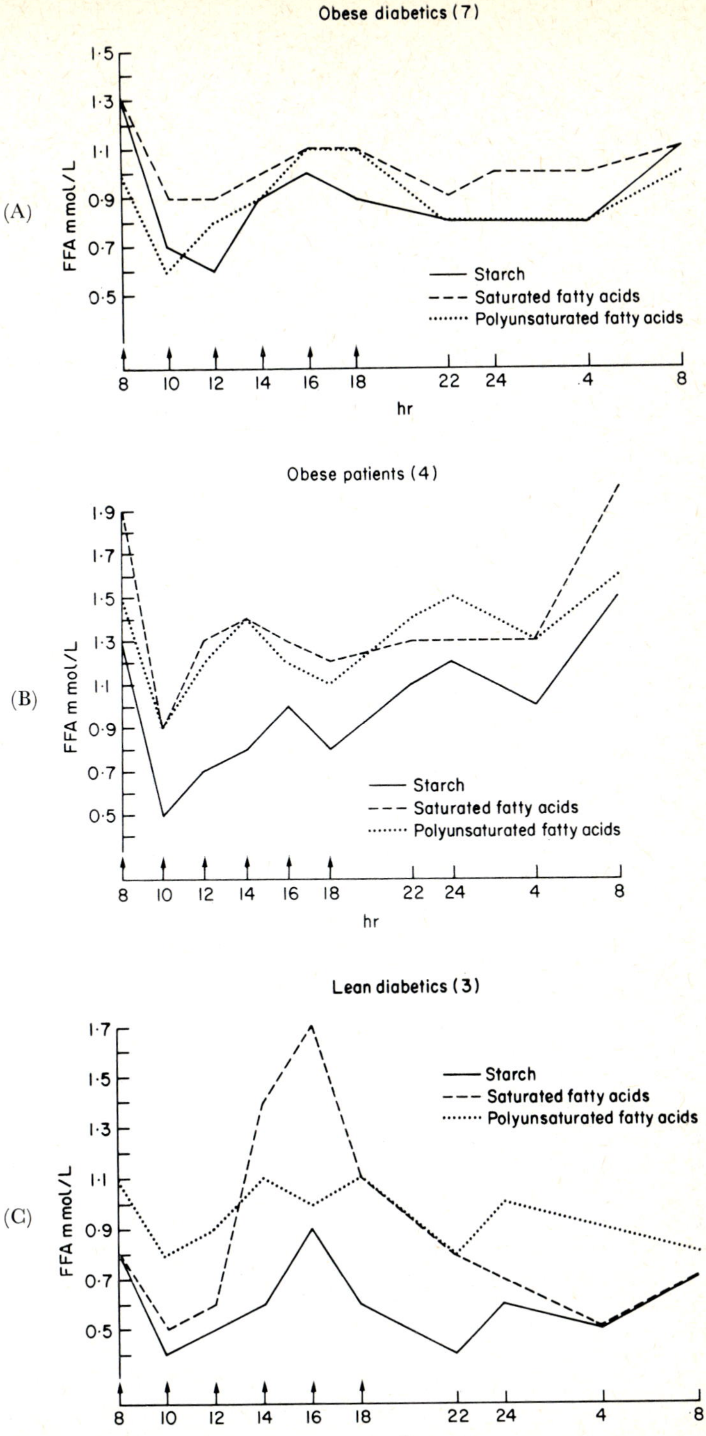


Fig. 15 A–C. 24-hr Plasma FFA levels in obese non-diabetic patients, and lean and obese diabetics. After the first meal a sharp decrease of the FFA levels appeared, followed by a gradual increase as feeding continued. Only in the obese non-diabetics did this increase continue after cessation of the feeding periods, suggesting a dominating lipolysis from the fat deposits. Isocaloric meals were given at the times indicated with arrows. During the starch period the FFA appeared to be the lowest in the three groups examined.

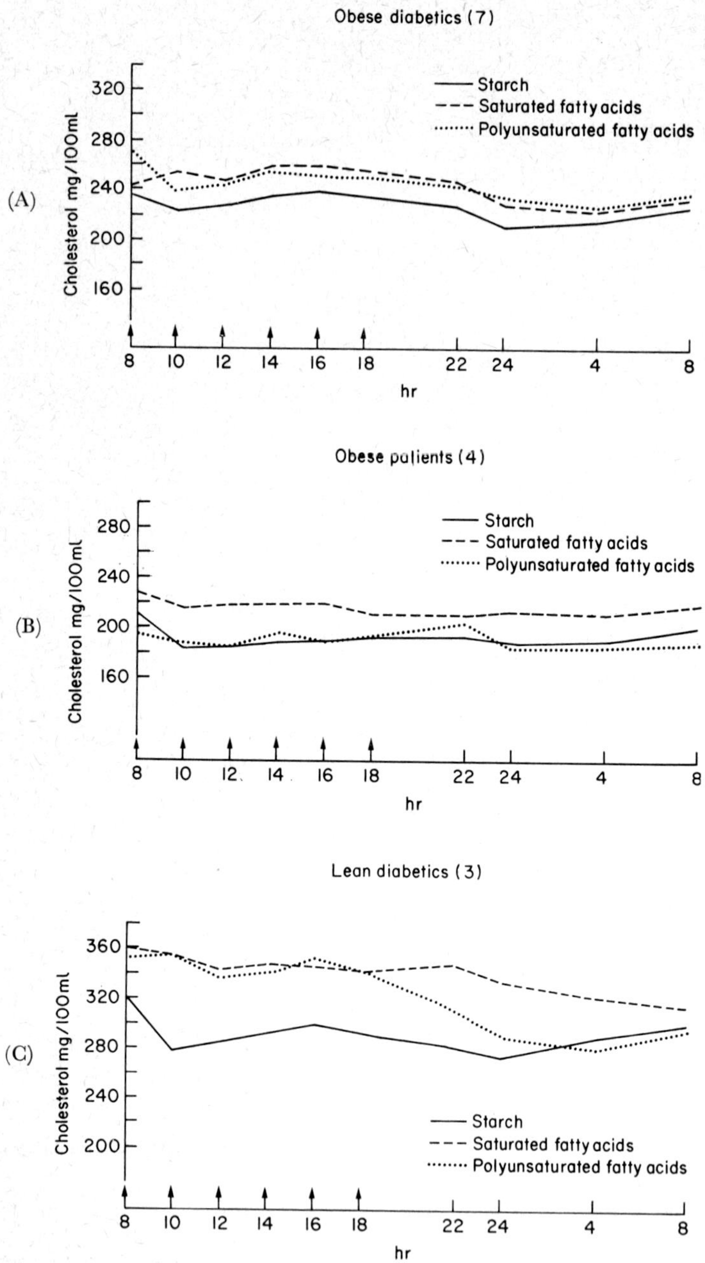


Fig. 16 A–C. 24-hr Plasma level of plasma cholesterol in obese non-diabetic patients and obese and lean diabetics. There is a significantly higher fasting cholesterol and 24-hr area for lean diabetics compared to obese diabetics and for obese diabetics compared to obese non-diabetics. Concerning the effect of the three diets (see text), in lean diabetics the 24-hr cholesterol area was significantly lower in the starch period. In obese diabetics and non-diabetics no significant differences were seen between the three diet periods. Isocaloric meals were given at the times indicated by arrows.

2. *Insulin* concentrations were highest for the obese diabetics, whereas the lean diabetics demonstrated the least insulin secretion during the whole period. Also the fasting insulin levels in this group were the lowest. All three groups had the highest insulin levels during the high carbohydrate diets and had—highly statistically significant—lower insulin levels during the high linoleic acid diets. The differences were most pronounced for the obese diabetics. The interesting observation that, especially in the obese diabetics, diets high in linoleic acid can induce both relatively low blood glucose and insulin concentrations suggests a possible insulin-sparing effect from linoleic acid which might have important therapeutic consequences for these patients.
3. *Serum–triglyceride* concentrations during the full 24 hours were higher for the obese diabetic group than for the obese non-diabetic patients. The concentrations were not clearly influenced by the three dietary treatments except for the high-carbohydrate diet which induced a significant rise in the obese group. A distinct feature was the enormous rise during daytime and the abrupt drop during the first four hours after the last meal.
4. *Fasting free fatty acid* concentrations (FFA) were highest for the obese patients and lowest in the lean diabetics. During the high carbohydrate diets these levels were lower than for the other diets, especially in the obese group. Another striking feature is the sharp decrease of FFA concentrations in the first two hours after breakfast as a result of the induced insulin secretion. Moreover it is remarkable after the last meal that the obese group displayed a distinct rise of the FFA levels as a result of lipolysis. In the lean diabetic patients no high degree of lipolysis can be expected because of the lack of subcutaneous fat. In the obese diabetics, however, although an excess of adipose tissue is present this is apparently counter-balanced by the still high nocturnal insulin levels.
5. Finally lipoprotein lipase activity appeared to be strongest during the starch periods in all experimental groups, suggesting an increased turnover of VLDL.

The above data suggest strongly that regulation of the levels of blood glucose and thus of insulin levels is decisive for the behaviour of blood lipids. Insulin secretion as measured over a 24-hr period is much greater in obese diabetic patients than in the non-diabetic obese group. Thus, the conclusion of most investigators that obese patients do produce less insulin than comparable obese controls (conclusions based on the non-physiological 100 g glucose challenge) is not true for the much more normal challenge of daily meal patterns which clearly show that obese diabetics produce the largest quantity of insulin. The following supposition seems justified: if food is supplied via the small intestine the $\beta$-cells of the pancreas are stimulated, although under comparable conditions this would seem to be different for saturated fat, unsaturated fat and starch. The insulin stimulation is strongest during the starch diet and weakest during the linoleic diet. As a result two mechanisms are much influenced by the starch diet, and even more so by sugar:

1. stimulation of the lipoprotein–lipase activity so that maximal fatty acid splitting from the triglycerides (pre-$\beta$-lipoproteins) occurs, which enables a maximal uptake of free fatty acids to the tissues, followed by maximal lipogenesis (especially visible in fatty tissue and liver but also in the large blood vessels);
2. maximal antilipolysis in the various tissues so that the release of free fatty acids from the intracellular glycerides deposits becomes minimal.

Conversely with the unsaturated fatty acid diet the insulin stimulation is lowest—as a result of which, on the one hand the lipolysis (e.g. of fatty tissue and liver) is highest, on the other hand the lipoprotein–lipase activity is lowest. When we recall the infiltration theory in the pathogenesis of atherosclerosis which assumes that an important part of the lipids found in the arterial walls penetrate from the plasma into the vessel walls, it is clear that the most unfavourable conditions are created by high triglyceride levels combined with high lipoprotein–lipase activity and high blood sugars, all stimulated by insulin—a combination which is often found in maturity-onset diabetes with its highest insulin levels. Thus it is vital to keep the plasma lipids as low as possible, although combined with optimal (and not maximal) insulin levels and as normal as possible blood sugars.

In the investigations mentioned previously it appeared that this could best be attained by polyunsaturated fatty acids by which the plasma insulin levels are the least stimulated.

In our opinion the current nutritional conditions in the treatment of patients with diabetes mellitus are far from optimal: general agreement exists concerning optimal caloric needs, but these however, are often difficult to attain. Thus in practice, especially in existing obesity, it is most vital to control the insulin levels to a point as optimal (and not maximal) as possible. As 70–80% patients with diabetes mellitus are insulin-independent and most are also obese, the need for accurate nutritional knowledge of these patients is fundamental. In this group of patients, in particular, it would be easy to overstimulate the $\beta$-cell system. It is clear that in this group of obese diabetics the practice of giving $\beta$-cell stimulating drugs, such as sulphonyl-urea derivatives, is very harmful. Concerning the nutritional stimuli it can be concluded from our results, that besides a low caloric intake short-chained carbohydrates must be avoided as much as possible, also those in fruit—an often underestimated source. With regard to proteins, one should remember that some amino acids such as arginine, etc., also stimulate the $\beta$-cells although sufficient proteins are needed in this catabolic disease. Concerning the nutritional fats, saturated fats must be avoided to a large extent, remembering that the hidden saturated fats are not to be neglected. In our opinion the fat concentration in diabetic diets should amount to 35–40 cal %, of which at least one-third should be in the form of linoleic acid, with proteins supplying about 15–20 cal %. The carbohydrate calorie requirement should be exclusively starch, allowing that these calories are in this respect not empty, as is too often believed, as they directly or indirectly stimulate insulin secretion.

## REFERENCES

Adlersberg, D. (1958). Angiopathy in diabetes: biochemistry and pathophysiology with special reference to lipid metabolism. Diabetes Mellitus: III. Cong. Int. Diab. Fed. Düsseldorf, p. 61.

Adlersberg, D. and Eisler, L. (1959). Circulating lipids in diabetes mellitus. *J. Am. Med. Ass.* **170,** 1261.

Adlersberg, D. and Wang, C. (1955). Syndrome of idiopathic hyperlipemia, mild diabetes mellitus and severe vascular damage. *Diabetes* **4,** 210.

Ahuja, M. M. S., Kumann, V. and Gossam, V. V. (1969). Interrelationship of vascular disease and blood lipids in young Indian diabetics. *Diabetes* **18,** 670.

Albrink, M. J. and Man, E. B. (1958). Serum triglycerides in health and diabetes. *Diabetes* **7,** 194.

Albrink, M. J., Mergs, J. W. and Granoff, M. A. (1962). Weight gain and serum triglycerides in normal men. *New. Engl. J. Med.* **266,** 484.

Albrink, M. J., Lavietes, P. M. and Man, E. B. (1963). Vascular disease and serum lipids in diabetes mellitus. Observations over thirty years (1931–1961). *Ann. Int. Med.* **58,** 305.

Albutt, E. C. and Chance, G. W. (1969). Plasma and adipose tissue fatty acids of diabetic children on long-term corn oil diets. *J. Clin. Invest.* **48,** 139.

Amherdt, M., Rufener, C., Scherrer, J. R. and Pometa, D. (1971). Early capillary changes in diabetes mellitus. *In* "Blood Vessel Disease in Diabetes Mellitus." V Capri Conference. (K. Lundbaeck, H. Keen, eds). *Acta Diabet. Lat.* **8,** Suppl. 1. 88.

Atwell, M. E. and Waterhouse, C. (1971). Glucose production from fructose. *Diabetes* **20,** 193.

Bagdade, J. D., Bierman, J. L. and Porte, D. (1967a). The significance of basal insulin levels in the evaluation of the insulin response to glucose in diabetic and non-diabetic subjects. *J. Clin. Invest.* **46,** 1549.

Bagdade, J. D., Porte, D. and Bierman, E. L. (1967b). Diabetic lipemia, a form of acquired fat-induced lipemia. *New Engl. J. Med.* **276,** 427.

Bagdade, J. D., Porte, D., and Bierman, E. L. (1968). Acute insulin withdrawal and the regulation of plasma triglyceride removal in diabetic subjects. *Diabetes* **17,** 127.

Baker, R. W. R., Joiner, C. L. and Trounce, J. R. (1955). A study by paperelectrophoresis of the serum lipoproteins in diabetics and non diabetic subjects. *Quart. J. Med.* **24,** 295.

Barter, P. J., Caroll, K. F. and Nestel, P. J. (1971). Diurnal fluctuations in triglyceride, free fatty acids and insulin during sucrose consumption and insulin infusion in man. *J. Clin. Invest.* **50,** 583.

Barach, H. and Lowy, A. D. (1952). Lipoprotein molecules, cholesterol and atherosclerosis in diabetes mellitus. *Diabetes* **1,** 441.

Beaumont, P., Schofield, P. J., Hollows, F. C., Williams, J. F. and Steinbeck, A. W. (1971). Growth hormone, sorbitol and diabetic capillary disease. *Lancet* **I,** p. 579.

Bierman, E. L. (1971). Insulin and hypertriglyceridemia, in impact of insulin on metabolic pathways. Int. Symp. Commemorating the 50th Anniversary of Insulin. Jerusalem 1971.

Bierman, E. L. (1972). The effect of a carbohydrate rich diet on glucose tolerance and insulin secretion in diabetic subjects. *In* "Nutrition and Diabetes Mellitus." VI Capri Conference. (E. R. Froesch, J. Yudkin, eds). *Acta Diabet. Lat.* **9.** Suppl. I, 377.

Bierman, E. L. and Hamlin, J. T. (1961). The hyperlipemic effect of a low-fat, high carbohydrate diet in diabetic subjects. *Diabetes* **10,** 432.

Bierman, E. L. and Porte, D. (1968). Carboyhdrate intolerance and lipemia. *Ann. Int. Med.* **68,** 4, 926.

Bierman, E. L., Porte, D., Bagdade, J. D. and Hasard, W. R. (1970). Lipoprotein lipase and plasma triglyceride, In "Atherosclerosis." Proc. Sec. Int. Symposium Chicago, p. 231. Springer Verlag, New York: Heidelberg: Berlin.

Bierman, E. L., Albrink, M. J., Arky, R. A., Connor, W. E., Dayton, S., Spritz, N. and Steinberg, D. (1971). Principles of nutrition and dietary recommendations for patients with diabetes mellitus. *Diabetes* **20,** 633.

Beitner, R. and Kalant, N. (1971). Stimulation of glycolysis by insulin. *J. Biol. Chem.* **246,** 500.

Bergen, S. S., Hashim, S. A. and van Itallı Th.B. (1966). Hyperketonemia induced in man by medium-chain triglyceride. *Diabetes* **15,** 725.

Boberg, J. and Hallberg, D. (1969). Application of a new intravenous fat tolerance test in the study of hypertriglyceridaemia in man. *J. Atheroscler. Res.* **9,** 159.

Boshell, B. R., Chandalia, H. B., Kreisberg, R. A. and Roddam, R. F. (1968). Serum insulin in obesity and diabetes mellitus. *Am. J. Clin. Nutr.* **21,** 1419.

Björntorp, P. and Karlsson, M. (1971). Triglyceride synthesis in human subcutaneous adipose tissue cells of different size. *Europ. J. Clin. Invest.* **1,** 112.

Björntorp, P. and Sjöström, L. (1971). Adipose tissue fat cell size and number in relation to metabolism. *In* "Impact of Insulin on Metabolic Pathways." Int. Symp. Commemorating the 50th Anniversary of Insulin. Jerusalem 1971, abstracts p. 33.

Björntorp, P., Karlsson, M. and Horden, A. (1969a). Quantitative aspects of lipolysis and reësterification in human adipose tissue *in vitro. Acta Med. Scand.* **185,** 89.

Björntorp, P., Berman, H. and Varnaushas, E. (1969b). Plasma free fatty acid turnover rate in obesity. *Acta Med. Scand.* **185,** 351.

Björntorp, P., Karlsson, M. and Hooden, A. (1969c). Quantitative aspects of lipolysis and reësterification in human adipose tissue *in vitro. Acta Med. Scand.* **185,** 89.

Braunsteiner, H., Di Pauli, R., Sailer, S. and Sandhofer, F. (1965). Hyperlipämie und latenter Diabetes mellitus. *Klin. Wsch.* **43,** 715.

Braunsteiner, H., Sailer, S. and Sandhofer, F. (1966). Plasmalipids bei Patienten mit Diabetes Mellitus. *Klin. Wschr.* **44,** 116.

Brunsell, J. D., Lerner, R. L., Hazzard, W. R., Pork, D. and Bierman, E. L. (1971). Improved glucose tolerance with high carbohydrate feeding in mild diabetes. *New Engl. J. Med.* **284,** 521.

Burns, Th.W. and Langley, P. E. (1970). Lipolysis by human adipose tissue: the role of cyclic 3′, 5′ adenosine monophosphate and adrenergic receptor sites. *J. Lab. Clin. Med.* **75,** 983.

Caird, F. J. (1968). Control of diabetes and diabetic retinopathy. Symposium on the treatment of diabetic retinopathy. Warrenton, 1968. Public Health Service publication no. 1890, p. 107.

Caird, F. J., Pirie, A. and Ramsell, T. G. (1969). "Diabetes and the Eye." Blackwell Scientific Publications, Oxford.

Catt, K. J. (1970). Insulin and glucose homoeostasis. *Lancet* **II,** 7668, 353.

Cerasi, E. (1967). An analogue computer model for the insulin response to glucose infusion. *Acta Endocrin.* (*Kobenhavn*) **55,** 163–183.

Cerasi, E. and Luft, R. (1967). "What is inherited—what is added": hypothesis for the pathogenesis of diabetes mellitus. *Diabetes* **16,** 615–627.

Chaikoff, J. L., Smyth, F. S. and Gibbs, G. E. (1936). The blood lipids of diabetic children. *J. Clin. Invest.* **15,** 627.

Clawson, B. J. and Bell, E. T. (1949). Incidence of fatal coronary disease in non-diabetic and diabetic persons. *Arch. Pathol.* **48,** 105.

Constam, G. R. (1965). Zur spätprognose des Diabetes mellitus. *Helv. Med. Acta.* **32,** 287.

Crespin, S. R., Greenough, W. B. and Steinberg, D. (1969). Stimulation of insulin secretion by infusion of free fatty acids. *J. Clin. Invest.* **48,** 1934.

Cruz, A. B., Amatusio, D. S., Grande, F. and Hay, L. J. (1961). Effect of intra-arterial insulin on tissue cholesterol and fatty acids in alloxan diabetic dogs. *Circulation Res.* **ix,** 39.

Dayton, S., Hashimoto, S. and Pearce, M. L. (1967). Adipose tissue linoleic acid as criterion of adherence to a modified diet. *J. Lipid Res.* **8,** 508.

Di Girolamo, M. and Rudman, D. (1968). Variations in glucose metabolism and sensitivity to insulin of the rats adipose tissue, in relation to age and body weight. *Endocrinology* **82,** 1133.

Ditschuneit, H. (1971). Obesity and diabetes mellitus, Diabetes. Proc. VII Congress Int. Diab. Fed. 1970. Int. Congress Series 231, p. 526.

Dollery, C. T. and Oakley, N. W. (1965). Reversal of retinal vascular changes in diabetes. *Diabetes* **14,** 121.

Drenich, E. J., Brichman, A. S. and Gold, E. M. (1972). Dissociation of the obesity-hyperinsulinism relationship following dietary restriction and hyperalimentation. *Am. J. Clin. Nutr.* **25,** 746.

Duff, G. L. and McMillan, G. C. (1949). The effect of alloxan diabetes on experimental cholesterol atherosclerosis in the rabbit:
I. the inhibition of experimental cholesterol atherosclerosis in alloxan diabetes.
II. the effect of alloxan diabetes on the retrogression of experimental cholesterol atherosclerosis. *J. Exp. Med.* **89,** 611.

Duff, G. L. and Payne, T. P. B. (1950). The effect of alloxan diabetes on experimental cholesterol atherosclerosis in the rabbit: III. the mechanism of the inhibition of

experimental cholesterol atherosclerosis in alloxan-diabetic rabbits. *J. Exp. Med.* **92,** 299.
Duff, G. L., Brechin, D. J. H. and Finkelstein, W. E. (1954). The effect of alloxan diabetes on experimental cholesterol atherosclerosis in the rabbit: IV. the effect of insulin therapy on the inhibition of atherosclerosis in the alloxan-diabetic rabbit. *J. Exp. Med.* **100,** 371.
Duncan, L. J. P., Cullen, J. F., Ireland, J. T., Nolan, J., Clarke, B. F. and Oliver, M. F. (1968). A three year trial of atromid therpy in exudative diabetic retinopathy. *Diabetes* **17,** 458.
Dunnigan, M. G., Fyfe, T., McKiddie, M. T. and Crosbie, S. M. (1970). The effects of isocaloric exchange of dietary starch and sucrose on glucose tolerance, plasma insulin and serum lipids in man. *Clin. Sci.* **38,** 1.
Eaton, R. P., Berman, M. and Steinberg, D. (1969). Kinetic studies of plasma free fatty acid and triglyceride metabolism in man. *J. Clin. Invest.* **48,** 1560.
Editorial (1971). Diabetes mellitus: disease or syndrome. *Lancet* **I,** p. 583.
Ejarque, P., Marble, A. and Tuller, E. (1959). Proteins, lipoproteins and protein bound carbohydrates in the serum of diabetic patients. *Am. J. Med.* **27,** 221.
Elkeles, R. S., Wyhle, A. D. H., Lowy, C., Young, J. L. and Fraser, T. R. (1971). Serum insulin, glucose and lipid levels among mild diabetics in relation to incidence of vascular complications. *Lancet* **I,** p. 880.
Engelberg, H., Gofman, J. and Jones, H. (1952). Serum lipids and lipoproteins in diabetic glomerulosclerosis. *Metabolism* **1,** 300.
Engerman, R. L., Davis, M. D. and Bloodworth, J. M. B. (1971). Retinopathy in experimental diabetes: its relevance to diabetic retinopathy in man. Diabetes Proc. VII Congress Int. Diab. Fed., Buenos Aires, Aug. 1970, Int. Congress Series 231, p. 261.
Entmacher, P. S. and Marks, H. H. (1965). Diabetes in 1964, a world survey. *Diabetes* **14,** 212.
Ernest, I., Lerner, E., Svanborg, A. (1965). Carbohydrate rich, fat poor diet in diabetes. *Am. J. Med.* **39,** 594.
Esmann, V., Jensen, H. J., Lundbaeck, K. (1963). Disappearance of waxy exudates in diabetic retinopathy during administration of *p*-amino-salicylate (PAS). *Acta Med. Scand.* **174,** 99.
Estrich, D. L., Fukayama, G., Kinsell, L. W. (1967). Diagnostic implications of plasma insulin, free fatty acids and glucose responses to protein and carbohydrate loads in normal and diabetic subjects. *Diabetes* **16,** 522.
Farquhar, J. W., Frank, A., Gross, R. C., Reaven, G. M. and Brown, E. P. (1966). Glucose, insulin and triglyceride responses to high and low carbohydrate diets in man. *J. Clin. Invest.* **45,** 1648.
Fanconi, G. (1955). Die sogenannte freie Kost (besser Normalkost) in der Behandlung des kindlichen Diabetes. *Schweiz. Med. Wschr.* **85,** 75
Floyd, J C., Fajans, S., Pek, S., Thiffault, Ch.A., Knopf, R. F. and Conn, J. W. (1970). Synergistic effect of essential amino acids and glucose upon insulin secretion in man. *Diabetes* **19,** 109.
Fredrickson, D. S., Levy, R. I. and Lees, R. S. (1967). Fat transport in lipoproteins. An integrated approach to mechanisms and disorders. *New Engl. J. Med.* **276,** 34.
Galton, D. J. and Wilson, J. P. D. (1970). Glycolitic enzymes in adipose tissue of adult diabetics. *Brit. Med. J.* **3,** 444.
Ghilchik, M. W. and Morris, A. S. (1971). Abnormal insulin response in patients with small vessel disease. *Lancet* **II,** 1227.

Glueck, C. J., Levy, R. J. and Fredrickson, D. S. (1969). Immunoreactive insulin, glucose tolerance and carbohydrate inducibility in types II, III, IV and V hyperlipoproteinemia. *Diabetes* **18,** 739.

Goldrick, R. B. (1967). Effects of insulin on glucose metabolism in isolated human fat cells. *J. Lip. Res.* **8,** 581.

Goldrick, R. B., McLoughlin, G. M. (1970). Lipolysis and lipogenesis from glucose in human fat cells of different sizes. *J. Clin. Invest.* **49,** 1213.

Gordon, E. S. (1962). Relationship between obesity and diabetes mellitus. *Met. Clin. Exper.* **11,** 819.

Greenhalgh, R. M., Rosengarten, D. S., Lewis, B., Calnan, J. S. and Martin, P. (1971). Serum lipids and lipoproteins in peripheral vascular disease. *Lancet* **II,** 947.

Greten, H., Levy, R. I., Eales, H. and Fredrickson, D. S. (1970). On the positional specificity of "lipoprotein lipase". *In* "Atherosclerosis." Proc. Soc. Int. Symposium Chicago, p. 200. Springer-Verlag, New York, Heidelberg, Berlin.

Grey, N. and Kipnis, D. M. (1971). Effect of diet composition on the hyperinsulinemia of obesity. *New Engl. J. Med.* **285,** 827.

Griffiths, J. D., Dymock, J. W., Davies, E. W. G., Hill, D. W. and Williams, R. (1971). Occurrence and prevalence of diabetic retinopathy in hemochromatosis. *Diabetes* **20,** 766.

Grodsky, G. M., Karam, J. H., Pavlatos, F. C. and Forsham, P. H. (1963). Reduction by phenformin of excessive insulin levels after glucose loading in obese and diabetic subjects. *Metabolism* **12,** 278.

Hales, C. N. and Randle, P. J. (1963). Effects of low carbohydrate diet and diabetes mellitus on plasma concentrations of glucose, non-esterified fatty acid and insulin during oral glucose tolerance tests. *Lancet* **i,** 1970.

Harrold, B. P., Marmion, V. J. and Gough, K. R. (1969). A double blind controlled trial of clofibrate in the treatment of diabetic retinopathy. *Diabetes* **18,** 285.

Hartman, A. D., Cohen, A. J., Richane, C. J. and Hsu, T. (1971). Lipolytic response and adenylcyclase activity of rat adipocytes as related to cell size. *J. Lipid. Res.* **12,** 4, 498.

Hashim, S. A. and Asfour, R. H. (1968). Tocopherol in infants fed diets rich in polyunsaturated fatty acids. *Am. J. Clin. Nutr.* **21,** 7.

Havel, R. J. (1965). Metabolism of lipids in chylomicrons and very low density lipoproteins. *In* "Handbook of Physiology." (A. E. Renold and G. F. Cahill, eds), p. 499. Williams and Wilkins, Baltimore.

Havel, R. J. (1970). Metabolism of plasma triglycerides. *In* "Atherosclerosis." Proc. of the second International Symposium, p. 210. Springer-Verlag, New York, Heidelberg, Berlin.

Havel, R. J., Naimark, A. and Borchgrevink, C. F. (1963). Turnover rate and oxidation of free fatty acids of blood plasma in man during exercise. Studies during continuous infusion of palmitate —1—$C^{14}$. *J. Clin. Invest.* **7,** 1054.

Heimberg, M. (1971). Effects of anti-insulin serum and insulin on hepatic metabolism of triglycerides and ketogenesis. *In* "Impact of Insulin on Metabolic Pathways." Int. Symp. Commemorating the 50th Anniversary of Insulin, Jerusalem.

Heimberg, M., Weinstein, I. and Kohout, M. (1969). Effects of glucagon, dibutyryl 3′, 5′ adenosine monpohosphate and concentration of free fatty acids on hepatic lipoid metabolism. *J. Biol. Chem.* **244,** 5131.

Herman, R. H. Zakim, D. and Stifel, F. B. (1970). Effect of diet on lipid metabolism in experimental animals and man. *Fed. Proc. Fed Am. Socs. Exp. Biol.* **29,** 1302.

Hodges, R. E. and Krehl, W. A. (1965). The role of carbohydrates in lipid metabolism. *Am. J. Clin. Nutr.* **17,** 334.

Houtsmuller, A. J. (1966). "The influence of Carbohydrates and Disturbances in Carbohydrate Metabolism upon the Lipoidspectrum in the Serum of Patients with Atherosclerosis; Results of some Investigations on Atherosclerosis," p. 20 (Van den Bergh and Jurgens, ed.), Rotterdam (Traduction).

Houtsmuller, A. J. (1967). Treatment of exudative diabetic retinopathy with atromid S. A double blind study. Diabetes Proc.; VI Congress Int. Diab. Fed. 1967. Excerpta Medica Inst. Congress series no. 140, p. 12.

Houtsmuller, A. J. (1968). Treatment of exudative diabetic retinopathy with atromid. *Ophtalmologica* **156,** 2.

Houtsmuller, A. J. (1969). "Agarose-Gel-Electrophoresis of Lipoproteins: A Clinical Screening Test," Van Gorcum, H. J. Prakke, Assen, Holland.

Houtsmuller, A. J. (1972). Einige internische Aspekte der zukünftigen therapie der diabetische Retinopathie. *Klin. Monatsblätter Augenheilk.* **160,** 521.

Houtsmuller, A. J. and Henkes, H. E. (1964). Clinical investigations of patients with diabetic retinopathy treated with anabolic steroids. V. Congress Int. Diab. Fed. Toronto, July 1964.

Houtsmuller, A. J., Van den Broek-Boot, M. M. A. and Peeters, G. A. M. (1973). Investigation of the influence of dietary fats and carbohydrates on the diurnal metabolic patterns of plasma glucose, insulin, growth hormone, and lipids in obese, non-insulin depending diabetic patients. Diabetes 8th Congress, Brussels.

Hirsch, J. and Gallian, E. (1968). Methods for determination of adipose cell size and cell number in man and animals. *J. Lip. Res.* **9,** 110.

Hirsch, J., Farquhar, J. W., Ahrens, E. H., Peterson, M. L. and Stoffel, W. (1960). Studies of adipose tissue in man. *Am. J. Clin. Nutr.* **8,** 499.

Hugh-Jones, P. (1955). Diabetes in Jamaica, *Lancet* **II,** 891.

Hulley, S. B., Burrows, M. J., Stan Wilson, W. and Nichaman, M. Z. (1972). Lipid and lipoprotein responses of hypertriglyceridaemic outpatients to a low-carbohydrate modification of the AHA fat controlled diet. *Lancet* **II,** 551.

Jackson, R. A., Moloney, M., Lowy, C., Wright, A. D. and Hartog, M. (1971). Differences between metabolic responses to fastening in obese diabetic and obese non-diabetic subjects. *Diabetes* **20,** 214.

Jacobson, Th., Kahanpäa A. and Nikkilä, E. A. (1965). Serum lipids and glucose tolerance in subjects with a family history of diabetes mellitus. *Acta Med. Scand.* **178,** 181.

Jahnke, K., Daweke, H., Liebermeister, H., Schilling, W. H., Hamer, G., Preiss, H. and Gries, F. A. (1967). Hormonal and metabolic aspects of obesity in humans. Diabetes. Proc. VI Congress Int. Diab. Fed. Int. Congress Series 172.

Jahnke, K., Gries, F. A., Engelhardt, A., Herberg, L., Berger, M., Koschinski, H., Claussen F. and Oberdisse, K. (1971). Adaptive and genetically determined regulation of metabolism in obesity. Diabetes. Proc. VII Congress Int. Diab. Fed. 1970. Int. Congress Series 231, p. 507.

Johnsson, S. (1960). Retinopathy and nephropathy in diabetes mellitus. *Diabetes* **9,** 1.

Joplin, G. F., Balck, R. K., Cheng, H., Elkeles, R. S., Fraser, T. R., Kohnen, E. M. and Oakley, N. W. (1971). Treatability of diabetic retinopathy. Diabetes. Proc. VII Congress Int. Diab. Fed., Buenos Aires, 1970. Int. Congress Series 231, p. 276.

Joslin, E. P. (1937). "The Treatment of Diabetes Mellitus." 6th ed. Kempton, London.

Joslin, E. P. and White, P. (1965). The dietary management of diabetes. *Med. Clin. N. Amer.* **49,** 905.

Joslin, E. P., Root, H. F., White, P. and Marble, A. (1952). The treatment of diabetes mellitus. Lea and Febiger, Philadelphia.

Kahil, M. E., McIlkaney, G. R. and Jordan, P. A. (1970). Effect of enteric hormones on insulin secretion. *Metabolism* **19,** 50.

Kahlenberg, A. and Kaland, N. (1964). The effect of insulin on human adipose tissue. *Can. J. Opthal.* **42,** 1623.

Karam, J. H., Grodsky, G. M. and Forsham, P. H. (1963). Excessive insulin response to glucose in obese subjects as measured by immunochemical assay. *Diabetes* **12,** 197.

Karam, J. H., Grodsky, G. M., Pavlatos, F. Ch. and Forsham, P. H. (1965). Critical factors in excessive serum-insulin response to glucose. Obesity in maturity-onset diabetes and growth hormone in acromegaly, *Lancet* **I,** 286.

Kaufmann, N. A., Poznanski, R., Blondheim, S. H. and Stein, Y. (1966). Effect of fructose, glucose, sucrose, and starch on serum lipids in carbohydrate induced hyper-triglyceridemia and in normal subjects. *Israel J. Med. Sci.* **2,** 715.

Keiding, N. R., Mann, G. V., Root, H. F., Lawry, E. J. and Marble, A. (1952a). Serum lipoproteins and cholesterol levels in normal subjects and in young patients with diabetes in relation to vascular complications. *Diabetes* **1,** 434.

Keiding, N. R., Rott, H. F. and Marble, A. (1952b.) Importance of control of diabetes in prevention of vascular complications, *J. Am. Med. Ass.* **150,** 964.

Keller, U., Froesch, E. R. (1972). Vergleichende untersuchungen über den Stoffwechsel von Xylit, Sorbit und Fruktose, *Schweiz. Med. Wschr.* **102,** 1017.

Kempner, W., Lohmann, Peschel R. and Sclayer, C. (1958). Effect of rice diet on diabetes mellitus associated with vascular disease. *Postgrad. Med.* **24,** 359.

Kent, P. W. (1971). Biochemical studies of basement membrane. *In* "Blood vessel disease in diabetes mellitus". V Capri Conference 1971. (K. Lundbaeck, H. Keen, eds). *Acta Diab. Lat.* **8,** Suppl. 1, 228.

Kilo, Ch., Vogler, N., Williamson, J. R. (1972). Muscle capillary basement membrane changes related to aging and diabetes mellitus. *Diabetes* **21,** 881.

King, R. C., Dobree, J. H., Kok, D. A., Foulds, W. S. and Dangerfields, W. G. (1963). Exudative diabetic retinopathy: spontaneous changes and effects of a corn oil diet. *Brit. J. Ophthal.* **47,** 666.

Kinsell, L. W. (1955). Prevention of vascular disease in diabetics. *Diabetes* **4,** 298.

Kinsell, L. W. (1967). Diet and diabetes. *In* "Vascular Complications of Diabetes Mellitus" (Kimura and Caygill, eds), p. 210. The C. V. Mosby Company, Saint Louis.

Kinsell, L. W. and Schlierf, G. (1965). Dietary fat in diabetes mellitus with particular reference to vascular disease. *In* "On the Nature and Treatment of Diabetes". Exerpta Medica. Intern. Congress Series no. 84, p. 430.

Kinsell, L. W., Partridge, J., Boling, L., Margen, S. and Michaels, G. D. (1952). Dietary modification of serum cholesterol and phospholipid levels. *J. Clin. Endocrin. Metab.* **12,** 909.

Kinsell, L. W., Walker, G., Michaels, G. D. and Alson, F. E. (1959a). Dietary fats and the diabetic patient. *New Engl. J. Med.* **261,** 431.

Kinsell, L. W., Michaels, G. D., Walker, G., Wheeler, P., Splitter, S. and Flynn, P. (1959). Dietary linoleic acid and linoleate. Effects in diabetic and nondiabetic subjects with and without vascular disease. *Diabetes* **8,** 179.

Kipnis, D. M. (1970). Studies of insulin secretion: radioimmunoassay of cyclic nucleotides and the role of cyclic AMP. On the pathogenesis of diabetes mellitus. IV Capri Conference 1970. *Acta Diabet. Lat.* **7.** Suppl. 1, 314.

Kipnis, D. M. (1969). Insulin antagonism and diabetes mellitus. International Congress Series no. 172, Diabetes: Proc. Sixth Congress Intern. Diab. Fed., 1967. Exerpta Med. 257–272.

Kjellberg, J. and Ostman, J. (1971). Lipolysis and glucose tolerance in obese subjects during prolonged starvation. *Acta Med. Scand.* **190,** 191.

Knowles, H. C. (1968). The control of diabetes mellitus and the progression of retinopathy, *In* "Treatment of Diabetic Retinopathy". Public Health Service Publication 2090, Symposium September 1968, Warrenton, Virginia.

Lassers, B. W., Kayser, L., Wahlqvest, M. L. and Carlson, L. A. (1971). Relationship in man between plasma free fatty acids and myocardial metabolism of carbohydrate substrates. *Lancet* **II,** p. 448.

Lenenberger, P., Cameron, D., Stauffacher, W., Renold, A. E. and Babel, J. (1971). Ocular lesions in rats rendered chronically diabetic with streptozotocin. *Ophthal. Res.* **2,** 189.

Levine, R. (1970). The mechanism of insulin secretion. *New Engl. J. Med.* **283,** 522.

Levine, R. and Haft, D. E. (1970). Carbohydrate homeostasis. *New Engl. J. Med.* **283,** 175.

Little, J. A., Birchwood, B. L., Simmons, D. A, Antar, M. A., Kallos, A., Buckley, G. C. and Csima, A. (1970). Interrelationship between the kinds of dietary carbohydrate and fat in hyperlipoproteinemic patients. Part I. Sucrose and starch with polyunsaturated fat. *Atherosclerosis* **11,** 173.

Lowy, A. D. and Barach, J. H. (1958). Predictive nature of lipoprotein and cholesterol determination in diabetic patients who developed cardiovascular complications. *Circulation* **17,** 14.

Lundbaek, K. and Keen, H. (1971). Blood vessel disease in diabetes mellitus. V Capri Conference. *Acta Diabet. Lat.* **8,** Suppl. 1.

Lundbaeck, K., Juel Christensen, N., Jensen, V. A., Johansen, K., Steen Olsen, T., Prange Hansen, A. S., Ørshof, R. and Østerby, R. (1971). The pathogenesis of diabetic angiopathy and growth hormone. *Dan. Med. Bull.* **18,** 1.

Macdonald, J. (1965). The lipid response of young woman to dietary carbohydrates. *Am. J. Clin. Nutr.* **16,** 458.

Macdonald, J. (1966). Dietary fructose and serum lipid levels in men. *Proc. Nutr. Soc.* **25,** 2.

Mahler, R. (1967). Insulin, diabetes and atheroma. *In* "Diabetes", Proc. VI Congress Int. Diab. Fed. Stockholm 1967. Int. Congress Series 172, p. 299.

Mahler, R. (1971). The effect of diabetes and insulin on biochemical reactions of the arterial wall in blood vessel disease in diabetes mellitus. *Acta Diabet. Lat.* **8,** Suppl. 1, 68.

Malherbe, C., de Gasparo, M., Berthet, P., de Hertogh, R. and Hoet, J. J. (1971). The pattern of plasma insulin response to glucose in patients with a previous myocardial infarction, the respective effects of age and disease. *Europ. J. Clin. Invest.* **1,** 265.

Marble, A. (1965). Relation of control of diabetes to vascular sequelae. *Med. Clin. N. Amer.* **49,** 1137.

McLean, P., Brown, J., Walters, E. and Greenslade, K. (1967). Effect of alloxan-diabetes on multiple forms of hexokinase in adipose tissue and lung. *Biochem. J.* **105,** 1301.

Mehnert, H. (1969). Diabetische Mikroangiopathie und Stoffwechselkontrolle. *Deut. Med. Wschr.* **94,** 42.

Melatti, A. M., Beck, J. C., Dupre, J. and Rubinstein, D. (1970). Conversion of glucose to lipid by human adipose tissue *in vitro*. *Metabolism* **19**, 988.

Merimee, H. J., Siperstein, M. D., Hall, J. D. and Fineberg, S. E. (1970). Capillary basement membrane structure: a comparative study of diabetics and sexual ateliotic dwarfs. *J. Clin. Invest.* **49**, 2161.

Montagne, W. and Taylor, K. W. (1968). Regulation of insulin secretion by short-chain fatty acids. *Nature* (*Lond.*) **217**, 853.

Moreau, P. G. and Pichon, P. (1970). Hyperlipidémie et retinopathie diabetique. *Arch. Opthal.* **30**, 11.

Morrison, A. D., Clements, R. S. and Winegrad, A. J. (1972). Effects of elevated glucose concentration on the metabolism of the aortic wall. *J. Clin. Invest.* **51**, 3114.

Mouratoff, G. J., Carroll, N. V., Scott, E. M. (1969). Diabetes mellitus in Alhabaskan Indians in Alaska. *Diabetes* **18**, 1, 29.

Muller, W. A., Faloona, G. R., Aquila-Paroda, E. and Unger, R. H. (1970). Abnormal alpha cell function in diabetes. *New Engl. J. Med.* **283**, 109.

Muller, W. A., Faloona, G. R. and Unger, R. H. (1971). Influence of antecedent diet upon glucagon and insulin secretion. *New Engl. J. Med.* **285**, 1450.

Nestel, P. J., Austin, W. and Foxman, C. (1969). Lipoprotein lipase content and triglyceride fatty acid uptake in adipose tissue of rats of different body weight. *J. Lipid. Res.* **10**, 383.

Nestel, P. J., Carroll, K. F. and Havenstein, N. (1970). Plasma triglyceride response to carbohydrates, fats and caloric intake. *Metabolism* **19**, 1.

New, M. J., Roberts, T. N., Burman, E. L. and Reader, G. G. (1963). The significance of blood lipid alterations in diabetes mellitus. *Diabetes* **12**, 208.

Nikkilä, E. A. and Ojala, K. (1966). Acute effects of fructose and glucose on the concentration and removal rate of plasma triglyceride. *Life Sci.* **5**, 89.

Nikkilä, E. A. and Taskinen, M. R. (1970). Hypertriglyceridemia and insulin secretion, a complex causal relationship. *In* "Atherosclerosis", p. 220. Proc. Second Intern. Symposium, Springer-Verlag, New York, Heidelberg, Berlin.

Numan, S., Bortz, W. M. and Lynen, F. (1965). Regulation of fatty acid synthesis at the acetyl CoA carboxylation step. *Adv. Enzym. Regulat.* **3**, 407.

Oakley, N., Hill, D. W., Joplin, G. F., Kohner, E. M. and Fraser, T. R. (1967). Diabetic retinopathy: I. the assessment of severity and prognosis by comparison with a set of standard fundus photographs. *Diabetologia* **3**, 402.

Østerby Hansen, R., Lundbaeck, K., Olson, T. S. and Orskow, H. (1966). Experimental diabetic glomerulopathy, some ultra-structural observations. *Diabetologia* **2**, 234.

Patel, J. C., Metha, A. B., Dhirawani, M. K., Juthani, V. J. and Aijer, L. (1969). High carbohydrate diet in the treatment of diabetes mellitus. *Diabetologica* **5**, 243.

Pelkonen, R., Miettinen, T. A., Taskinen, M. R. and Nikkilä, E. A. (1968). Effect of acute elevation of plasma glycerol, triglyceride and EFA levels on glucose utilization and plasma insulin. *Diabetes* **17**, 76.

Perley, M. and Kipnis, D. (1966). Plasma insulin responses to glucose and tolbutamide of normal weight and obese diabetic and nondiabetic subjects. *Diabetes* **15**, 867.

Peterson, D. T. and Reaven, G. M. (1971). Evidence that glucose load is an important determinant of plasma insulin response in normal subjects. *Diabetes* **30**, 729.

Pi-Sunyer, F. X., Hashim, S. A. and Van Italli, Th. B. (1969). Insulin and ketone responses to ingestion of medium and long-chain triglycerides in man. *Diabetes* **18**, 96.

Pollack, H. (1960). Fat content of the diabetic diet. *Diabetes* **9**, 145.

Pomerance, J. and Kunkel, H. G. (1950). Serum lipids in diabetes mellitus. *Proc. Am. Diab. Ass.* **10,** 217.

Porte, D., O'Hara, D. D. and Williams, R. H. (1965). Low post heparin lipolytic activity in myxoedema (abstract). *Clin. Res.* **13,** 108.

Rabinowitch, J. N. (1935). Arteriosclerosis in diabetes: I. relationship between plasma cholesterol and arteriosclerosis. *Ann. Int. Med.* **8,** 1436.

Rabinowitz, D. and Zierler, K. L. (1962). Forearm metabolism in obesity and its response to intraarterial insulin: characterization of insulin resistance and evidence for adaptive hyperinsulinism. *J. Clin. Invest.* **12,** 2173.

Randle, P. J., Hales, C. N., Garland, P. B. and Newholme, E. A. (1963). The glucose fatty acid cycle: Its role in insulin sensitivity and the metabolic disturbances of diabetes mellitus. *Lancet* **I,** 7285.

Reaven, G. M., Lerner, R. L., Stern, M. P., Farquhar, J. F. and Nakinishi, R. (1967). Role of insulin in endogenous hypertriglyceridemia. *J. Clin. Invest.* **46,** 1756.

Reaven, G. M., Shen, S. W., Silvers, A. and Farquhar, J. W. (1971). Is there a delay in the plasma insulin response of patients with chemical diabetes mellitus? *Diabetes* **20,** 416.

Renold, A. E. (1971). Metabolism in spontaneous and experimental hyperglycemic animal syndromes. *In* "Impact of Insulin on Metabolic Pathways". Int. Symp. commemorating the 50th anniversary of Insulin. Jerusalem Oct. 1971.

Ricketts, H. T. (1965). The influence of diabetic control on angiopathy. *In* "On the Nature and Treatment of Diabetes". p. 588. Excerpta Medical Foundation Amsterdam.

Righetti, A., Scherrer, J. R., Micheli, H. and Pomella, D. (1973). Etude clinique des relations entre le diabète, les hyperlipoprotéinémies et l'athéromatose. *Schweiz. Med. Wschr.* **103,** 668.

Root, H. F., Sinden, R. H. and Zanca, R. (1950). Factors in the rate of development of vascular lesions in the kidneys, retinae and peripheral vessels in the youthful diabetic. *Am. J. Diet. Ass.* **17,** 179.

Rozen, P. and Shafrir, E. (1972). Comparison of changes in plasma free fatty acids, glycerol and insulin following glucose and fructose loads. *Israel J. Med. Sci.* **8,** 75.

Ryan, J. R., Baladimos, M. C., Charan, B. I., Root, H. F., Marble, A., White, P. and Joslin, A. P. (1970). Quarter century victory medal for diabetes: a follow up of patients one to twenty years later. *Metabolism* **19,** 493.

Sageld, U., Littauer, H., Jesperen, C. S. and Aendersen, S. (1966). Diabetes mellitus in Eskimos. Epidemiological studies in Greenland. *Acta Med. Scand.* **179,** 29.

Salans, L. B. (1973). Effect of dietary carbohydrate intake on plasma glucose and insulin concentration. Diabetes Proc. VIII Congress Int. Diab. Fed. 1973. Excerpta Med. Int. Congress series No. 280, p. 128.

Salans, L. B. and Dougherty, J. W. (1971). The effect of insulin upon glucose metabolism by adipose cells of different size. *J. Clin. Invest.* **50,** 1399.

Salans, L. B. and Reaven, G. M. (1966). Effect of insulin pretreatment on glucose and lipid metabolism of liver slices from normal rats. *Proc. Soc. Exp. Biol. Med.* **122,** 1208.

Salans, L. B., Knittle, J. L. and Hirsch, J. (1968). The role of adipose cell size and adipose tissue insulin sensitivity in the carbohydrate intolerance of human obesity. *J. Clin. Invest.* **47,** 153.

Salans, L. B., Horton, E. and Sims, E. (1970). Influence of fat cell size and dietary carbohydrate intake on adipose tissue insulin sensitivity in adult onset obesity. *Clin. Res.* **18,** 463.

Salans, L. B., Horton, E. S. and Sims, E. A. H. (1971). Experimental obesity in man: cellular character of the adipose tissue. *J. Clin. Invest.* **50,** 1005.

Scherf, D. and Boyd, L. J. (1955). "Herzkrankheiten und Gefässerkrankungen". Springer-Verlag, Wien.

Schettler, F. G. and Wahl, P. (1969). Diabetes mellitus and atherosclerosis, *In* "Atherosclerosis", p. 367. (Schettler and Boyd, eds). Elsevier, Amsterdam.

Schlierf, G., Reinheimer, W. and Stossberg, V. (1971). Diurnal patterns of plasma triglycerides and free fatty acids in normal subjects and in patients with endogeneous (type IV) hyperlipoproteinemia. *Nutr. Metabol.* **13,** 80.

Schöflıng, K. and Graeve, R. (1956). Über die Todesursachen bei der Zuckerkrankheit. *Med. Welt* **25,** 627.

Schrade, W., Boehle, E., Biegler, R. and Harmuth, E. (1963). Fatty acid composition of lipid fractions in diabetic serum. *Lancet* **I,** 285.

Schwartz, J. P. and Jurigas, R. L. (1971). Studies on the hormone-sensitive lipase of adipose tissue. *J. Lipid. Res.* **12,** 553.

Seltzer, H. S. and Smith, W. L. (1959), Plasma insulin activity after glucose. An index of insulogenic reserve in normal and diabetic man. *Diabetes* **8,** 417.

Seltzer, H. S., Allen, W. E., Herron, A. L. and Brennan, M. T. (1967). Insulin secretion in response to glycemic stimulus: relation of delayed initial release to carbohydrate intolerance in mild Diabetes mellitus. *J. Clin. Invest.* **46,** 323.

Seyffert, W. A. and Madison, L. L. (1967). Physiologic effect of metabolic fuels on carbohydrate metabolism. *Diabetes* **16,** 765.

Shrago, E., Glennon, J. A. and Gordon, E. S. (1971). Comparative aspects of lipogenesis in mammalian tissues. *Metabolism* **20,** 54.

Singh, J. (1955). Low-fat diet and therapeutic doses of insulin in diabetes mellitus. *Lancet* **I,** 268, 422.

Siperstein, M. D., Unger, R. H. and Madison, L. L. (1968). Studies of muscle capillary basement membranes in normal subjects, diabetic and prediabetic patients, *J. Clin. Invest.* **47,** 1973.

Sjöström, L. (1972). Adult human adipose tissue cellularity and metabolism. *Acta Med. Scand.*, suppl. 544.

Sjöström, L., Stern, N., Hollander, S., Batchelor, B. R., Cohn, C. K. and Hirsch, J. (1972). Adipose-cell size and immunoreactive insulin levels in obese and normal-weight adults. *Lancet* **II,** 948.

Sloan, J. M., Mackay, J. S. and Sheridan, B. (1970). Glucose tolerance and insulin response in atherosclerosis. *Brit. Med. J.* **4,** 586.

Smith, U. (1971). Effect of cell size on lipid synthesis by human adipose tissue in vitro. *J. Lipid. Res.* **12,** 65.

Soskin, S. and Levine, R. (1952). "Carbohydrate Metabolism", p. 8. University of Chicago Press.

Spiro, R. G. (1959). Role of insulin in two pathways of glucose metabolism in vivo glucosamine and glycogen synthesis. *Ann. N.Y. Acad. Sci.* **82,** 366.

Stephan, F., Reville, Ph., Thierry, R. and Schlienger, J. L. (1972). Correlations between plasma insulin and body weight in obesity, anorexia nervosa and diabetes mellitus. *Diabetologia* **8,** 196.

Stout, R. W. (1970). Development of vascular lesions in insulin treated animals fed a normal diet. *Brit. Med. J.* **3,** 685.

Stout, R. W. (1971). The effect of insulin on the incorporation of sodium (1–$^{14}$C)-Acetate into the lipids of the rat aorta. *Diabetologia* **7,** 367.

Sutherland, E. W. and Robinson, G. A. (1969). The role of cyclic AMP in the control of carbohydrate metabolism. *Diabetes* **18,** 797.

Tripathy, B. B. and Kar, B. C. (1965). Observations on clinical patterns of diabetes mellitus in India. *Diabetes* **14,** 404.

Tuna, N., Frankhauser, S. and Goetz, F. C. (1968). Total serum fatty acids in diabetes. Relative and absolute concentrations of individual fatty acids. *Am. J. Med. Sci.* **255,** 120.

Tzagournis, M., Serdensticker, J. F. and Hamwi, G. J. (1967). Serum insulin, carbohydrate and lipid abnormalities in patients with premature coronary heart disease. *Ann. Int. Med.* **67,** 1, 42.

Unger, R. H. (1971). Glucagon physiology and pathophysiology. *New Engl. J. Med.* **285,** 443.

Van Eck, W. F. (1959). The effect of a low-fat diet on the serum lipids in diabetes and its significance in diabetic retinopathy. *Am. J. Med.* **27,** 196.

Wessels, M., Gries, F. A., Irmcher, K., Liebermeister, H., Buchenau, H. and Viehweger, I. (1970). Metabolische Konsequenzen einer kohlenhydratarmen Diät (Punkt Diät) bei Normalpersonen. *Deut. Med. Wschr.* **95,** 382.

West, K. M. and Kalbfleisch, J. M. (1966). Glucose tolerance, nutrition and diabetes in Uruguay, Venezuela, Malaya and East Pakistan. *Diabetes* **15,** 1, 9.

West, K. M. and Kalbfleisch, J. M. (1971). Influence of nutritional factors on prevalence of diabetes. *Diabetes* **20,** 99.

Williamson, J. R. (1971). V Capri Conference April 7–8, 1971. *Acta Diab. Lat.* **8,** 527.

Williamson, J. R., Vogler, N. J. and Kilo, C. (1970). Muscle capillary basement membrane changes in diabetes mellitus. *Diabetes,* **19,** 356 (abstract).

Zinder, O., Arad, R. and Shapiro, B. (1962). Effect of cell size on the metabolism of isolated fat cells. *Israel J. Med. Sci.* **3,** 787.

6

# Specific Effects of Types of Dietary Fat on Arterial Thrombosis

G. HORNSTRA

*Unilever Research, Vlaardingen, The Netherlands*



## I. INTRODUCTION

Arterial thrombosis is the main lethal complication of atherosclerosis (Owren, 1964; Harland, 1969). Moreover, there is increasing morphological (Duguid, 1946; Heggtveit, 1968; Likar *et al.*, 1969) and experimental (Friedman and Byers, 1961; Hand and Chandler, 1962; Sumiyoshi *et al.*, 1973) evidence that it also plays a role in atherogenesis. However, biochemical studies on the type and origin of lipid in atherosclerotic plaques (Newman and Zilversmit, 1962; Smith, 1967; Weigensberg *et al.*, 1972; Craig *et al.*, 1973a, 1973b) show convincingly that this role is only a contributing one. Morphological work on monkeys has given the same indication (Prathap, 1973) and therefore the thrombogenic theory should not be considered as exclusive (see also Born *et al.*, 1971). Nonetheless there are sufficient grounds to include arterial thrombosis as a topic when investigating the physiological effects of dietary fats. It is therefore surprising that up till now it has received little attention, which may be due to the fact that so far no

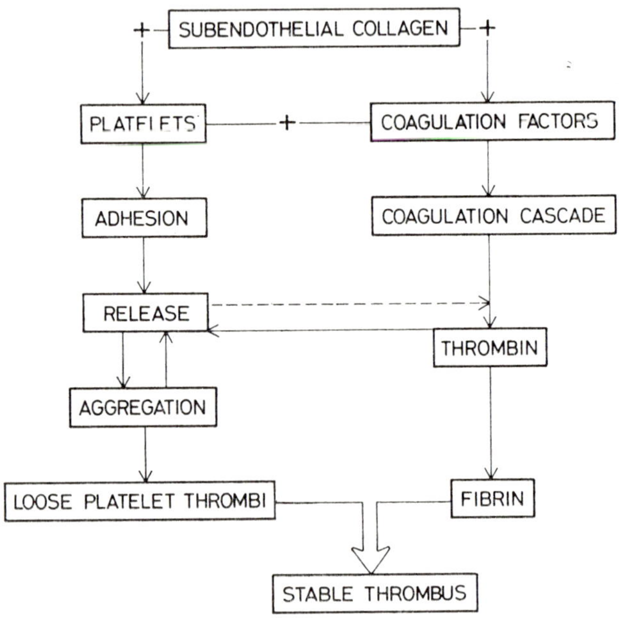


Fig. 1. Diagram of thrombus formation (simplified).

suitable techniques have been available for induction and exact quantification of experimental arterial thrombosis and moreover, such studies could start only after the pathways for arterial thrombus formation had been elucidated. Present knowledge now meets these conditions and in view of the great clinical importance of arterial thrombosis, extensive systematic research is required on the effects of type and amount of dietary fat on arterial thrombus formation.

The processes leading to the formation of a stable thrombus, are schematically outlined in Fig. 1. These processes have been described in detail (French, 1969; Mustard and Packham, 1970). Briefly, circulating platelets adhere to subendothelial tissue—collagen, microfibrils, basement membrane—which may become blood-exposed after vessel trauma, rupturing of an atherosclerotic plaque, etc. Adhered platelets release some of their constituents such as adenine nucleotides, serotonin, $Ca^{++}$ and adrenalin. Adenosine diphosphate (ADP), made available by this release reaction, causes blood platelets to aggregate: passing platelets stick to the adhered ones, thus forming a mural platelet thrombus which, being unstable, is easily embolized. The platelet release reaction is also induced by platelet aggregation, so the formation of mural and circulating platelet thrombi is a self-propagating process.

Collagen, while interacting with one of the contact factors, factor XII (Niewiarowski *et al.*, 1965), or with platelets (Walsh, 1972b), triggers the intrinsic coagulation system, which is also initiated by platelets *per se*, especially when a low amount of ADP is present (Walsh, 1972a). Coagulation is accelerated by platelet factor 3 ($PF_3$, platelet phospholipids) which is normally inactive (Fantl and Ward, 1958) but which becomes available concommittant with the platelet release reaction (Sixma and Nijessen, 1970). The end product of the clotting process, fibrin, reinforces the unstable platelet thrombus, leading to a stabilized thrombus. Thus thrombus formation comprises two main processes: formation of loose platelet thrombi and fibrin formation. There is good evidence that haemodynamic factors determine which process prevails: at high flow rates the platelet thrombotic functions are prominent, leading to white thrombus formation, whereas at stasis and low flow velocities coagulation is dominant, leading to the formation of a red clot, containing relatively few platelets (Rosenberg, 1970; Wells, 1970; Rieger *et al.*, 1973). These findings explain why in the venous system mainly red blood clots are formed, whereas the arterial thrombi are fibrin-poor and platelet-rich. Consequently, the latter cannot be prevented by anticoagulants (Michaels, 1972; Sherry, 1972), as can venous thrombi (Sharnoff and DeBlasio, 1970; Kakkar *et al.*, 1971).

Dietary oils and fats have long been thought to influence arterial thrombosis. A recent literature review (Hornstra, 1973/74) shows that there is no unanimity as to the effect of dietary fats on *in vitro* platelet thrombotic functions, no matter whether the fats are administered as a single oral load, by intravenous infusion, or by continuous feeding. The conflicting results cannot be ascribed to differences in fatty acid composition but are most probably from methodological origin. The rather few experiments concerning the effects of dietary fats on arterial thrombosis suggest that saturated fats enhance thrombus formation, whereas unsaturated fats do not or are even antithrombotic. Our own research, which will be reviewed below, agrees with this.

# II. ARTERIAL THROMBUS FORMATION IN RATS

## A. Experimental Model

The technique of inducing and quantifying an arterial thrombus in the rat has been described previously (Hornstra and Vendelmans, 1973). A loop-shaped polyethylene cannula—the aorta loop—is inserted into the abdominal aorta of male rats in such a way that it projects from the body. Endothelial damage and flow disturbances result in the production and growth of a fibrin-poor, platelet-rich mural thrombus, which reaches an occlusive state after about five days. The structures of these experimental thrombi in comparative phases of development are similar to those of natural arterial thrombi in man and animal. Loop obstruction can be observed by a change in colour of the translucent loop from light red to dark blue. The period between insertion and total obstruction of the loop, the obstruction time (OT), is a measure of the thrombosis tendency, as was checked by demonstrating the known antithrombotic effects of prostaglandin $E_1$ and aspirin (Fig. 2).

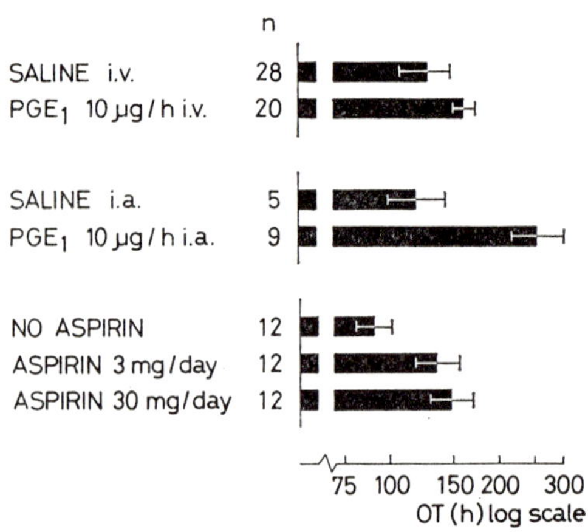


Fig. 2. Effect of prostaglandin $E_1$ ($PGE_1$), administered either intravenously or intra-arterially, and of aspirin, mixed with the diet, on arterial thrombus formation in rats (OT $\pm$ SEM).

## B. Effect of Amount of Dietary Fat

OT-Measurements in young male rats fed for four months adequate diets containing 2·5–60 cal% sunflowerseed oil (SO) at the expense of sucrose revealed that arterial thrombosis tendency decreased with increasing dietary SO content (Fig. 3). Since similar effects were not found with increasing amounts of hydrogenated coconut oil (HCO) and

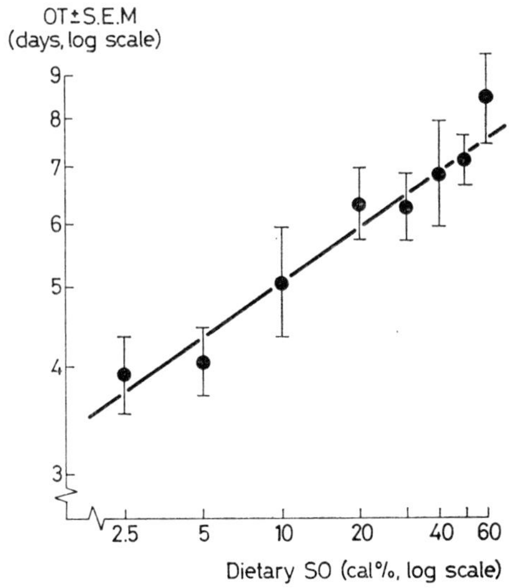


Fig. 3. Effect of dietary sunflowerseed oil (SO) on arterial thrombosis tendency (OT) in rats.

butterfat (BF), it is highly probable that the observed effect is not due to the different amounts of sucrose in the various diets. This is confirmed by experiments in which the dietary fat and carbohydrate contents were kept constant at 60 and 17 cal% respectively. The fat was composed of various mixtures of SO and HCO or of SO and BF. The results of both experiments show a significant, rectilinear, positive relationship between log OT and the amount of SO in the diet (Fig. 4).

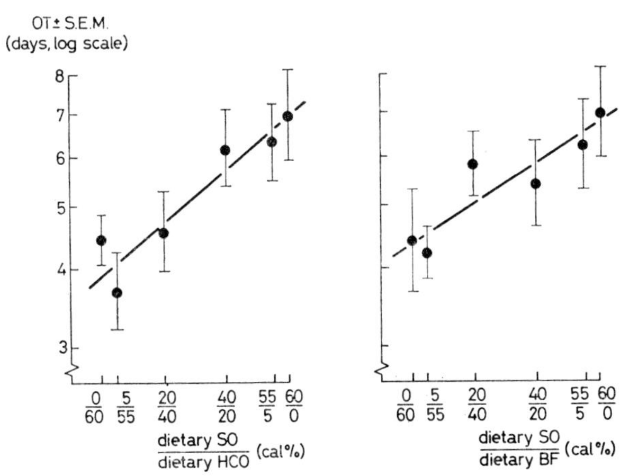


Fig. 4. Effect of mixtures of sunflowerseed oil (SO) with hydrogenated coconut oil (HCO) or butterfat (BF) in the diet on arterial thrombosis tendency in rats.

Although the amount of dietary carbohydrate does not seem to have a significant effect on arterial thrombosis tendency, the type of carbohydrate definitely has. This is shown in Fig. 5, in which the SO-induced OT-change is shown with diets containing either saccharose or corn starch. In both cases SO increased the OT to a comparable

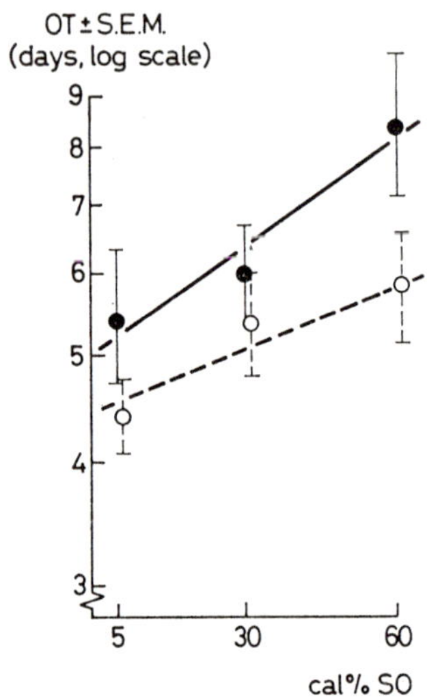


Fig. 5. Effect of saccharose (●–●) and corn starch (○–○) on arterial thrombosis tendency (OT) induced by three dietary levels of sunflowerseed oil in rats.

extent, but as the general OT-level for the saccharose-fed animals was significantly higher than that for the rats fed the corn starch diets, it can be concluded that in this arterial thrombosis model, saccharose is less thrombogenic than corn starch.

## C. Effect of Different Types of Dietary Fat

The differences in thrombogenicity between SO, HCO and BF suggest that SO contains some antithrombotic factor which is missing in HCO and BF. The main constituents of SO are palmitic, stearic, oleic and linoleic acid (Table 1). As the former three fatty acids occur in comparable amounts in both HCO and BF, it is tempting to speculate that linoleic acid is the anti-thrombotic fraction in SO. This indication is supported by the significant, positive relationship that exists between dietary linoleic acid content and thrombogenicity, no matter whether SO is the only dietary fat or whether it is mixed with HCO or BF

Table 1

Average fatty acid composition of some oils and fats (%)[a]

| Fatty acid | Butter fat | Canbra oil | Coconut oil | Coconut oil, hydrogenated | Linseed oil | MCT oil | Olive oil | Palm oil | Rapeseed oil | Soyabean oil, hydrogenated | Sunflowerseed oil | Triglyceride mixture | Whale oil |
|---|---|---|---|---|---|---|---|---|---|---|---|---|---|
| ⩽10:0 | 6 | | 14 | 14 | | 94 | | | | | | | |
| 12:0 | 4 | | 44 | 44 | | 1 | | | | | | 32 | |
| 14:0 | 12 | | 19 | 19 | | | | 1 | | | | 57 | 8 |
| 14:1 | 2 | | | | | | | | | | | | |
| 15:0 | 1 | | | | | | | | | | | | |
| 16:0 | 26 | 5 | 10 | 10 | 6 | 1 | 13 | 44 | 3 | 11 | 6 | 10 | 20 |
| 16:1 | 3 | | | | | | 1 | | | | | | 12 |
| 17:0 | 1 | | | | | | | | | | | | 1 |
| 17:1 | | | | | | | | | | | | | 2 |
| 18:0 | 11 | 1 | 3 | 11 | 5 | | 3 | 5 | | 12 | 4 | | 4 |
| 18:1 | 25 | 50 | 8 | 2 | 20 | 1 | 70 | 38 | 12 | 68[b] | 25 | | 17 |
| 18:2 | 2 | 19 | 2 | | 13 | | 10 | 10 | 14 | 7[b] | 63 | | 3 |
| 18:3 | 1 | 9 | | | 55 | | | | 10 | | | | |
| 18:4 | | | | | | | | | | | | | 4 |
| 20:0 | 2 | | | | | | | | 1 | | | | |
| 20:1 | | 4 | | | | | | | 7 | | | | |
| 20:poly | | | | | | | | | | | | | 16 |
| 22:0 | | | | | | | | | | | 1 | | |
| 22:1 | | 8 | | | | | | | 50 | | | | |
| 22:poly | | | | | | | | | 1 | | | | 3 |
| 24:0 | | | | | | | | | 1 | | | | |
| 24:1 | | | | | | | | | | | | | 6 |
| Σ saturated | 63 | 6 | 90 | 98 | 11 | 96 | 16 | 50 | 5 | 23 | 11 | 99 | 33 |
| Σ monoenoic | 30 | 62 | 8 | 2 | 20 | 1 | 71 | 38 | 69 | 68[b] | 25 | | 37 |
| Σ polyenoic | 3 | 28 | 2 | | 66 | | 10 | 10 | 25 | 7[b] | 63 | | 26 |

[a] Only fractions ⩾ 1% are given.

[b] About 58% *trans* fatty acids.

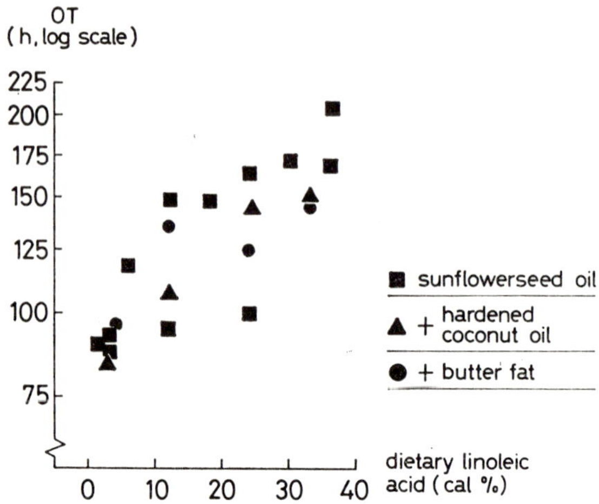


Fig. 6. Relationship between dietary linoleic acid content and thrombogenicity (OT).

(Fig. 6). The relationship between linoleic acid content and dietary thrombogenicity was investigated further by feeding rats diets containing 50 cal% fats with highly different fatty acid spectra (Table 1). The OT values after two months of feeding are shown in Fig. 7. The

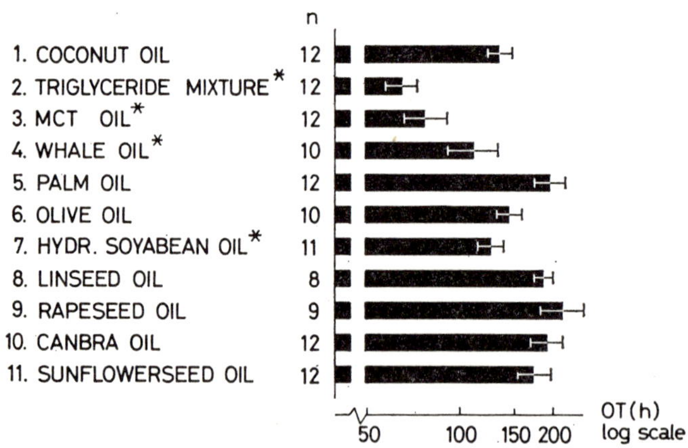


Fig. 7. Effect of different dietary fats on arterial thrombus formation (OT ± SEM).

fats are sequenced on the basis of their linoleic acid content; those marked with an asterisk were supplied with sufficient glyceryl trilinolate to prevent EFA deficiency. As can be seen from Table 1, all fats contain palmitic, stearic, oleic and linoleic acid (except the mixture of medium-chain triglycerides (MCT oil) and rapeseed oil, which do not contain 18:0). When the proportional amounts of each of these fatty acids in the various dietary fats are plotted against the OT values induced by those fats (Fig. 8), the palmitic acid content seems to be negatively related to the OT, whereas the linoleic acid content seems to be positively related to the OT. This latter relationship indeed appeared

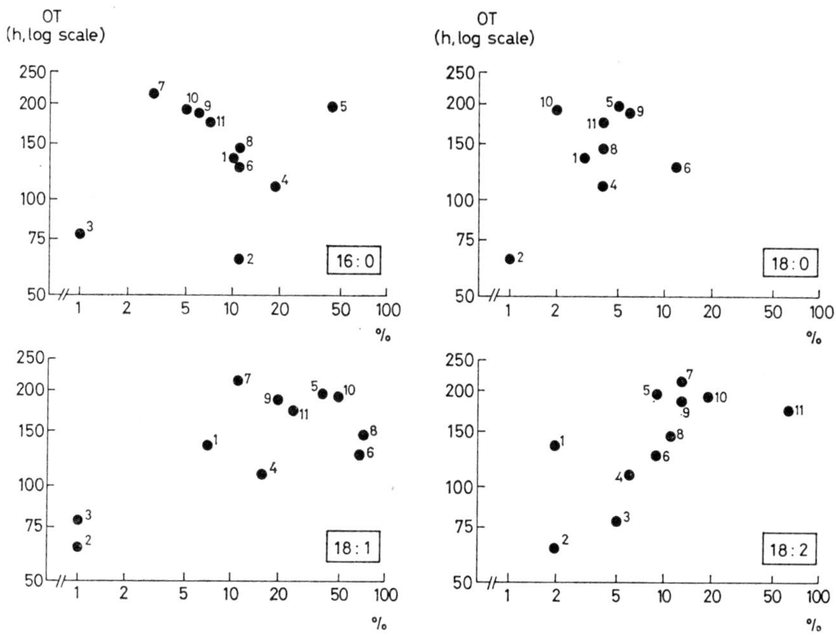


Fig. 8. Relationship between fatty acid composition (%) and thrombogenicity (OT) of different dietary fats (log scales). Numbers refer to fats mentioned in Fig. 7.

to be significant ($r = 0{\cdot}72$, $P < 0{\cdot}05$, Spearman's rank correlation test), confirming the assumed antithrombotic effect of linoleic acid. No clear relationship of the OT with the stearic or oleic acid content of the dietary fats could be observed.

Since food intake and fatty acid absorption are considerably influenced by the type of dietary fatty acid (Carroll, 1958; Carroll and Richards, 1958; Hornstra, 1972) we tried to describe the average log OT per dietary fat as a function of the average amounts of the different fatty acids absorbed (Hornstra and Lussenburg, to be published). As can be seen from Fig. 9, log OT is very well related with half the amount of absorbed myristic acid plus the total amount of absorbed palmitic and stearic acid. Only MCT (No. 3) and PO (No. 5) do not fit this relationship. MCT contains mainly C 8:0 and C 10:0, which are metabolized quite differently from longer-chain fatty acids. Absorption and metabolism of these fatty acids seem to be more related to carbohydrates and from this consideration MCT feeding can be considered as low-fat feeding, which was shown to induce a low OT (Section II B). Why PO is an exception is not known.

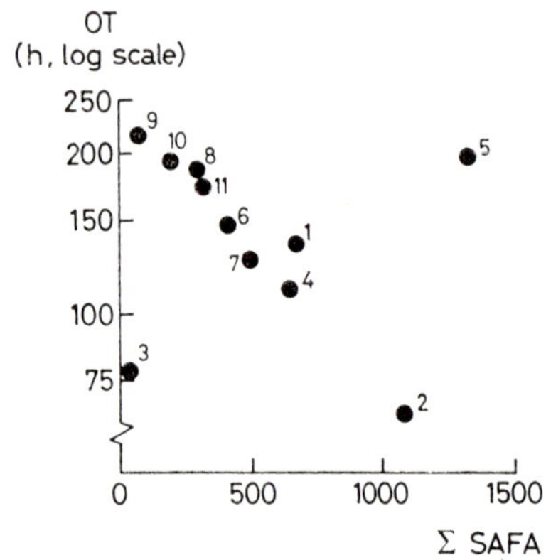


Fig. 9. Relationship between the amount of dietary fatty acids absorbed (Σ SAFA: (C 14:0)/2 + C 16:0 + C 18:0, mg/animal/day) and arterial thrombosis tendency (OT) in rats.

This experiment indicates that dietary long-chain saturated fatty acids (SAFAs) with 14 or more carbon atoms are thrombogenic. This implies that their replacement by unsaturated fatty acids will decrease dietary thrombogenicity. In order to investigate whether all unsaturated fatty acids are equally effective in this antithrombotic effect, a comparative study was performed with oleic and linoleic acid. Rats were fed diets containing 60 cal% fat, the dietary fats consisting either of 10 or 40% SAFA, mainly palmitic and stearic acid. The linoleic acid content was either 30 or 50%, the rest being oleic acid (Fig. 10). If oleic and linoleic acid are equally antithrombotic, there will be no difference in OT between the two low-SAFA diets and between the two high-SAFA diets. This was, however, not the case: at both SAFA levels the OT is significantly longer (thrombosis tendency lower) in the group receiving the high linoleic acid dose ($P_2 < 0{\cdot}05$). Correction for differences in food intake and fatty acid absorption did not change this result; hence it can be concluded that linoleic acid has a stronger antithrombotic effect than oleic acid.

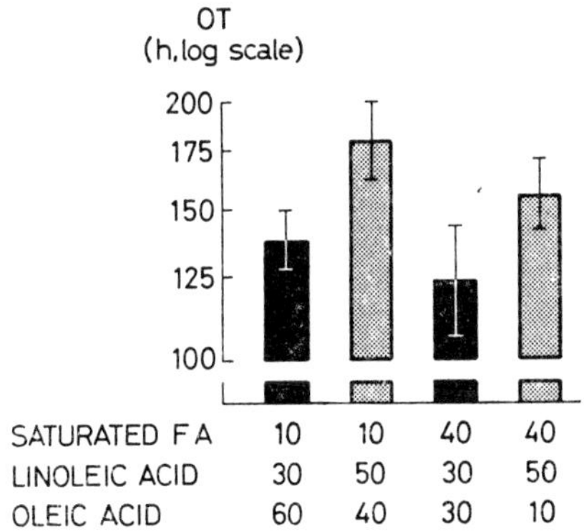


Fig. 10. Effect of fatty acid composition (%) of dietary fat (60 cal%) on dietary thrombogenicity (OT ± SEM).

Combining the findings shown in Figs 7–10 it is highly probable that:

1. saturated fatty acids with 14 or more carbon atoms promote arterial thrombus formation;
2. oleic acid is neutral as to arterial thrombus formation. Since rapeseed- and canbra oil differ mainly in their erucic and oleic acid contents (Table 1) and induce about the same OT (Fig. 7, Nos. 9 and 10), all long-chain monoenoic fatty acids may be non-thrombogenic;
3. linoleic acid has a specific antithrombotic effect. Most probably this is also the case with linolenic acid, since linseed oil and sunflowerseed oil, differing mainly in their C 18:2 and C 18:3 content (Table 1), induce about the same thrombosis tendency (Fig. 7, Nos. 8 and 11).

There are no indications that the molecular configuration around the double bonds influence the effect of unsaturated fatty acids on thrombogenesis. Hydrogenated soyabean oil, as used in the experiment shown in Fig. 7 (No. 7), contained about 58% *trans* fatty acids. Nevertheless it fits perfectly in the curve showing the relationship between SAFA absorption and arterial thrombosis tendency (Fig. 9). Moreover, *trans* oleic acid in a 1:1 mixture with *cis* oleic acid induced an OT (105 hr) which is not significantly different from that induced by *cis* oleic acid alone (124 hr, 60 cal% fat, 80% C 18:1).

## D. Mechanism of the Dietary Fat Effect

All experiments concerning the mechanism by which dietary fats exercise their (anti-) thrombotic effects were performed with rats fed diets containing 50 cal% SO (SO-diet) or 45 cal% HCO supplemented with 5 cal% SO in order to prevent EFA deficiency (HCO diet). These dietary regimens induce OTs of about 170 hr (SO) and 100 hr (HCO), the effect of both fats depending on the feeding period. The anti-thrombotic effect of the SO diet is maximal after 3–5 weeks feeding (Fig. 11); this period is not significantly influenced by a pre-experi-

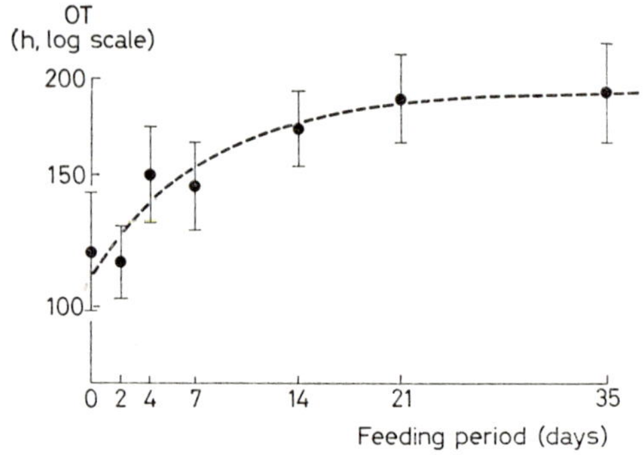


Fig. 11. Course of OT-increasing effect of a diet containing 50 cal% SO, observed in rats (OT ± SEM) $n = 12$.

mental 4-week fat-free period. The course of the thrombosis-promoting effect of HCO depends greatly on the pre-experimental feeding conditions. The effect is maximal within one week if the animals are pre-fed SO for one week, whereas after a 4-week pre-experimental SO period, it takes about 3–4 weeks to obtain a maximum thrombotic response (Fig. 12). When rats, pre-fed a commercial stock diet, are given diets

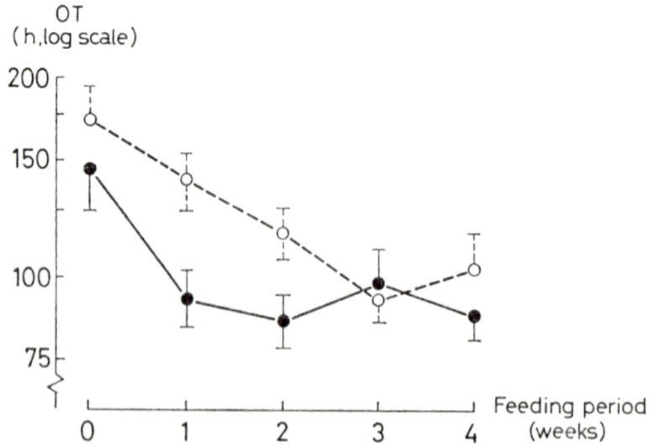


Fig. 12. Effect of pre-experimental SO-feeding (●–● 1 week, ○–○ 4 weeks) on the course of the thrombotic effect of HCO (45 cal%) in rats (OT ± SEM).

containing 5 cal% SO, either or not supplemented with 55 cal% HCO, the OT decreases in both groups to the same final value. This OT decrease occurs, however, more rapidly in the HCO-fed group (Fig. 13), which suggests that HCO has a specific thrombotic effect. These kinetic studies indicate that arterial thrombosis tendency depends on the presence of certain (anti-) thrombotic substances in the platelets or their

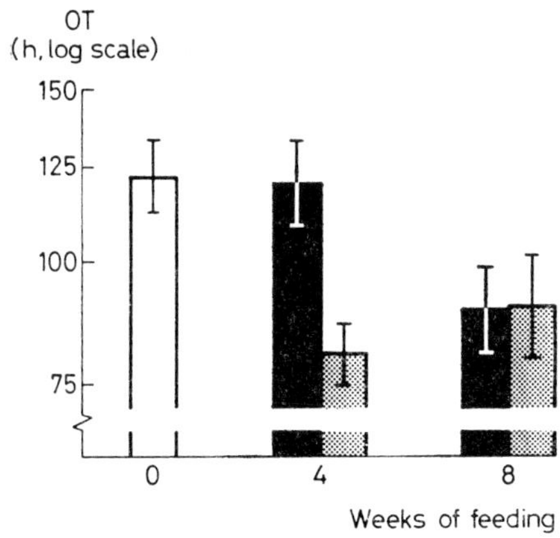


Fig. 13. Accelerating effect of saturated fat on the increase of thrombosis tendency in rats, following dietary changes (OT ± SEM). □ = stock diet, ■ = 5 cal% SO, ::: = 5 cal% SO + 55 cal% HCO.

environment, the concentrations of which seem to depend on the content of particular dietary fatty acids. These substances are probably linoleic acid and long chain SAFAs, which in the previous paragraph were demonstrated to be antithrombotic and thrombosis-promoting substances respectively. This hypothesis is supported by the observations that the dietary fatty acid composition influences the fatty acid spectrum of platelet lipids in rats (Renaud *et al.*, 1970), pigs (Andreoli *et al.*, 1974) and man (Nordøy and Rødset, 1971). However, to our surprise, we could not find striking differences in the fatty acid spectra of platelet total lipids and only minor changes in that of plasma total lipids (Table 2), although the fatty acid composition of SO and HCO differs greatly (Table 1).

Similar findings were observed in rats fed six different oils and fats which induce highly different thrombosis tendencies. It, therefore, seems evident that any further research into the possible participation of platelet fatty acid composition in platelet thrombotic function should be directed towards the several lipid classes (cholesteryl esters and phospholipids in particular) and towards special platelet organelles

Table 2

Fatty acid spectra of plasma and platelet total lipids of rats fed diets containing 50 cal% SO or 45 cal% HCO + 5 cal% SO for 8 weeks (%)[a]

| Fatty acid | plasma (4 pools of 3 animals) | | platelets (2 pools of 6 animals) | |
|---|---|---|---|---|
| | SO | HCO | SO | HCO |
| 14:0 | — | 1·3 | — | 4·2 |
| 16:0 | 13·1 | 13·9 | 29·6 | 25·6 |
| 16:1 | — | — | 1·7 | 1·8 |
| 18:0 | 21·5 | 18·4 | 19·2 | 19·9 |
| 18:1 *n*–9 | 5·0 | 6·5 | 12·5 | 13·1 |
| 18:2 *n*–6 | 11·9 | 10·0 | 8·4 | 6·2 |
| 20:3 *n*–6 | — | — | 1·0 | 1·5 |
| 20:4 *n*–6 | 38·7 | 39·8 | 18·2 | 22·9 |
| 22:4 *n*–6 | 3·3 | 2·5 | 2·9 | 2·2 |

[a] Only fractions $\gg$ 1% are mentioned.

(membranes). As far as the platelet environment is concerned, special attention should be paid to the fatty acid spectra of plasma free fatty acids, which are considerably influenced by the dietary fatty acid composition. Work in these fields is now in progress, from which it is already evident (Table 3) that there are no differences between rats fed SO and HCO as to the concentrations of plasma protein and plasma-free fatty acids and to the phospholipid (total and classes) and cholesterol content of the platelets. A significant difference was found only in the plasma cholesterol content, but further investigations with six other dietary fats and oils showed that there is no significant relationship between plasma cholesterol content and arterial thrombosis tendency.

Another approach to elucidate the mechanism by which arterial thrombogenesis is affected by dietary fats is to investigate which of the steps of the thrombotic process (Fig. 1) is influenced. Up till now our investigations were restricted to platelet aggregation and to coagulation.

An important role of coagulation in thrombogenesis as affected by dietary fat was suggested by Gautheron and Renaud (1972), but the thrombosis model they use is more comparable to venous thrombosis in which process the importance of enhanced coagulation is generally acknowledged. Using the same technique as Renaud for measuring the clotting time in platelet-rich plasma after recalcification (Renaud,

Table 3

Some biochemical parameters in plasma and platelets of rats fed either an antithrombotic (50 cal% SO) or a thrombogenic (45 cal% HCO + 5 cal% SO) diet[a]

| Parameter | Unit | SO | HCO |
|---|---|---|---|
| plasma cholesterol | mmol/l | 1·52 ± 0·11 | 1·84 ± 0·06 |
| plasma FFA | μmol/l | 422·1 ± 30·44 | 454·4 ± 33·61 |
| plasma protein | g/l | 46·5 ± 0·36 | 48 ± 1·16 |
| platelet total lipids | mg/$10^9$ pl. | 0·343 | 0·352 |
| platelet cholesterol | mg/$10^9$ pl. | 0·083 | 0·079 |
| | % of pl. lip. | 24·4 | 22·5 |
| platelet phospholipids | mg/$10^9$ pl. | 0·223 | 0·220 |
| | % of pl. lip. | 64·9 | 62·5 |
| phospholipid classes: | | | |
| start | | 3·0 | 2·2 |
| SPH | | 27·1 | 25·9 |
| PI + PS | % of ph. lip. | 4·1 | 4·4 |
| PC | | 37·5 | 38·0 |
| PE | | 28·5 | 29·9 |

[a] Plasma analyses : mean ± S.E.M., $n = 12$.
Platelet analyses : mean value of 2 pools comprising 6 animals each.

1969), we indeed observed a significant negative correlation between PCT and log OT in a study comprising five different oils and fats. This finding indicates an association between increased coagulability and increased arterial thrombosis tendency, but because of the very low correlation coefficient ($r = -0·29$) such a correlationship can hardly be of any functional importance. Nevertheless this test was repeated in SO- and HCO-fed rats, together with measurement of clot formation in the Chandler loop (Chandler, 1958; Engelberg, 1969) and of platelet factor 3 activity and availability (Spaet and Cintron, 1965) in whole blood.

The results of this very recent study revealed it highly improbable that changes in coagulability contribute to the enhanced arterial thrombosis tendency on feeding a thrombogenic, saturated-fat diet: neither whole blood coagulability (Chandler loop) nor clotting time of platelet rich and platelet poor plasma after recalcification were significantly different in both groups whereas $PF_3$-availability in response to collagen appeared even to be significantly reduced in the group receiving the thrombogenic diet as compared to the other group (Hornstra, to be published).

The next thrombotic property of the platelets we investigated in relation to dietary fat and arterial thrombosis tendency was platelet aggregation. To be able to measure this process in circulating arterial rat blood, we developed the "filter-loop technique" (Hornstra, 1970). This technique is based on the continuous measurement of the blood pressure before and after a metal filter with pores of 20 $\mu$m in diameter. This pore size permits the passage of red and white cells and of single platelets, but not of platelet aggregates. The filter is extracorporeally taken up into the arterial blood stream by means of an aorta loop. When circulating aggregates obstruct the filter, a pressure difference develops,

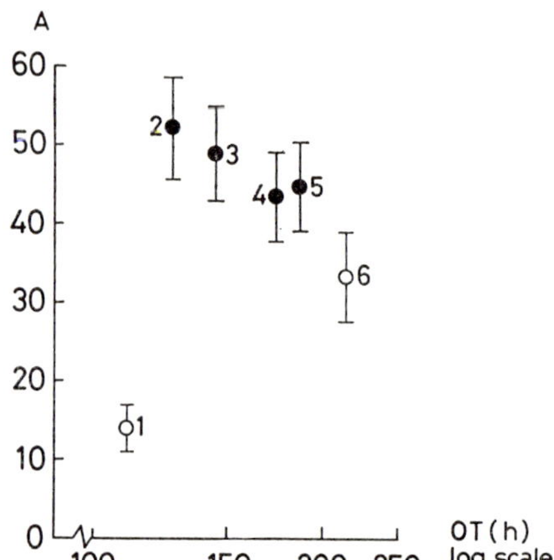


Fig. 14. Relationship between ADP-induced aggregation in circulating blood (A ± SEM) and arterial thrombosis tendency (OT) in rats fed diets containing 50 cal%: 1. whale oil; 2. hydrogenated soyabean oil; 3. olive oil; 4. sunflowerseed oil; 5. linseed oil; 6. rapeseed oil. Aggregation values indicated by open circles differ significantly from the other values.

from the time course of which the degree of aggregation, the aggregation index A, is calculated. Most of the time aggregation has to be induced by infusing adenosine diphosphate (ADP) in the blood stream in front of the filter; sometimes, however, spontaneous aggregation develops immediately after connecting the extracorporeal system. Both types of aggregation are reversible, disaggregation occurring either after termination of ADP infusion or spontaneously. The filter-loop technique appeared to be a very suitable technique to quantify the effect of drugs on platelet aggregation, not only in rats (Hornstra, 1971; Muirhead, 1973) but also in dogs (Broersma *et al.*, 1973). An effect of dietary fats on platelet aggregation was suggested from experiments in which platelet aggregation and arterial thrombosis tendency was measured in rats fed different dietary fats (Fig. 14). With one inexplicable exception (whale oil), a high aggregation index was associated with a low OT, so a high thrombosis tendency. When comparing the effect of SO- and HCO-feeding on ADP-induced platelet aggregation, in 15 out of 16 cases aggregation was higher in the HCO-group than in the SO-group ($P_2 < 0{\cdot}01$, sign test), although the difference was not always as pronounced as shown in Fig. 15. A more consistent difference

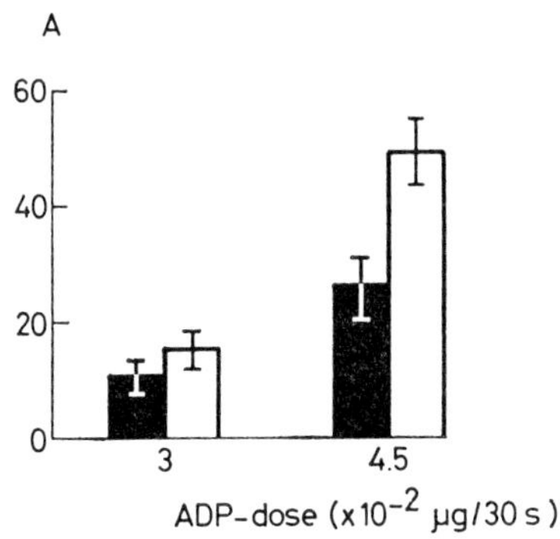


Fig. 15. ADP-induced platelet aggregation (A ± SEM) in circulating blood of rats fed either an antithrombotic diet (50 cal% SO, ■) or a thrombogenic diet (45 cal% HCO + 5 cal% SO, □) $n = 13$.

was obtained as to the effect of both dietary fats on frequency and degree of spontaneous aggregation which, retrospectively, was much higher in the HCO-fed animals than in the SO-fed rats. This observation was convincingly confirmed in two subsequent prospective studies ($P_2 < 0{\cdot}01$). The combined results are given in Fig. 16. Thus,

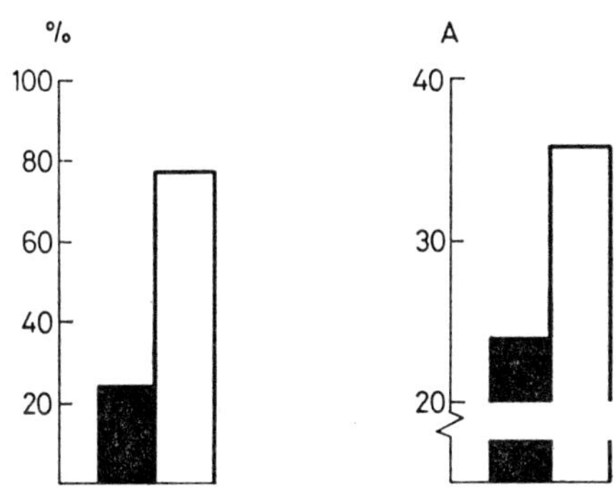


Fig. 16. Frequency (%) and degree (A) of spontaneous aggregation in rats fed either an antithrombotic diet (50 cal% SO, $n = 103$, ■) or a thrombogenic diet (45 cal% HCO + 5 cal% SO, $n = 93$, □).

spontaneous aggregation seems to be a more suitable criterion than ADP-induced aggregation for investigating the effect of dietary fats on platelet aggregation. Therefore an apparatus has been developed to quantify this type of aggregation in man, with which the effect of dietary linoleic acid has been assessed (Section III).

According to Renaud *et al.* (1970) thrombosis tendency, as measured with their model, is very well correlated with platelet aggregatibility in response to thrombin. Thrombin-induced aggregation cannot be measured with the filter loop because in this system the animals are heparinized. Therefore it was measured in citrated platelet-rich plasma (PRP), using the turbidimetric technique of Born (1962) and O'Brien (1962). However, no differences were found on feeding SO or HCO, neither with thrombin, nor with ADP or collagen as inducers of aggregation. Since ADP did give different results in the filter-loop technique, we considered the turbidimetric technique in our hands to be unsuitable for further research on the effects of dietary fats on platelet aggregation.

## III. EFFECT OF DIETARY LINOLEIC ACID ON PLATELET AGGREGATION AND CORONARY THROMBOSIS IN MEN

In a 12-year study carried out in Helsinki, Finland, comprising two groups of 400 mental patients, the use of a diet containing 12 cal% linoleic acid was found to reduce mortality from coronary heart disease (CHD) in males considerably and significantly as compared with a diet containing 4 cal% linoleic acid (Miettinen *et al.*, 1972). Since mortality from CHD is for the greater part the result of occlusion of a coronary artery by a thrombus (Harland and Holburn, 1966; Haerem, 1974; Sinapius, 1972), this finding is in line with the antithrombotic effect of dietary linoleic acid observed in rats (Section II C). As in these animals thrombosis tendency seemed to be associated with intravascular aggregation (Section II D), an apparatus, the Filtragometer,* was developed to measure this type of spontaneous aggregation in flowing venous blood (Fig. 17). With a motor ($M$), driven syringe ($S$), blood from a cubital vein is drawn through a nickel filter ($F$) having square pores of 20 $\mu$m. Pressures are measured on both sides of the filter and subtracted electronically to obtain the pressure difference across the filter ($\Delta P$), which is monitored. The pressure between arm and filter ($P_2$) is recorded to check blood supply. Heparin ($H$) is infused just behind the needle and mixed with the blood in a mixing

* Patent applied for.

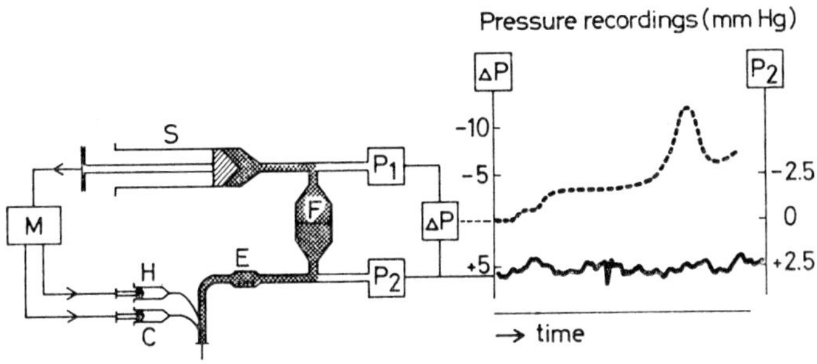


Fig. 17. Diagram of Filtragometer.

chamber ($E$) to an end concentration of 5 IU/ml. It anticoagulates the blood and stabilizes intravascular aggregates which therefore obstruct the filter, resulting in a change in pressure difference, the course of which is shown schematically in Fig. 18. At the start of the experiment,

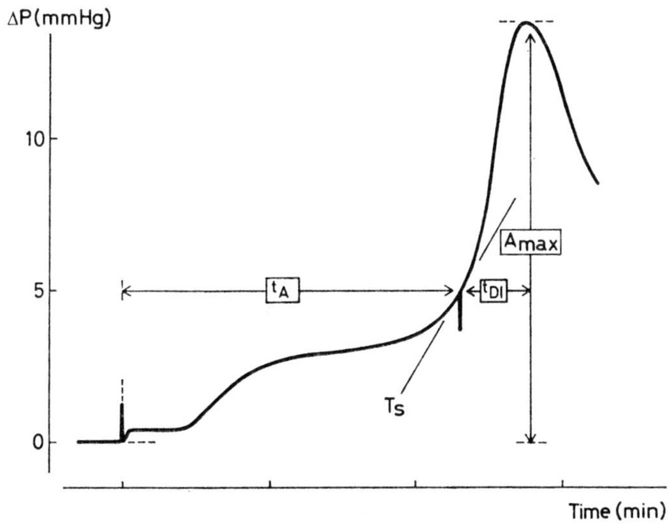


Fig. 18. Recording of the pressure difference across the filter ($\Delta P$, mm Hg) obtained during an aggregation measurement (schematic).

indicated by an upward deflection of the tracing, blood is drawn from the arm and heparin administered. Due to the internal resistance of the system a very small pressure difference builds up, which increases when the viscous blood replaces the priming saline. A further increase in $\Delta P$ indicates that aggregates are obstructing the filter. A downward deflection marks the moment when $\Delta P$ equals 5 mm Hg. At this moment heparin is replaced by sodium citrate ($C$) and after a short period the decrease of $\Delta P$ indicates that the filter is being cleaned by disaggregation. From this tracing the following parameters are calculated:

1. the aggregation time, $t_A$, being the time in sec needed to reach a $\Delta P$ of 5 mm Hg;
2. the aggregation slope, $T_s$, being the slope of the tangent to the curve at the moment $\Delta P$ equals 5 mm Hg;
3. the maximal aggregation, $A_{max}$, being the maximal height of the aggregation curve in mm Hg;
4. the disaggregation induction time, $t_{DI}$, being the time between termination of the heparin infusion (at $\Delta P = 5$ mm Hg) and the beginning of disaggregation.

Platelet aggregation, as measured with the Filtragometer, is increased by venous compression and decreased by ingestion of aspirin. Prostaglandin $E_1$, infused extracorporeally, also decreased platelet aggregation. These results are in line with findings obtained with other aggregation techniques (Hornstra and ten Hoor, to be published).

The Filtragometer was used in measuring platelet aggregation in a random selection of the male participants in the Helsinki trial (Hornstra *et al.*, 1973) not showing differences in mean age, body weight, smoking habits, blood pressure and medication. As might be expected, the serum cholesterol content was significantly lower in the group high in linoleic acid (5·8 versus 6·5 mmol/l, $P_2 < 0·001$); no significant difference existed in the serum triglyceride content (1·90 versus 1·83 mmol/l) of the two groups. The results of the aggregation measurements are given in Fig. 19. In the group high in linoleic acid the aggregation time is longer, the aggregation slope flatter and the maximum height of the aggregation curve lower. Moreover, the disaggregation induction time is shorter. These findings indicate a decreased platelet aggregation and enhanced tendency to disaggregation of the formed aggregates in the high linoleic-acid group as compared with the subjects receiving the normal diet, low in linoleic acid. This is consistent with the lower arterial thrombosis tendency found in the former group (Miettinen *et al.*, 1972). It is conceivable that this lower platelet aggregation has contributed to the lower CHD-mortality observed. These findings show that the Filtragometer is a useful device to measure thrombosis tendency in humans, preferably in groups. Furthermore, these human results are in complete agreement with the results of our animal studies.

The anti-aggregating effect of a diet high in linoleic acid has also been observed in children with type II-hyperlipoproteinaemia (unpublished work carried out in cooperation with Dr T. Zurcher and

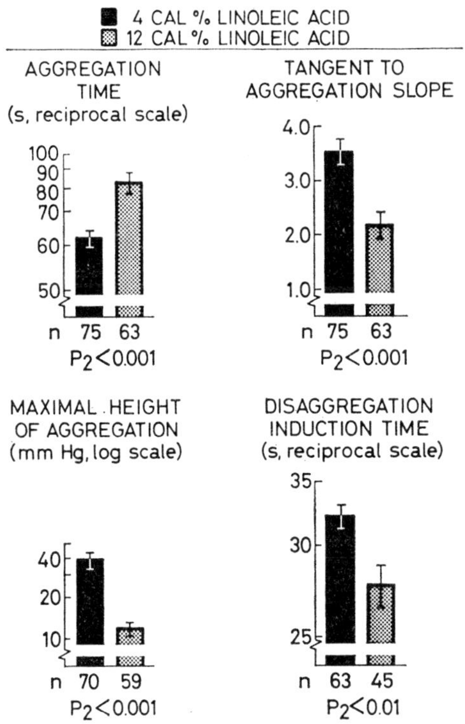


Fig. 19. Effect of dietary linoleic acid content on platelet aggregation (Filtragometer). Mean values ± SEM. Figures under bars represent number of observations.

Dr J. Fernandez, Sophia Children Hospital, Rotterdam) and in geriatric patients with a high incidence of CHD and/or diabetes mellitus (Fleischmann *et al.*, 1973), the beneficial effect in the latter investigation being evident after two weeks of feeding. When subsequently the normal diet was given again, the initial level of aggregation was reached within two weeks (Bierenbaum, unpublished work).

## IV. ESSENTIAL FATTY ACID DEFICIENCY AND ARTERIAL THROMBUS FORMATION

As shown in Section II, rats receiving a low-fat diet show a high arterial thrombosis tendency, which can be reduced by administering SO. When feeding a fat-free diet, thrombosis tendency increases first, but decreases afterwards (Fig. 20). It is known that a fat-free diet causes essential fatty acid (EFA) deficiency in a great number of animal species (Aaes-Jørgensen, 1961) and determination of the triene/tetraene ratio of the plasma lipids, according to Holman (1960), revealed that the rats under investigation were indeed EFA deficient. Supplementation of the diet with 5 cal% SO, which rectifies EFA deficiency, increased the thrombosis tendency, whereas supplementation with 50 cal% HCO, which hardly contains any essential fatty acids and

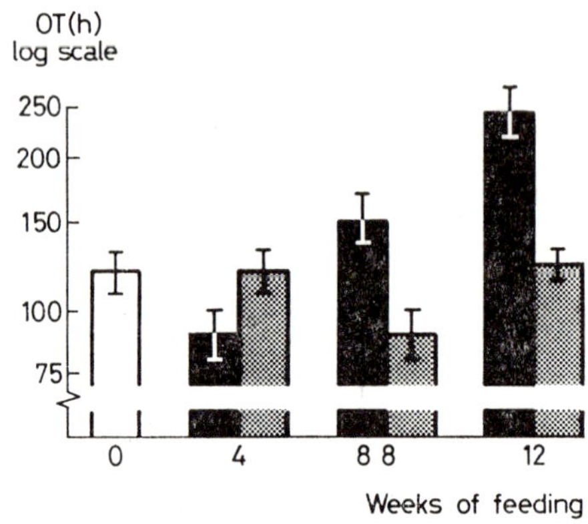


Fig. 20. Effect of fat-free feeding on arterial thrombosis tendency in rats (OT ± SEM) $n = 12$. □ = stock diet, ■ = fat-free diet, ::: = 5 cal% SO.

which increases the EFA requirement (Deuel *et al.*, 1955; Peifer and Holman, 1959) decreased the thrombosis tendency further, in spite of HCO being a highly thrombogenic fat (Fig. 21). It can therefore be concluded that in EFA-deficient rats the normal thrombotic functions are impaired.

To investigate which of the thrombotic processes (Fig. 1) are affected by EFA deficiency, adhesion, release and aggregation of platelets were measured in EFA-deficient and control rats fed diets containing

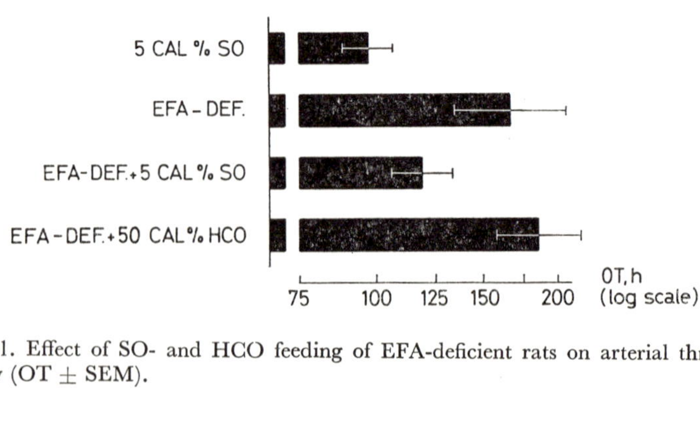


Fig. 21. Effect of SO- and HCO feeding of EFA-deficient rats on arterial thrombosis tendency (OT ± SEM).

Table 4

Effect of EFA deficiency on some blood platelet properties (mean ± SEM)

| Criterion | Unit | $n$ | EFA deficiency | Control | $P_2$ |
|---|---|---|---|---|---|
| Adhesion | pl./micro. field | 12 | 5 ± 1·3 | 48 ± 14·2 | <0·05 |
| Aggregation (blood, ADP) | Aggr. index | 12 | 30·3 ± 6·11 | 32·4 ± 5·70 | >0·1 |
| Aggregation (PRP, ADP) | ΔOD (75″) | 8 | 30·7 ± 1·78 | 28·8 ± 2·17 | >0·1 |
| Aggregation (PRP, Collagen) | ΔOD (180″) | 5 | 5·4 ± 1·92 | 40·0 ± 3·88 | <0·01 |
| Release (Collagen) | % (180″) | 5 | 13·8 ± 1·70 | 34·7 ± 2·12 | <0·01 |
| Release (ADP) | % (75″) | 8 | 2·6 ± 0·67 | 1·1 ± 0·22 | <0·1 |
| 18:2 $n$–6 | % of total | 1[a] | 0·7 | 7·0 | |
| 20:3 $n$–9 | platelet | 1[a] | 18·5 | 0·0 | |
| 20:4 $n$–6 | lipids | 1[a] | 1·6 | 22·0 | |

[a] Pool of 6 animals.

5 cal% HCO (EFA def.) or SO (control) for at least three months (Table 4). No significant differences were observed in the ADP-induced platelet aggregation in circulating blood, nor in platelet-rich plasma. The collagen-induced platelet aggregation in PRP, however, was considerably reduced in the EFA-deficient animals, as was the collagen-induced serotonin release in PRP (Spaet and Zucker, 1964) and the adhesion of blood platelets to glass. The latter platelet function was measured in circulating blood, using a flow chamber as devised by Lyman *et al.* (1970), connected to the arterial blood stream by means of an aorta loop. Since the release reaction is secondary to platelet adhesion (Fig. 1), the impairment of the latter may be the primary cause of the decreased arterial thrombosis tendency in EFA deficiency.

Platelet adhesion is a membrane-located phenomenon (O'Brien, 1969; Jamieson *et al.*, 1971) and may therefore be diminished following any disturbance of membrane integrity. EFAs and their metabolites are important membrane constituents and of vital importance for membrane function. In EFA-deficiency membrane fatty acid composition is considerably altered, leading to functional disturbances (Seiler and Haselbach, 1971). It is conceivable that this may also occur in the platelet membranes of EFA-deficient rats, resulting in impaired platelet adhesion. The decreased release reaction of platelets of EFA-deficient rats may also be mediated by two other mechanisms, namely, impaired energy and prostaglandin production.

For proper functioning, platelets require energy which is obtained through anaerobic and aerobic glycolysis (Chernyak, 1965). The latter process is of major importance (Gross and Schneider, 1971), although platelets contain only few mitochondria which, moreover, are morphologically underdeveloped (Schulz, 1968). In EFA deficiency oxidative phosphorylation in liver mitochondria is uncoupled (Klein and Johnson, 1954), consequently, ATP production is impaired. It may, therefore, be assumed that also in platelets of EFA-deficient rats the mitochondrial ATP production is insufficient for normal functioning. Since the energy requirement is highest for the release reaction (Holmsen *et al.*, 1973) as compared to adhesion and aggregation it is conceivable that this function will be affected first. This may explain why ADP-induced aggregation is normal in EFA deficiency.

It has been suggested (Salzman *et al.*, 1973) that the platelet release reaction is mediated by prostaglandin $E_2$ ($PGE_2$), synthesized following platelet stimulation (Clausen and Srivastava, 1972; Smith *et al.*, 1973). The precursor of $PGE_2$ is arachidonic acid (Van Dorp *et al.*, 1964). One of the intermediates in $PGE_2$-synthesis is reported to have very strong aggregating properties (Willis and Kuhn, 1973; Smith *et al.*, 1974). PG production is suggested to depend on the level of its precursor (Vogt and Distelkötter, 1967) and was reported to be diminished in several tissues of EFA-deficient rats (Van Dorp, 1971). Since we found the arachidonic acid (C 20:4) content in EFA-deficient platelets to be very much lower than that of platelets of control animals (Table 4), a decreased $PGE_2$-synthesis and, consequently, a decreased release reaction and diminished pro-aggregant production in EFA-deficient platelets is very likely. Further research is required to elucidate which of the proposed mechanisms is effective in decreasing the platelet release reaction in EFA deficiency.

## REFERENCES

Aaes-Jørgensen, A. (1961). Essential fatty acids. *Phys. Rev.* **41,** 1–51.

Andreoli, V. M., Maffei, F., Tonon, G. C. (1973/74). Platelet lipid modifications induced by fatty acids: experimental studies and correlations with human neuropathology. *Haemostasis* **2,** 118–140.

Born, G. V. R. (1962). Aggregation of blood platelets by adenosine diphosphate and its reversal. *Nature* **194,** 927–929.

Born, G. V. R. *et al.* (1971). Thrombogenic mechanisms in atherosclerosis. *In* "The Artery and the Process of Arteriosclerosis: Pathogenesis". (S. Wolfe, ed.), Advances in Experimental Medicine and Biology". Vol. 16A, pp. 175–184. Plenum Press, New York, London.

Broersma, R. J., Dickerson, G. D., Sullivan, M. S. (1973). The determination of platelet aggregation by filtration pressure in circulating dog blood. *Thromb. Diath. Haemorrh.* **29**, 201–210.

Carroll, K. K. (1958). Digestibility of individual fatty acids in the rat. *J. Nutr.* **64**, 399–410.

Carroll, K. K., Richards, J. F. (1958). Factors affecting digestibility of fatty acids in the rat. *J. Nutr.* **64**, 411–424.

Chandler, A. B. (1958). *In vitro* thrombotic coagulation of blood. *Lab. Invest.* **7**, 110–115.

Chernyak, N. B. (1965). Processes of formation and utilization of energy in human blood platelets. *Clin. Chim. Acta* **12**, 244–257.

Clausen, J. and Srivastava, K. C. (1972). The synthesis of prostaglandins in human platelets. *Lipids* **7**, 246–250.

Craig, I. H., Bell, F. P. and Schwartz, C. J. (1973a). Thrombosis and atherosclerosis: the organization of pulmonary thromboemboli in the pig. Individual phospholipids, fatty acid composition of lecithin, sphingomyelin, esterified cholesterol and $^3$H-cholesterol specific activity. *Exp. Mol. Pathol.* **18**, 290–304.

Craig, I. H., Bell, F. P., Goldsmith, C. H. and Schwartz, C. J. (1973b). Thrombosis and atherosclerosis: the organization of pulmonary thromboemboli in the pig. Macroscopic observations, protein, DNA and major lipids. *Atherosclerosis* **18**, 277–300.

Deuel, H. J., Jr, Alfin-Slater, R. B., Wells, A. F., Kryder, G. D. and Aftergood, L. (1955). The effect of fat level of the diet on general nutrition XVI. Further studies of the effect of hydrogenated coconut oil on essential fatty acid deficiency in the rat. *J. Nutr.* **55**, 337–346.

Duguid, J. B. (1946). Thrombosis as a factor in the pathogenesis of coronary atherosclerosis. *Am. J. Pathol. Bacteriol.* **58**, 207–212.

Engelberg, H. (1969). Studies with the Chandler Rotating Loop—Evidence that thrombin generation is responsible for the formation of the artificial *in vitro* thrombi. *Thromb. Diath. Haemorrh.* **22**, 344–350.

Fantl, P. and Ward, H. A. (1958). The thromboplastic component of intact blood platelets is present in masked form. *Austr. J. Exp. Biol. Med. Sci.* **36**, 499–504.

Fleischman, A. L., Simpkins, H. and Bierenbaum, M. (1973). Beneficial effect of increased dietary linoleate upon *in vivo* platelet function in man. *Circulation* **48**, Suppl. 4, 55.

French, J. E. (1969). The fine structure of experimental thrombi. *In* "Thrombosis" (S. Sherry, K. M. Brinkhous, E. Genton, J. M. Stengle, eds), pp. 300–320. National Academy of Sciences, Washington D.C., U.S.A.

Friedman, M. and Byers, S. O. Experimental thrombo-atherosclerosis. *J. Clin. Invest.* **40**, 1139–1152.

Gautheron, P. and Renaud, S. (1972). Hyperlipemia induced hypercoagulable state in rat. Role of increased activity of platelet phosphatidyl serine in response to certain dietary fatty acids. *Thromb. Res.* **1**, 353–370.

Gross, R. and Schneider, W. (1971). Energy metabolism. *In* "The Circulating Platelet" (S. A. Johnson, ed.), pp. 123–188. Academic Press, New York and London.

Hand, R. A. and Chandler, A. B. (1962). Atherosclerotic metamorphosis of autologous pulmonary thromboemboli in the rabbit. *Am. J. Pathol.* **40**, 469–486.

Haerem, J. W. (1974). Platelet aggregates and mural microthrombi in early stages of acute, fatal coronary disease. *Thromb. Res.* **5**, 243–249.

Harland, W. A. (1969). The pathogenesis of myocardial infarct and coronary thrombosis. *In* "Thrombosis" (S. Sherry, K. M. Brinkhous, E. Genton, J. M. Stengle, eds), pp. 126–131. National Academy of Sciences, Washington D.C., U.S.A.

Harland, W. A. and Holburn, A. M. (1966). Coronary thrombosis and myocardial infarction. *Lancet* **II,** 1158–1159.

Heggtveit, H. A. (1968). Atheromatous transformation of intracardiac mural thrombi. *Am. J. Pathol.* **52,** 70a.

Holman, R. T. (1960). The ratio of trienoic/tetraenoic acids in tissue lipids as a measure of essential fatty acid requirement. *J. Nutr.* **70,** 405–410.

Holmsen, H., Setkowsky, C. A. and Day, H. J. (1973). Correlation between platelet function and level of metabolic ATP. Proc. IV Int. Congr. Haem. Thromb. Vienna, 1973, pp. 49.

Hornstra, G. (1970). Method to determine the degree of ADP-induced platelet aggregation in circulating rat blood (Filter loop technique). *Brit. J. Haematol.* **19,** 321–329.

Hornstra, G. (1971). Degree and duration of prostaglandin $E_1$-induced inhibition of platelet aggregation in the rat. *Eur. J. Pharmacol.* **15,** 343–349.

Hornstra, G. (1972). Digestibility, efficiency and other metabolic effects of dietary rapeseed oil in rats. *Nutr. Metab.* **14,** 282–297.

Hornstra, G. (1973/74). Dietary fats and arterial thrombosis. *Haemostasis* **2,** 21–52.

Hornstra, G. and Vendelmans, A. (1973). Introduction of experimental arterial occlusive thrombi in rats. *Atherosclerosis* **17,** 369–382.

Hornstra, G., Lewis, B., Chait, A., Turpeinen, O., Karvonen, M. J. and Vergroesen, A. J. (1973). Influence of dietary fat on platelet function in men. *Lancet* **i,** 1155–1157.

Jamieson, G. A., Urban, C. L. and Barber, A. J. (1971). Enzymatic basis for platelet: collagen adhesion as the primary step in hemostasis. *Nature* (*New Biol.*) **234,** 5–7.

Kakkar, V. V., Nicolaides, A. N., Field, E. S., Flute, P. T., Wessler, S. and Yin, E. T. (1971). Low doses of heparin in prevention of deep vein thrombosis. *Lancet* **ii,** 669–671.

Klein, P. D. and Johnson, R. M. (1954). Phosphorus metabolism in unsaturated fatty acid deficient rats. *J. Biol. Chem.* **211,** 103–110.

Likar, I. N., Likar, L. J., Robison, R. W. and Gouvelis, A. (1969). Microthrombi and intimal thickening in bovine coronary arteries. *Arch. Pathol.* **87,** 146–153.

Lyman, D. J., Klein, K. G., Brash, J. L. and Fritzinger, B. K. (1970). The interaction of platelets with polymer surfaces: I. Uncharged hydrophobic polymer surfaces. *Thromb. Diath. Haemorrh.* **23,** 120–128.

Michaels, L. (1972). Heparin administration in acute coronary insufficiency. Its value in the initial stages of treatment. *J. Am. Med. Ass.* **221,** 1235–1239.

Miettinen, M., Turpeinen, O., Karvonen, M. J., Elosuo, R. and Paavilainen, E. (1972). Effect of cholesterol-lowering diet on mortality from coronary heart disease and other causes. A twelve year clinical trial in men and women. *Lancet* **ii,** 835–838.

Muirhead, C. R. (1973). The filter loop technique as a method for measuring platelet aggregation in the flowing blood of the rat; the inhibitory activity of 5-oxo-1-cyclopentene-1-heptanoic acid (AY-16,804) on platelet aggregation. *Thromb. Diath. Haemorrh.* **30,** 138–147.

Mustard, J. F. and Packham, M. A. (1970). Factors influencing platelet function: adhesion, release, and aggregation. *Pharmacol. Rev.* **22,** 97–187.

Newman, H. A. I. and Zilversmit, D. B. (1962). Quantitative aspects of cholesterol flux in rabbit atheromatous lesions. *J. Biol. Chem.* **237,** 2078–2084.

Niewiarowski, S., Bańkowski, E. and Rogowicka, I. (1965). Studies on the adsorption and activation of the Hageman factor (Factor XII) by collagen and elastin. *Thromb. Diath. Haemorrh.* **14,** 387–400.

Nordøy, A. and Rødset, J. M. (1971). The influence of dietary fats on platelets in man. *Act. Med. Scand.* **190,** 27–34.

O'Brien, J. R. (1962). Platelet aggregation II. Some results from a new method of study. *J. Clin. Pathol.* **15,** 452–455.

O'Brien, J. R. (1969). The properties of the platelet membrane. *In* "Dynamics of Thrombus Formation and Dissolution" (S. A. Johnson and M. Mason, eds), pp. 121–148. J. B. Lipincott Co., Philadelphia and Toronto.

Owren, P. A. (1964). Nutrition and thrombosing atherosclerosis. *Bibl. Nutritio Dieta,* **6,** 156–182.

Peifer, J. J. and Holman, R. T. (1959). Effect of saturated fat upon essential fatty acid metabolism in the rat. *J. Nutr.* **68,** 155–168.

Prathap, K. (1973). The natural history of platelet-rich mural thrombi in systemic arteries of hypercholesterolaemic monkeys: light- and electron microscope observations. *J. Pathol.* **110,** 203–212.

Renaud, S. (1969). The recalcification plasma clotting time. A valuable general clotting test in man and rats. *Can J. Physiol. Pharmacol.* **47,** 689–693.

Renaud, S., Kinlough, R. L. and Mustard, J. F. (1970). Relationship between platelet aggregation and the thrombotic tendency in rats fed hyperlipemic diets. *Lab. Invest.* **22,** 339–343.

Renaud, S., Kuba, K., Goulet, C., Lemire, Y. and Allard, C. (1970). Relationship between fatty acid composition of platelets and platelet aggregation in rat and man. *Circ. Res.* **26,** 553–564.

Rieger, H., Schmid-Schönbein, H., Klose, H. J. and Heinich, L. Recording and quantification of shear induced platelet aggregation in humans. *Eur. J. Physiol.* **343,** Suppl., R 33.

Rozenberg, M. C. (1970). Experimental thrombosis and prevention by drugs that interfere with platelet aggregation. *Austr. Ann. Med.* Suppl. to 1970: 9–11.

Salzman, E. W., Stead, N. and Deykin, D. (1973). Interrelations of Platelet Prostaglandin Synthesis and Cyclic AMP Metabolism. Proc. IVth Int. Congr. Thromb. Haem., Vienna, pp. 46.

Schulz, H. (1968). "Thrombocyten und Thrombose in Elektronenmikroskopischen Bild", pp. 38. Springer-Verlag, Berlin, Heidelberg, New York.

Seiler, D. and Haselbach, W. (1971). Essential fatty acid deficiency and the activity of the sarcoplasmic calcium pump. *Eur. J. Biochem.* **21,** 385–387.

Sharnoff, J. G. and DeBlasio, G. (1970). Some implications in the successful heparin prophylaxis of sudden cardiopulmonary arrest by thrombosis and embolism. *Am. Heart J.* **80,** 848–850.

Sherry, S. (1972). Prospects in antithrombotic therapy. *Am. J. Cardiol.* **29,** 81–89.

Sinapius, D. (1972). Beziehungen zwischen Koronarthrombosen und Myocardinfarkten. *Deut. Med. Wschr.* **97,** 443–448.

Sixma, J. J. and Nijessen, J. G. (1970). Characteristics of platelet factor 3 release during ADP-induced aggregation. Comparison with 5 Hydroxytryptamine release. *Thromb. Diath. Haemorrh.* **24,** 206–213.

Smith, E. B. (1967). Quantitative and qualitative comparisons of the lipids in platelets, aortic intima and mural thrombi. *Cardiovasc. Res.* **1,** 111–115.

Smith, J. B., Ingerman, C., Kocsis, J. J. and Silver, M. J. (1973). Formation of prostaglandins during the aggregation of human blood platelets. *J. Clin. Invest.* **52,** 965–969.

Smith, J. B., Ingerman, C., Kocsis, J. J. and Silver, M. J. (1974). Formation of an intermediate in prostaglandin biosynthesis and its association with the platelet release reaction. *J. Clin. Invest.* **53,** 1468–1472.

Spaet, T. H. and Cintron, J. (1965). Studies on platelet factor-3 availability. *Brit. J. Haematol.* **11,** 269–275.

Spaet, T. H. and Zucker, M. B. (1964). Mechanism of platelet plug formation and role of adenosine diphosphate. *Am. J. Physiol* **206,** 1267–1274.

Sumiyoshi, A., More, R. H. and Weigensberg, B. I. (1973). Aortic fibrofatty type atherosclerosis from thrombus in normolipidemic rabbits. *Atherosclerosis* **18,** 43–57.

Van Dorp, D. A. (1971). Recent developments in the biosynthesis and the analyses of prostaglandins. *Ann. N.Y. Acad. Sci.* **180,** 181–199.

Van Dorp, D. A., Beerthuis, R. K., Nugteren, D. H. and Vonkeman, H. (1964). Enzymatic conversion of all-cis polyunsaturated fatty acids into prostaglandins. *Nature* **203,** 839–841.

Vogt, W. and Distelkötter, B. (1967). Release of prostaglandin from frog intestine. *In* "Prostaglandins" (S. Bergström, B. Samuelson, eds), pp. 237–240. Almqvist and Wiksell. Stockholm.

Walsh, P. N. (1972a). The role of platelets in the contact phase of blood coagulation. *Brit. J. Haematol.* **22,** 237–254.

Walsh, P. N. (1972b). The effects of collagen and kaolin on the intrinsic coagulant activity of platelets. Evidence for an alternative pathway in intrinsic coagulation not requiring Factor XII. *Brit. J. Haematol.* **22,** 393–405.

Weigensberg, B. I., More, R. H., Sumiyoshi, A. and Mullen, B. (1972). Evolution of the lipid profiles of thromboatherosclerotic lesions in normolipidemic rabbits. *Lab. Invest.* **26,** 495.

Wells, R. E. (1970). Quantification of hydrodynamic factors in arterial thrombus formation. *Circulation* **41** and **42,** Suppl. III, 49.

Willis, A. L. and Kuhn, D. C. (1973). A new potential mediator of arterial thrombosis, whose biosynthesis is inhibited by aspirin. *Prostaglandins* **4,** 127–130.

# 7 Specific Biological Effects of Polyunsaturated Fatty Acids

U. M. T. HOUTSMULLER

*Unilever Research, Vlaardingen, The Netherlands*



## I. INTRODUCTION

It is not the objective of this chapter to be a review of the literature on essential fatty acids. Readers are referred for that purpose to articles of other authors, particularly the series of Holman (1968, 1970). This contribution will stress the point that polyunsaturated fatty acids in general and essential fatty acids in particular seem to have several functions in the living animal.

These functions may require diverging specificities and different amounts of the fatty acids. It will be argued that some of the existing discrepancies concerning the essentiality of linolenic acid are due to this differentiation in biological activity.

It is generally accepted that essential fatty acids (EFA) have a structural function as an integral part of phospholipids, the building stones of biomembranes. This is inferred from the specific composition of the fatty acids in phospholipids—the β-position being esterified with the highly unsaturated members of the EFA families—and the observation that in EFA deficiency these fatty acids are replaced by 5, 8, 11 eicosatrienoic acid (20:3 *n*–9) with a concomitant deleterious effect on the function of the membranes. However, it has not been ascertained whether these structural requirements can also be fulfilled by other polyunsaturated fatty acids.

Moreover, the eicosapolyenoic members of the EFA families apparently have a dynamic function as well in so far as they are substrates for the biosynthesis of prostaglandins. These biologically very potent compounds seem to play a regulatory role in many cellular processes. It may well be that several of the functional disorders observed in EFA deficiency are due to an insufficient release from phospholipids of the precursor fatty acids for prostaglandin synthesis rather than a structural insufficiency of those phospholipids.

A first indication that this may be the case is obtained from the work of Ziboh and Hsia (1972) who have shown that prostaglandin $E_2$ applications on the skin of EFA-deficient rats cure the scaly lesions. Recently Ziboh (1973) has shown that in human skin—as has been observed previously in other tissues—phospholipase A, which releases the β-fatty acid from phospholipids, may be involved in the production of the substrate fatty acids for prostaglandin synthesis.

In an attempt to discriminate between the structural and dynamic functions, the effects of a series of polyunsaturated fatty acids were investigated on four symptoms of EFA deficiency in rats:

1. decreased growth rate, a parameter for the general condition of the animals;
2. increased skin permeability for water, which might be related, as outlined above, to prostaglandin synthesis;
3. increased spontaneous swelling of liver mitochondria *in vivo*, which may be regarded as a parameter for membrane integrity;
4. the altered fatty acid pattern of liver mitochondria. Together with the previous parameter the incorporation of the dietary fatty acids into phospholipids of the mitochondria will give quantitative information on the suitability of the particular fatty acid for a structural function.

## II. THE BIOASSAY

The symptoms of EFA deficiency were investigated in two types of curative bioassays (Fig. 1). In the first method according to Deuel (1951) newly weaned rats are raised on a fat-free diet for about 14 weeks, causing a retardation in their growth rate. If the diet is then supplemented with a known amount of linoleic acid, e.g. by the addition of sunflowerseed oil, the growth rate accelerates. A difference in body weight compared with the deficient control group ensues, which can be used as a standard for the estimation of the biological activity of an unknown fatty acid.

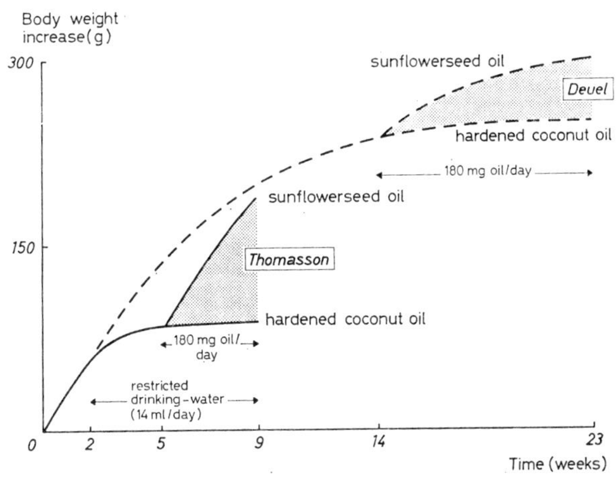


Fig. 1. Comparison of the bioassays according to Deuel and Thomasson. The effect on growth of restricted drinking water and subsequent feeding of 180 mg of either coconut oil or sunflowerseed oil is shown.

In the bioassay according to Thomasson (1953) the rats also receive a fat-free diet but in addition the supply of drinking water is restricted to 14 ml/day. The result is that the body weight levels off rapidly. In this test sunflowerseed oil causes a much larger increase in body weight than the same amount in the bioassay according to Deuel. This makes a more accurate estimation possible of the unknown biological activity of other fatty acids.

## III. COMPARISON OF (*n*–3) AND (*n*–6) FATTY ACIDS

### A. Body Weight

Both bioassay methods were used for comparing the activities of linoleic and linolenic acid (Figs 2 and 3). Simultaneously the effects were tested

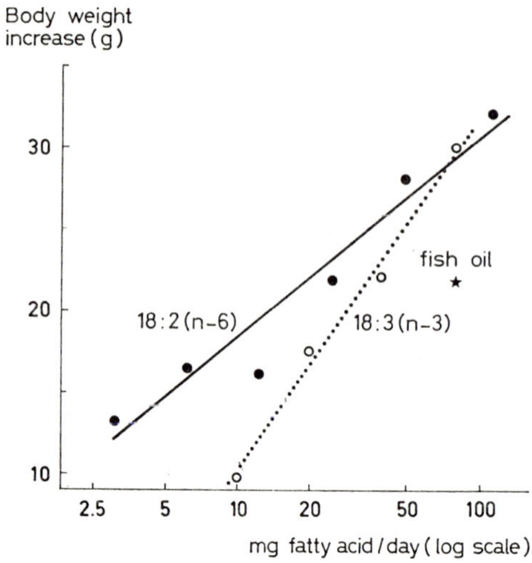


Fig. 2. Bioassay according to Deuel. Increase in body weight of rats after four weeks of feeding various doses linoleic or linolenic acid or a fish oil to EFA-deficient rats. For composition of the fish oil see Table 1.

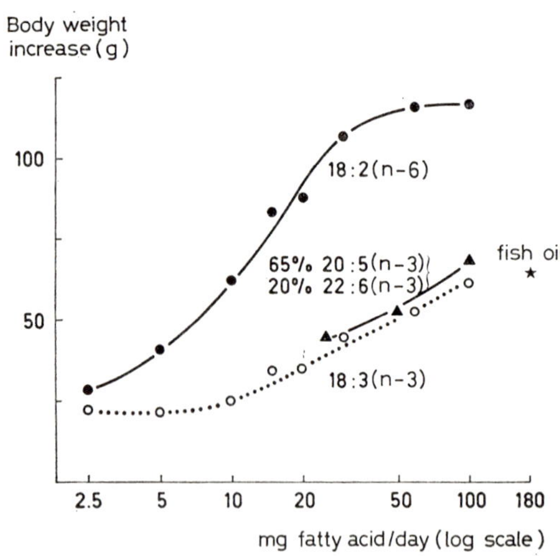


Fig. 3. Bioassay according to Thomasson (restricted drinking water). Increase in body weight of rats after four weeks of feeding various doses linoleic or linolenic acid, a fish oil and a concentrate of 20:5 (*n*-3) and 22:6 (*n*-3) to EFA-deficient rats. For composition of the fish oil see Table 1.

Table 1

Fatty acid composition of fish oil.
(Components present in traces only are omitted)

| Fatty acid | % of total fatty acids |
|---|---|
| 14:0 | 10 |
| 15:0 | 0·5 |
| 16:0 | 23·5 |
| 16:1 | 12·5 |
| 17:0 | 1·0 |
| 17:1 | 1·5 |
| 18:0 | 3·5 |
| 18:1 | 16·0 |
| 18:2 (*n*–9) | 1·0 |
| 18:2 (*n*–6) | 0·4 |
| 18:3 (*n*–3) | 0·5 |
| 20:0 | 2·0 |
| 20:1 | 2·5 |
| 20:4 (*n*–6) | 0·4 |
| 20:4 (*n*–3) | 2·0 |
| 20:5 (*n*–3) | 13·5 |
| 22:5 (*n*–3) | 1·5 |
| 22:6 (*n*–3) | 5·5 |

of a fish oil, containing very low amounts of fatty acids from the linoleic acid type (<0·8%, Table 1), and of a concentrate of timnodonic (20:5 *n*–3) and clupanodonic acid (22:6 *n*–3), which was prepared from a fish oil.

In the Deuel assay (Fig. 2) linoleic and linolenic acid induced about the same change in body weight, although linolenic acid tended to be somewhat less potent at low doses. Neither fatty acid appears to have induced maximal growth rate with 100 mg fatty acid/day. In sharp contrast to these findings the Thomasson assay (Fig. 3) shows much less potency for linolenic acid. Increase in body weight with linolenic acid is maximal at about 30 mg/day, whereas it seems that a dose of 100 mg/day of linolenic acid is not yet optimal. The concentrate of the pentaenoic and hexaenoic members of the linolenic acid family exhibits the same activity as the parent fatty acid and the effect of the fish oil is also in accordance with its content of *n*–3 fatty acids. A calculation of the biological activity of linolenic acid in the Thomasson assay depends on the ingested amount because the slopes of the graphs are not parallel. At low doses an activity of about 15% relative to linoleic acid is found whereas this figure decreases to 6% at higher doses. In the Deuel assay the activity was found to be 100%. Obviously the differences between both methods are caused by the restriction of drinking water in the Thomasson assay. Therefore it seemed relevant to study the increased skin permeability for water of the deficient rats in order to explain this apparent discrepancy.

## B. Skin Permeability

This criterion may be measured in three different ways (giving essentially the same results):

1. the loss of water by the anaesthetized rat;
2. the permeation of water through an isolated piece of skin *in vitro* (Thomasson, 1961);
3. the consumption of water when freely available (cannot be used in the Thomasson assay).

The first method was used in the comparison of linoleic and linolenic acid.

A linear relationship between the loss of water by the anaesthetized rat and the amount of fatty acid administered was found for linoleic as well as for linolenic acid (Fig. 4). However, the slope of the line is much steeper for linoleic acid. From these differences in slope an activity of 10% for linolenic acid can be calculated. Normal skin permeability was obtained with 30 mg/day of linoleic acid which was also the amount that caused almost maximal growth in the Thomasson assay (Fig. 3).

For linolenic acid, on the other hand, a maximal effect was not obtained with the doses used, neither with respect to growth, nor with respect to skin permeability. Therefore, it seemed appropriate to use much higher doses in a subsequent experiment. As, however, an adequate supply of the pure fatty acids was not available, use was made in a Deuel assay of sunflowerseed oil and the fish oil that had been tested in the previous experiments; the very small amount of linoleic acid in this oil apparently can be neglected. Skin permeability has been measured with the *in vitro* method (Thomasson, 1961). The dotted lines in Fig. 5 show that the body weight of the rats, recovering from EFA deficiency never reached the level of the rats fed a normal diet from weaning (the scales of Fig. 5 have been adjusted in such a way that the lines at the bottom and at the top depict for both criteria the EFA-deficient and the normal values). Maximal growth was obtained for both fats with about 180 mg/day which in the case of sunflowerseed oil corresponded with 110 mg/day of linoleic acid. The actual amount of effective fatty acids in the fish oil cannot be given, due to the complexity

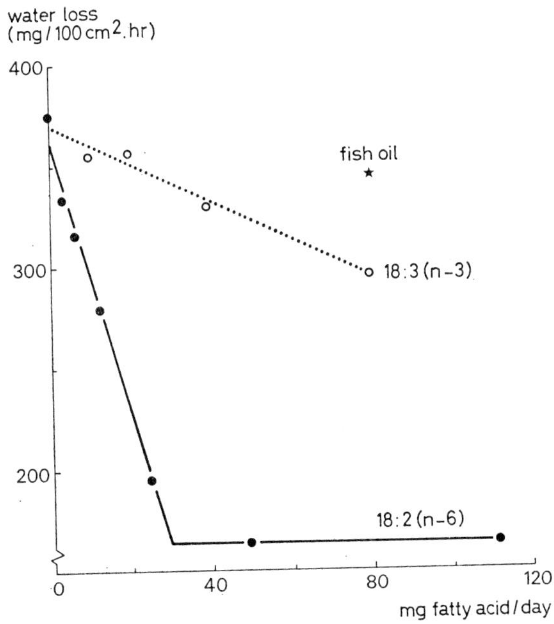


Fig. 4. Loss of water by the anaesthetized rat as a function of the fatty acid doses given for four weeks to EFA-deficient rats. Dry air is passed through a cylinder containing the anaesthetized animal; the water, evaporated in 30 min. is absorbed on silicic acid, weighed and expressed as mg water lost per 100 $cm^2$ body surface per hour.

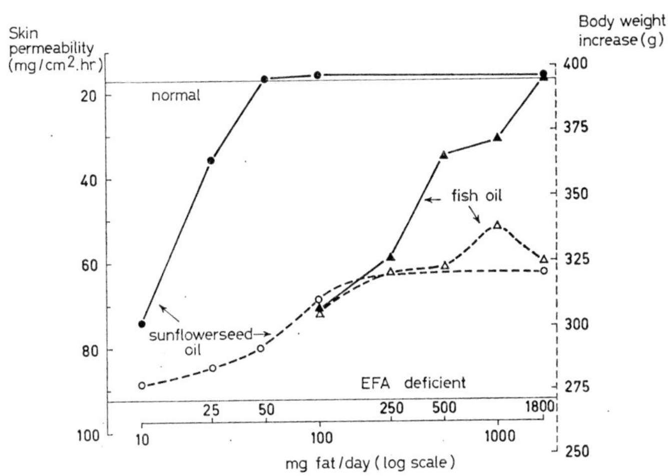


Fig. 5. Bioassay according to Thomasson, using a wide range of doses of sunflowerseed oil (60% linoleic acid) and fish oil (for composition see Table 1); rat skin permeability for water is measured *in vivo* as the amount of water permeating during three consecutive days through a biopsy of shaved skin 1·5 cm in diameter.

of the fatty acid composition (Table 1) and the uncertainty which of these fatty acids contribute to what extent to the effects; however, 180 mg of the fish oil contains a total of about 45 mg of ($n$–3) and ($n$–6) fatty acids.

Skin permeability, measured *in vitro*, is restored to normal with 50 mg/day of sunflowerseed oil which is the same amount of linoleic acid (30 mg/day) as found in the previous experiments. With very high doses of fish oil the skin becomes normal also. This effect cannot be ascribed to the small amount of ($n$–6) fatty acids in this oil; therefore the ($n$–3) fatty acids must also have contributed. In this context it is interesting to note that prostaglandin $E_3$, which is derived from timnodonic acid (20:5 $n$–3), is much less potent than prostaglandin $E_1$ and $E_2$ in various biological tests (Bergström, 1966; Bygdeman, 1966). This suggests that in rat skin linolenic acid is converted into prostaglandin $E_3$ after chain elongation and desaturation of the fatty acid, which supports the hypothesis of Ziboh and Hsia (1972), discussed before, that skin permeability may be a criterion for adequate prostaglandin synthesis. One possibility to substantiate this hypothesis seems to be comparison of the potencies of prostaglandins $E_2$ and $E_3$ upon application on the EFA-deficient skin.

The diverging results obtained with linoleic and linolenic acid on skin permeability make an explanation possible of the discrepancies between the two bioassays: The increase in body weight in the Thomasson bioassay compares very well with the improvement of the skin permeability (30 mg/day of linoleic acid is optimal in both criteria; linolenic acid has only 10% activity), whereas in the Deuel assay much higher doses of both types of fatty acids are needed for optimal growth. Obviously the differences between the bioassays are caused by the restriction of drinking water in the Thomasson assay: 14 ml/day is a minimal supply, even for normal rats. As EFA-deficient rats lose a considerable part of this water through their skin, a water deficiency ensues next to the EFA deficiency. And since animal tissues contain about 70% water, tissue proliferation cannot take place in the absence of sufficient water. Therefore growth stops rapidly. When linoleic acid is administered, the skin permeability decreases, so that more water can be retained in the animal and growth becomes possible. Optimal growth will be attained at that dose of linoleic acid which completely cures the skin (30 mg/day). Linolenic acid, which has only 10% of the potency of linoleic acid in curing the skin, will alow only a limited growth.

Moreover in the Thomasson bioassay the change in mean body weight of the groups was found to be a function of food consumption (Fig. 6), which again appeared to be a function of the amount of

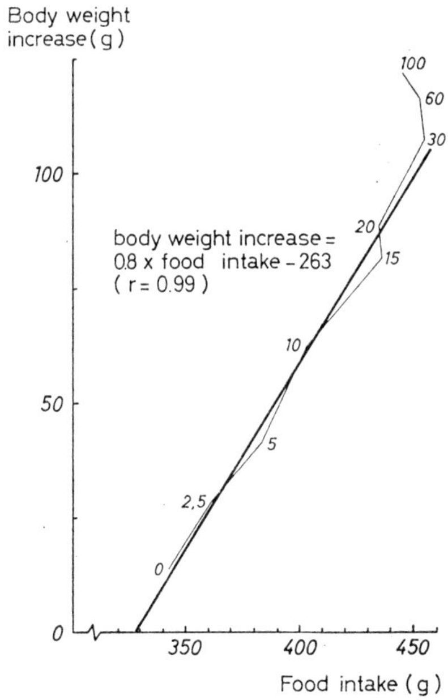


Fig. 6. Correlation between growth and increase in food consumption of EFA-deficient rats as induced by various doses of linoleic acid (figures along graph represent mg linoleic acid administered per day).

linoleic acid administered to the rats, but only so up to 30 mg/day. Obviously, the start of tissue proliferation, made possible by the sparing effect of linoleic acid on available water, can only be effectuated if more food is consumed. However, the slight additional growth (Fig. 6), at constant food consumption, when more than 30 mg/day of linoleic acid is administered apparently can not be attributed to the water sparing effect. Neither can the growth in the Deuel assay be thus explained, as water is available *ad libitum* and the food consumption is equal in all groups. This increase in body weight is rather the result of increased food efficiency, which means that the body needs less substrate for energy production and therefore a larger fraction is available for the synthesis of new tissues.

Underlying the decreased food efficiency of EFA-deficient animals must be a process that uses the energy contained in the dietary substrates with diminished efficiency. Such a process may be the partial uncoupling of the oxydative phosphorylation in mitochondria, which has been observed in isolated liver mitochondria from EFA-deficient rats (Klein and Johnson, 1954).

Ordinarily mitochondria conserve the energy available from the oxidation of substrates with high efficiency in the energy-rich bonds of ATP by coupling the phosphorylation of ADP onto the oxidative process (overall reaction: substrate + $O_2$ + ADP + phosphate → oxidized substrate + ATP). However, this phosphorylation is readily dissociated of the oxydation process—releasing the energy as heat which is subsequently lost to the environment—by a number of agents, such as long-chain fatty acids, substituted benzenes, etc. These agents cause damage to the structural integrity of the mitochondrial membranes. Since the lipid fraction of these membranes consists mainly of phospholipids it is often reasoned that a change in the fatty acid composition of these phospholipids, such as is observed in EFA deficiency, will affect the coupling of the phosphorylation to the oxidation. The observation of Klein and Johnson (1954) seem to support this hypothesis. However, it remains to be investigated whether this inefficient phosphorylation is brought about by the isolation procedure —implying increased fragility of the mitochondria—or exists also in the intact liver cells.

## C. Swelling of Liver Mitochondria

The increased swelling properties of isolated liver mitochondria might be relevant with respect to the structural integrity of the mitochondrial membranes. As shown in Fig. 7 the spontaneous swelling of the liver mitochondria, measured as the change in optical density, is proportional to the amount of linoleic acid administered to the rats. It has been shown (Houtsmuller *et al.*, 1969) that the curves representing the change in optimal density can be described by

$$E_t\,(\%) = A.\mathrm{e}^{-\alpha t} + B.\mathrm{e}^{-\beta t}$$

in which $E_t\,(\%)$ = optimal density at time $t$,

expressed as a percentage of the initial value. $A$, $B$, $\alpha$ and $\beta$ are parameters which are correlated with the amount of linoleic acid fed to the rats. For practical purposes only $\alpha$ has been used as a criterion of EFA deficiency. When $\alpha$ is plotted as function of the dose of linoleic or linolenic acid both show the same linear correlation (Fig. 8). At a dose of 100 mg/day the optimal effect is not yet reached. Also the results obtained with the fish oil and the 20:5 and 22:6 concentrate fit well within the correlation. Therefore, this criterion parallels in every respect the increase in body weight in the Deuel assay, which suggests that the latter is due to changes in mitochondrial properties, resulting in better food efficiency. In contrast the bioassay with restricted drinking water

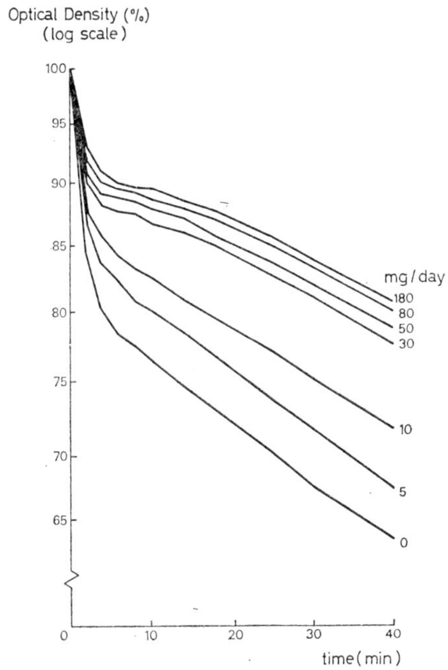


Fig. 7. Spontaneous swelling of rat liver mitochondria *in vitro* after feeding various doses of sunflowerseed oil (60% linoleic acid) to EFA-deficient rats for four weeks.

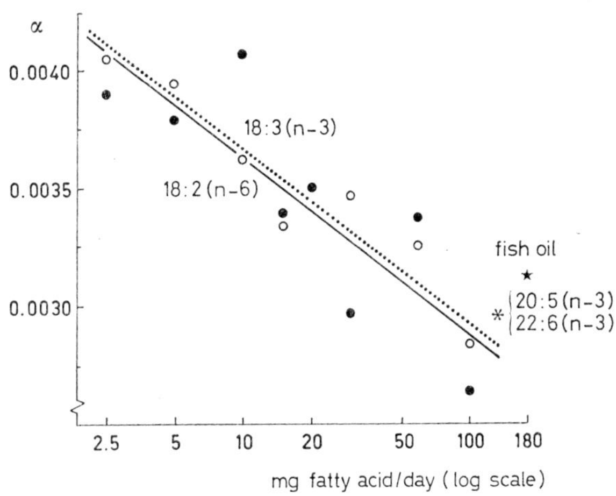


Fig. 8. Relation between parameter $\alpha$, derived from the equation $E_t$ (%) $= A.\mathrm{e}^{-\alpha} + B.\mathrm{e}^{-\beta t}$ describing the spontaneous swelling of rat liver mitochondria *in vitro* and the doses of linoleic or linolenic acid, a concentrate of 20:5 (*n*–3) and 22:6 (*n*–3) or a fish oil (for composition see Table 1) fed for four weeks to EFA-deficient rats.

mainly measures the skin permeability. But also some effect of improved food efficiency is observed, particularly the additional increase in body weight at equal food consumption upon administration of doses of linoleic acid larger than necessary for complete restoration of skin permeability (Fig. 6, doses > 30 mg/day).

## D. Fatty Acid Pattern

It is well known that in EFA deficiency the fatty acids of the linoleic acid family are partially replaced by those of the oleic acid group, particularly arachidonic acid by eicosatrienoic acid. Holman (1960) has introduced the triene/tetraene ratio as a criterion of EFA deficiency. This criterion implies that arachidonic acid has properties that cannot be met by eicosatrienoic acid. These properties, as argued before, may either be structural, e.g. in phospholipids, or dynamic, such as the production of prostaglandins. In mitochondria a structural function seems preponderant as these organelles have a high content of polyunsaturated fatty acids in their membranes, but prostaglandin synthesis has not been demonstrated in these organelles. Moreover, the proper functioning of mitochondria is strongly dependent on the integrity of the membranes. Therefore they seem to be especially suited for the study of the structural properties of dietary polyunsaturated fatty acids. However, a problem that arises is that the dietary fatty acid may be converted in the animal into other fatty acids with another number of carbon atoms and/or double bonds. If more than one of these fatty acids is incorporated into the mitochondria it becomes problematic to which of these the effects have to be ascribed. For example after feeding 100 mg/day of linoleic or linolenic acid the percentages of these fatty acids and their derivatives in liver mitochondria are as shown in Table 2. After feeding linoleic acid the main fatty acid is arachidonic

Table 2

Fatty acids of the *n*–6 and *n*–3 fatty acid families found in liver mitochondria after feeding 100 mg/day of linoleic or linolenic acid

| 18:2 (*n*–6) | | 18:3 (*n*–3) | |
|---|---|---|---|
| 18:2 (*n*–6) | 5·6% | 18:3 (*n*–3) | 0·6% |
| 20:3 (*n*–6) | 1·8% | 20:5 (*n*–3) | 12·0% |
| 20:4 (*n*–6) | 17·3% | 22:5 (*n*–3) | 1·9% |
| 22:4 (*n*–6) | 0·6% | 22:6 (*n*–3) | 13·0% |
| 22:5 (*n*–6) | 5·3% | | |

acid, but also appreciable amounts of docosapentaenoic and linoleic acid itself are found. On the other hand dietary linolenic acid is hardly incorporated, while 20:5 (*n*–3) and 22:6 (*n*–3) are abundant. Analogous results were obtained with the concentrate of the latter two fatty acids. With respect to the linoleic acid family it is generally accepted that those with 20 and 22 carbon atoms, especially arachidonic acid, are the structurally important ones. Supporting evidence for this assumption will be presented in Section IV. As these fatty acids replace 20:3 (*n*–9)

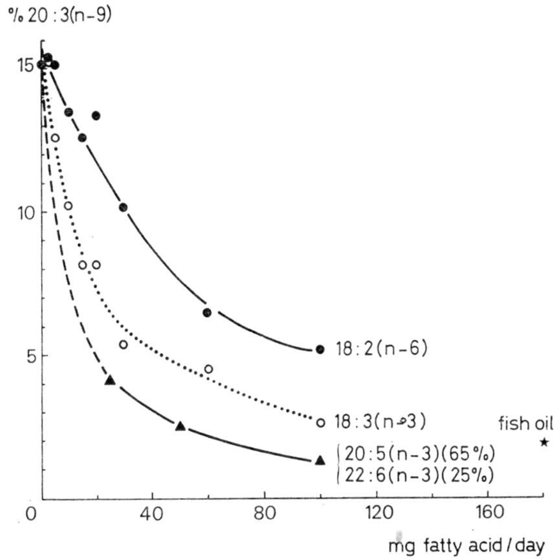


Fig. 9. Decrease in content of 20:3 (*n*–9) in liver mitochondria after feeding linoleic or linolenic acid, a concentrate of 20:5 (*n*–3) and 22:6 (*n*–3) or a fish oil (for composition see Table 1) for four weeks to EFA-deficient rats.

at the $\beta$-position in the phospholipids the latter seems to be the proper parameter for comparing the affinities of various fatty acid families for mitochondrial phospholipids. Figure 9 shows the decrease of this fatty acid after feeding increasing doses of the experimental oils.

The fatty acids of the (*n*–3) family are incorporated 3 times more readily than the (*n*–6) fatty acids and the mitochondria have even higher "affinity" for the fatty acids of the 20:5 and 22:6 concentrate. However, in normalizing the swelling properties of the mitochondria, linoleic and linolenic acid showed the same activity (Fig. 7). This means that three times as many fatty acids of the linolenic acid type are needed for the same structural effect, or in other words that with respect to this criterion linolenic acid has only 30% of the biological activity of linoleic acid. As has been shown in Section III.B the potency of linolenic acid with regard to alleviating the skin symptoms of EFA deficiency was only 10%. This difference in potency with respect to the two criteria may be due to the different functions of polyunsaturated fatty acids—structural in the mitochondria and dynamic (prostaglandin) in the skin.

On the other hand it could be that *n*–3 fatty acids have a sparing effect on *n*–6 fatty acids in so far as the latter are replaced in the mitochondria (a decrease in arachidonic acid was observed after feeding linolenic acid) and become available for their dynamic function in the skin.

## IV. OTHER POLYUNSATURATED FATTY ACIDS

A series of synthetic polyunsaturated fatty acids* of variable chain-length and different degrees of unsaturation were tested for EFA activity in the bioassay with restricted drinking water. At the end of the four-week feeding periods the mitochondrial fatty acid pattern and swelling properties were established and in some instances also the skin permeability *in vitro*. The fatty acids comprised a series of odd and even numbered trienes and tetraenes ($C_{18}$–$C_{22}$). All of these had *cis* double bonds on the 8, 11 and 14 position, the tetraenes having an additional double bond at the 5 position. In addition 19:4 (*n*–6) and two isomers of arachidonic acid were synthesized in which the first or the last double bond was shifted one position [(*n*–15) → (*n*–16) and (*n*–3) → (*n*–2)]. Figure 10 shows the effects of these fatty acids on the three criteria. Only 22:3 (*n*–8), 22:4 (*n*–8) and 18:3 (*n*–4) show no activity at all. The other fatty acids all normalize the swelling properties of the mitochondria to a greater or lesser extent. Particularly the eicosatetraenoic acids are very potent in this respect. With regard to growth only three fatty acids show an appreciable activity: arachidonic acid, its isomer 20:4 (*n*–6, 9, 12, *16*) and 21:4 (*n*–7). The remaining fatty acids have minor or no activity. In these assays with restricted drinking water the skin permeability again parallels growth: arachidonic acid and the (*n*–6, 9, 12, *16*) isomer have high potency, the third isomer (*n*–*2*, 6, 9, 12) low potency.

Unfortunately the skin permeability of 21:4 (*n*–7) was not measured, but it can be inferred from the high growth rate in this test where drinking water was limited that this fatty acid must have improved the

* Synthetized in the department of organic chemistry of Unilever Research Laboratories, Vlaardingen/Duiven (Struijk *et al.*, 1966; Beerthuis *et al.*, 1968, 1971).

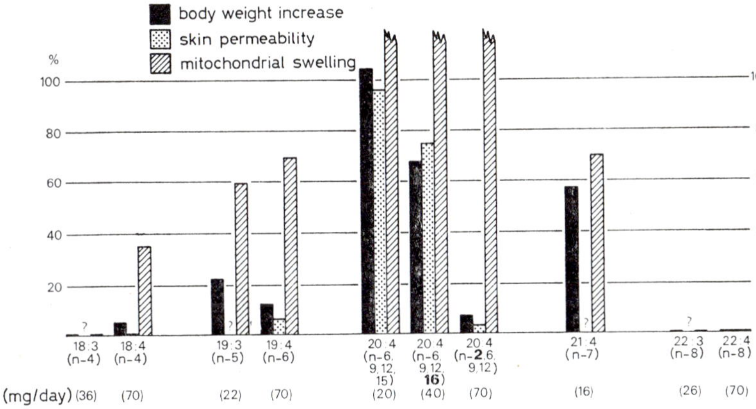


Fig. 10. The curative effects on growth, skin permeability for water and spontaneous swelling of liver mitochondria *in vitro* after feeding different synthetic fatty acids for four weeks to EFA-deficient rats. The effects are expressed as percentage of linoleic acid.

skin condition. Possibly also 19:3 (*n*–5) has some activity (not measured), but the other fatty acids hardly affect the skin. The production of prostaglandins from these fatty acids has also been investigated (for a review on this matter see Van Dorp, 1971). In complete agreement with the postulation that EFA have a dynamic (i.e. prostaglandin producing) function in skin, it was found that only those fatty acids which produced biologically active prostaglandins had a beneficial effect on skin lesions in the rat. Moreover quantitatively the rate of prostaglandin formation *in vitro* corresponds very well with the biological activity in the Thomasson bioassay, i.e. with the potency to restore skin permeability to normal.

With regard to the structural function of the synthetic fatty acids, it is interesting to investigate which fatty acids occur in the mitochondria (Table 3).

When the incorporation of (*n*–6) fatty acids is compared after feeding linoleic acid (100 mg/day) or arachidonic acid (10 mg/day) it appears that in the latter case only fatty acids with 20 or more C-atoms and more than four double bonds increased, but not 18:2 (*n*–6) or 20:3 (*n*–6), the precursor of $PGE_1$. As arachidonic acid cures abnormal swelling properties even more effectively than linoleic acid (Fig. 10) it must be concluded that for the structural function in mitochondria only the tetraenoic and pentaenoic members of this family are essential. With regard to the 20:4 isomers, 20:4 (*n*–6, 9, 12, *16*) behaves like arachidonic acid, while 20:4 (*n–2*, 6, 9, 12) seems to have the properties of the (*n*–3) family. This holds for the type of fatty acids incorporated (20:4

Table 3

Fatty acids incorporated into liver mitochondria, after feeding different fatty acids for four weeks to EFA-deficient rats

| Dietary fatty acid | Amount mg/day | Derivative found in mitochondria | | % of total fatty acid |
|---|---|---|---|---|
| — | — | 18:2 | (n–6) | 2·7 |
| | | 20:3 | | — |
| | | 20:4 | | 5·9 |
| | | 22:4 | | 0·2 |
| | | 22:5 | | 1·4 |
| 18:2 (*n*–6) | 100 | 18:2 | (*n*–6) | 5·6 |
| | | 20:3 | | 1·8 |
| | | 20:4 | | 17·3 |
| | | 22:4 | | 0·6 |
| | | 22:5 | | 5·3 |
| 20:4 (*n*–6, 9, 12, 15) | 10 | 18:2 | (*n*–6) | 2·4 |
| | | 20:3 | | — |
| | | 20:4 | | 13·2 |
| | | 22:4 | | 0·4 |
| | | 22:5 | | 2·4 |
| 18:3 (*n*–4) | 36 | 18:3 | (*n*–4) | 3·5 |
| | | 18:4 | | 1·0 |
| | | 20:5 | | 1·5 |
| 18:4 (*n*–4) | 70 | 18:4 | (*n*–4) | 10·7 |
| | | 20:4 | | 1·6 |
| | | 20:5 | | 8·3 |
| | | 22:5 | | 0·7 |
| 19:3 (*n*–5) | 22 | 19:3 | (*n*–5) | 2·5 |
| | | 19:4 | | 7·5 |
| | | 21:5 | | 5·5 |
| 19:4 (*n*–6) | 70 | 19:3 | (*n*–6) | 1·0 |
| | | 19:4 | | 16·8 |
| | | 21:4 | | 5·0 |
| 20:4 (*n*–6, 9, 12, *16*) | 40 | 20:4 | (*n*–6, 9, 12, *16*, . . .) | 20·7 |
| | | 22:4 | | 1·5 |
| | | 22:5 ? | | 2·0 |
| 20:4 (*n*–*2*, 6, 9, 12) | 70 | 20:4 | (*n*–*2*, 6, 9, . . .) | 2·1 |
| | | 20:5 | | 16·0 |
| | | 22:5 | | 0·8 |
| | | 22:6 | | 5·8 |
| 21:4 (*n*–7) | 16 | 21:4 | (*n*–7) | 16·5 |
| 22:3 (*n*–8) | 26 | 22:3 | (*n*–8) | 1·5 |
| | | 22:4 | | 0·5 |
| 22:4 (*n*–8) | 70 | 22:4 | (*n*–8) | 13·4 |

in the former versus 20:5 and 22:6 in the latter) as well as for the biological effects (the former is active in all criteria, while the latter has an appreciable effect on mitochondria only).

The lack of activity of 22:3 (*n*–8) is the consequence of the fact that this fatty acid is not incorporated into the mitochondria. On the other hand 22:4 (*n*–8) is readily incorporated but still has no effect on the mitochondria. An analogous situation is found for 18:3 (*n*–4) and 18:4 (*n*–4), both are incorporated, but only the tetraene shows a minor effect

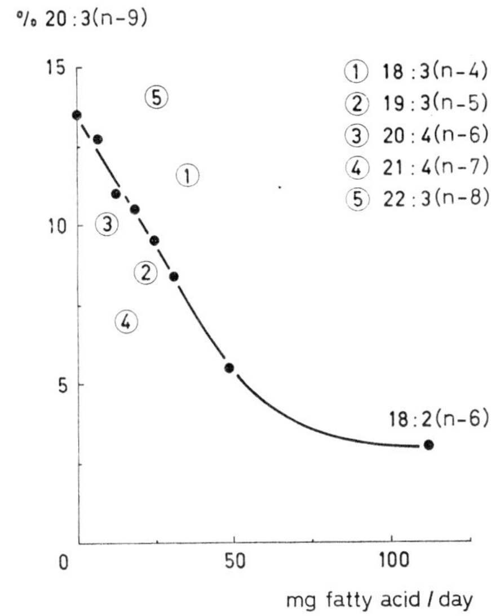


Fig. 11. Decrease in content of 20:3 (*n*–9) in liver mitochondria after feeding a series of homologous polyunsaturated fatty acids for four weeks to EFA-deficient rats.

on swelling. This effect most probably has to be ascribed to the eicosapentaenoic acid (8·3 %) produced in the body. 19:3 (*n*–5) is dehydrogenated and elongated into the tetraene and heneicosapentaenoic acid. To which of these the improvement of mitochondrial swelling must be ascribed cannot be decided. The same applies also for 19:4 (*n*–6), which is also elongated, but only to a tetraene as a fifth double bond would be too close to the carboxyl group.

In order to compare quantitatively the biological effects of the various fatty acids with their affinity for incorporation into the liver mitochondria, irrespective which of the derivatives contributes and to what extent, use can be made again of the 20:3 (*n*–9) content of the mitochondria. The decrease of this fatty acid upon feeding of linoleic acid or the synthetic fatty acids is shown in Figs 11 and 12, each

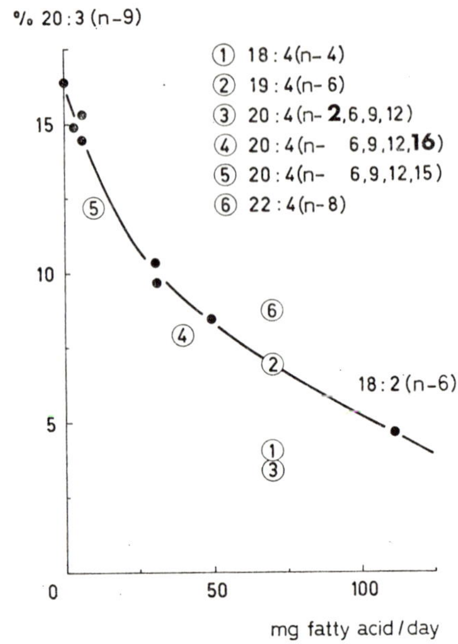


Fig. 12. Decrease in content of 20:3 (*n*–9) in liver mitochondria after feeding several polyunsaturated fatty acids for four weeks to EFA-deficient rats.

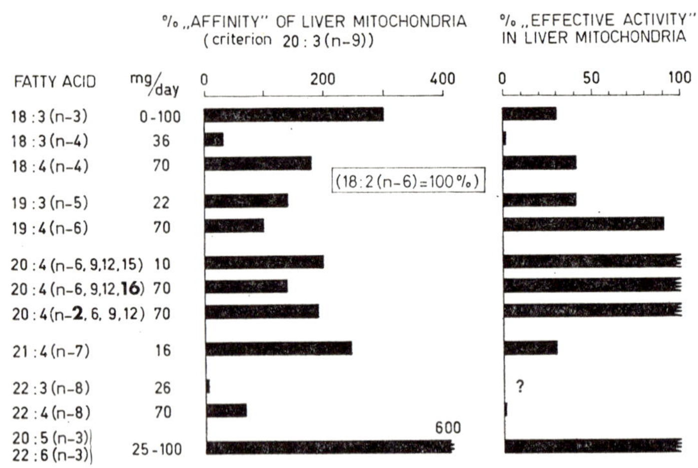


Fig. 13. Left hand side: the "affinity" of liver mitochondria from EFA-deficient rats for different fatty acids, using the decrease of 20:3 (*n*–9) after feeding the fatty acids for four weeks as a criterion. Right hand side: the "effective activity" of these fatty acids in liver mitochondria, i.e. the normalization of mitochondrial swelling relative to the extent of replacement of 20.3 (*n*–9) in the mitochondria by these fatty acids.

representing the results of separate experiments. As expected the replacement of 20:3 (*n*–9) correlates inversely with the incorporation of the dietary fatty acids and their derivatives.

Using the amount of 20:3 (*n*–9) as a criterion of incorporation, the "affinity" of the fatty acids for incorporation into the mitochondria can now be calculated (Fig. 13, left hand side). Except both (*n*–8) fatty acids and 18:3 (*n*–4) all fatty acids have higher affinity than linoleic acid, the linolenic acid family being particularly potent. From these affinities and the potency of the fatty acids to normalize mitochondrial swelling the "effective activity" of the fatty acids can be derived (Fig. 13, right hand side). This "effective activity" expresses the suitability of the incorporated fatty acid to function as a structural element in the mitochondria.

The "effective activity" of linolenic acid has been discussed in Section III.D. From 22:3 (*n*–8) no value could be calculated, because this fatty acid was not incorporated. 22:4 (*n*–8) is reasonably incorporated, but nevertheless it has no "effective activity", which indicates that the configuration of this type of fatty acid is unsuited for a structural function in mitochondria. An analogous conclusion cannot be drawn for 18:3 (*n*–4) because in this case the observed low "effective activity" may be due to the combination of low potency and slight incorporation as a result of the relatively low dietary dose. 19:4 (*n*–6) is almost as suited for the mitochondria as linoleic acid. Arachidonic acid and both its isomers as well as the fatty acids of the concentrate (derivatives of linolenic acid) are even more adequate than linoleic acid but the actual values were too high to be accurately calculated. The three remaining fatty acids (18:4 (*n*–4), 19:3 (*n*–5) and 21:4 (*n*–7)) all have an "effective activity" around 40%.

## V. CONCLUSIONS

Reviewing these results in relation to comparable published data (Holman, 1968, 1970) it appears that for a proper structural function in liver mitochondria the incorporated fatty acid should have 19 or preferably 20 carbon atoms and at least 4 double bonds, two of which have to be in the *cis* configuration and on the *n*–6 and *n*–9 position; the remaining double bonds should be in a methylene interrupted or isolated position with respect to these double bonds (Fig. 13, right hand side). Shifting of the skipped double bond system from positions *n*–6, 9 progressively decreases the "effective activity". It follows from this generalization that any dietary fatty acid which can be converted in the animal into a fatty acid as defined above will be suited for structural functions (e.g. linoleic acid).

These requirements resemble the rule proposed by Thomasson, which, however, is much more exacting as it states that the ($n$–6) as well as the ($n$–9) double bond (both in *cis* configuration) are prerequisites for EFA activity. Additional *cis* double bonds toward the carboxyl end of the fatty acid chain ($n$–12, 15, etc.) increase the EFA activity, while extra double bonds at the terminal end ($n$–3) decrease activity. It should be realized, however, that Thomasson based his rule on results obtained with the bioassay with restricted drinking water. As discussed in Section II such results refer mainly to skin permeability and therefore are indicative of the dynamic function of polyunsaturated fatty acids. Apparently the requirements for a structural function of fatty acids are less specific as for the dynamic function, e.g. the production of prostaglandins. It is not within the scope of this contribution to define requirements for prostaglandin synthesis. Readers are referred for a discussion of this problem to the review of Van Dorp (1971). Presently it may only be inferred that skin and its permeability seem to be suitable instruments for quantitative studies of prostaglandins and their synthesis, a conclusion that very recently has also been put forward by Ziboh (1973).

## REFERENCES

Beerthuis, R. K., Nugteren, D. H., Pabon, H. J. J. and Van Dorp, D. A. (1968). Biologically active prostaglandins from some odd-numbered essential fatty acids. *Receuil* **87,** 461–480.

Beerthuis, R. K., Nugteren, D. H., Pabon, H. J. J., Steenhoek, A. and Van Dorp, D. A. (1971). Synthesis of a series of polyunsaturated fatty acids, their potencies as essential fatty acids and as precursors of prostaglandins. *Receuil* **90,** 943–960.

Bergström, S. (1966). Isolation, structure and action of the prostaglandins. *In* "Prostaglandins; Nobel Symposium 2" (S. Bergström and B. Samuelsson, eds), pp. 21–30. John Wiley and Sons, London.

Bygdeman, M. (1966). Studies on the effects of prostaglandins in seminal plasma on human myometrium *in vivo*. *In* "Prostaglandins; Nobel Symposium 2" (S. Bergström and B. Samuelsson, eds), pp. 71–77. John Wiley and Sons, London.

Deuel, H. J. (1951). The effect of fat level of the diet on general nutrition: VIII. The essential fatty acid content of margarines, shortenings, butters and cottonseed oil as determined by a new biological assay method. *J. Nutr.* **45,** 535–549.

Holman, R. T. (1960). The ratio of trienoic: tetraenoic acids in tissue lipids as a measure of essential fatty acid requirement. *J. Nutr.* **70,** 405–410.

Holman, R. T. (1968). Essential fatty acid deficiency. *In* "Progress in the Chemistry of Fats and other Lipids" (R. T. Holman, ed), Vol. IX, part 2, pp. 279–348. Pergamon Press.

Holman, R. T. (1970). Biological activities of and requirement for polyunsaturated acids. *In* "Progress in the Chemistry of Fats and other Lipids" (R. T. Holman, ed), Vol. IX, part 5, pp. 611–682. Pergamon Press.

Houtsmuller, U.M.T., Van der Beek, A. and Zaalberg, J. (1969). A new criterion in the bioassay of essential fatty acids: the spontaneous swelling of rat liver mitochondria *in vitro*. *Lipids* **4,** 571–574.

Klein, P. D. and Johnson, R. M. (1945). Phosphorus metabolism in unsaturated fatty acid deficient rats. *J. Biol. Chem.* **211,** 103–110.

Struijk, C. B., Beethuis, R. K., Pabon, H. J. J. and Van Dorp, D. A. (1966). Specificity in the enzymic conversion of polyunsaturated fatty acids into prostaglandins. *Receuil* **85,** 1233–1250.

Thomasson, H. J. (1953). Biological standardization of essential fatty acids (a new method). *Int. Z. Vitaminforsch.* **25,** 26–82.

Thomasson, H. J. (1961). Acidi Grassi Essenziale. *Rivista Italiana Sostanze Grasse* **12,** 541–548.

Van Dorp, D. A. (1971). Essentielle Fettsäuren und Prostaglandine. *In* "Fettstoffwechselstörungen, ihre Erkennung und Behandlung" (Gotthard Schettler, ed), pp. 152–177. Georg Thieme Verlag, Stuttgart.

Ziboh, V. A. (1973). Biosynthesis of prostaglandin $E_2$ in human skin: subcellular localization and inhibition by unsaturated fatty acids and anti-inflammatory drugs. *J. Lipid Res.* **14,** 377–384.

Ziboh, V. A. and Hsia, S. L. (1972). Effects of prostaglandin $E_2$ on rat skin: inhibition of sterol ester biosynthesis and clearing of scaly lesions in essential fatty acid deficiency. *J. Lipid Res.* **13,** 458–467.

# 8 Cholesterol Absorption

G. S. BOYD

*Department of Biochemistry, Edinburgh University Medical School, Edinburgh, Scotland*



## I. INTRODUCTION

Cholesterol is the principal sterol found in mammalian tissues. It is present in all cells, subcellular organelles and membranes. The sterol is sparingly soluble in water, and hence in cells and body fluids; cholesterol appears to be effectively solubilized by an interaction with other lipids and proteins yielding macromolecular complexes termed "lipoproteins". Cholesterol is synthesized from simple precursors such as acetate by most mammalian cells and the rate of cholesterol synthesis in different mammalian tissues varies markedly. However, two tissues, the liver and the small intestine, by virtue of their size and high rate of cholesterol synthesis stand out from all other mammalian tissues. These organs play an important part in the overall complex dynamics of cholesterol absorption and metabolism in mammalian systems. The subject of cholesterol metabolism has been reviewed (Bloch, 1965; Taylor and Ho, 1967).

Since cholesterol is present in all mammalian tissues it follows that carnivores must ingest appreciable quantities of cholesterol. The average human subject eating a varied diet consumes amounts of cholesterol which vary, depending upon the foodstuffs selected, from 0·5–3·0 g/day. On the one hand, foods such as eggs, liver, kidneys and brain are relatively rich in this sterol, while lean meat and vegetable products are relatively low in cholesterol (Okey, 1945; Pihl, 1952). The cholesterol content of some common foodstuffs is shown in Table 1.

Table 1

Cholesterol content of some common foodstuffs

| Food item | Cholesterol content mg/100 g | Cholesterol content mg/standard unit |
|---|---|---|
| Lean meat | 80 | 360 mg/lb |
| Bacon | 200 | 900 mg/lb |
| Liver | 300 | 1350 mg/lb |
| Kidneys | 200 | 900 mg/lb |
| Brain | 3000 | 13500 mg/lb |
| Egg | 460 | 300 mg/egg |
| Butter | 250 | 1100 mg/lb |
| Lard | 100 | 450 mg/lb |
| Cheese | 100 | 450 mg/lb |
| Fish (white) | 60 | 270 mg/lb |
| Milk | 10 | 540 mg/pint |
| Chicken | 80 | 360 mg/lb |

Of all the lipids encountered in biological material, cholesterol is one of the simplest substances to identify and measure. Specific and sensitive colorimetric methods for the determination of cholesterol have been available for many years and a large number of gas–liquid chromatographic methods are also available. As the concentration of cholesterol in most tissues and body fluids is quite high, this has resulted in large numbers of observations being made on various facets of cholesterol metabolism in mammals.

Long before the "isotopic era" considerable evidence had accumulated regarding the ability of mammals to absorb cholesterol from the diet, by the so-called "balance technique". This involves a combination of accurate cholesterol assays of the sterol content of the diet, the carcasses of the animals and the faeces. It was possible by the balance technique to show that animals such as rabbits, rats and mice absorbed cholesterol from the diet, see reviews (Cook, 1958; Deuel, 1951).

When rabbits receive a cholesterol supplement in the diet these animals exhibit an increase in the plasma cholesterol concentration (Keigs, 1953). However, when man receives a dietary cholesterol supplement there may be only a minor increment to the plasma cholesterol concentration (Conner *et al.*, 1961).

There is now little doubt that in normal animals and in man, a portion of the dietary cholesterol will undergo physico-chemical change in the small intestine—which will result in absorption of a fraction of this dietary sterol load. Consequently some of the dietary cholesterol will enter the plasma compartment and then be distributed throughout all the tissues of the body in varying degrees (Chevallier, 1953; Borgstrom *et al.*, 1958).

The mechanism by which cholesterol is absorbed from the gut has been under investigation for many years. After feeding a cholesterol-rich diet it was shown that the cholesterol concentration of the lymph was markedly increased (Mueller, 1916). A large number of experiments have supported the concept that the absorption of cholesterol from the gut via the lymph is influenced by the amount of triglyceride in the diet (Pihl, 1955; Swell *et al.*, 1955). It is, of course, well known that the enzyme cholesteryl ester hydrolase (cholesterol esterase) is present in the intestinal mucosa and hence the ingestion of cholesterol, as the free alcohol, or cholesterol esterified to long-chain fatty acids, results in a similar response with regard to the intestinal absorption of the sterol. Analyses of the cholesterol content of the lymph have shown that 50–80% of the lymph cholesterol is esterified to long-chain fatty acids while the remainder is present as free or non-esterified cholesterol (Vahouny and Treadwell, 1957).

As a consequence of the introduction of the isotopic method it was possible to investigate the absorption of cholesterol from the gut by the use of tracer dosages of cholesterol as opposed to the cholesterol loading techniques which had to be employed in previous studies on cholesterol absorption. It was shown that when a small dose of [$^{14}$C]-cholesterol was dissolved in corn oil and administered to rats, about 25–50% of the administered radioactive cholesterol was absorbed by these animals. Furthermore, it was shown that almost all of the absorbed cholesterol could be accounted for in terms of the radioactive cholesterol recovered from the thoracic duct lymph (Chaikoff *et al.*, 1952).

Accepting the physiological fact that when cholesterol is fed to normal mammals it is absorbed from the small intestine via the lymph and hence delivered into the plasma compartment then a number of facets of the absorptive process remain to be elucidated. The cholesterol content of the small intestine originates from four main sources. These are, the cholesterol content of the foodstuffs imbibed by the animal, the cholesterol content of the bile secreted by the liver into the small intestine, the cholesterol secreted by the intestinal cells and the cholesterol arising from epithelial cells shed as part of the normal turnover of intestinal cells. These four main sources of cholesterol form the "pool of intestinal cholesterol", or "cholesterol load", confronting the mammal. This is shown in Fig. 1.

It might be deduced that these four sources of cholesterol under the influence of chemical and mechanical factors in the gut would be rendered into a single homogeneous cholesterol pool. There is experimental work suggesting that the intestinal cholesterol pool is heterogeneous in that biliary cholesterol is more effectively absorbed than dietary cholesterol. The cholesterol found in bile is mainly free cholesterol (non-esterified cholesterol) but the cholesterol originating from intestinal cells and from the diet may contain variable amounts of esterified cholesterol.

The pancreatic secretions contain the enzyme, cholesterol ester hydrolase or cholesterol esterase which is capable of splitting cholesterol esters into the free sterol and fatty acids. This hydrolytic enzyme is activated by bile salts (Hernandez and Chaikoff, 1957; Swell *et al.*, 1953), and hence eventually most of the material presented to the small intestine for absorption will consist of free or non-esterified cholesterol (Vahouny and Treadwell, 1964). The other lipids consumed along with cholesterol in the usual mixed diet are also subjected to enzymatic modification in the presence of bile salts in the small intestine. Thus the triglyceride content of the diet is degraded to diglycerides and monoglycerides with the release of free fatty acids. It has been demonstrated that the combination of monoglycerides, bile salts, phospholipids and cholesterol results in the production of an aqueous micellar phase provided the molar ratios of the various components fall within certain specific ranges. It appears therefore that the diet containing cholesterol is exposed to conditions in the small intestine which initially resulted in the production of a fine emulsion and as the components of this emulsion are attacked by various hydrolytic enzymes, the products of hydrolysis are able to combine in a non-covalent form to yield water soluble mixed micelles. Thus the cholesterol content of the small intestine is present both in an emulsion phase and in a micellar phase. Since there is no evidence that cholesterol can be absorbed from the emulsion phase it seems likely that one of the rate-limiting factors in the absorption of cholesterol by the small intestine is the ultimate conversion of cholesterol into the micellar phase prior to sterol uptake by the intestinal cells.

A large number of studies have been performed on the quantitative

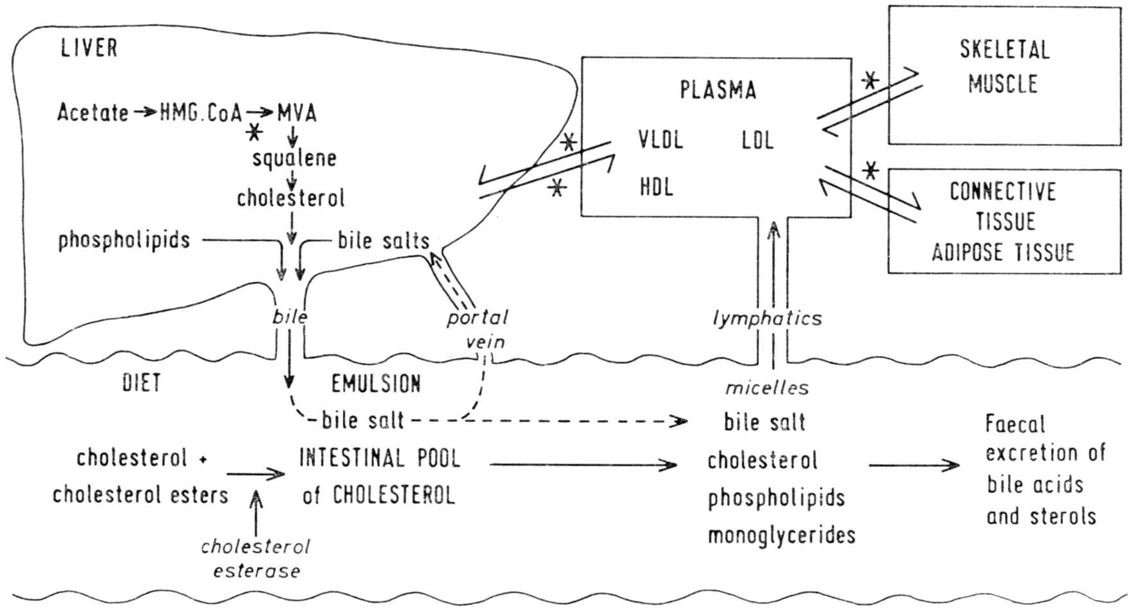


Fig. 1. This is a diagrammatic representation of the interrelationship between the liver, small intestines, plasma and extra-hepatic tissues with regard to cholesterol exchanges. The liver and the small intestine both have the ability to synthesize cholesterol from simple precursors such as acetate. In the case of liver, one of the principal controlling points is the enzyme system involved in the reduction of HMG.CoA—MVA. The liver is the only known source of the enzymes involved in degrading cholesterol to bile salts. The bile salts are discharged into the small intestine and activate cholesterol esterase and other lipases and participate in the formation of micelles. The plasma is the vehicle for the exchange of cholesterol between liver, small intestine and various extra-hepatic tissues. The cholesterol which is contained in plasma is present as VLDL, LDL, HDL or/and chylomicrons.

aspects of sterol absorption in various animals. From a kinetic standpoint the uptake of cholesterol into the intestinal cells from micelles has the characteristics of a passive diffusion process (Sylven and Borgstrom, 1969a). Hence the limiting factor for the rate of absorption of cholesterol is related to the concentration of cholesterol in the micellar phase within the small intestine. Micelles however, are of variable composition depending upon the other components in the diet.

It has been shown that the extent of lymphatic transport of cholesterol is dependent upon the type of triglyceride administered in the diet along with the sterol. In some species more cholesterol is absorbed when the sterol is fed along with long-chain fatty acids than when fed with short-chain fatty acids, and in fact, the lymphatic transport of cholesterol increased proportionally with the fatty acid chain length in the range $C_6$ to $C_{18}$ (Sylven and Borgstrom, 1969b). It has been suggested that the effect of the fatty acid chain length of the glyceride fed on the uptake of cholesterol into the intestinal cells may be mediated through an effect of the hydrolytic products of the glyceride on the transfer of the sterol to the micellar phase of the intestinal contents (Sylven and Borgstrom, 1969b). These results then suggest that the concentration of cholesterol is higher in micelles generated in the presence of the long-chain fatty acids, leading to an increased uptake of cholesterol into the intestinal cells.

There is now considerable evidence to support the concept that most of the cholesterol absorbed by the small intestine from the micellar phase is, in fact, accomplished in the upper part of the small intestine (Simmonds *et al.*, 1967; Borgstrom, 1960). After an appropriate test meal containing radioactive cholesterol it can be shown that most of the radioactivity can be found in the thoracic duct lymph in the period six to nine hours after the administration of the test substance (Chaikoff *et al.*, 1952).

## II. ABSORPTION OF STEROLS STRUCTURALLY RELATED TO CHOLESTEROL

Although the precise mechanism by which intestinal cells take up cholesterol from the micellar phase has not been fully established it has been shown that the intestinal cells do in fact have a fairly high degree of specificity with regard to the type of sterol absorbed. Plant sterols such as sitosterol and campesterol which differ only slightly from cholesterol in that they have additional groups in the side chain at position $C_{24}$ are in fact poorly absorbed by comparison with cholesterol (Gould *et al.*, 1955, 1956). Saturation of the double bond of cholesterol to give cholestanol results in a decrease in the absorption of this compound relative to cholesterol; however the two sterols appear to be absorbed by the same mechanism (Gould *et al.*, 1956). On the other hand, saturation of the double bond of cholesterol to give coprostanol produces a sterol which is not absorbed to any significant extent. Introduction of an additional double bond into the B ring of cholesterol to give 7-dehydro-cholesterol also decreases the efficiency of absorption of this sterol relative to cholesterol (Peterson *et al.*, 1954; Cook *et al.*, 1954). The structure of a few sterols related to cholesterol is shown in Figs 2 and 3. The relative absorption rates are shown in Table 2. Since

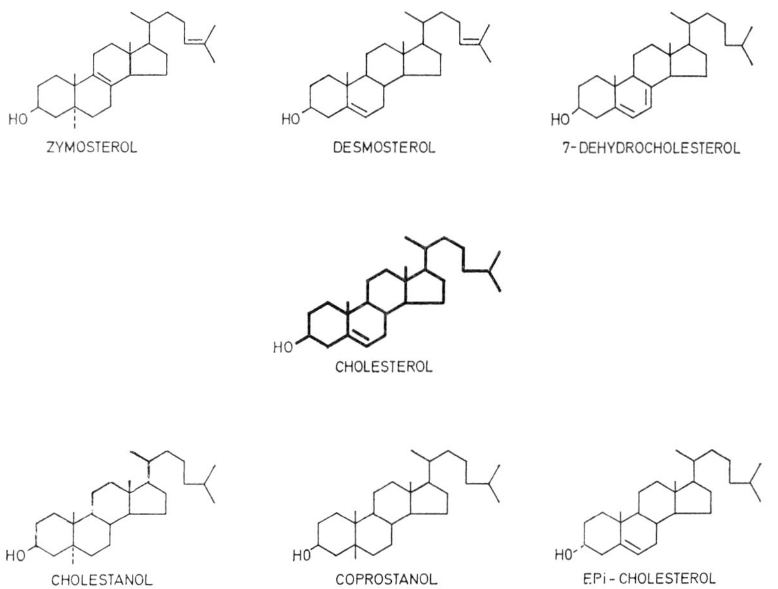


Fig. 2. The structures of various sterols related to cholesterol and which may be present in tissues as precursors of cholesterol, reduction products of cholesterol or metabolites of cholesterol.

the plant sterols such as sitosterol are only poorly absorbed by comparison with cholesterol, these sterols can be used as markers in cholesterol absorption studies. This will be discussed in a later part of this chapter devoted to the quantitative assessment of cholesterol absorption.

The uptake of cholesterol from the micellar phase into the intestinal cells is followed by a poorly understood mechanism whereby the sterol crosses the epithelial cell and is then extruded as chylomicrons or lipoprotein particles into the lymph. During the active phase of cholesterol

Table 2

Sterols related to cholesterol and found in the diet

| Trivial name | Chemical name | Source | Absorption from the gut |
|---|---|---|---|
| 7-dehydro-cholesterol | Cholest-5,7-diene-3β-ol | mammalian tissues | appreciable |
| Cholesterol | Cholest-5-en-3β-ol | mammalian tissues | appreciable |
| Cholestanol | 5α-cholestan-3β-ol | minor sterol in mammalian tissues and in faeces | little |
| Coprostanol | 5β-cholestan-3β-ol | faeces of carnivores | negligible |
| Ergosterol | Cholest-5,7,22-triene-24-methyl-3β-ol | yeast | little |
| Stigmasterol | Cholest-5,22-diene-24-ethyl-3β-ol | soya bean | not absorbed |
| Sitosterol | Cholest-5-en-24-ethyl-3β-ol | plants, grain, beans, etc. | negligible |
| Campesterol | Cholest-5-en-24-methyl-3β-ol | minor sterol in plants, grain, etc. | negligible |
| Epi-cholesterol | Cholest-5-en-3α-ol | synthetic | negligible |
| Fucosterol | Cholest-5-en-24-vinyl-3β-ol | algae | |
| Desmosterol | Cholest-5,24-diene-3β-ol | minor sterol in mammalian tissues | |
| Zymosterol | 5α-cholest-8(9), 24-diene-3β-ol | minor sterol in yeast | |
| Brassicasterol | Cholest-5,22-diene-24-methyl-3β-ol | minor component of rape seed oil | little |

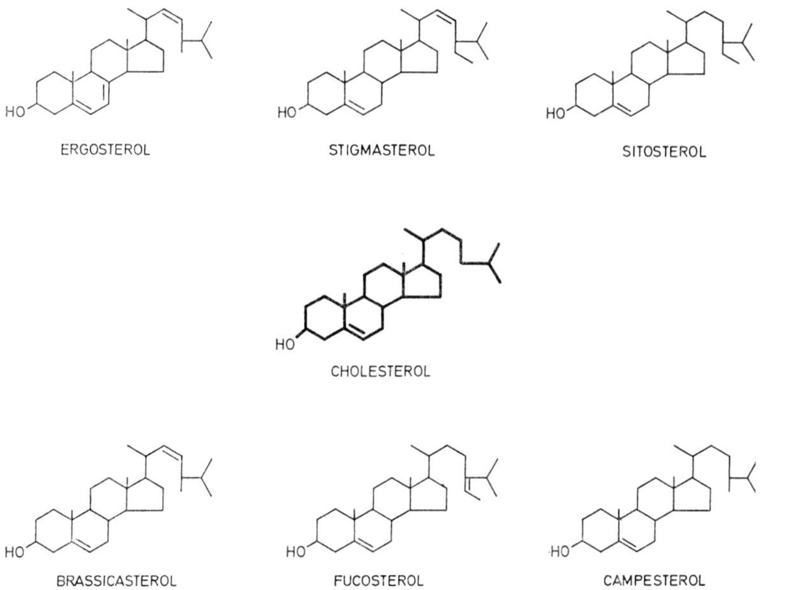


Fig. 3. The structures of various sterols related to cholesterol and which are found in various plants and unicellular organisms.

absorption there is a rise in the cholesterol content of the intestinal cells (Glover and Morton, 1958). The sterol which is found as chylomicrons or lipoproteins in the lymph is in part esterified and it seems likely that the esterification reaction has occurred within the intestinal cells. There is evidence to suggest that the degree of esterification of cholesterol in lymph may be related to the dietary cholesterol load because the activity of the cholesterol esterifying system in rat intestinal mucosa may be increased by the administration of diets rich in cholesterol (Murthy *et al.*, 1961).

The lymphatic cholesterol, cholesterol esters, phospholipids and triglycerides which compose the chylomicrons are transported via the thoracic duct to the plasma. These chylomicrons survive for a variable time in the circulation and due to the action of the "clearing factor lipase" (lipoprotein lipase) much of the triglyceride content of these large particles is hydrolysed at various extra-hepatic capillary sites (Robinson, 1964). As a consequence of the removal of triglycerides from the chylomicron particles the residual chylomicron particles or chylomicron remnants are proportionally much richer in cholesterol esters (Redgrave, 1970). These cholesterol-rich chylomicron remnants are taken up by the liver where the cholesterol ester is hydrolysed, *trans*-esterified and stored or incorporated into various lipoprotein macromolecules. A portion of this hepatic cholesterol will be secreted by the liver into the plasma as very low density lipoproteins (VLDL). Thus the result of the administration of a cholesterol-rich meal to a normal subject is the elevation of the liver cholesterol ester concentration followed by a later secretion of VLDL by that organ.

A large number of other factors present in the diet can, of course, modify the rate and extent of cholesterol absorption from a test meal. Apart from the triglyceride composition and content of the diet, previously discussed, substances which influence the intestinal bile salt concentration exert a profound effect upon cholesterol absorption processes. Thus, the inclusion in the diet of substances such as anionic exchange resins of the cholestyramine type, which will bind bile salts and hence decrease or totally inhibit the activity of the intestinal lipases and cholesterol esterases will prevent the formation of micelles and effectively block cholesterol absorption (Wilson and Reinke, 1968). A number of other physiological components in the diet appear to act like cholestyramine in that they also sequester bile salts and decrease their effectiveness. These compounds include components in the roughage of the diet and substances such as lignin (Eastwood and Hamilton, 1968).

It is self-evident that the total cholesterol present in the carcass of an adult animal (or human) must be controlled by the interplay of factors such as cholesterol absorption, cholesterol synthesis and cholesterol excretion or breakdown.

A considerable number of studies have been performed in attempts to establish the limits of cholesterol absorption in man. In the older balance-type experiments it was shown that cholesterol was relatively poorly absorbed by man. In fact, many of these investigations suggested that not more than about 10 mg of cholesterol/kg body weight/day could be effectively absorbed. Much of the older literature on this subject has been reviewed (McIntyre, 1971; Treadwell and Vahouny, 1968).

Using modern methods for the study of the regulation of total body cholesterol in man, it has been shown that the absorption of dietary cholesterol is related to the intake. In some subjects up to 1 g of cholesterol was absorbed when 3 g of cholesterol were fed. In these studies it has been shown that with increased absorption of cholesterol there occurred two compensatory mechanisms. On the one hand, there was an increased excretion of cholesterol and on the other hand there may be a variable decrease in the total body synthesis of cholesterol (Quintao *et al.*, 1971). The evidence which has been collected in man suggests that the daily transport of cholesterol circulating through the lymphatics, plasma, liver, bile and back to the small intestine is of the order of several grammes of cholesterol per day. However the normal intake of cholesterol only accounts for a small fraction of the total cholesterol transported; consequently the exogenous dietary cholesterol mixes in the intestine with endogenous cholesterol forming the total intestinal cholesterol pool from which absorption via micelles takes place. From this total intestinal cholesterol pool a fraction is absorbed and as long as the dietary cholesterol contribution to the pool is small, relative to the total cholesterol pool, no saturation will be apparent for the absorption of the dietary cholesterol. However, with a limited total absorption of cholesterol any large increase in the dietary cholesterol load leads to an increased faecal excretion of cholesterol. Thus some of the endogenous cholesterol will be exchanged for exogenous cholesterol with little effect on the total cholesterol absorption (Quintao *et al.*, 1971).

The gastro-intestinal tract in man has only a limited ability to absorb dietary cholesterol. Consequently this organ plays an important part with regard to cholesterol metabolism in the whole animal. Such a control over cholesterol absorption, in man, is thought to be a significant protection against dietary induced hypercholesterolaemia. Furthermore, the small intestine is one of the major sites of synthesis of cholesterol which is contributed to the circulating plasma cholesterol pool.

When cholesterol is fed to a normal, healthy animal, the sterol is absorbed as described previously and much of the cholesterol is deposited in the liver. This organ responds at once, in some species, by an almost complete suppression of cholesterologenesis (Gould *et al.*, 1953; Tomkins *et al.*, 1953). When these studies have been extended to man it has been found that while hepatic cholesterologenesis does respond to dietary cholesterol intake, nevertheless the quantitative response to this dietary constraint is much less in man than has been observed in certain experimental animals (Taylor and Ho, 1967; Davis, 1959). By contrast, cholesterol feeding has little effect on the rate of cholesterol synthesis by the small intestine in all species. Thus during a cholesterol loading type of experiment much of the circulating plasma cholesterol arises from the dietary cholesterol together with the cholesterol synthesized *de novo* by the small intestine (Kaplan *et al.*, 1963; Wilson and Dietschy, 1966).

When animals are subjected to interruption of the enterohepatic circulation of bile salts, by biliary drainage or by feeding a bile salt sequestering agent such as cholestyramine, there is a decreased content of cholesterol in the lymph. The animal responds by increasing the rate of cholesterol synthesis in the liver and by increasing the rate of cholesterol degradation to bile acids in the liver (Eriksson, 1957; Bergstrom and Danielsson, 1958; Myant and Eder, 1961). The increased hepatic cholesterol biosynthesis observed in this situation is due to the direct (or indirect) activation of the liver $\beta$-hydroxy-$\beta$-methyl glutaryl coenzyme A reductase, which is one of the key enzymes in the conversion of acetate to cholesterol in living cells (Bucher *et al.*, 1960). This rate limiting step is considerably activated in the absence of bile salts and hence when [$^{14}$C]-acetate is used to assess rates of cholesterol synthesis, interruption of the enterohepatic circulation of bile salts is observed to activate cholesterol synthesis. Similarly, decreasing the feedback of bile salts to the liver activates the hepatic microsomal cholesterol 7$\alpha$-hydroxylase enzyme system (Danielsson *et al.*, 1967; Boyd *et al.*, 1967). This enzyme is thought to be a key enzyme in the breakdown of cholesterol to bile acids. Consequently, there is an increased overall catabolism of cholesterol to bile acids in the bile fistula animal. In the absence of bile salts the decreased concentration of cholesterol in lymph is due to the intestinal lipases and cholesterol esterases lacking activation by this surface active agent (Vahouny *et al.*, 1965). The absence of bile salts in the gut therefore prevents the formation of suitable micelles required in sterol absorption (Siperstein *et al.*, 1952; Watt and Simmonds, 1971). In animals subjected to biliary obstruction there are, of course, virtually no bile salts in the small intestine. The cholesterol content of the lymph is again decreased and studies have shown that the rate of cholesterol synthesis in liver as judged by the conversion of [$^{14}$C]-acetate into cholesterol is again increased (Eastwood, 1973).

When animals are subjected to drainage of the thoracic duct lymph this situation appears to be associated with an increased rate of cholesterol synthesis by the liver (Bloomfield, 1963).

A large number of attempts have been made within recent years to produce accurate measurements of the cholesterol balance in man and in experimental animals. As discussed in an earlier section in this chapter, using simple chemical methods, it was possible to establish from "input" versus "output" of cholesterol and by direct measurement of the carcass cholesterol, that this sterol could be absorbed by most animals. Similar indirect methods applied to man, such as measuring the cholesterol intake and the faecal cholesterol output and measurement of the plasma cholesterol concentration suggested that man behaved like many experimental animals, in that he was capable of absorbing an appreciable quantity of a "cholesterol load".

The increase in interest in cholesterol metabolism which has occurred over the last three decades prompted a number of investigators to suggest that elevated plasma cholesterol concentrations seen in certain subjects might be correlated with the dietary cholesterol load. This necessitated the development of sophisticated methods for the accurate measurement of cholesterol absorption in man.

## III. THE PLASMA–ERYTHROCYTE–LIVER–BILE–CHOLESTEROL POOL

By application of the isotopic tracer method and the availability of specifically labelled cholesterol it was possible to show that when [$^{14}$C]-cholesterol was administered to mammals by the intravenous route, the radioactive cholesterol distributed itself almost instantly throughout the plasma compartment, equilibrated rapidly with the liver cholesterol and appeared in bile. It was also possible to show that the plasma cholesterol rapidly equilibrated with the erythrocyte membrane cholesterol and this equilibration between plasma–erythrocyte–liver–bile occurred within a few hours (Gould *et al.*, 1955; Kurland *et al.*, 1954). Thus the specific activity of the radioactive cholesterol administered intravenously, dropped very rapidly during about ten hours. Accepting that the equilibration of labelled cholesterol amongst these different organelles occurs rapidly, the question then arises as to the explanation for the continuing decline in specific activity of the plasma cholesterol over the period of 1–100 days. This is shown in Fig. 4.

It has been shown in animals and to a lesser degree in man that the cholesterol contained within the plasma compartment is available to a variety of other tissues. It is relatively simple to demonstrate that many extra-hepatic tissues take up cholesterol from the plasma compartment. This uptake of cholesterol by these extra-hepatic tissues is much slower than the uptake of cholesterol by liver or erythrocytes. Thus for practical purposes it is possible to divide the tissues of the body into two main divisions those which take up cholesterol very rapidly from the plasma–liver compartment and the other tissues which take up cholesterol at a slower rate. Of the tissues which take up cholesterol slowly, these again can be further subdivided into those which take up this sterol at a measurable rate, albeit a slow rate, and tissues which take up cholesterol at a rate which is so slow that accurate determination of the uptake becomes almost impossible. Examples of tissues in this slow uptake class would be skeletal and cardiac muscle which take up cholesterol at a slow but measurable rate, whereas the central nervous system and peripheral nerve which contain considerable

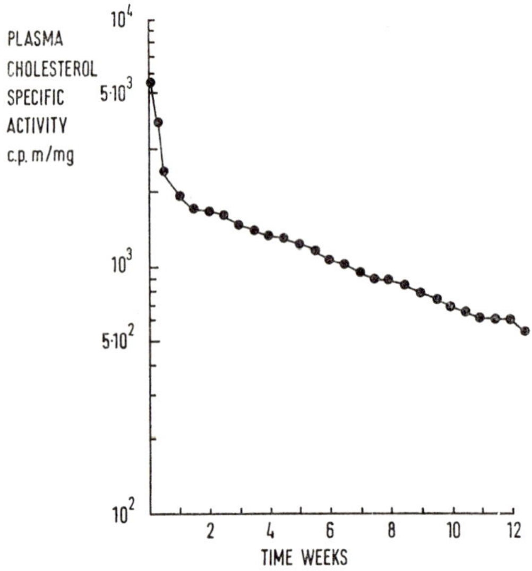


Fig. 4. A typical example of a radioactive plasma cholesterol decay curve. The subject was injected with [4-$^{14}$C]-cholesterol, intravenously at time 0. Thereafter, the specific activity of the plasma cholesterol was determined at various intervals from 0–100 days. It may be noted that over a substantial portion of the experiment the rate of decay of the radioactive cholesterol is linear on this semi-logarithmic plot. It is assumed by certain workers that if the specific activity of the plasma cholesterol is sampled at a specific period during this linear phase of the decay curve then the value obtained for the specific activity of the plasma cholesterol will be identical to the specific activity of the cholesterol secreted into the gut at that time. These workers then use this information in order to estimate the amount of cholesterol secreted into the gut of known specific activity. This establishes a value for the endogenous secretion of sterols.

amounts of cholesterol appear to take this sterol from the plasma compartment at a rate which is almost immeasurable. For practical purposes many workers consider that the uptake of cholesterol by the central nervous system should be considered to be zero. The distribution of cholesterol between the various organs in man is shown in Table 3 from which it can be seen that some tissues have a much larger cholesterol content than others. It is interesting to note that the rate of cholesterol turnover by any specific tissue is not related to the cholesterol content of that tissue.

Various 2- and 3-pool models of cholesterol metabolism have been devised (Goodman and Noble, 1968; Wilson, 1970). In the 3-pool model, one considers that the body consists of various tissues, which, from the standpoint of cholesterol metabolism, can be grouped into three distinct entities (Wilson, 1970). There are tissues which are classified as having cholesterol non-exchangeable with the plasma pool

Table 3
Cholesterol content of various mammalian tissues

| | | mg/100 g wet weight of tissue | Organ cholesterol as a percentage of the total body cholesterol |
|---|---|---|---|
| Liver | | 300–400 | 4·0 |
| Kidney | | 200–300 | 0·4 |
| Lung | | 100–200 | 0·8 |
| Spleen | | 200–300 | 0·3 |
| Muscle | Cardiac | 100–200 | 0·4 |
| | Skeletal | 80–150 | 23·0 |
| Brain | White matter | 4000 | 26·0 |
| | Grey matter | 1000 | |
| Adipose tissue | | 100–200 | 12·0 |
| Skin | | 200–400 | 10·0 |
| Adrenal cortex | | 7000–9000 | 1·0 |
| Blood plasma | | 200–300 | 5·0 |
| Connective tissue | | 100–200 | 9·0 |
| Intestine | | 100–200 | 2·0 |

meaning that the cholesterol content of these tissues may not equilibrate with the plasma compartment even over a period of six to twelve months. Secondly, there is the pool of cholesterol associated with tissues such as muscle, kidney and skin, where equilibration with the plasma cholesterol may take from 10–40 days. Thirdly, there is the rapidly exchanging pool of cholesterol within the plasma–erythrocyte–bile and small intestine where intravenous radioactive cholesterol very rapidly attains identical specific activity values (Kurland *et al.*, 1954). This is shown in Fig. 5.

In the usual physiological situation in which the concentration of a metabolite in a particular pool may remain fairly constant it is usually possible to demonstrate by the isotopic technique that the particular metabolite under study in the biological system is being generated and degraded (or excreted) at rates which are identical but opposite in value and thus, the concentration of the metabolite within the pool remains almost constant. This concept of the "turnover" of a metabolite in a homogenous pool has been acceptable for many years. The usual definition of "turnover" refers to that fraction of the total pool of available metabolite which is replaced or renewed per unit time. The rate of disappearance of labelled cholesterol from the pool with respect to time is a function of the concentration of radioactive cholesterol in the pool.

When an attempt is made to determine the turnover of the plasma

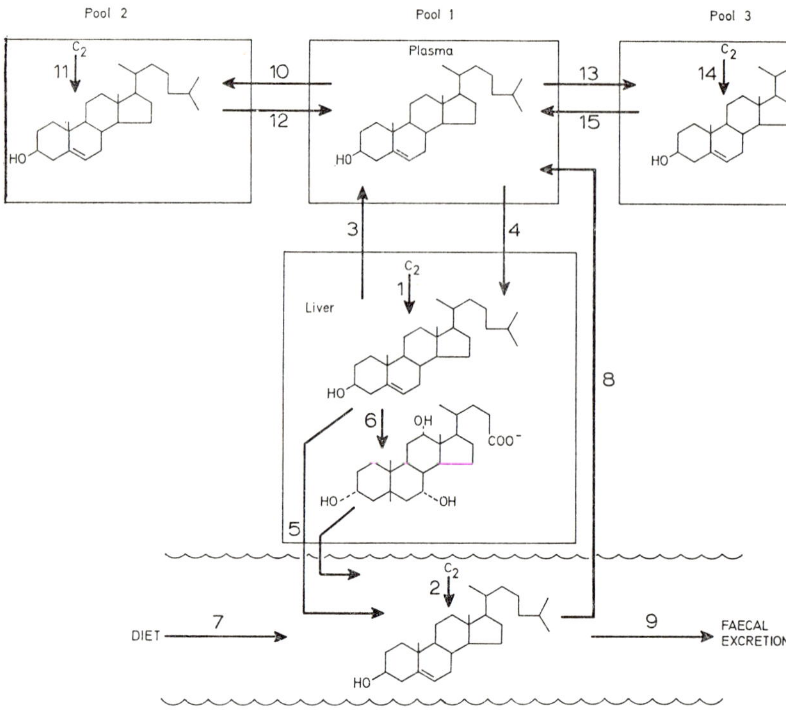


Fig. 5. This is a diagrammatic version of a typical three pool system for the description of cholesterol dynamics in a mammal. Pool 1 contains the plasma, liver, small intestine and the erythrocyte cholesterol. It is assumed that the cholesterol in pool 1 very rapidly equilibrates so that after the administration of cholesterol isotopically labelled into the plasma, most of the cholesterol in the liver, small intestine and erythrocyte will achieve a uniform specific activity. Pool 2 represents the cholesterol in a variety of other tissues such as cardiac and skeletal muscle with which the plasma cholesterol equilibrates more slowly than it equilibrates with liver but nevertheless equilibrates with these tissues to a measurable degree. Pool 3 includes all the tissues which equilibrate with cholesterol very slowly and this pool includes the cholesterol in brain, nerve, etc. A complete description of the dynamics of cholesterol in this simplified system would require an accurate assessment of the following rate constants. (1) The rate of synthesis of cholesterol from acetate in liver. (2) The rate of synthesis of cholesterol from acetate in the small intestine. (3) The rate of transference of newly synthesized cholesterol from the liver to the plasma compartment. (4) The rate of transference of cholesterol from the plasma compartment into the liver. (5) The rate of transference of cholesterol from the liver into the small intestine via the bile. (6) The rate of conversion of cholesterol into bile acids in the liver. (7) The rate of addition of cholesterol from the diet into the rapidly exchanging pool. (8) The rate of absorption of cholesterol from the small intestine into the plasma via the lymph. (9) The rate of faecal excretion of cholesterol from the rapidly exchanging pool. (10) The rate of transference of cholesterol from the plasma compartment into the tissues grouped together as pool 2. (11) The rate of synthesis of cholesterol from acetate in pool 2. (12) The rate of transference of cholesterol from the tissues grouped together as pool 2 into the plasma compartment. (13) The rate of transference of cholesterol from the plasma compartment into the very slowly exchanging pool 3. (14) The rate of synthesis of cholesterol from acetate in the very slowly turning-over pool 3. (15) The rate of transference of cholesterol from the very slowly turning-over pool 3 into the plasma compartment.

cholesterol in man using the radioactive method, this may be performed by the intravenous administration of, for example [$^{14}$C]-cholesterol to a subject at zero time followed by the subsequent removal of samples of plasma at intervals thereafter for the determination of the specific activity of the plasma cholesterol. The result which is obtained is usually similar to that shown in Fig. 4. Thus there is a rapid decline in specific activity for the first few hours continuing into the first few days and thereafter the specific activity of the "plasma cholesterol–liver cholesterol–biliary cholesterol–intestinal cholesterol" proceeds to decline at a fairly uniform rate. If the logarithm of the specific activity of the plasma cholesterol is plotted against time, a linear decline in the specific activity of the plasma cholesterol is obtained over the second phase of the experiment (Kurland *et al.*, 1954). This implies therefore that if the concentration of cholesterol in plasma is constant and if the concentration of cholesterol in the liver, bile and small intestine are also held constant then cholesterol must be leaving the plasma at a constant rate. This rate can be determined from these specific activity measurements in association with a knowledge of the concentration of cholesterol in the pool.

Thus, in order to perform a meaningful experiment on the turnover of the plasma cholesterol in man, it would be necessary to ensure that the dietary intake of cholesterol remained at a constant value because the dietary cholesterol, as discussed previously in this chapter, mixes with the biliary and intestinal cholesterol and forms the basis of the cholesterol load to which the organism is subjected and from which the organism absorbs a proportion. The absorbed cholesterol is then, as discussed previously, transported via the lymph and delivered into the plasma compartment from whence it is taken up by the liver. It is therefore necessary to establish a cholesterol steady-state in a subject by ensuring a constant dietary intake of cholesterol and by maintaining the diet isocaloric to the subject's requirements during such an experiment. This isocaloric control is required because the rate of cholesterol synthesis in tissues exhibits a diurnal variation and is affected by periods of fasting and feeding. Consequently by controlling the cholesterol content and adjusting the calorie intake to the subject's needs it may be possible to hold the plasma cholesterol concentration fairly constant and so arrive at an accurate figure for the rate of turnover of the plasma cholesterol.

This ideal situation is very difficult to achieve in practice. Some investigators have used the technique of feeding a fixed amount of cholesterol labelled with an isotope such as tritium, at a constant specific activity to the experimental subject or the experimental animal in a diet of constant cholesterol composition. The organism absorbs this labelled dietary cholesterol and after a time the specific activity of the rapidly turning-over cholesterol compartment (containing the plasma) and the specific activity of the more slowly turning-over cholesterol compartments achieve isotopic equilibrium. It is then possible to calculate the ratio of the specific activity of the dietary cholesterol to the specific activity of the plasma cholesterol. If all the plasma cholesterol were derived from the dietary cholesterol the ratio of the specific activity of the plasma cholesterol to the specific activity of the dietary cholesterol would be 1:0. Conversely if none of the plasma cholesterol were derived from the dietary cholesterol this ratio would be zero. This ratio of specific activity of the plasma cholesterol to the specific activity of the dietary cholesterol gives an index of the rate of *de novo* synthesis of the plasma cholesterol. When this steady-state has been achieved it is then possible to administer intravenously to the animal, cholesterol labelled with a different isotope, for instance, [$^{14}$C]-cholesterol. The administered [$^{14}$C]-cholesterol mixes with the cholesterol in the rapidly exchanging pool and by analysis of the change in specific activity of the [$^{14}$C]-cholesterol compared to the specific activity of the tritiated cholesterol it is possible to obtain a more accurate evaluation of the rate of turnover of cholesterol within the plasma pool. This refinement allows corrections to be made for changes in the plasma cholesterol pool size or changes in the rate of cholesterol synthesis which may arise during biological experiments whose duration may be many weeks. In addition, it allows studies to be made of the possible mechanisms by which certain procedures, such as dietary changes, affect cholesterol metabolism (Wilson, 1970).

## IV. METHODS FOR THE INVESTIGATION OF CHOLESTEROL ABSORPTION

The application of the isotopic balance technique coupled to chromatographic methods for separation, isolation and quantitation of faecal neutral sterols and bile acids has proved to be a powerful tool for the accurate assessment of cholesterol absorption. A large number of studies have been made within recent years in many laboratories to devise techniques for the accurate measurement of cholesterol absorption under various experimental conditions. It is hardly surprising that these different studies have given rise to widely differing results and when one considers that many of the studies have been conducted in man with his inherent variability, coupled to the limitations of experimentation in man, it will be obvious why many workers have devoted much time and effort to the production of a possible simplified technique for accurate evaluation of cholesterol absorption in man.

The fundamental premise on which all studies on cholesterol absorption are dependent is that exogenous cholesterol absorbed equals exogenous cholesterol (dietary cholesterol) minus unabsorbed exogenous cholesterol. As discussed elsewhere in this paper the dietary cholesterol or exogenous cholesterol is mixed with a large pool of endogenously secreted cholesterol which reaches the gut via the bile from the plasma–liver pool. This means that if a radioactive tracer dose of cholesterol is administered orally to the subject and faecal analyses are performed on neutral sterols and bile acids, then after a few days the isotopic label will appear in the sterol and acids in the faeces. The isotopically-labelled dietary cholesterol will have been absorbed in part, mixed with the plasma–liver–bile–intestinal cholesterol pool, some of the cholesterol will have been degraded to bile acids and excreted in the bile as bile salts and some of the cholesterol will be re-excreted in the bile as unchanged cholesterol and this entero-hepatic circulation will occur repeatedly.

This method is possibly one of the simplest to conduct because all that is required is that radioactive cholesterol be administered to the subject and the absorption of this dietary cholesterol is calculated as the percentage of the dose which is not recovered in the faeces. This simple approach appears to be extremely effective in practice but suffers from the complication that within the large intestine there is a wide spectrum of micro-organisms some of which appear to have the ability to degrade the sterol nucleus. When one considers the bacterial spectrum of the large intestine and the almost infinite capacity of microbial systems to adapt to their environment it is not surprising that some members of the microbial population have acquired the ability to exploit part of the potential energy locked up within the steroid nucleus. While the specific organisms which are capable of scission of the sterol skeleton have not been isolated and characterized there is experimental work to support their existence. As discussed elsewhere in this chapter, sterols with a "cholesterol-type" nucleus but with additional substituents at $C_{24}$ such as $\beta$-sitosterol are much less readily absorbed than is cholesterol. These plant sterols are also "lost" during transit through the gastro-intestinal tract and it is then assumed that since sitosterol is poorly absorbed and since the amount of sitosterol ingested per day can be measured and the amount of sitosterol or sitosterol reduction products in the faeces can also be measured then the percentage sitosterol degraded by the intestinal flora can be used as an approximate index of the amount of cholesterol degraded by the same flora. Thus, in this method, the percentage of the dose of radioactive cholesterol not recovered in the faeces is corrected for the calculated amount of cholesterol which had undergone bacterial degradation and this gives an approximation to the amount of the radioactive cholesterol which has been absorbed. In this technique the absorption of cholesterol is determined after the administration of a single oral dose of radioactive cholesterol. The absorption is calculated as the percentage of the oral dose which is not recovered in the faeces.

Percentage of the dietary cholesterol absorbed =

$$= \frac{(\text{Radioactive cholesterol admin.} - \text{Radioactive faecal cholesterol})}{\text{Radioactive cholesterol admin.}} \times 100$$

$$= \left(1 - \frac{\text{Radioactive faecal cholesterol}}{\text{Radioactive cholesterol admin.}}\right) \times 100$$

In this method it is usually a requirement to correct for the cholesterol "destroyed" in the intestinal tract—by micro-organisms. This is sometimes performed by the use of a radioactive tracer dose of sitosterol—a sterol which is poorly absorbed compared to cholesterol but which may be degraded by microbial systems at a rate comparable to the rate of destruction of cholesterol. Thus by a knowledge of the radioactivity of the dietary sitosterol and the radioactivity in the faecal sitosterol it is possible to correct the cholesterol absorption data for this microbial cholesterol degradative loss.

Percentage cholesterol absorption =

$$= \left[\left(1 - \frac{\text{Faecal cholesterol}}{\text{Admin. cholesterol}}\right) \times 100\right] - \left[\left(1 - \frac{\text{Faecal sitosterol}}{\text{Admin. sitosterol}}\right) \times 100\right]$$

This method only requires the administration of about 1 $\mu$Ci of radioactively-labelled cholesterol to be given on one occasion.

In this instance, it is possible to measure accurately the amount of cholesterol in the diet and the radioactivity administered. It is possible to measure accurately the faecal excretion of sterol over a finite period, say eight days, and also determine the radioactivity of the faecal sterols. As discussed previously, it is possible from the percentage of plant sterols degraded to estimate the cholesterol degraded by bacteria in the individual under study. This leaves unresolved the two components, cholesterol absorbed, plus cholesterol secreted into the gut.

Using this basic approach it is possible to produce other methods which enable these basic premises to be extended to give, for example, an estimate of the endogenous sterol secreted by a subject. Since the plasma–liver–biliary–intestinal cholesterol rapidly achieves isotopic equilibrium then any neutral sterol secreted into the gut via the bile will have a specific activity identical to the specific activity of the plasma cholesterol at that instant. It is for this reason that many investigators interested in the absorption of cholesterol make use of the intravenous administration of radioactive cholesterol and study the specific activity of the plasma cholesterol of the subject with respect to time in order to obtain an accurate assessment of the specific activity of neutral sterols secreted into the gut at any finite time throughout their experiment.

In this case, the dietary cholesterol intake and the total faecal neutral sterols can be directly determined. The endogenous neutral sterol contribution to the cholesterol load in the intestine can be determined by introducing a radioactive label into the plasma compartment —in man this would need about 50 $\mu$Ci [$^{14}$C]-cholesterol. Some time later when the rate of decline of the specific activity of the plasma cholesterol becomes constant, the specific activity of the plasma cholesterol at a specific instant is identical to the specific activity of the neutral sterols secreted into the small intestine. By making certain assumptions about the faecal flow rate and by measuring the specific activity of the faecal neutral sterols, knowing that the labelled sterols had all originated from the plasma cholesterol pool of known specific activity, it is possible to calculate how much of the total faecal neutral sterols has arisen from the endogenous sterol secretion. Hence it is possible to calculate the dietary cholesterol absorbed.

$$\underset{\text{mg/day}}{\begin{bmatrix}\text{Dietary}\\ \text{cholesterol}\\ \text{absorbed}\end{bmatrix}} = \underset{\text{mg/day}}{\begin{bmatrix}\text{Dietary}\\ \text{cholesterol}\\ \text{intake}\end{bmatrix}} + \underset{\text{mg/day}}{\begin{bmatrix}\text{Endogenous}\\ \text{neutral}\\ \text{sterols}\end{bmatrix}} - \underset{\text{mg/day}}{\begin{bmatrix}\text{Total}\\ \text{faecal neutral}\\ \text{sterols}\end{bmatrix}}$$

The only assumptions which need be made in this instance are that the faecal sterols which are excreted and derived from the endogenous cholesterol pool were derived from this pool about 48 hours previously in that this is the time delay between equilibration of the plasma–liver–bile–intestinal cholesterol compared to the time of excretion of the faecal sterols.

Another variant on the methods for studying the absorption of cholesterol is as follows. The subject is continuously dosed with radioactively-labelled cholesterol. Thus the specific activity of the dietary cholesterol is known and this will give the specific activity of the unabsorbed dietary cholesterol. The plasma cholesterol will become labelled and hence the specific activity of the endogenous neutral sterols will be identical to the specific activity of the plasma cholesterol at the same instant. The specific activity of the faecal neutral sterols can be determined directly. This method again requires that about 50 $\mu$Ci [$^{14}$C]-cholesterol be administered to the subject to achieve an adequate labelling of the main cholesterol pool. The unabsorbed dietary cholesterol can be calculated as follows

$$\underset{\text{mg/day}}{\begin{bmatrix}\text{Total faecal}\\ \text{neutral sterols}\end{bmatrix}} = \underset{\text{mg/day}}{\begin{bmatrix}\text{Endogenous}\\ \text{neutral sterols}\end{bmatrix}} + \underset{\text{mg/day}}{\begin{bmatrix}\text{Unabsorbed}\\ \text{dietary sterols}\end{bmatrix}}$$

One other method which has been used calculates the cholesterol absorbed from turnover data. In this approach the subject receives a constant oral dose of radioactive cholesterol. When the subject is in an isotopic steady state, the daily cholesterol turnover can be determined from the specific activity of the plasma cholesterol–time curves while the fraction of the plasma cholesterol derived from the absorbed cholesterol is computed from the specific activity of the plasma cholesterol divided by the specific activity of the dietary cholesterol. This method requires the administration of about 200 $\mu$Ci of radioactive cholesterol.

$$\underset{\text{mg/day}}{\begin{bmatrix}\text{Dietary cholesterol}\\ \text{absorbed}\end{bmatrix}} = \underset{\text{mg/day}}{\begin{bmatrix}\text{Daily cholesterol}\\ \text{turnover}\end{bmatrix}} \times \begin{bmatrix}\text{Fraction of the}\\ \text{plasma cholesterol}\\ \text{derived from the}\\ \text{absorbed}\\ \text{cholesterol}\end{bmatrix}$$

The absorption of cholesterol from the small intestine presents the organism with certain complex problems because this molecule is very sparingly soluble in electrolyte solutions. The recent developments in our understanding of the production and structure of micelles have greatly aided our concepts on the mechanism of cholesterol absorption. The investigation of the optimum environment and supply of materials for effective synthesis of cholesterol micelles has emphasized that cholesterol absorption requires an adequate supply of bile salts to activate the lipases and cholesterol esterases, enzymes which are essential for cholesterol uptake by mucosal cells. The pH of the gut must be maintained within fairly narrow limits for effective action of these enzymes and the cholesterol ester hydrolase which operates in the small intestine apparently originates in the pancreas. Thus, cholesterol absorption demands normal pancreatic function with respect to the external secretions of this organ.

There is still a great deal to learn regarding the precise mechanism by which the micelles are taken up by the mucosal cells. The subsequent events occurring in the intestinal cells will certainly merit further biochemical investigations. The reactions by which cholesterol in the mucosal cells is esterified, associated with phospholipids and triglycerides before being assembled into macro-molecular chylomicron-like structures prior to extrusion into the lymph will certainly be a challenging area for future developments. The subtle regulatory function of the small intestine with respect to cholesterol dynamics cannot be overstated. This organ plays an important role in the wider aspects of cholesterol metabolism by directly affecting cholesterologenesis in the liver, while the liver interacts directly with the small intestine by acting as the sole organ involved in the breakdown of cholesterol to bile salts. These surface active bile salts in turn are delivered into the small intestine to play a key role in the cholesterol absorption process.

There are obviously marked species differences in the ability of mammals to absorb cholesterol. In restricting our considerations to cholesterol absorption in man one of the major problems to which we have to address ourselves is "what is the nature of the controlling factor which appears to operate at the gut to control the intake of cholesterol?" It seems likely from a large number of studies that there are in fact marked differences in cholesterol absorption in man. Thus, within a heterogeneous population there appear to be those individuals who are capable of absorbing a much greater fraction of the normal dietary cholesterol load and this raises the problem of what happens to the additional cholesterol absorbed. Until we have some quantitative data on the feed-back control of hepatic cholesterologenesis it will be impossible to predict whether those individuals who are efficient cholesterol absorbers do in fact also have an efficient feed-back control on cholesterol biosynthesis. If the feed-back of dietary cholesterol on cholesterologenesis is sluggish or ineffective then in certain individuals the dietary cholesterol intake may markedly affect the tissue and plasma cholesterol concentrations.

As a result of extensive experimental work it is now adequately established that the cholesterol absorption process is markedly affected by the presence of other lipids in the diet particularly the amount and type of triglyceride in the diet. Consequently, in assessing the amount of cholesterol absorbed by an individual it is essential to consider the quantitative and qualitative aspects of the other lipid components in the diet.

In this paper considerable attention has been devoted to comparing and contrasting the various methods which experimental workers have used in attempts to accurately assess cholesterol absorption in man. A considerable range of experimental approaches have been devised and some of the snags associated with attempting to determine cholesterol absorption have been outlined in this chapter. It is tempting to establish cholesterol absorption in subjects under metabolic ward conditions and with the use of a liquid-formula diet. Under these circumstances it is possible to control the other lipids in the diet and to control accurately the protein, carbohydrate and caloric content of the intake with a very high degree of precision. While these results produce informative data obtained under these metabolic ward conditions in subjects consuming this liquid-formula diet, this situation is quite different from that which prevails in the normal population eating a mixed diet and consequently it is difficult to extrapolate the results obtained under metabolic ward conditions to the normal dietary situation of humans eating a mixed diet. A large number of factors present in the average mixed diet obviously influence the bile salt content of the gut, the water content of the gut, the efficiency of the cholesterol ester hydrolase, the efficiency of lipases and other factors which may be of considerable significance in the generation of the cholesterol micelles required in the absorption of cholesterol. Thus, the so called roughage in the diet influences cholesterol and bile salt metabolism to a significant degree.

In many procedures for the determination of cholesterol absorption it is necessary to assess the magnitude of the cholesterol "lost" in the large intestine as a result of microbial transformation of the sterol molecule into nonsterol, as yet non-detectable metabolites. It is obvious that a fruitful line of investigation associated with cholesterol absorption will be the assessment of the qualitative and quantitative aspects of the intestinal flora in different individuals. In many of the studies reported so far it is obvious that there are wide discrepancies between the amount of cholesterol which is presumably being degraded by the intestinal flora in different individuals. Thus, the microbial population may be degrading from 10–500 mg of cholesterol/day and this is a sizeable proportion of the total cholesterol load.

The accurate assessment of cholesterol absorption in man presents the clinical investigator with a challenging problem. With the development of many new techniques and with the assessment of these different methods in a large number of centres it may be possible to arrive at a precise evaluation of cholesterol absorption in man in the not too distant future.

## V. SUMMARY

The absorption of cholesterol from the small intestine presents the organism with certain complex problems because this molecule is very sparingly soluble in electrolyte solutions. Recent developments in our understanding of the production and structure of micelles has greatly aided studies on cholesterol absorption. The investigation of the optimum environment and supply of materials for effective synthesis of cholesterol micelles has emphasized that cholesterol absorption requires an adequate supply of bile salts to activate the lipases and cholesterol esterases which are essential for cholesterol uptake by mucosal cells. The pH of the gut must be maintained within fairly narrow limits for effective action of these enzymes and the cholesterol ester hydrolase which operates in the small intestine apparently originates in the pancreas. Thus cholesterol absorption demands normal pancreatic exocrine function.

There is still a great deal to learn regarding the precise mechanism by which micelles are taken up by the mucosal cells and the subsequent events occurring in the intestinal cells will no doubt merit further biochemical investigations. The mechanism by which cholesterol in the mucosal cells is esterified, and then associated with phospholipids, and triglycerides before being assembled into macromolecular chylomicron-like structures prior to extrusion into the lymph will certainly be a challenging area for future developments. The regulatory function of the small intestine with respect to the cholesterol dynamics of the whole organism cannot be overstated. This organ plays an important role in cholesterol metabolism by affecting cholesterologenesis in the liver, while the liver in turn interacts directly with the small intestine by acting as the sole organ involved in the breakdown of cholesterol to bile salts. These detergent-like molecules are delivered into the small intestine to play a key role in the cholesterol absorptive processes.

The complex array of micro-organisms in the gut adds to the complexity of studies on cholesterol absorption. We have as yet little quantitative data on the amount of cholesterol degraded to non-steroidal structures by microbial attack. The variations in the magnitude of the "lost sterols" shown on cholesterol absorption balance sheets may reflect qualitative or quantitative differences in the bacterial flora of the gut. This may prove to be an important area of investigation in the future.

## REFERENCES


Bergstrom, S. and Danielsson, H. (1958). On the regulation of bile acid formation in the rat liver. *Acta Physiol. Scand.* **43,** 1–7.

Bloch, K. (1965). The biological synthesis of cholesterol. *Science* **150,** 19–28.

Bloomfield, D. K. (1963). Dynamics of cholesterol metabolism. *Proc. Natn Acad. Sci.* 117–124.

Borgstrom, B. (1960). Studies in intestinal cholesterol absorption in the human. *J. Clin. Invest.* **39,** 809–815.

Borgstrom, B., Lindhe, B. A. and Wlodawer, P. (1958). Absorption and distribution of cholesterol-4-$C^{14}$ in the rat. *Proc. Soc. Exptl Biol. Med.* **99,** 365–368.

Boyd, G. S., Mitton, J. R., Simpson, E. R. and Sulimovici, S.I. (1967). The hydroxylation of cholesterol by various mammalian tissues. Proc. 7th Int. Congress Biochemistry Tokyo V-2.

Bucher, N. L. R., Overath, P. and Lynen, F. (1960). $\beta$-Hydroxy-$\beta$-methylglutaryl coenzyme A reductase cleavage and condensing enzymes in relation to cholesterol formation in rat liver. *Biochem. Biophys. Acta* **40,** 491–501.

Chaikoff, I. L., Bloom, B., Siperstein, M. D., Kiyasu, J. Y., Reinhardt, W. O., Dauben, W. G. and Eastham, J. F. (1952). Lymphatic transport of absorbed cholesterol-4-$C^{14}$. *J. biol. Chem.* **194,** 407–412.

Chevallier, F. (1953). Le cholesterol: données chimiques et apport des méthodes isotopiques dans la connaissance de son metabolisme. *Ann. Nutrit. alimentation* **7,** 305–338.

Connor, W. E., Hodges, R. E. and Bleiler, R. E. (1961). The serum lipids in men receiving high cholesterol and cholesterol-free diets. *J. Clin. Invest.* **40,** 894–901.

Cook, R. P. (1958). "Cholesterol: Chemistry, Biochemistry and Pathology." Academic Press, New York.

Cook, R. P., Kliman, A. and Fieser, L. F. (1954). The absorption and metabolism of cholesterol and its main companions in the rabbit—with observations on the atherogenic nature of the sterols. *Arch. Biochem. Biophys.* **52,** 439–450.

Danielsson, H., Einarsson, K. and Johansson, G. (1967). Effect of biliary drainage on individual reactions in the conversion of cholesterol to taurocholic acid. *Eur. J. Biochem.* **2,** 44–49.

Davis, C. B., Cox, G. E., Taylor, C. B. and Cross, S. L. (1959). Cholesterol synthesis in human liver. *Surg. Forum* **9,** 486–489.

Deuel, H. J. Jr. (1951). "The Lipids", Vol. 1–3. Interscience, New York.

Eastwood, M. A. (1973). Dietary fibre and gastroenterology. *Digestion* **8,** 368–371.

Eastwood, M. A. and Hamilton, D. (1968). Studies on the adsorption of bile salts to non-absorbed components of diet. *Biochem. Biophys. Acta* **152,** 165–173.

Eriksson, S. (1957). Bilary excretion of bile acids and cholesterol in bile fistula rats, bile acids and steroids. *Proc. soc. Exptl Biol. Med.* **94,** 578–582.

Glover, J. and Morton, R. A. (1958). The absorption and metabolism of sterols. *Brit. Med. Bull.* **14,** 226–233.

Goodman, D. S. and Noble, R. P. (1968). Turnover of plasma cholesterol in man. *J. Clin. Invest* **47,** 231–241.

Gould, R. G., Taylor, C. B., Hagerman, J. S., Warner, I. and Campbell, D. J. (1953). Effect of dietary cholesterol on the synthesis of cholesterol in dog tissue *in vitro. J. biol. Chem.* **201,** 519–528.

Gould, R. G. and others (1955). Absorbability of $\beta$-sitosterol. *Trans. N.Y. Acad. Sci.* **18,** 129–134.

Gould, R. G., Lotz, L. V. and Lilly, E. M. (1956). Absorption and metabolism of dihydrocholesterol and $\beta$-sitosterol. *In* "Biochemical Problems of Lipids". (Popjak and Le Breton, eds), pp. 353–358. Butterworth, London.

Hernandez, H. H. and Chaikoff, I. L. (1957). Purification and properties of pancreatic cholesterol esterase. *J. biol. Chem.* **228,** 447–457.

Kaplan, J. A., Cox, G. E. and Taylor, C. B. (1963). Cholesterol metabolism in man. *Arch. Path.* **76,** 359–368.

Keigs, A. (1953). *J. Mount Sinai Hosp.* **20,** 118.

Kurland, G. S., Lucas, J. L., Freedberg, A. S. (1954). The metabolism of intravenously infused $C^{14}$-labelled cholesterol in man. *J. Clin. Invest.* **33,** 950.

McIntyre, N. (1971). Sterol absorption—from lumen to liver. *Gut* **12,** 411–416.

Mueller, J. H. (1916). The mechanism of cholesterol absorption. *J. biol. Chem.* **27,** 463–480.

Murthy, S. K., Mahadevan, S. and Ganguly, J. (1961). High cholesterol diet and esterification of cholesterol by the intestinal mucosa of rats. *Arch. Biochem. Biophys.* **95,** 176–180.

Myant, N. B. and Eder, H. A. (1961). The effect of biliary drainage upon the synthesis of cholesterol in the liver. *J. Lipid Res.* **2,** 363–368.

Okey, R. (1945). *J. Am. Dietet. Ass.* **21,** 341–344.

Peterson, D. W., Shneour, E. A. and Peek, N. F. (1954). Effects of dietary sterols and sterol esters on plasma and liver cholesterol in the chick. *J. Nutr.* **53,** 451–459.

Pihl, A. (1952). The cholesterol content of food. *Scand. J. Clin. Lab. Invest.* **4,** 115–121.

Pihl, A. (1955). The effect of dietary fat on the intestinal cholesterol absorption and on the cholesterol metabolism in the liver of rats. *Acta Physiol. Scand.* **34,** 183–196.

Quintao, E., Grundy, S. M. and Ahrens, E. H. (1971). Effects of dietary cholesterol on the regulation of total body cholesterol in man. *J. Lipid Res.* **12,** 233–247.

Redgrave, T. G. (1970). Formation of cholesteryl ester-rich particulate lipid during metabolism of chylomicrons. *J. Clin. Invest.* **49,** 465–471.

Robinson, D. S. (1964). The physiological significance of the plasma triglycerides in fat transport. *In* "Metabolism and Physiological Significance of Lipids" (R. M. C. Dawson and D. N. Rhodes, eds), pp. 275–288. John Wiley, New York.

Sinmonds, W. J., Hoffmann, A. F. and Theodor, E. (1967). Absorption of cholesterol from a micellar solution: intestinal perfusion studies in man. *J. Clin. Invest.* **46,** 874–890.

Siperstein, M. D., Chaikoff, I. L. and Reinhardt, W. O. (1952). Obligatory function of bile in intestinal absorption of cholesterol. *J. biol. Chem.* **198,** 111–114.

Swell, L., Field, H. and Treadwell, C. R. (1953). Role of bile salts in activity of cholesterol esterase. *Proc. Soc. Exptl Biol. Med.* **84,** 417–420.

Swell, L., Flick, D. F., Field, H. Jr. and Treadwell, C. R. (1955). Role of fat and fatty acid in absorption of dietary cholesterol. *Am. J. Physiol.* **180,** 124–128.

Sylven, C. and Borgstrom, B. (1969a). Absorption and lymphatic transport of cholesterol and sitosterol in the rat. *J. Lipid Res.* **10,** 179–182.

Sylven, C. and Borgstrom, B.,(1969b). Intestinal absorption and lymphatic transport of cholesterol in the rat: influence of the fatty acid chain length of the carrier triglyceride. *J. Lipid. Res.* **10,** 351–355.

Taylor, C. B. and Ho, K-J. (1967). A review of human cholesterol metabolism. *Arch. Path.* **84,** 3–14.

Treadwell, C. R. and Vahouny, G. V. (1968). Cholesterol absorption. *In* "Handbook of Physiology"—Section 6, Vol. 3. Chapter 72, pp. 1407–1438. American Physiological Society, Washington, D.C.

Tomkins, G. M., Sheppard, H. and Chaikoff, I. L. (1953). Cholesterol synthesis by liver: its regulation by ingested cholesterol. *J. Biol. Chem.* **201,** 137–141.

Vahouny, G. V. and Treadwell, C. R. (1957). Changes in lipid composition of lymph during cholesterol absorption in rat. *Am. J. Physiol.* **191,** 179–184.

Vahouny, G. V. and Treadwell, C. R. (1964). Absolute requirement for free sterol for absorption by rat intestinal mucosa. *Proc. Soc. Exptl Biol. Med.* **116,** 496–498.

Vahouny, G. V., Weersing, S. and Treadwell, C. R. (1965). Function of specific bile acids in cholesterol esterase activity *in vitro. Biochim. Biophys. Acta* **98,** 607–616.

Watt, S. M. and Simmonds, W. J. (1971). Uptake and efflux by everted intestinal sacs of micellar cholesterol in bile salts and in non-ionic detergents. *Biochim Biophys. Acta* **225,** 347–355.

Wilson, J. D. (1970). The measurement of the exchangeable pools of cholesterol in the baboon. *J. Clin. Invest.* **49,** 655–665.

Wilson, J. D. and Dietschy, J. M. (1966). The biosynthetic origin of serum cholesterol in the monkey. *J. Clin. Invest.* **45,** 1086.

Wilson, J. D. and Reinke, R. T. (1968). Transfer of locally synthesised cholesterol from intestinal wall to intestinal lymph. *J. Lipid Res.* **9,** 85–92.

# 9 Linoleic Acid Intake and Vitamin E Requirement

F. C. JAGER

*Unilever Research, Vlaardingen, The Netherlands*



## I. INTRODUCTION

Edible fats contain small amounts of non-glyceride components, one of which is vitamin E. This vitamin occurs mainly in fats of vegetable origin; the richest source is wheatgerm oil. Animal fats, in general, have a low vitamin E content.

Vitamin E was discovered by Evans and Bishop (1922), when they concluded that the resorption gestation occurring in their feeding experiments with rats was due to a deficiency of a fat-soluble factor in the food. Since this discovery was related to reproduction, vitamin E was long regarded as a special "fertility vitamin". However, rats later proved to be an exceptional case: most animals would have died from myopathy, anaemia or encephalomalacia, long before reproduction could have occurred. The resorption gestation occurs because the embryo dies after 12–14 days due to affection of the vascular tissue. Although the females remain fertile, male rats may become sterile after prolonged feeding on a diet deficient in vitamin E, because of testis degeneration. A review of the early history of vitamin E research has been given by Evans (1962).

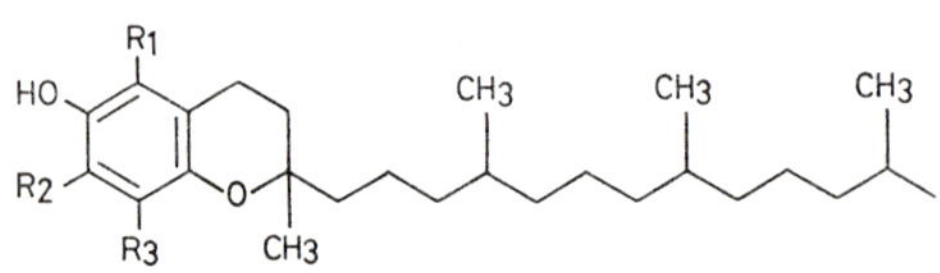


| R1 | R2 | R3 | tocopherol | Biopotency I.U./mg |
|---|---|---|---|---|
| $CH_3$ | $CH_3$ | $CH_3$ | α | 1.5 |
| $CH_3$ | H | $CH_3$ | β | 0.4 |
| H | $CH_3$ | $CH_3$ | γ | 0.2 |
| H | H | $CH_3$ | δ | 0.02 |

Fig. 1. Structure and biopotency of naturally occurring tocopherols. One mg DL-α-tocopherol acetate has a biopotency of 1 international unit (I.U.) by definition. The biopotencies mentioned are those of the natural D-forms.

The name vitamin E refers to a group of tocopherols (Fig. 1), which differ in structure, biopotency and antioxidant capacity. The latter is supposed to be the natural function of vitamin E in oils, especially in relation to polyunsaturated fatty acids (PUFA). Vitamin E most commonly occurs as D-α- or as D-γ-tocopherol. The other tocopherols occur so rarely, or have such low biopotencies, that they are not of practical value. Synthetic vitamin E is usually D-α- or DL-α-tocopheryl acetate. The biopotencies of the acetate esters are about 9% less than those of the corresponding free tocopherols (Brubacher and Weiser, 1967).

The vitamin E requirement may be influenced by different dietary factors, the effect being dependent on the species studied and the tissue affected. Such factors are: synthetic antioxidants (encephalomalacia, embryonic degeneration, *in vitro* haemolysis), selenium (exudative diathesis, liver necrosis, myopathy), the amino acids, cystine and menthionine (myopathy) and polyunsaturated fatty acids (encephalomalacia, *in vitro* haemolysis, myopathy) (see also Scott, 1970). Most factors have a beneficial effect, but polyunsaturated fatty acids may increase the need for vitamin E. The term PUFA comprises both the highly unsaturated hexaenes and pentaenes from fish oils as well as linoleic acid. The PUFA contained in edible fats and margarines relates almost exclusively to linoleic acid.

In recent years there has been a growing interest in the consumption of vegetable oils with a high content of linoleic acid, such as sunflower, safflower or maize oil. Much confusion has existed as to whether or not the vegetable oils rich in linoleic acid naturally contain sufficient vitamin E to balance their PUFA content. Harris (1962) calculated that in natural oils a positive correlation exists between the content of total tocopherols and the content of linoleic acid plus linolenic acid. From data obtained from human studies by Horwit (1960) and from a literature review of animal studies, Harris and Embree (1963) were led to suggest a vitamin E requirement of 0·6 mg D-α-tocopherol/g of linoleic acid ingested. This E/PUFA ratio of 0·6 means that most vegetable oils which are rich in linoleic acid do not contain sufficient vitamin E.

Some experimental work designed to obtain quantitative information on the relation between linoleic acid intake and vitamin E requirement was done by Weber *et al.* (1964) on rats and by Søndergaard and Dam (1966) on chickens. The former found that linoleic acid had a profound effect on the vitamin E requirement, whereas no such effect was noted by the latter.

In view of these and other confusing results, we carried out experiments with rats and ducklings in order to quantify the effect of linoleic acid intake on vitamin E requirement. In this work, vitamin E was not given in single doses, but incorporated into the food, in order to ensure good absorption (Pudelkiewicz and Nakiya, 1969). Care was taken that the diets contained sufficient essential fatty acids (EFA), as much confusion has arisen from the fact that many researchers did not realize they were working with EFA-deficient diets.

## II. DETERMINATION OF VITAMIN E REQUIREMENT

The principle of the determination of vitamin E requirement is simple. Animals are for some time given diets containing increasing amounts of vitamin E. The amount of vitamin E that is found to be just sufficient to prevent deficiency symptoms may be regarded as the actual requirement for this vitamin. The difficulty is to find an animal species that develops a suitable deficiency symptom within a short time and to express the degree of disease quantitatively. Moreover, it is important that no other deficiency symptoms occur at the same time. The *in vitro* haemolysis in rats (Jager, 1968) and the myopathy in ducklings (Jager *et al.*, 1969; Jager and Vles, 1970; Jager and Verbeek-Raad, 1970) were found to fulfil these requirements. In addition to these methods the use of some other deficiency criteria will be discussed.

## A. *In vitro* Haemolysis

Rose and György (1950a) discovered that the erythrocytes of rats kept for some time on diets deficient in vitamin E, haemolysed *in vitro*, after the addition of dialuric acid. Vitamin E is supposed to act as an antioxidant and, therefore, oxidizing agents such as hydrogen peroxide might have the same haemolytic action on red cells (*in vitro*) of vitamin E deficient animals as dialuric acid. This was indeed found to be true (Rose and György, 1952). It was found later (Christensen *et al.*, 1956) that *in vitro* haemolysis of vitamin E deficient erythrocytes may also occur spontaneously. This phenomenon of spontaneous *in vitro* haemolysis was used by Jager (1968) to determine the vitamin E requirement of rats. It proved to offer a better sensitivity and reproducibility than the dialuric acid method (Christensen *et al.*, 1956; Jager, 1968; Draper and Saari Csallany, 1969). Horwitt *et al.* (1956) showed that the hydrogen peroxide haemolysis may give widely varying results, dependent on the way in which the test is carried out.

Some insight into the cause of *in vitro* haemolysis was given by Tsen and Collier (1960), who demonstrated that it is associated with lipid peroxidation and that addition of α-tocopherol to the erythrocyte suspension decreased or completely prevented haemolysis.

Jacob and Lux (1968) studied the mechanism by which hydrogen peroxide causes *in vitro* haemolysis of vitamin E deficient red cells of rats. They demonstrated that the locus of attack by hydrogen peroxide was the red cell membrane, in which especially one phospholipid, i.e. phosphatidyl ethanolamine was destroyed prior to the onset of haemolysis. Phosphatidyl ethanolamine is presumably so vulnerable to oxidative destruction, because it contains the largest proportion of unsaturated fatty acids in red cell membranes (Ways and Hanahan, 1964). An initial sequence of fatty acid destruction in phosphatidyl ethanolamine may lead to membrane disorganization, which results in the observed haemolysis.

The relation between *in vitro* haemolysis and fatty acids in the red cell membrane was clearly demonstrated by Bieri and Poukka (1970). They found in (EFA-deficient) rats a linear relationship between the peroxidizable index—calculated after Holman (1954) and Witting and Horwitt (1964a)—of the erythrocyte polyunsaturated fatty acids and the α-tocopherol content of the red cells required to prevent ten per cent *in vitro* haemolysis by dialuric acid.

The spontaneous haemolysis of washed red cells incubated at 37°C may be attributed to small amounts of hydrogen peroxide generated continuously during aerobic incubation (Jacob and Jandl, 1966). The hydrogen peroxide may be eliminated by glutathione peroxidase (Mills, 1957; Cohen and Hochstein, 1963) and under certain conditions by catalase (Theorell and Ehrenberg, 1952; Nitowski and Tildon, 1956; Gross *et al.*, 1967). The glutathione peroxidase pathway, however, requires the presence of glucose to maintain adequate levels of reduced glutathione (Wittels and Hochstein, 1966), as otherwise the initiated reaction chain of lipid-free radicals may be broken by a lipid-soluble antioxidant as is vitamin E (Witting, 1965). There is no proof so far that dietary selenium has any effect of practical importance upon the results of the *in vitro* haemolysis test (Christensen *et al.*, 1958; Gitler *et al.*, 1958; Krishnamurty and Bieri, 1961), nor is this the case with cystine or methionine or the dietary protein level (Gitler *et al.*, 1958; Scott, 1970; Jager, unpublished results).

Leonard and Losowski (1967) studied the relationship between the plasma vitamin E level and the results of the hydrogen peroxide haemolysis test in human subjects. They found that a negative correlation exists between the plasma tocopherol level and the percentage *in vitro* haemolysis. This found confirmation in the work of Silber *et al.* (1969) and Poukka and Bieri (1970), who showed that the tocopherol content of the erythrocyte membrane depends upon the tocopherol concentration of the blood plasma and that a complete exchange takes place between plasma and red cells within a few hours.

Besides tocopherol, the red cells take up fatty acids from the surrounding medium and incorporate them in the phospholipids of the erythrocyte membrane (Oliveira and Vaughan, 1964; Jacob and Lux, 1968). The fatty acid pattern of the red cell membrane is a reflexion of the fatty acid composition of the blood plasma (Waku and Lands, 1968).

Jacob and Lux (1968) observed that the *in vivo* survival time of $^{59}$Fe-labelled red cells was identical for vitamin E deficient and vitamin E supplemented rats. This initially somewhat unexpected observation means that *in vivo* the destruction of vitamin E deficient red cells is not increased. The destruction is most probably prohibited by a reparative mechanism in the erythrocyte membrane; damaged fatty acids in the phosphoethanolamine are exchanged for intact fatty acids from the plasma. When the $^{51}Cr$-method was used it was found that in the case of vitamin E deficiency the red cells survival time was decreased (Horwitt *et al.*, 1963; Marvin, 1963). Binder and Spiro (1967) showed that this was due to a labelling artefact.

Erythrocytes of vitamin E deficient rats have been found to be no more sensitive to haemolysis by hypotonic solutions than were those of normal controls, when examined by the usual saline osmotic resistance test. At the same time, however, the *in vitro* haemolysis test may be strongly positive (Christensen *et al.*, 1956; Walker and Kummerow, 1964). Porter *et al.* (1962) found that in vitamin E deficient monkeys, despite a severe degree of anaemia, the erythrocytes of the vitamin E deficient animals did not differ significantly from the controls in the osmotic resistance test. Remarkable was the finding that when in two monkeys the red cell osmotic fragility test was repeated, some days after vitamin E administration, an increased fragility could be demonstrated.

### 1. *In Rats*

#### *a. Dose-response effect*

(i) Experimental design. In order to determine the dose-response effect of vitamin E intake on the percentage spontaneous haemolysis *in vitro*, newly weaned male albino Wistar rats (SPF) were kept for 16 months on vitamin E deficient diets (see Table 1) to which increasing doses of

Table 1

Composition (weight%) of vitamin E deficient diets containing 35 cal% fat for rats and ducklings

| Components | Rats | Ducklings |
|---|---|---|
| Casein | 29·3 | 36·0 |
| Sucrose | 48·5 | |
| Maize starch | | 34·6 |
| Fat | 17·8 | 14·4 |
| Salt mixture | 4·0 | 5·8 |
| Cellulose powder | | 8·9 |
| Vitamin mixture[a] | 0·4 | 0·3 |

[a] See Jager and Houtsmuller (1970) and Jager and Vles (1970).

vitamin E (DL-α-tocopheryl acetate) had been added. The diet contained 35 cal % lard. Male rats were chosen as test animals because, according to Ward (1963), they are more susceptible to vitamin E deficiency than the females. The 48 rats were divided into six groups of eight animals in each. The successive groups received 3, 8, 13, 18, 23 and 43 mg DL-α-tocopheryl acetate/kg food, respectively. Food and drinking-water were given *ad libitum*. Regular determinations of the food intake of all animals revealed that the intake of all dietary components, other than vitamin E, was the same for all groups. Determinations of vitamin E requirement in rats by means of an *in vitro* haemolysis test had been done before by Rose and György (1950b), Friedman *et al.* (1958) and Ward (1963). In all these cases, vitamin E was administered in single doses daily or weekly per os. According to Ward (1963), however, under these circumstances the result of the haemolysis test is dependent on the time elapsing between the vitamin E administration and the moment at which the test is carried out. For this reason in the experiment presented here the vitamin E was taken up in the food in graded levels, to ensure an almost constant plasma tocopherol level for each group (Jager, 1968).

(ii) The spontaneous haemolysis test. This test was performed with the following reagents: stock solution (1); buffer, pH 7·4; 136 g $KH_2PO_4$ + 30 g solid NaOH was made up to 1000 ml with distilled water. Stock solution (2): physiological saline: 170 g NaCl, was made up to 1000 ml with distilled water. The test solution was made by: 50 ml solution (1) + 75 ml solution (2), made up to 2000 ml with aq. dest., and saturated with oxygen before use by shaking with air; the pH was adjusted at 7·4, if necessary. 0·1 ml blood was taken from the rats' tails, immediately suspended in 7·5 ml test solution and centrifuged for 10 min at 500 × *g* at 15°C. The supernatant was removed by suction and the red cells were re-suspended in 7·5 ml test solution. After homogenization, 1·0 ml suspension was pipetted into: (A) 4·0 ml test solution (determination 1), (B) 4·0 ml test solution (determination 2), (C) 4·0 ml aq. dest. (total haemolysis). The tubes (A), (B) and (C) were incubated for 4 hr at 38°C, homogenized and centrifuged for 10 min at 500 × *g* at 15°C. The degree of haemolysis in the supernatant was determined colorimetrically at 543 nm, setting the test solution at 100 % transmission. The percentage haemolysis was calculated from: extinction of the determination × 100, divided by the extinction from the total haemolysis test. The animals were not previously fasted, as is usual in a blood test, because it was found that after they had been fasted for 24 hr the degree of haemolysis had decreased (Jager, unpublished results). In some cases, besides the spontaneous method, dialuric acid haemolysis was performed (Moore *et al.*, 1957).

(iii) Results. The relationship between the dietary vitamin E content and the percentage *in vitro* haemolysis is a somewhat sigmoid-shaped curve (Fig. 2).

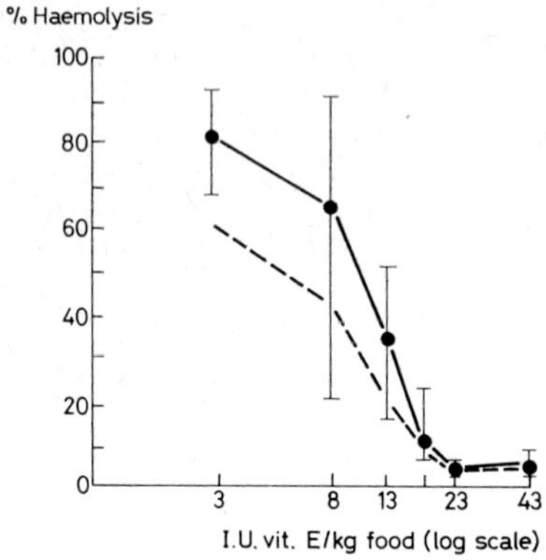


Fig. 2. (Jager, 1968.) Relationship between vitamin E content of food and *in vitro* haemolysis. Drawn line: spontaneous haemolysis. Dotted line: dialuric acid haemolysis.

A linear relationship appeared to exist from 8–18 I.U. (international units) of vitamin E (DL-α-tocopheryl acetate)/kg food. Within one dosing group, considerable differences in percentages of haemolysis could be observed. When the individual percentages of haemolysis within one dosing group were compared over a certain period, there were no clear indications that invariably the same animals had a high or low percentage of haemolysis. There was a certain individual level, but its significance in comparison with the total of the variations within a dosing group was slight. Vitamin E requirement, as determined by spontaneous haemolysis *in vitro*, was somewhat arbitrarily defined as the amount needed to prevent 10% haemolysis. This amount was determined from the steeply-descending part of the dose-response curve, where necessary, by linear extrapolation. In view of the fact that with higher doses of vitamin E 4–6% haemolysis is still observed, the 10% mentioned has to be considered as an initial haemolysis. The percentages of haemolysis by dialuric acid were somewhat less than those found by the spontaneous method, as is indicated in Fig. 2. The spontaneous haemolysis test was found to have a better reproducibility.

The influence of the incubation time is illustrated in Fig. 3. Since the dose–response relationship did not change appreciably after 4 hr, this incubation time was maintained in further experiments.

The value of the spontaneous *in vitro* haemolysis test will be highly dependent on the extent to which vitamin E requirement, as calculated from this test, is found to remain constant throughout the lifetime of the rat. The results of such an investigation are given in Fig. 4. The initially high level can be explained by the fact that during the first 14 days the animals received no vitamin E. Apparently it took some weeks before a steady level was reached after the administration of vitamin E. After the 262nd day, the level again increased and, until the 408th day, all measuring points were higher than those over the entire preceding period.

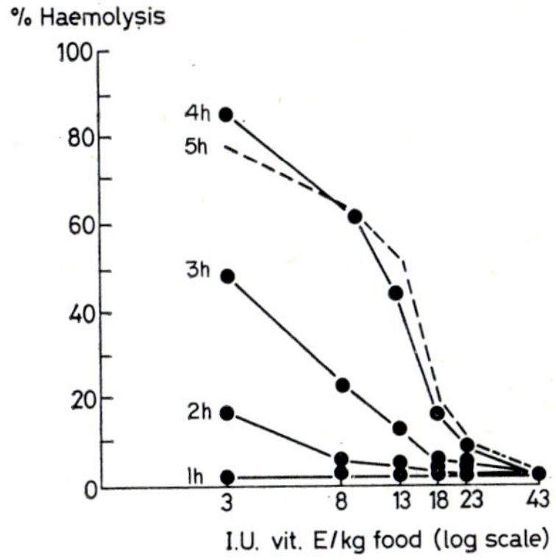


Fig. 3. (Jager, 1968.) Influence of the incubation time (at 38°C) on the dose-response relationship between *in vitro* haemolysis and dietary vitamin E content.

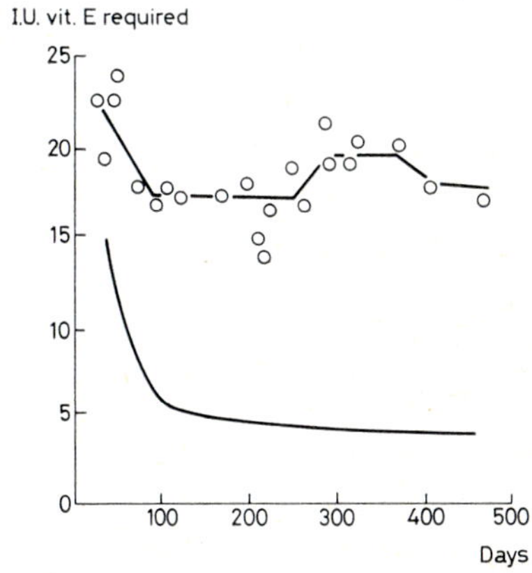


Fig. 4. (Jager, 1968.) Influence of the duration of the experiment on the amount of vitamin E required to prevent 10% haemolysis *in vitro*. Measured points: found amounts (per kg food). Drawn line (×10): calculated amounts per kg body weight per day.

From the 263rd until the 375th day, a different batch of lard was used; however, analysis of this lard with respect to fatty acid composition and tocopherol content gave no indication whatsoever to explain this increase. Nevertheless it can be stated that over a period of 15 months no major changes occurred in the vitamin E requirement calculated/kg food (mean 19·0 I.U./kg). When calculated/kg body-weight, however, there was a continuous decrease in the requirement for vitamin E, for the food intake remained fairly constant, whereas the mean body-weight increased from 200 g on the 35th day to 660 g on the 480th day. From these results we may conclude that vitamin E requirement is related to food intake (or perhaps, better, calorie intake) and not to body-weight.

(iv) Calculation of human requirement for vitamin E. A mean vitamin E requirement of 19 I.U./kg food for the rat, corresponds with 4·0 I.U./1000 kcal in the diet applied in this experiment. Extrapolation to man with a consumption of 2500 cal/day gives a daily requirement of 10·0 I.U. vitamin E. One mg DL-α-tocopheryl acetate (= 1·0 I.U. vitamin E, by definition) is equivalent to 0·65 mg D-α-tocopherol (Fig. 1), and therefore man would need 6·5 mg D-α-tocopherol/day. Harris and Embree (1963) calculated that the average diet in the USA supplied 14·9 mg D-α-tocopherol/day. Bunnell *et al.* (1965), however, calculated from their analysis of different foods that the daily intake of D-α-tocopherol in the USA varied between 2·6–15·4 mg with average of 7·4 mg/day.

These calculations were based on an analysis of raw materials. For processed foods (cooked, fried, etc.), Losowsky and Kelleher (1970) and Smith *et al.* (1971) found that in the UK in about 70% of the cases investigated the food supplied less than 5·0 mg D-α-tocopherol/day.

Dayton *et al.* (1965) performed the hydrogen haemolysis test on a group of seven men each of whom received 2·4 mg D-α-tocopherol/day from a diet containing 40 cal% saturated fat. The degree of haemolysis was 12% and therefore their daily intake must be considered insufficient.

Considering all these facts together, we must conclude that, based on the *in vitro* haemolysis test, a rather high percentage of human beings are, in fact, border-line cases of vitamin E deficiency.

*b. Relation to other criteria.* Significance of the haemolysis test. A positive haemolysis test is generally considered to indicate a state of vitamin E deficiency. However, it is not clear so far to what extent the results of an *in vitro* test may be indicative of an actual pathological condition (Weber and Weiser, 1967; Anonymous, 1969). Therefore, in male rats, long-term, dose-response effects of vitamin E in relation to different possible deficiency symptoms were studied in order to correlate these with the degree of spontaneous *in vitro* haemolysis (Jager, 1972a).

(i) Experimental design. Forty-eight newly-weaned male albino Wistar rats (SPF), divided into six groups of eight animals in each, were kept for 22 months on vitamin E deficient diets, as indicated in Table 1. Lard was used as a source of fat. Vitamin E was added to the diet as D-α-tocopheryl acetate. The six groups received 0·5, 1·5, 2·5, 4·5, 8·5 and 16·5 mg D-α-tocopheryl acetate/kg food respectively.

After 22 months the surviving animals were killed by decapitation, dissected and observed for gross pathology. The musculi gastronemii, liver and testicles were removed and examined microscopically. In the cross-section of the muscles, the affected fibres were counted with a maximum count of ten per section. Testis degeneration was also evaluated in a cross-section, using a score ranging from 0–4. Score 0 was given if less than three tubuli were affected (excluding the outer border, because on the outside of the testis some degenerated tubuli were frequently found, independent of the vitamin E dose). Scores 1, 2, 3 and 4 indicate that up to 25, 50, 75 and 100% respectively of the tubuli were degenerated. The scores of both testicles were added (total score 0–8).

(ii) Results and discussion. Although about 25% of the animals died before the end of the experimental period, no relation between the vitamin E content of the diet and mortality was observed.

Only the group receiving the lowest dose of vitamin E (0·5 mg D-α-tocopheryl acetate/kg food) showed a decreased weight gain, this becoming significant after about one year.

Liver necrosis was not observed; this is, however, only to be expected if the diet not only has a very low vitamin E content, but is also deficient in selenium (Schwarz and Foltz, 1957; Bonetti and Stirpe, 1962).

The leg muscles showed myopathy. The amount of hyaline-degenerated fibres showed the best response to the dose of vitamin E and was therefore regarded as a typical result of vitamin E deficiency. The relation between the three most important deficiency symptoms, that is, myopathy, testis degeneration and *in vitro* haemolysis is given in Table 2 (Vles and Jager, 1970).

No signs of disability in locomotion were observed. Obviously, an amount of 0·5 mg D-α-tocopheryl acetate/kg food was already enough to protect the animals in this respect.

According to Table 2, even 1·5 mg D-α-tocopheryl acetate/kg food was sufficient to prevent testis degeneration. Some degeneration was, it is true, found in the groups receiving 1·5 mg or more vitamin E, but this is likely to be the result of old age (Berg, 1967).

Table 2

Relation between myopathy, testis degeneration and spontaneous *in vitro* haemolysis in vitamin E deficient rats

| | D-α-tocopheryl acetate (mg/kg food) | | | | | |
|---|---|---|---|---|---|---|
| | 0·5 | 1·5 | 2·5 | 4·5 | 8·5 | 16·5 |
| Number of animals studied | 7 | 8 | 6 | 6 | 6 | 4 |
| Mean number of hyaline degenerated fibres per leg muscle cross-section | 10·0 | 7·8 | 5·6 | 2·4 | 0·8 | 0·4 |
| Testis degeneration (score 0–8) | 7·6 | 0·9 | 0·7 | 0·7 | 0 | 0·5 |
| Spontaneous *in vitro* haemolysis (%) | 90 | 87 | 80 | 41 | 19 | 3 |

Over a period of 22 months, the vitamin E requirement to prevent more than 10% haemolysis was practically constant (12 mg D-α-tocopheryl acetate/kg food). This was in good agreement with the results mentioned previously (Jager, 1968). In Fig. 5, the individual

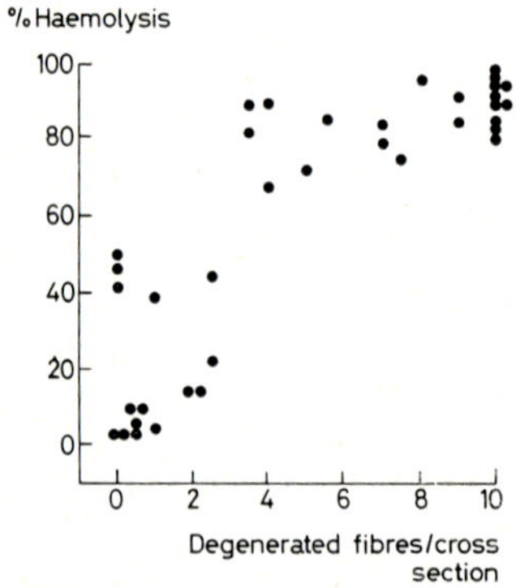


Fig. 5. Relation between number of hyaline-degenerated fibres per muscle cross-section and degree of *in vitro* haemolysis in rats.

relation between the number of hyaline-degenerated fibres per muscle cross-section and the percentage spontaneous haemolysis *in vitro* is expressed. An haemolysis of less than 50% is accompanied by hardly any myopathy.

Severe myopathy may be expected if the haemolysis is more than 70%. We might conclude, therefore, in contrast with the opinion of Alfin Slater *et al.* (1969a), that the *in vitro* haemolysis test is a valid indicator of vitamin E nutriture. A high percentage of haemolysis indicates that the vitamin E status is so low that it may predispose to myopathy (Jager, 1969a).

*2. In Other Species*

In the case of vitamin E deficiency, *in vitro* haemolysis, either by the addition of dialuric acid or hydrogen peroxide or spontaneously, is to be expected in all mammalian erythrocytes. In man *in vitro* haemolysis is often found in new-born or premature infants; in the latter case it is mostly associated with some degree of anaemia (György *et al.*, 1952; Gordon and Nitowsky, 1956; Hanna *et al.*, 1965; Oski and Barness, 1967). Obviously only little tocopherol passes the placenta as the plasma tocopherol level of the new-borns is mostly very low, whereas the mother has normal values. After administration of vitamin E to the children, the haemolysis disappears and the haemoglobin levels become normal within two weeks (Oski and Barness, 1967). *In vitro* haemolysis in adult men, under experimental vitamin E deficiency, has been reported by Horwitt *et al.* (1956). In patients with gastro-intestinal diseases, associated with severe steatorrhoea, a positive haemolysis test is often found, frequently concomitant with creatinuria (Binder *et al.*, 1965). A true nutritional vitamin E deficiency was found in some Jordanian children by Majaj *et al.* (1963). The disease, however, was complicated by a protein malnourishment. Also Whitaker *et al.* (1967) cured anaemia in protein-malnourished children by the additional administration of vitamin E.

Vitamin E deficiency, as expressed in a positive haemolysis test, has been reported in various animals: monkeys (Fitch *et al.*, 1964), pigs (Hill, 1963), rabbits (Draper, 1959; Ringler and Abrams, 1971) and dogs (Haynes and Rousseau, 1970). In mammals, a positive haemolysis test may occur for a long time, without any concomitant changes in histological structures, indicative for vitamin E deficiency. The *in vitro* haemolysis test is therefore regarded as the most sensitive criterion for vitamin E deficiency in mammals. In contrast to this, the erythrocytes of birds seem to be very resistant to *in vitro* haemolysis. Christensen *et al.* (1956) noticed that chickens on diets that produced severe encephalomalacia, showed almost no *in vitro* haemolysis, whether spontaneous or induced by adding dialuric acid. The same phenomenon was observed by Jager and Vles (1970) in ducklings, where despite serious myopathy of leg muscles and gizzard, the spontaneous *in vitro* haemolysis remained very low. These findings are probably related to the difference in erythrocyte structure between birds and mammals. The red cells from the first still contain a nucleus and those from the latter do not.

Although *in vitro* haemolysis has been found to occur in a wide variation of different animals, it has only been used in rats for the actual determination of vitamin E requirement (Rose and György, 1950b; Friedman *et al.*, 1958; Ward, 1963; Jager, 1968).

## B. Myopathy

Myopathy of the skeletal muscles is the most frequently occurring manifestation of vitamin E deficiency in mammals and birds. This general occurrence would make it suitable for the determination of vitamin E requirement. However, this is only possible when myopathy is a rather sensitive criterium for all the animal species studied and when the myopathy is not complicated by other vitamin E deficiency symptoms at the same time.

Myopathy may be studied by direct microscopical observation of the diseased muscle cells, but also by recording secondary effects as the increased excretion of creatine in the urine (creatinuria) (Gerber *et al.*, 1952) or the elevated level of different serum enzymes, which are supposed to leak from the diseased muscle cell into the bloodstream (Jager *et al.*, 1969). Gerber *et al.* (1952) concluded that creatinuria in rats was not caused by a release of creatine by the diseased muscle cell, but that the uptake of creatine by the muscle was diminished in the vitamin E deficient animal, so that, in consequence, the size of the free creatine pool increases and creatinuria results.

Although the skeletal muscles are in general the most sensitive to vitamin E deficiency, myopathy may also be found in heart muscle (Bowman and Dyer, 1960) and in the smooth muscles of stomach (Jungherr and Pappenheimer, 1937) and intestine (Jager, 1972b).

The study of myopathy in vitamin E deficient animals is somewhat complicated by the fact that the disease may be prevented in part or completely by the addition of cystine or menthionine to the diet (Dam *et al.*, 1952; Machlin and Shalkop, 1956; Scott and Calvert, 1962; Witting and Horwitt, 1964b). Another complication is formed by selenium, which was originally discovered as the factor giving protection against dietary liver necrosis in rats (Schwarz and Foltz, 1957). It was also found that only trace amounts in the diet are needed to prevent almost completely myopathy in vitamin E deficient chicks (Dam and Søndergaard, 1957; Scott, 1962) ducklings (Jager, 1972b) and rats (Moore and Sharman, 1964). It was, however, found ineffective in rabbits (Hove *et al.*, 1958; Proctor *et al.*, 1961).

Jager (1972b) found that for the protection of ducklings against myopathy the activity of 0·1 mg selenium is equivalent to at least 20 mg D-α-tocopheryl acetate. This effect of selenium could not be explained by a raised blood tocopherol level as Desai and Scott (1965) concluded from their experiments on chickens. Already 0·1 mg selenium/kg food protected ducklings fully against myopathy, despite a serum tocopherol level of only 1·2 μg/ml. In ducklings not receiving selenium, a serum tocopherol level of 5·3 μg/ml was needed.

A survey of selenium treatment against myopathy in a wide range of different animals has been given by Wolf *et al.* (1963).

The function of vitamin E in the prevention of myopathy is still not quite clear. Zalkin *et al.* (1962) found a release of lysozomal enzymes in vitamin E deficient rabbit muscle and advanced the theory that for lack of antioxidant the primary damage would consist of free radical damage to lipoprotein membranes of the cell and its subcellular organelles. Macrophages and phagocytic leucocytes, which are particularly rich in lysozomes, enter the regions of lipid peroxidation and could undergo rupture due to peroxidation damage. This process would set free lysozomal enzymes, leading to cell necrosis. Morphologic studies on rats (Howes *et al.*, 1964), chickens (Cheville, 1966) and rabbits (van Vleet *et al.*, 1968) indicated that the primary injury involves mitochondria. Van Vleet *et al.* (1968) draw attention to their observation that although lysozomes were numerous in degenerated muscle cells, they were not observed in skeletal muscle fibres during the early stages of degeneration; they therefore concluded that lysozomes served a secondary role in muscle cell lysis. Jager (1972a) found that vitamin E deficient rat muscle fibres at an early stage of degeneration frequently showed an increased activity of succinic dehydrogenase (SDH), just as was noted by Cheville (1966) for chicken muscle. But the most conspicuous feature in these rat muscle fibres was the very strong activity of lactic dehydrogenase (LDH). It was found (Jager, 1972a) that as the state of degeneration increased, the SDH-activity decreased and finally disappeared, whereas LDH activity increased and remained highly active until complete myolysis of the fibre set in. This is demonstrated in Fig. 6: strong LDH activity is especially found in the swollen fibres, a stage just preceding complete myolysis. These phenomena indicate that apparently an increasing part of the required cell energy is taken up by glycolysis when the mitochondria fail to supply sufficient energy by normal oxidation.

When the glycolysis, as a last source of energy, also fails, myolysis

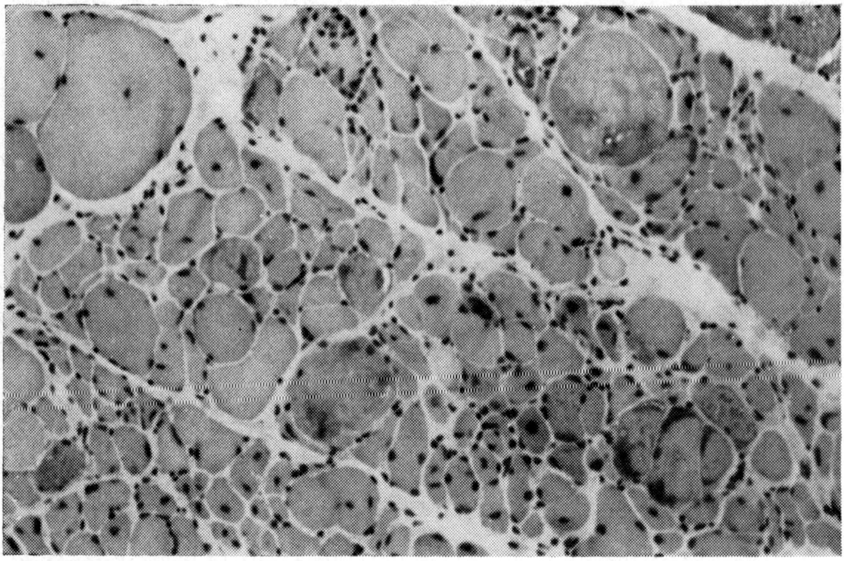

(a)

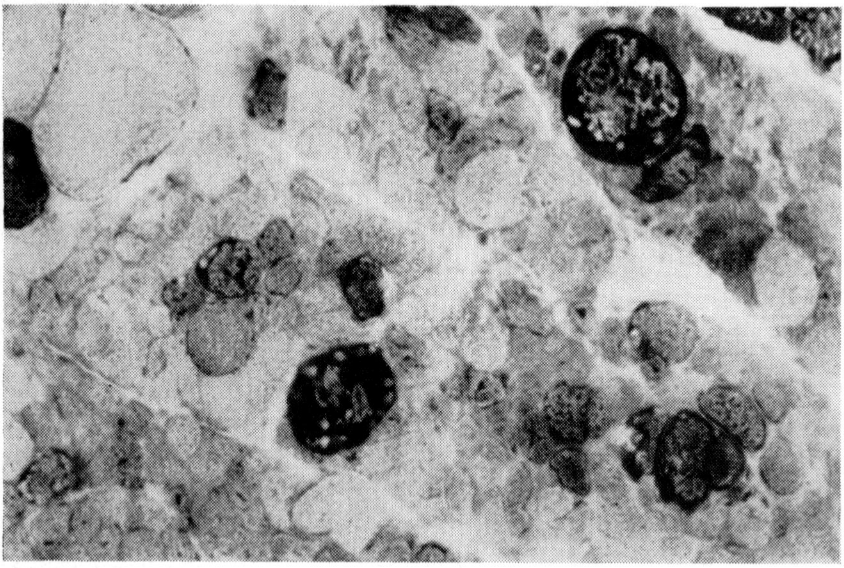

(b)

Fig. 6. (a) Cryostat section (140×) of muscle of vitamin E deficient rat showing hypertrophic and atrophic fibres and an increase of interstitial cells. Staining: haematoxylin-eosin. (b) Alternate section of Fig. 5. Swollen fibres show strong LDH-activity.

starts. Therefore, muscle degeneration obviously finds its cause in a failure of cellular energy production.

With respect to the mitochondria, indications have been found that in some way vitamin E is involved in oxidative phosphorylation (Corwin, 1965; Naito *et al.*, 1966; Carabello *et al.*, 1971). Another phenomenon that might be related to mitochondrial disfunction has been found by Molenaar *et al.* (1968, 1970), who observed in electron microscopy of intestinal epithelial cells of man and ducklings a decreased membrane contrast in state of vitamin E deficiency. This was most distinctly observed in the outer mitochondrial membrane. This contrast-loss in membranes was explained as a critical loss of double bonds and therefore probably represented a visualization of lipid peroxidation. In agreement with this explanation, Vos *et al.* (1972), who found an analogous loss of contrast in liver tissue of vitamin E deficient ducklings, demonstrated that on analysing the fatty acids of these liver mitochondria the largest decrease in arachidonic acid was found in the outer membranes (Vos, 1972; Molenaar *et al.*, 1972).

These observations strongly suggest that vitamin E may function in some way as an antioxidant *in vivo*. This view on vitamin E has found support by many researchers (Tappel, 1962, 1965, 1970; Horwitt, 1965; Witting, 1965). Bunyan *et al.* (1967), however, were not able to detect an increase in lipid peroxides in different parenchematous tissues of vitamin E deficient rats. Such an increase may, however, in some instances be found in adipose tissue of vitamin E deficient animals (Glavind *et al.*, 1971; Green, 1972). Several observations have been reported (Diplock *et al.*, 1968; Green, 1972) that do not quite fit in with an *in vivo* antioxidant function of vitamin E and it is quite obviously not the only function of this vitamin (Gilbert and Birky, 1971). The antioxidant concept still remains the most widely accepted view on vitamin E function.

### *1. Dose-response Effects in Ducklings*

*a. Introduction.* Ducklings are suitable animals for vitamin E research: when placed, after hatching, on a vitamin E deficient diet, the animals develop, within a few weeks, a severe myopathy. The disease is characterized by a hyaline degeneration of the striated muscles; symptoms of encephalomalacia or exudative diathesis are not observed (Pappenheimer and Goettsch, 1934; Pappenheimer, 1940).

The suitability of the duckling for determination of vitamin E requirement was investigated by studying the dose–response effects of vitamin E intake versus different criteria. It was found by Jager and

Table 3

Dose-response effects of vitamin E in ducklings after four weeks (mean values)

| Criterion (* = in survivors) | Vitamin E (mg/kg diet) 1·7 | 2·5 | 3·8 | 5·0 | 9·5 | 15·5 |
|---|---|---|---|---|---|---|
| Myopathy score (0–24) ($n = 10$) | 10·0 | 9·2 | 6·2 | 4·8 | 3·7 | 1·1 |
| Myopathy score* | 7·2 | 5·5 | 5·8 | 4·8 | 4·0 | 1·1 |
| Gizzard myopathy (number of animals) ($n = 10$) | 4 | 4 | 3 | 0 | 0 | 0 |
| Heart lesions (number of animals) ($n = 10$) | 4 | 1 | 0 | 0 | 0 | 0 |
| Mortality (number of animals) ($n = 10$) | 4 | 5 | 1 | 0 | 1 | 1 |
| Weight gain (g)* | 820 | 840 | 860 | 980 | 1000 | 910 |
| C.P.K. (Wroblewski units)* | 1900 | 1900 | 2400 | 2900 | 1800 | 800 |
| G.O.T. (Karmen units)* | 149 | 138 | 121 | 55 | 49 | 45 |
| L.D.H. (Wroblewski units)* | 2090 | 2120 | 1670 | 1400 | 1200 | 700 |
| Albumin (mg/ml)* | 13·9 | 17·1 | 20·2 | 22·0 | 22·7 | 25·8 |
| Tocopherol ($\mu$g/ml)* | 0·6 | 1·7 | 2·6 | 4·2 | 4·7 | 7·6 |
| Differential leucocyte count:* | | | | | | |
| heterophilic granulocytes (%) | 53 | 38 | 38 | 28 | 41 | 33 |
| heterophils with rods (%) | 20 | 12 | 7 | 6 | 7 | 4 |

Vles (1970) that the myopathy itself could be best expressed by awarding a score after microscopical examination of a muscle cross-section. The myopathy score of each section ranged from 0–4, indicating that less than 3 fibres (0), up to 25% (1), 50% (2), 75% (3) and 100% (4) of the muscle fibres were affected. The myopathy score of an individual animal was obtained by adding together the myopathy scores of all the muscles examined. This myopathy score was found to give better

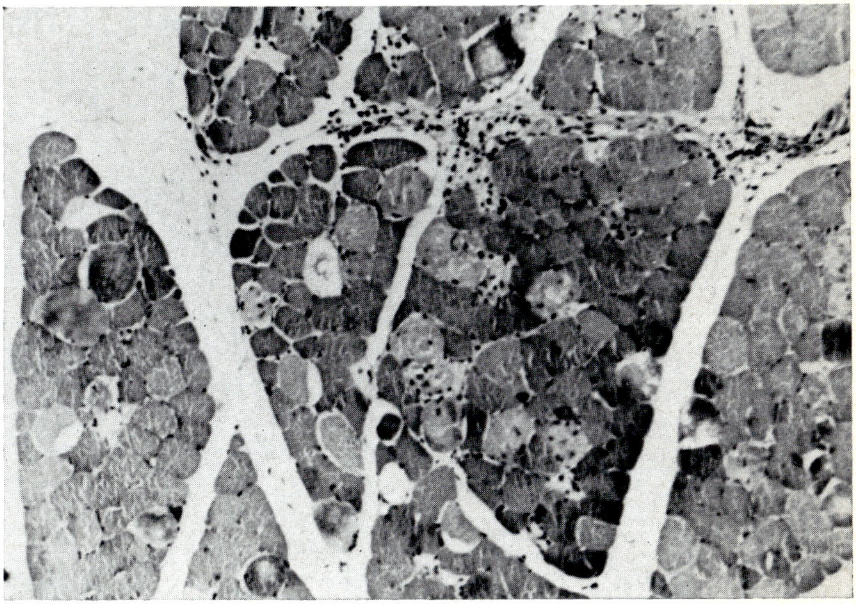

Fig. 7. Cross-section (140×) of leg muscle of vitamin E deficient duckling, showing hyaline necrosis of scattered muscle cells, associated with infiltration of macrophages and cellular reaction in perimysium. Staining: Masson trichrome.

results than the often used incidence of myopathy (percentage of animals affected) or even than the precise determination of the percentage of affected fibres per muscle cross-section.

Concomitant with myopathy, several other changes are to be expected in the case of vitamin E deficiency that might be suitable criteria for determining the vitamin E requirement. An increased activity of the following serum enzymes might be observed; aspartate amino-transferase (GOT) (Walter and Jensen, 1964; Anonymous, 1966), lactic dehydrogenase (LDH) (Giese, Erzoy and Hill, 1965; Anonymous, 1966) and creatine phosphokinase (CPK) (Bird and Carabello, 1966). Besides leucocytosis (Dinning, 1952), a change in serum protein composition should be expected (Goldstein and Scott, 1956).

*b. Experimental design.* Six groups of ten male Peking ducklings were kept from the day of hatching on a lard diet, as indicated in Table 1. Vitamin E was added to the diet in increasing doses as D-α-tocopheryl acetate. After four weeks the survivors were killed by decapitation, but

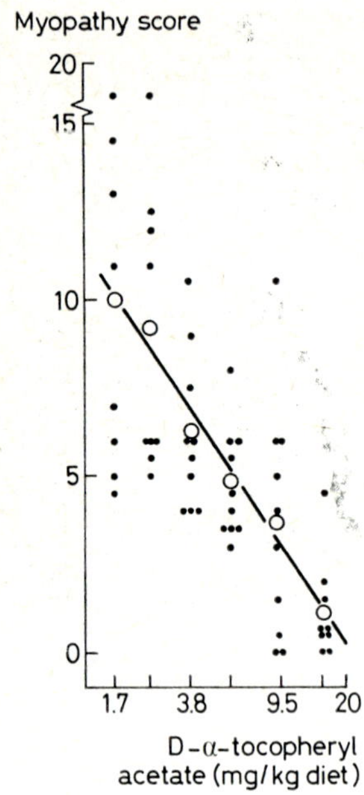


Fig. 8. Effect of vitamin E on myopathy in ducklings, four weeks after hatching. O = mean value.

just before that, blood was obtained by heart puncture for differential leucocyte counts and serum determinations of proteins, enzyme activities and total tocopherol. At autopsy, the bodies were observed for gross pathology and parts of the heart and gizzard removed for microscopical examination. The myopathy score was determined by taking three pairs of muscles from the legs, namely, M. gastrocnemious pars interna, M. sartorius and M. semimembranosus. Since six cross-sections were examined the maximum score per animal was 24.

*c. Results.* The dose–response effects of vitamin E according to different criteria are summarized in Table 3. The myopathy of the skeletal muscles manifested itself at autopsy by longitudinal, white striations and a waxy appearance. Concomitant with the severest cases of myopathy of the legs, occasionally haemorrhage and a greenish exudate were found. Microscopically the disease was characterized by the typical Zenker's degeneration (Fig. 7) as described by Pappenheimer and Goettsch (1934).

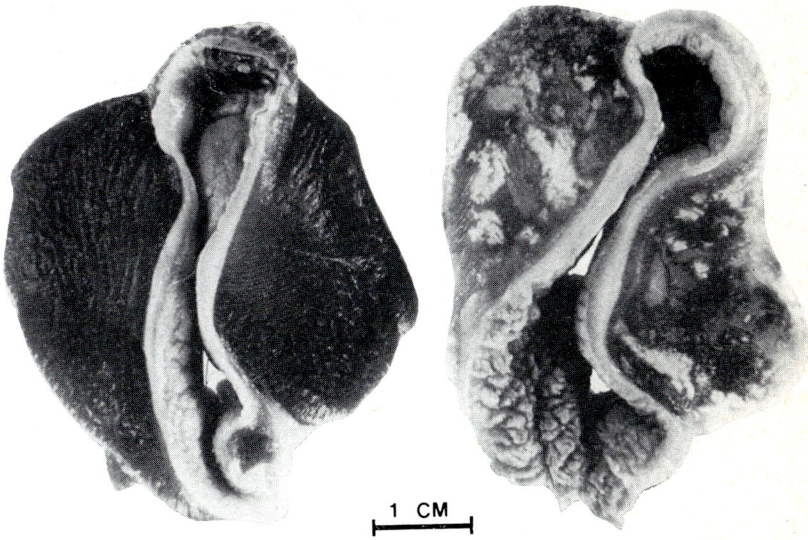


Fig. 9. Gizzard of vitamin E deficient (right) and of control (left) ducklings. Severe calcinosis is shown by the white areas in the cross-section of the left gizzard.

Even at high doses of vitamin E, some affected fibres may occasionally be found. Vitamin E requirement was therefore defined as the amount needed to prevent a myopathy score of more than one. A linear relationship was found between the logarithm of the vitamin E dose and the myopathy score (Fig. 8). It was estimated that 16 mg D-$\alpha$-tocopheryl acetate/kg food were required to prevent myopathy of the skeletal muscles (Jager and Verbeek-Raad, 1970).

The lesions in the gizzard were recognizable macroscopically as circumscribed white areas (Fig. 9). The histological picture showed necrocalcinosis and proliferation of muscle nuclei. This picture was different from that observed by Scott *et al.* (1967) in the gizzard of turkey poults, where, besides proliferation of muscle nuclei, oedema with infiltration of heterophilic leucocytes and fibrosis were the main features; calcinosis was not found. Obviously as little as 6 mg D-α-tocopheryl acetate/kg food was sufficient to protect the smooth muscles of the gizzard from myopathy, while even less (4 mg) was needed to protect the heart musculature. The heart lesions were also characterized by necrocalcinos (Figs 10 and 11). In addition, proliferation of muscle nuclei, oedema and haemorrhage were observed.

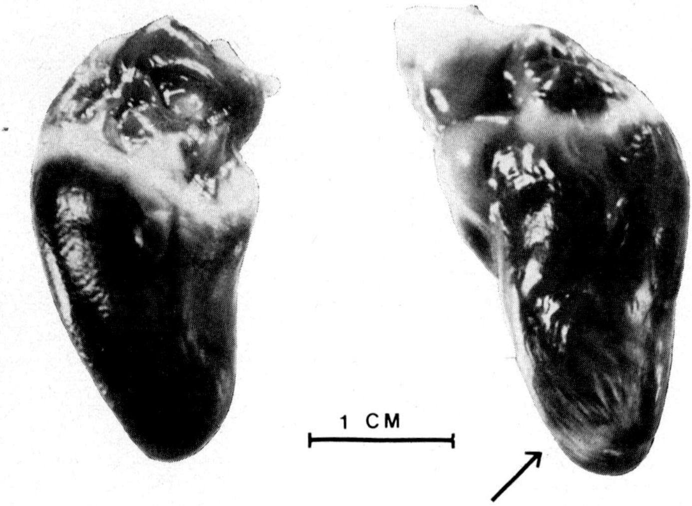


Fig. 10. Heart of vitamin E deficient (right) and of control (left) ducklings. Site of calcinosis is indicated by arrow.

Besides in heart and gizzard of vitamin E deficient ducklings, necrocalcinosis may also occur in the smooth musculature of the intestine, as was found by Jager (1972b) in a later experiment on ducklings (see also Table 6). The disease is illustrated in Figs 12 and 13.

Mortality occurred for the most part during the third experimental week. Practically all animals with a low body weight (<800 g) showed gizzard myopathy or severe myopathy of the legs (score >6). Jager and Vles (1970) found a significant correlation between the mean food consumption and weight increase per vitamin E dosing group. The decreased weight gain in the groups with the lower vitamin E doses seems to be a secondary effect, caused by a reduced food intake as a result of myopathy of the gizzard. Further, an impaired mobility and reduced food and water intake was observed, due to weakness of the skeletal muscles. The disease seems to reach a critical point rather suddenly, as during the first two weeks no differences in weight gain

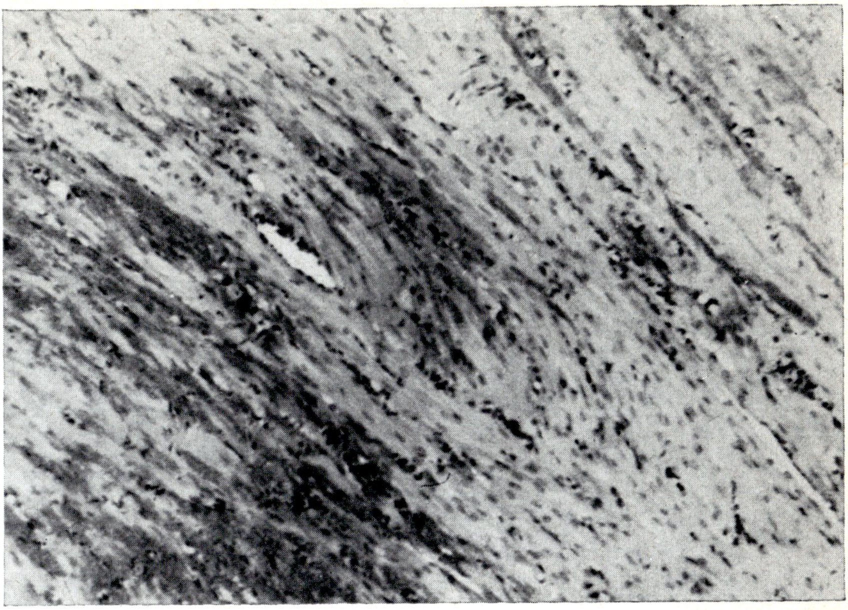

Fig. 11. Heart-muscular tissue (140×) of vitamin E deficient duckling. Areas of necro-calcinosis are characterized by dark, coarse granular appearance and pycnotic nuclei. Staining: haemotoxylin-eosin.

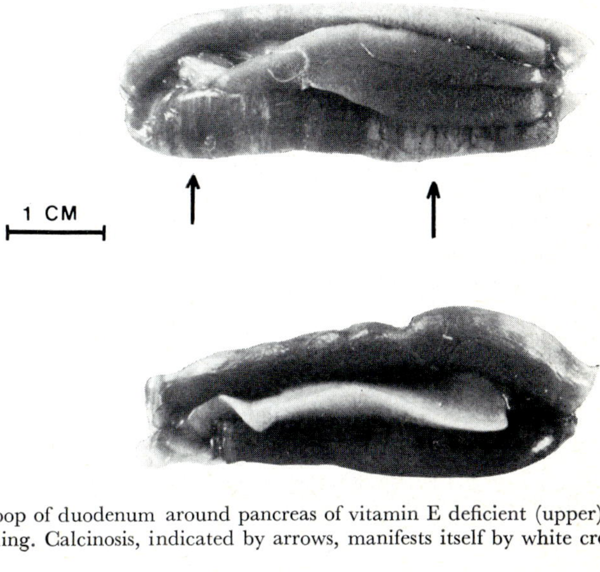


Fig. 12. Loop of duodenum around pancreas of vitamin E deficient (upper) and control (lower) duckling. Calcinosis, indicated by arrows, manifests itself by white cross striations.

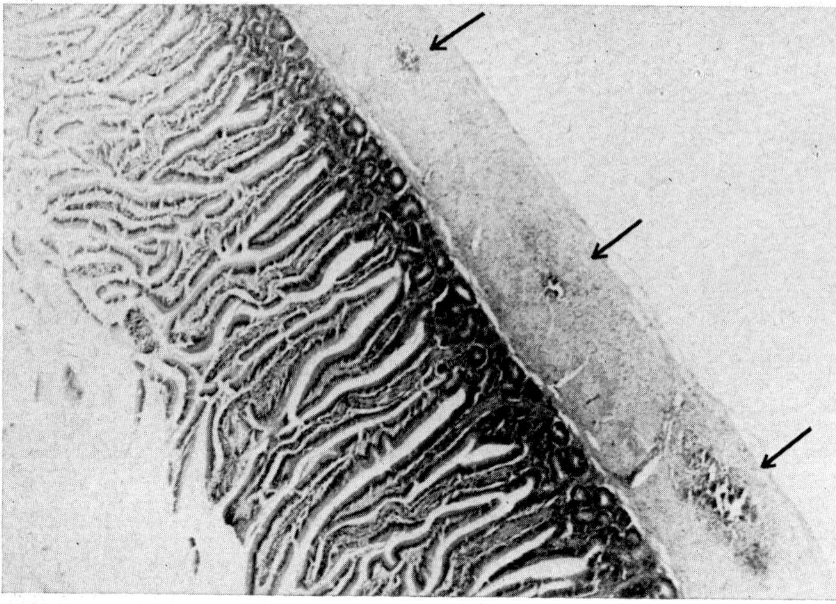

Fig. 13. Duodenum (55×) of vitamin E deficient duckling. Sites of necrocalcinosis are indicated by arrows. Staining: haemotoxylin-eosin.

or food intake were observed between the groups. Within each group the increase in weight varied greatly. An amount of 6 mg D-α-tocopheryl-acetate/kg food appeared to be sufficient for a normal growth response.

An increased CPK activity is considered typical of muscular diseases. The general concept is that the serum enzyme is of muscular origin and enters into the bloodstream as a result of an increased permeability of the muscle cell membrane (Bird and Carabello, 1966). On the basis of this concept, an increase in CPK activity in the blood could be expected, the ultimate activity being the result of an equilibrium between release and breakdown of the enzyme. A positive correlation was indeed found between the myopathy score and the CPK activity.

However, at the lowest vitamin E doses, where high myopathy scores prevailed, the CPK level—in contrast to GOT and LDH—was low. This is probably explained by the earlier onset of myopathy at the lowest vitamin E doses and the faster disappearance of CPK from the blood than the GOT and LDH (as known to occur after myocardial damage).

A significant negative relationship was found to exist between the logarithm of the vitamin E dose and the GOT activity, suggesting an

S-shaped curve, although there was no proof of a significant deviation from a linear relationship because of the great variations within the groups.

The LDH activity showed a linear relationship to the log dose vitamin E. The serum level of this enzyme seems to offer a sensitive criterion for establishing vitamin E deficiency (myopathy), in addition to the advantage of a linear relationship to determine vitamin E requirement.

The serum protein concentrations appeared to be linearly related to the log dose vitamin E (Fig. 14). The albumin concentrations decreased,

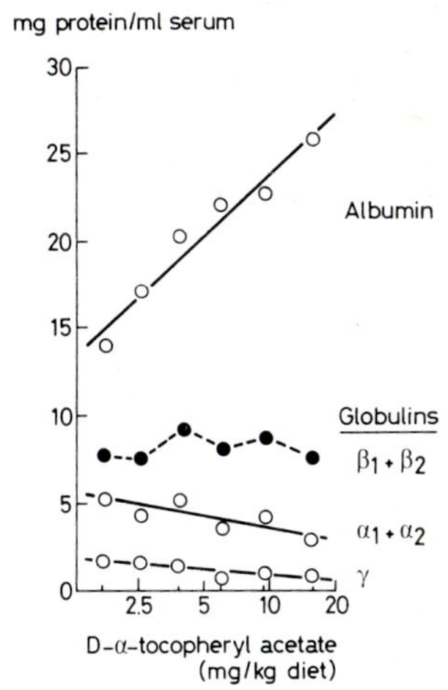


Fig. 14. Effect of vitamin E on serum-protein concentration in ducklings ($n = 5$–10).

whereas those of $\alpha_1 + \alpha_2$-globulin and $\gamma$-globulin increased at low vitamin E doses. These results suggest that vitamin E is, in some way, involved in protein metabolism, although for the lowest vitamin E doses, the low serum albumin content might be partly caused by a reduced food intake.

A linear relationship was found between the log dose vitamin E and the serum tocopherol level, but the tocopherol concentrations varied greatly within one group, e.g. for the group receiving 5·9 mg vitamin E/kg food from 0·4 to 10·0 $\mu$g/ml serum.

Statistical analysis revealed that there was no significant influence of vitamin E on total white blood cell count (number/$\mu$l) or on the percentages of heterophils with granular eosinophilic bodies, eosinophils, basophils and monocytes, but from 1·7 to 5·9 mg vitamin E there was a significant increase of lymphocyte percentage and a decrease of the percentage of total heterophils and of heterophils with rod-shaped eosinophilic bodies. Severe granulocytosis, as found by Dinning (1952) in rabbits and by Nafstad (1965) in pigs, was only occasionally observed in the vitamin E deficient ducklings. Obviously the differential white blood cell count does not offer a criterion sensitive enough for the determination of vitamin E requirement in ducklings.

*d. Conclusions.* Myopathy of the skeletal muscles proves to be the most sensitive and reliable criterion for vitamin E deficiency studies in ducklings. As in fact, as far as known, myopathy in any form is the only disease occurring in vitamin E deficient ducklings, the importance of the criteria investigated in the serum depends upon their relation to the myopathy. The correlation coefficients between the myopathy score and the criteria investigated were as follows:

| | |
|---|---|
| LDH | +0·71 |
| log GOT | +0·70 |
| log CPK | +0·55 |
| albumin (mg/ml) | −0·52 |
| tocopherol (μg/ml) | −0·49 |
| heterophilic granulocytes | +0·53 |

LDH and GOT showed good correlation with the myopathy score. It must, however, be realized that perhaps better correlations would be obtained if the skeletal muscles were the only source of these enzymes, as it may be expected that at the lowest doses of vitamin E the gizzard and heart muscles also contribute to the enzyme levels in the blood. The correlation with CPK was low, as might be expected for reasons explained previously.

Although both serum albumin concentration and the myopathy score showed a linear relationship to the log dose vitamin E, the correlation between both was poor. The explanation is that the changes in serum protein concentrations must be considered a vitamin E deficiency phenomenon, independent of myopathy and are probably caused by some disfunction of the liver.

The serum tocopherol level appeared to give only a rough indication of the state of muscular disease. The correlation coefficients between the serum tocopherol level and the above criteria, determined in the same way as for the myopathy score, were either much lower or entirely absent.

Although in this experiment the correlation coefficient between the myopathy score and the percentages of heterophilic granulocytes was only poor (+0·53), in another experiment on vitamin E deficient ducklings by Jager and Vles (1970) a much better correlation of +0·67 was found. This suggests that the granulocytosis is the direct result of the muscle disease.

The ultimate conclusion from this experiment must be that, in ducklings, the histologically assessed score of myopathy of the skeletal muscles offers the best criterion for determining vitamin E requirement. It was ultimately found (Jager, 1972b) that when, concomitant with degeneration of the skeletal muscles, severe myopathy of gizzard, heart and intestine occurs, the determination of serum LDH activity does not offer a suitable criterion for the determination of vitamin E requirement. The differential serum protein determination appeared to offer a far less accurate and sensitive criterion than the myopathy score.

Myopathy has been used only incidentally as a criterion for the determination of vitamin E requirement. Most work on myopathy in relation to dietary vitamin E has been done on chickens. Vitamin E requirement of chickens in relation to dietary selenium was determined by Scott (1962), using the incidence of myopathy as a criterium in combination with a score for the severity of the disease. This score was assessed by gross observation of the skeletal muscles at autopsy. The same method in vitamin E deficient chickens was used by Jenkins *et al.* (1962) and by Søndergaard and Dam (1970).

Another method is to determine the time needed until the onset of creatinuria, as has been done by Witting and Horwitt (1964a).

*2. Dose-response Effects in Rats*

The pathology of vitamin E deficient rats is mainly characterized by damage of the testicles and the skeletal muscles. The muscular disease in young rats has been described by Olcott (1938) and Pappenheimer (1939), while Evans *et al.* (1938) described the degeneration of cross-striated musculature in vitamin E deficient old rats. Vitamin E deficiency diseases in young rats may be observed by taking the offspring from vitamin E deficient (or nearly deficient) mother animals. When the experiment starts with young from mothers on normal diets, it may take several months before any histological changes due to vitamin E deficiency are observed.

Long-term, dose-response effects of vitamin E in relation to myopathy, as found by Jager (1972a), are given in Table 4. Besides myopathy of the skeletal muscles, degeneration of the testis was found (Table 2). As appears from Table 4, not all phenomena mentioned

Table 4

Effect of vitamin E on morphology of both the musculi gastrocnemii in rats, after 22 months. Nunber of affected fibres observed per cross-section (maximum count = 10)

| D-α-tocopheryl acetate (mg/kg) | 0·5 | 1·5 | 2·5 | 4·5 | 8·5 | 16·5 |
|---|---|---|---|---|---|---|
| *n* | 7 | 8 | 7 | 6 | 6 | 4 |
| Fibre with one or more centrally-located sarcolemmic nuclei | 10·0 | 10·0 | 10·0 | 10·0 | 10·0 | 10·0 |
| Swollen fibre | 10·0 | 5·4 | 8·0 | 8·8 | 3·2 | 4·5 |
| Swollen fibre with one or more centrally-located sarcolemmic nuclei | 9·0 | 4·5 | 5·6 | 3·4 | 1·1 | 1·5 |
| Hyaline-degenerated fibre, infiltrated with histiocytes | 10·0 | 7·8 | 5·6 | 2·4 | 0·8 | 0·4 |
| Degenerated fibre with centrally-located myoblasts | 10·0 | 1·3 | 2·6 | 1·7 | 0·0 | 0·0 |
| Fibre with centrally-degenerated cylinder | 0·6 | 0·3 | 0·3 | 0·0 | 0·0 | 0·0 |
| Interfibrilar fat cells | 10·0 | 8·4 | 6·3 | 9·6 | 5·1 | 4·2 |
| Atrophied fibre, associated with increase of interstitial cells or with centrally-located nuclei in the fibre | 6·4 | 2·5 | 3·7 | 1·0 | 1·0 | 1·8 |

showed clear dose–response effects. Some phenomena occur, almost to the same extent, at all doses of vitamin E. This is most probably due to the old age of the rats. Dystrophic changes, resembling those occurring in vitamin E deficiency may then be observed (Berg, 1967).

The amount of the hyaline degenerated fibres (Table 4) showed the best response to the dose of vitamin E and this degeneration can therefore be regarded as a typical result of vitamin E deficiency. Besides the different types of diseased muscle fibres mentioned in Table 4, an increase in interstitial cells was observed at decreasing doses of vitamin E.

The results obtained indicate quite clearly that myopathy in rats is not a sensitive enough criterium to serve the determination of vitamin E requirement.

#### 3. *Effects in Other Species*

Except in ducklings and rats, nutritional myopathy, caused by vitamin E deficiency has been found in many different species: monkeys (Dinning and Day, 1957), cows (Vawter and Records, 1947), horses (Jones and Reed, 1948), sheep (Metzger and Hagan, 1927), pigs (Adamstone *et al.*, 1949; Forbes and Draper, 1958), goats (Madsen *et al.*, 1933), dogs (Anderson *et al.*, 1939), minks (Mason and Hartsough, 1951), guinea-pigs and rabbits (Goettsch and Pappenheimer, 1931), hamsters (Houchin and Mattill, 1942), chickens (Dam *et al.*, 1952), turkeys (Jungherr and Pappenheimer, 1937) and guppy fish (Cumings, 1942).

Although severe myopathy may occur in monkeys, the most important symptom of vitamin E deficiency in these animals is formed by anaemia (Dinning and Day, 1957). In chickens the myopathy is complicated by the occurrence of encephalomalacia and exudative diathesis at the same time (Cheville 1966; Scott, 1970).

Pure nutritional myopathy caused by vitamin E deficiency has not been reported to occur in man. But tocopherol deficiency, manifested by creatinuria and lesions in the skeletal muscles, was found in patients who suffered from severe steatorrhea of long duration (Binder *et al.*, 1965).

## C. Encephalomalacia and Dose-Response Effects in Chickens

Of all other symptoms of vitamin E deficiency (encephalomalacia, exudative diathesis, liver necrosis, anaemia, resorption gestation, testis degeneration and diminished fertility) only the incidence of encephalomalacia in chickens has actually been used for the determination of vitamin E requirement (Dam and Søndergaard, 1964; and Søndergaard and Dam, 1966). The dose-response showed a sigmoid shaped curve (Fig. 15) that pointed to a vitamin E requirement (for a diet containing 50 cal% lard) of the same order as found by Jager (1968, 1972b) in rats (*in vitro* haemolysis test) and in ducklings (myopathy score).

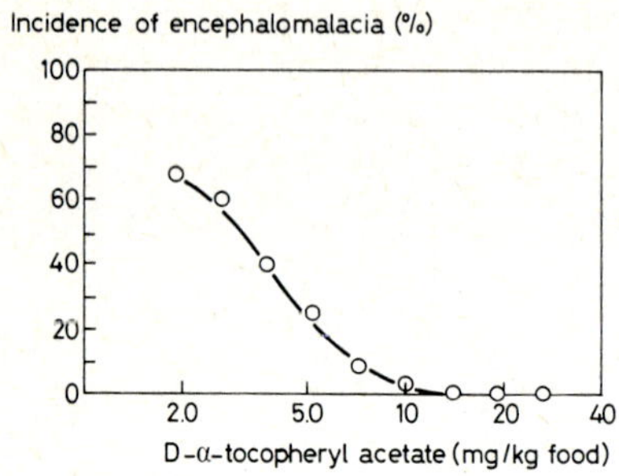


Fig. 15. (Søndergaard and Dam, 1966.) Effect of dietary vitamin E on incidence of encephalomalacia in chickens ($n = 10$).

## III. EFFECT OF HIGH LINOLEIC ACID INTAKE ON VITAMIN E REQUIREMENT

Even in the early days of vitamin E research it was known that the intake of polyunsaturated fatty acids (PUFA) may increase vitamin E requirement. The addition of cod liver oil to vitamin E deficient diets was a known procedure to speed up the appearance of vitamin E deficiency symptoms. Although the effect of highly unsaturated PUFA and also linolenic acid on vitamin E requirement may be interesting from a theoretical point of view, PUFA in edible fats and oils consist almost exclusively of linoleic acid. For this reason the experiments mentioned here will relate only to this fatty acid.

Weber *et al.* (1964) calculated from their experiments on rats, using *in vitro* haemolysis as a criterion, that 0·5 mg DL-α-tocopheryl acetate per extra gram of linoleic acid would be needed. In contrast with these results, Søndergaard and Dam (1966), in their experiments on chickens in which the incidence of encephalomalacia was used as a criterion, did not find any effect of linoleic acid intake on vitamin E requirement.

Weber *et al.* (1964) used single oral doses of vitamin E. This procedure may give too high values for the requirement, as the absorption of vitamin E is expected to be better, when incorporated in small quantities in the food (Pudelkiewicz and Nakiya, 1969). Moreover, the coconut-oil diet which they used as a control has to be considered EFA deficient.

## A. Experiments on Rats (*in vitro* haemolysis)

### 1. *Experimental Design*

Ninety-six newly-weaned male albino Wistar rats (SPF) were kept for four weeks on a vitamin E deficient lard diet (Table 1), in order to allow the animals to use up their vitamin E reserves. In a second period of three weeks, the animals were divided in four groups each of 24 animals, receiving increasing doses of vitamin E (D-α-tocopheryl acetate) in their diets as indicated in Fig. 16. In the third period of nine

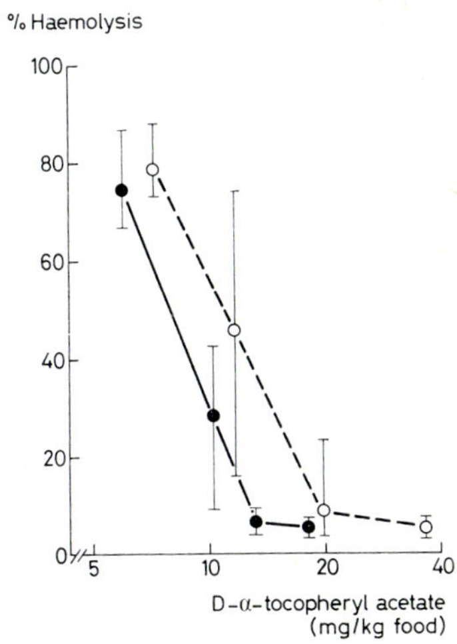


Fig. 16. (Jager, 1969c.) Effect of type of diet on dose-response curves of vitamin E ($n = 12$); ● lard; ○ maize oil.

weeks, half the animals of each group of the second period received tocopherol-free maize oil (Jager, 1969b) instead of lard in their diets.

Spontaneous *in vitro* haemolysis (Jager, 1968) was used as a criterium to indicate vitamin E requirement.

The fatty acid composition of the lard and maize oil is given in Table 5.

### 2. *Results*

The mean results of weekly determinations during the experimental period are presented in Fig. 16. The difference in vitamin E requirement between the lard and maize oil group appeared to be very significant.

Table 5

Fatty acid composition (%) of lard and maize oil

| Fatty acid | Lard | Maize oil |
|---|---|---|
| C 14:0 | 2·0 | — |
| C 16:0 | 29·5 | 13·0 |
| C 17:0 | 0·5 | — |
| C 18:0 | 18·0 | 1·7 |
| C 18:1, $\omega 9$ | 36·0 | 27·0 |
| C 18:2, $\omega 6$ | 10·5 | 56·7 |
| C 18:3, $\omega 3$ | — | 1·1 |
| C 20:0 | 1·5 | — |
| C 20:1 | 0·5 | — |
| C 20:2 | 0·5 | — |
| Iodine value | 58 | 125 |

For both diets a linear relationship was found between log vitamin E content of the diet and the haemolysis percentage. The regression coefficients of the two dose–response curves, however, differed significantly and therefore the lines in Fig. 16 do not run parallel.

According to the haemolysis test, the vitamin E requirement for the lard diet (4·0 cal% linoleic acid) was 12·4 mg D-α-tocopheryl acetate/kg food and that for the maize oil diet (20·2 cal% linoleic acid) was 19·0 mg; this is 2·4 and 3·7 mg D-α-tocopherol/1000 kcal of food.

*3. Conclusion*

Table 5 shows that the great difference in PUFA content between lard and maize oil almost exclusively concerns linoleic acid. Calculated per kg food, the difference in linoleic acid content between the lard and the maize oil diet is 81·2 g, and the difference in need of vitamin E is 6·6 mg D-α-tocopheryl acetate. This difference is (Brubacher and Weiser, 1967) equivalent to $136/149 \times 6{\cdot}6 = 6{\cdot}0$ mg D-α-tocopherol. On the assumption that the need of vitamin E increases linearly with increasing linoleic acid content, this need is $6{\cdot}0/81{\cdot}2 = 0{\cdot}074$ mg D-α-tocopherol per extra gram of linoleic acid. We may therefore conclude that the intake of vegetable oils with a high linoleic acid content, such as sunflower, maize and safflower oil, may cause an increased requirement for vitamin E, but that this increase is amply covered by the natural vitamin E content of these oils, as 74 mg D-α-tocopherol/kg linoleic acid would itself be sufficient to cover this extra need.

## B. Myopathy in Ducklings

### *1. Experimental Design*

Newly-hatched male Peking ducklings were given diets as indicated in Table 1, the dietary fat being lard or stripped maize oil (tocopherol-free). The division into groups ($n = 8$) with respect to the dietary vitamin E content is given in Table 6. After four weeks, the surviving animals were killed by decapitation. All animals were examined for gross pathology and different organs were removed for microscopic examination. The myopathy of the leg muscles was expressed in a score (0–24) as described before (Section II B, 1). Just before killing the survivors at the end of the experiment, blood was obtained by heart puncture for determination of the serum tocopherol level (Jager, 1972b).

Table 6

Number of affected ducklings per group ($n = 8$), after four weeks on diets containing lard (L) or tocopherol-free maize oil (M)

| Criterion | Fat | D-α-tocopheryl acetate (mg/kg) | | | | | |
|---|---|---|---|---|---|---|---|
| | | 2·5 | 4·0 | 6·5 | 11·0 | 18·0 | 34·0 |
| Mortality | L | 8 | 6 | 1 | 0 | 1 | 0 |
| | M | 4 | 5 | 7 | 2 | 1 | 1 |
| Fatty liver | L | 3 | 5 | 2 | 2 | 0 | 0 |
| | M | 0 | 2 | 1 | 0 | 0 | 0 |
| Necro-calcinosis: | | | | | | | |
| Heart | L | 1 | 3 | 1 | 0 | 0 | 0 |
| | M | 4 | 5 | 1 | 3 | 0 | 0 |
| Intestine | L | 4 | 7 | 6 | 2 | 0 | 0 |
| | M | 4 | 3 | 4 | 4 | 3 | 0 |
| Gizzard | L | 8 | 8 | 1 | 2 | 0 | 0 |
| | M | 8 | 8 | 8 | 7 | 2 | 0 |

### *2. Results*

The result of the assessment of the score of myopathy of the leg muscles is shown in Fig. 17. After square-root transformation, a linear relationship was found between dietary vitamin E content and myopathy score for both the lard and the (stripped) maize oil diet. The lines in Fig. 17 were found to run parallel. Twice as much vitamin E was needed for the maize oil diet (21·8 cal% linoleic acid) as for the lard diet (3·0 cal%

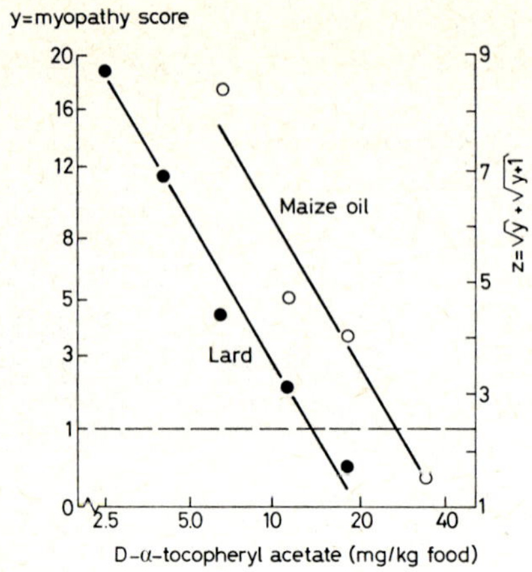


Fig. 17. Effect of dietary fats with low (lard) and high (maize oil) linoleic acid content on the need for vitamin E to prevent myopathy (score 1) of the skeletal muscles in ducklings

linoleic acid); 27·0 and 13·5 mg D-α-tocopheryl acetate/kg diet respectively, or 6·4 and 3·2 mg D-α-tocopherol/1000 kcal of food.

The effects of linoleic acid intake on criteria other than the skeletal muscles, are indicated in Table 6. Although the values found were not so suitable for an exact calculation of vitamin E requirement as the myopathy score of the leg muscles, the general trend is the same. An exception is the occurrence of fatty liver, which showed a higher frequency in the lard groups than in the maize oil groups.

Figure 18 illustrates the effect of a high linoleic acid intake on the

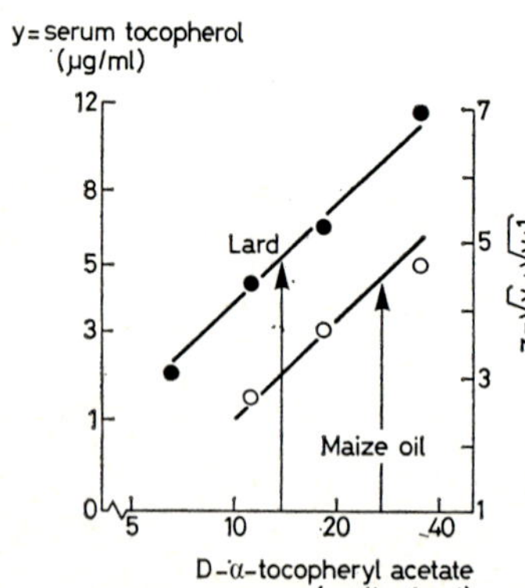


Fig. 18. Effect of dietary fats with low (lard) and high (maize oil) linoleic acid content on the serum–tocopherol level of ducklings. Arrows indicate amount of vitamin E needed to prevent myopathy (score 1).

serum tocopherol level. As for the myopathy score, a linear relationship was found with the vitamin E content of the diet, for both the lard and maize oil groups. The lines in Fig. 18 appeared to run parallel. The serum tocopherol levels of the maize oil groups were 43% of that of the lard groups. This means that the increased vitamin E requirement caused by the maize oil can be completely explained by the drop in blood-tocopherol level.

Obviously, the lard diet needed a somewhat higher serum-tocopherol level to avoid skeletal-muscle myopathy than the maize oil diet (5·3 and 4·6 $\mu$g/ml serum respectively). This difference might have been due to a difference in selenium content of the fats, although no selenium could be detected in any of the dietary fats used (thus, the concentration must have been below 0·1 mg/kg fat).

*3. Conclusions*

The important conclusion from this experiment is that high linoleic acid intake does not induce an increased need for vitamin E in the tissues, as the required blood-tocopherol level of the maize oil diet was not higher than that of the lard diet. The increased need for dietary vitamin E on the maize oil diet is obviously caused by destruction of vitamin E in the gastro-intestinal tract and perhaps by a decreased absorption, which results in a drop in the blood-tocopherol level.

For both the lard and maize oil diet, ducklings needed more vitamin E than rats, which is indeed to be expected for such rapidly growing animals as far as the basic requirement is concerned. Furthermore, at high dietary linoleic acid concentrations their feeding habits favour oxidation of the food components much more than is the case with rats.

The dietary fats are to be considered the natural sources of vitamin E. From this point of view it could be calculated that in order to cover the need for vitamin E, the lard should contain at least 86 mg D-$\alpha$-tocopherol/kg fat. However, lard contains by nature seldom more than about 10 mg/kg fat. The maize oil should contain twice as much, i.e. 172 mg D-$\alpha$-tocopherol/kg fat, which is indeed amply covered by the natural vitamin E content of this oil. This conclusion was experimentally confirmed; ducklings on a lard diet all died within three weeks because of severe myopathy, when no extra vitamin E was added to the diet. On the other hand, ducklings on a diet containing natural maize oil did not need extra vitamin E. After four weeks on the (natural) maize oil diet all animals were in good condition and no signs of myopathy were observed.

Obviously, a mainly saturated animal fat such as lard must be considered inadequate in its vitamin E content, whereas a mainly unsaturated vegetable oil like maize oil is more than adequate.

The same conclusion can be drawn from an experiment by Dayton *et al.* (1965) who found that a group of men on a diet containing 40 cal% saturated fat showed a positive haemolysis test. This test, however, remained negative on an identical diet containing unsaturated vegetable fat.

## C. Encephalomalacia in Chickens

From the day of hatching, chickens were given, for one week, a ration free of vitamin E, followed by a diet containing 50 cal% fat for six weeks. The fat was one of a series of mixtures of lard and (tocopherol-free) sunflower oil, which provided 3·3 cal% linoleic acid for the diet lowest, and 9·7 cal% for the diet highest, in linoleic acid. Each group at one dietary linoleic acid level was subdivided into eight groups ($n = 10$) receiving increasing doses of D-α-tocopheryl acetate in order to determine vitamin E requirement by means of the incidence of encephalomalacia (Fig. 15 (Søndergaard and Dam, 1966).

Increasing the level of dietary linoleic acid from 3·3 to 9·6 cal%, proved to have no effect upon the requirement for vitamin E, which remained 2·3 mg D-α-tocopherol/1000 kcal of food. Obviously, within this range of linoleic acid intake, no relationship with vitamin E requirement exists. An increase in the latter might, however, be seen at linoleic acid intakes above 9·7 cal%. This is, at least, strongly suggested by the results of Vogtmann and Prabucki (1971), who found that the liver vitamin E level of chickens after three weeks on a sunflower oil diet (22·5 cal% linoleic acid) was 67% of that of chickens on a lard diet (3·8 cal% linoleic acid). The dietary fats were tocopherol-free and vitamin E was added to both diets in equal doses of 4·0 mg DL-α-tocopheryl acetate/1000 kcal of food.

## D. Serum Tocopherol Level and *in vitro* Haemolysis in Man

Information on vitamin E requirement of man is scarce. No direct facts with regard to vitamin E requirement of man are available. Horwitt (1960), in experiments on man ($n = 6$), found that when a daily ingestion of 30 g lard was replaced by 30 g tocopherol-free maize oil, this caused a slight drop in the serum-tocopherol level (about 5%), which again fell by about 10% when the maize oil intake was increased to 60 g/day. From these facts it could be calculated that at linoleic acid intakes of about 3, 9 and 15 cal% of the diet the corresponding serum-tocopherol levels were: 10, 9·5 and 8·0 μg/ml respectively, at a constant vitamin E intake of 15 mg D-α-tocopheryl acetate/day (+2 mg free tocopherol, contained in the food). At these serum-tocopherol levels, the *in vitro* haemolysis test remained negative.

## IV. DOSE-RESPONSE EFFECTS OF LINOLEIC ACID INTAKE

### A. Vitamin E Requirement

For three weeks, 192 newly-weaned male rats were given a vitamin E deficient lard diet (Table 1) in order to deplete them of their vitamin E reserves. Thereafter the animals were divided into six groups of 32 that received for five weeks lard diets to which increasing doses of D-α-tocopheryl acetate were added; 2·5, 4·0, 6·5, 10·0, 15·5 and 23·5 mg/kg food respectively. In this period a steady state between vitamin E intake and the blood tocopherol level was reached.

Finally each group of 32 animals was split into 4 subgroups of eight animals that received, for five weeks, increasing doses of linoleic acid in their diets: 0·5, 2·0, 7·0 and 25·6 cal% respectively. For this reason the lard in the diet was replaced by four different mixtures of coconut oil and tocopherol-free safflowerseed oil. In fact, the group receiving only 0·5 cal% linoleic acid, was on an essential fatty acid deficient diet (Holman, 1960), but an EFA deficient status was not attained during this period of five weeks, as the preceding periods on lard diets had supplied enough linoleic acid to build up sufficient reserves. During this last period, vitamin E requirement was determined weekly by the spontaneous haemolysis test *in vitro* (Jager, 1968).

The mean results over the experimental period are given in Table 7, together with those of other previously mentioned experiments.
They indicate, that up to an intake of about 10 cal%, linoleic acid has no effect on vitamin E requirement or status. Between 10 and 20 cal% dietary linoleic acid, the vitamin E requirement may increase up to 200% (Jager and Houtsmuller, 1970).

It is obvious that there exists a basic need for vitamin E, unaffected by linoleic acid intake. The increased requirement for vitamin E above 10 cal% linoleic acid intake is apparently caused by an increased destruction (and/or decreased absorption) of tocopherol in the intestinal tract, as shown by a decreased tocopherol level in liver and blood. Weber *et al.* (1964) made the remarkable observation that linoleic acid

Table 7

Relation between linoleic acid intake and vitamin E requirement or status

| Dietary linoleic acid (cal%) | Vitamin E requirement: mg D-α-tocopherol/ 1000 kcal of food | Vitamin E requirement: Percentage of basic need | |
|---|---|---|---|
| 0·5 | 2·5 | 100[a] | Rat; haemolysis test (Jager and Houtsmuller, 1970) |
| 2·0 | 2·5 | 100 | |
| 7·0 | 2·5 | 100 | |
| 25·6 | 3·5 | 140 | |
| 4·0 | 2·4 | 100 | Rat; haemolysis test (Jager, 1969c) |
| 20·2 | 3·7 | 154 | |
| 3·0 | 3·2 | 100 | Duckling; myopathy score (Jager, 1972) |
| 21·8 | 6·5 | 200 | |
| 3·3 | 2·3 | 100 | Chickens; incidence of encephalomalacia (Søndergaard and Dam, 1966) |
| 5·7 | 2·3 | 100 | |
| 8·1 | 2·3 | 100 | |
| 9·7 | 2·3 | 100 | |
| | Tocopherol concentration in liver[b] (μg/g) | | Chickens |
| 3·8 | 52·2 ± 3·2 | | (Vogtmann and Prabucki, 1971) |
| 22·8 | 35·3 ± 4·4 | | |
| | Serum-tocopherol level[b] (μg/ml) | | |
| 3 | 10·0 | | Man (Horwitt, 1960) |
| 9 | 9·5 | | |
| 15 | 8·0 | | |

[a] Animals were not yet EFA-deficient because of a preceding period on a diet containing 4·0 cal% linoleic acid.
[b] At equal vitamin E intake (see text).

intake in rats had no effect on different tissue tocopherol levels, when vitamin E was administered intraperitoneally in contrast to peroral administration. Green *et al.* (1967) also showed that linoleic acid has no effect on tissue tocopherol levels, when interaction of this fatty acid with tocopherols in the gut was avoided, by giving them at separate times. When tocopherol and fatty acids were given together and interaction in the gut could take place, only about half as much tocopherol was recovered from rats given linoleate as from those given oleate. This was attributed to loss of tocopherol in the gut by increased peroxidation due to the presence of linoleate.

## B. Vitamin E Requirement and Dietary E/PUFA Ratio

It has been suggested by many researchers that PUFA intake should be balanced by a concomitant intake of vitamin E. Harris and Embree

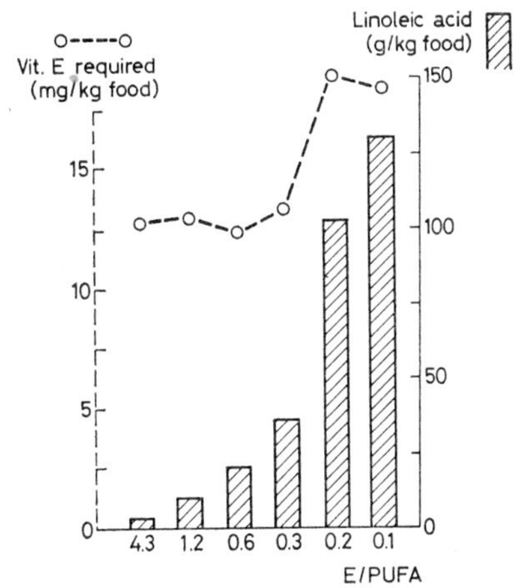


Fig. 19. Effect of intake of linoleic acid on vitamin E requirement of rats. E/PUFA = intake of D-α-tocopherol (mg) divided by intake of linoleic acid (g).

(1963) were led to calculate, that the dietary E/PUFA ratio should be at least 0·6. That is, the intake of each gramme of PUFA would need a concomitant intake of at least 0·6 mg D-α-tocopherol, as otherwise symptoms of vitamin E deficiency could be expected. For this reason the results of the (spontaneous *in vitro*) haemolysis test in rats in relation to the effect of linoleic acid intake on vitamin E requirement (Jager, 1969b, c; Jager and Houtsmuller, 1970) have been compiled in Fig. 19. They indicate quite clearly that as no fixed critical dietary E/PUFA ratio exists, any attempts to calculate such a ratio for the evaluation of the vitamin E adequacy of a certain diet, is pointless.

## C. Vitamin E Requirement and EFA Deficiency (E/PUFA ratio in membranes)

Literature data concerning the relation between linoleic acid intake and vitamin E requirement often seem contradictory. We find, on the one hand, experiments in which the addition of even small amounts of linoleic acid to the diet caused an increase in vitamin E requirement (Dam *et al.*, 1958; Hutcheson *et al.*, 1963; Calvert *et al.*, 1964; Weber *et al.*, 1964; Bieri and Poukka, 1970), and on the other, experiments in which linoleic acid had no such effect (Søndergaard and Dam, 1966;

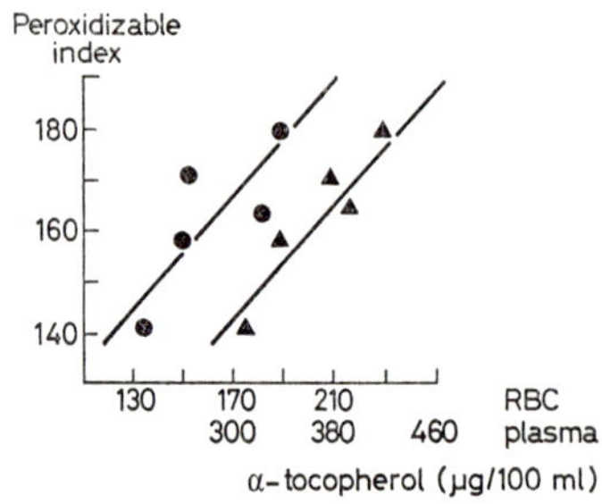


Fig. 20. (Bieri and Poukka, 1970.) Relationship between the peroxidizable index of the erythrocyte polyunsaturated fatty acids and the α-tocopherol content of the red cells (●) or plasma (▲) required to prevent 10% haemolysis in EFA-deficient rats.

Jager and Houtsmuller, 1970). This discrepancy is due to the fact that in the first series of experiments, all diets used were EFA deficient. In this case the addition of linoleic acid to the diet causes an increase in the PUFA content (mainly arachidonic acid) of the bio-membranes, which is reflected by an increase in the need for vitamin E. This is, for instance, clearly demonstrated by the experiments of Bieri and Poukka (1970), who used the *in vitro* haemolysis test to determine vitamin E requirement. They found in their EFA-deficient rats a linear, positive relationship between the peroxidizable index of the erythrocytes and the required plasma α-tocopherol level needed to prevent haemolysis (Fig. 20).

The peroxidizable index (PI) is used to indicate the sensitivity to oxidative destruction of the erythrocyte lipids. The index represents an estimate of the relative peroxidizability of the PUFA and is obtained by multiplying the percentages of the various fatty acids by the following factors: 1, 2, 4, 6 and 8 for fatty acids containing: 2, 3, 4, 5 and 6 double bonds respectively (Holman, 1954; Witting and Horwitt, 1964a).

A case comparable to that in Fig. 20 was mentioned by Witting (1972), who found that in EFA- and vitamin E deficient rats, the time needed to produce creatinuria decreased as the percentage $\omega$6-fatty acids in the muscle fatty acids was increased by the addition of linoleic acid to the diet.

These examples show that although the E/PUFA ratio is not critical in diets, it is very probably critical in the biomembranes of erythrocytes and muscle. In other words, a certain amount of PUFA incorporated in biomembranes needs a circumscribed amount of $\alpha$-tocopherol for protection against (oxidative) destruction. This view fits in quite well with a hypothesis by Diplock *et al.* (1971) and Lucy (1972) put forward on the basis of studies with molecular models. Lucy (1972) suggested that polyunsaturated lipids can be packed in an orderly manner in a bilayer membrane by association with either vitamin E or cholesterol molecules. A special relation is assumed to exist between arachidonic acid and $\alpha$-tocopherol. The position of two methyl groups of the alkyl-side chain of the $\alpha$-tocopherol molecule is thought here to be opposite ("space filling") to the system of double bonds of arachidonic acid. In the light of this special relation between $\alpha$-tocopherol (which would fit in better than the other tocopherols) and arachidonic acid, it is easy to explain the increased need for vitamin E of EFA-deficient animals given additional dietary linoleic acid, as a proportional increase in arachidonic acid in the biomembranes results from linoleic acid intake in EFA-deficient animals (Holman, 1960). In nonEFA-deficient animals, however, the increase in dietary linoleic acid has no effect upon the vitamin E requirement, because the biomembranes are already "saturated" with arachidonic acid, and there is at least no important increase in PUFA. As shown in Table 8 (Jager, 1972c), the erythrocyte lipids increase their linoleic acid content, mainly at the expense of oleic acid (Jager and Houtsmuller, 1970). The increased need for vitamin E at an intake of 25·6 cal% linoleic acid is obviously not due to a change in the fatty acid composition of the erythrocyte membrane, but is the result of a lowered blood tocopherol level, as explained previously. The PIs are lower than those found by Bieri and Poukka (1970), but this must be due to differences in the strains of rats used.

In order to get enough essential fatty acids, male rats would need 1–2 cal% linoleic acid in their diets (Holman, 1960). For chickens these figures are 3·6 and 1·8 cal% for males and females respectively (Menge, 1970).

Table 8

Dietary linoleic acid content, fatty-acid composition of erythrocyte lipids and vitamin E requirement (haemolysis test) of rats

| Linoleic acid | | Erythrocyte lipids (%) | | | | |
|---|---|---|---|---|---|---|
| Weight % | Cal% | C 18:1 ω9 | C 18:2 ω6 | C 20:4 ω6 | PI[a] | Vitamin E requirement[b] |
| 0·27[c] | 0·5 | 13·7 | 5·2 | 18·8 | 128 | 12·9 |
| 0·98 | 2·0 | 12·2 | 7·9 | 19·5 | 130 | 12·8 |
| 3·6 | 7·0 | 9·9 | 9·4 | 20·9 | 135 | 12·7 |
| 13·0 | 25·6 | 9·0 | 13·3 | 20·7 | 145 | 18·5 |

[a] PI = peroxidizable index of erythrocyte lipids.
[b] D-α-tocopheryl acetate (mg/kg food).
[c] This diet was in fact deficient in essential fatty acids, but no important decrease in erythrocyte arachidonic acid was found because of a preceding period of eight weeks on a diet containing 4 cal% linoleic acid.

## V. VITAMIN E ADEQUACY OF FATS AND OILS

For the calculation of the vitamin E adequacy of a fat, it should be noted that in a diet containing a normal amount of fat (40 cal%) the fat component must contain sufficient tocopherol to cover the total dietary requirement for vitamin E.

Table 7 shows that dietary linoleic acid up to an intake of about 10 cal% does not affect the basic requirement for vitamin E. This corresponds with a linoleic acid content of $100/40 \times 10 = 25\%$ in the dietary fat.

As a general conclusion from Table 7, we may state that 3 mg D-α-tocopherol/1000 kcal of food will be sufficient to meet the basic need for vitamin E, which need may increase to 200% at linoleic acid intakes above 10 cal%. Calculated on this basis we may say that a dietary fat (9·4 kcal/g) at an intake of 40 cal%, needs $100/40 \times 3 \times 9{\cdot}4 \approx 70$ mg D-α-tocopherol/kg fat, in order to contain enough vitamin E, if the fat contains more than 25% linoleic acid, the need may increase to 140 mg/kg fat.

More vitamin E per kg fat would be needed at a lower dietary fat level. For a diet containing 30 cal% fat, the basis need would be 93 and 186 mg D-α-tocopherol/kg fat, for fats containing less or more than 25% linoleic acid respectively. For the sake of convenience we might state that at a normal range of fat intake (30–40 cal%), 100 mg D-α-tocopherol/kg fat will be sufficient, an amount that will increase to 200 mg, if the dietary fat contains more than 25 cal% linoleic acid.

The vitamin E "adequacy" of different fats and oils are compiled in Fig. 21, based on a dietary fat intake of 35 cal%. The vitamin E content of the (refined) oils is based on data obtained from Weber *et al.* (1962), Herting and Drury (1963), Swern (1969) and Slover (1971). The total of different tocopherols has been expressed as equivalents of mg D-α-tocopherol, according to the bio-potencies given by Brubacher and Weiser (1967) (see Fig. 1).

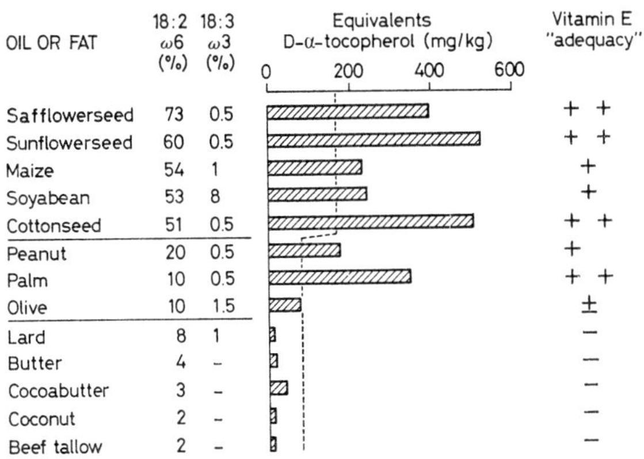


Fig. 21. Linoleic and linolenic acid contents and vitamin E adequacy of several oils and fats. Dotted line: amount of vitamin E required.

The most striking fact to appear from Fig. 21 is that obviously all highly saturated fats are deficient in vitamin E, whereas most vegetable oils with a high linoleic acid content must be considered natural sources of vitamin E. This was not only found from the experiment of Jager (1972b, c), but was also supported by the work of Dayton *et al.* (1965) and Alfin-Slater *et al.* (1969a, b), who found linoleic-rich vegetable oils to be adequate in vitamin E.

An exact evaluation of soybean oil meets with some difficulty because of its relatively high content of linolenic acid. Quantitative experimental data, with respect to the effect of dietary linolenic acid on vitamin E requirement in non-EFA-deficient diets, are not available.

It was noted in several cases (in EFA- and vitamin E-deficient animals) that whereas dietary linoleic acid aggravated symptoms of vitamin E deficiency, dietary linolenic acid did not; these symptoms were encephalomalacia in chicks (Dam *et al.*, 1958), myopathy in chicks (Hudcheson *et al.*, 1963) or testicular degeneration in rats (Witting *et al.*, 1967; Witting, 1970).

In a border-line case of dietary-EFA deficiency, however, it was noted that ample dietary linolenic acid increased the onset of creatinuria in rats (Witting and Horwitt, 1964a; Witting, 1970). This was associated with an increase of ω3-fatty acids in the muscle phospholipids.

Therefore, although dietary linolenic acid might affect the fatty acid composition of biomembranes and consequently the requirement for vitamin E, this effect will be relatively unimportant in circumstances where the diet supplies ample linoleic acid. This may be concluded from feeding experiments on rats by Walker (1972), when the PI of different organ lipids is calculated from their fatty acid compositions.

For this reason linolenic acid must be judged on its peroxidizability, i.e. on the extent to which an increased destruction of vitamin E in the intestinal tract (as is supposed to occur at high linoleic acid intake) may be expected. The PI of soyabean oil is not higher than that of safflowerseed oil and therefore soyabean oil must be regarded as adequate in vitamin E.

## VI. CONCLUSIONS

In the study of the effect of linoleic acid intake on vitamin E requirement, much confusion has arisen from the fact that many researchers did not realize that they were working with EFA-deficient animals.

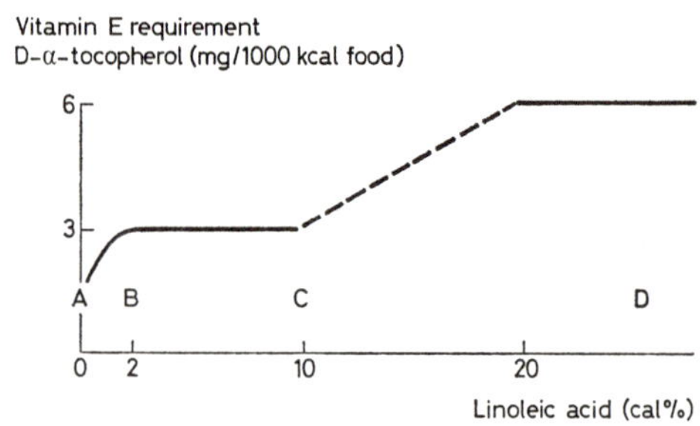


Fig. 22. Relationship between dietary content of linoleic acid and vitamin E requirement.

Under the conditions of EFA deficiency, the addition of only small amounts of dietary linoleic acid results in an increased PUFA content (especially arachidonic acid) of membrane structural lipids, which is obviously associated with a proportionally increased need for vitamin E (Fig. 22; phase AB).

In normal animals, when biomembrane systems are "saturated" with essential fatty acids, dietary linoleic acid has no effect on the vitamin E requirement (Fig. 22; phase BC) except when very high intakes of linoleic acid are involved (Fig. 22; phase CD), which appears to be associated with a lowered blood tocopherol level, probably because of an increased destruction of tocopherol in the intestinal tract.

A critical dietary E/PUFA ratio, which might otherwise be used for evaluating the vitamin E adequacy of a given diet, does not exist.

Most saturated fats are inadequate in vitamin E; vegetable oils rich in linoleic acid may be considered the natural sources of vitamin E.

At a normal range of fat intake (30–40 cal %), 100 mg D-α-tocopherol/kg fat is sufficient to meet the need for vitamin E, but if the dietary fat contains more than 25% linoleic acid this value increases to a maximum of 200 mg/kg fat.

## REFERENCES


Adamstone, F. B., Krider, J. L. and James, M. F. (1949). Response of swine to vitamin E-deficient rations. *Ann. N.Y. Acad. Sci.* **52**, 260.

Alfin-Slater, R. B., Hansen, H. and Marris, R. S. (1969a). Dietary fat composition and tocopherol requirement: I. Lack of correlation between nutritional indices and results of *in vitro* peroxide haemolysis tests. *J. Am. Oil Chem. Soc.* **46**, 563.

Alfin-Slater, R. B., Morris, R. B. and Aftergood, L. (1969b). Dietary fat composition and tocopherol requirement: II. Nutritional status of heated and unheated vegetable oils of different ratios of unsaturated fatty acids and vitamin E. *J. Am. Oil Chem. Soc.* **46**, 657.

Anderson, H. D., Elvehjem, C. A. and Gonce, J. E. (1939). Vitamin E deficiency in dogs. *Proc. Soc. Exp. Biol. Med.* **42**, 750.

Anonymus (1966). Experimental nutritional dystrophy and isozymes. *Nutr. Rev.* **24**, 337.

Anonymus (1969). A syndrome of vitamin E deficiency? *Lancet* **i**, 405.

Berg, B. N. (1967). *In* "Pathology of Laboratory Rats and Mice" (E. Cothin and F. J. Roe, eds), p. 749. Blackwell, Oxford.

Bieri, J. G. and Poukka, R. K. H. (1970). *In vitro* haemolysis as related to rat erythrocyte content of α-tocopherol and polyunsaturated fatty acids. *J. Nutr.* **100**, 557.

Binder, H. J. and Spiro, H. M. (1967). Tocopherol deficiency in man. *Am. J. Clin. Nutr.* **20**, 594.

Binder, H. J., Herting, D. C., Hurst, V., Finch, S. C. and Spiro, H. M. (1965). Tocopherol deficiency in man. *New Engl. J. Med.* **273**, 1289.

Bird, J. W. C. and Carabello, F. (1966). Serum ATP creatine phosphotransferase activity in guinea-pigs with experimental muscular dystrophy. *Nature* **210**, 95.

Bonetti, E. and Stirpe, F. (1962). Conditions affecting dietary liver necrosis and liver regeneration in rats. *J. Nutr.* **77**, 179.

Bowman, O. and Dryer, I. A. (1960). Experimentally induced muscular dystrophy; blood creatine levels and histopathology in dystrophic rabbits. *J. Nutr.* **72**, 289.

Brubacher, G. and Weiser, H. (1967). Biologische Wirksamkeit von Tocopherol und von Antioxydantien. *Wissensch. Veröffent. Deut. Ges. Ern.* **16**, 50. Steinkopff Verlag, Darmstadt.

Bunnell, R. H., Keating, J., Quaresimo, A. and Parman, G. K. (1965). Alpha-tocopherol content of foods. *Am. J. Clin. Nutr.* **17**, 1.

Bunyan, J., Murrell, E. A., Green, J. and Diplock, A. T. (1967). On the existence and significance of lipid peroxides in vitamin E deficient animals. *Brit. J. Nutr.* **21**, 475.

Calvert, C. C., Desai, I. D. and Scott, M. L. (1964). Effect of linoleic acid on nutritional muscular dystrophy in the chick. *J. Nutr.* **83,** 307.

Carabello, F., Liu, F., Eames, C. and Bird, J. (1971). Effect of vitamin E deficiency on mitochondrial energy transfer. *Fed. Proc. Fedn. Am. Socs. Exp. Biol.* **30,** 639.

Cheville, N. F. (1966). The pathology of vitamin E deficiency in the chick. *Path. Vet.* **3,** 208.

Christensen, F., Dam, H., Gortner, R. A. and Søndergaard, E. (1956). *In vitro* haemolysis of erythrocytes from vitamin E deficient rats and chicks. *Acta Physiol. Scand.* **35,** 215.

Christensen, F., Dam, H., Prange, I. and Søndergaard, E. (1958). The effect of selenium on vitamin E deficient rats. *Acta Pharmacol. Toxicol.* **15,** 181.

Cohen, G. and Hochstein, P. (1963). Glutathione peroxidase. The primary agent for the elimination of hydrogen peroxide in erythrocytes. *Biochemistry* **2,** 1420.

Corwin, L. M. (1965). Further studies on the regulation of succinate oxidation by vitamin E. *J. Biol. Chem.* **240,** 34.

Cumings, H. W. (1942). The effects of vitamin E deficiency in the guppy Lebistis reticulatus. *Anat. Rec.* **84,** 499.

Dam, H. and Søndergaard, E. (1957). Prophylactic effect of selenium dioxide against degeneration (white striation) of muscles in chicks. *Experientia* **13,** 494.

Dam, H. and Søndergaard, E. (1964). Comparison of the acetates of D-, DL- and L-α-tocopherols against encephalomalacia in chicks. *Z. Ernährungswiss.* **5,** 73.

Dam, H., Prange, I. and Søndergaard, E. (1952). Muscular degeneration (white striation of muscles) in chicks reared on vitamin E deficient low fat diets. *Acta Path. Microbiol. Scand.* **31,** 172.

Dam, H., Kofoed Nielsen, G., Prange, I. and Søndergaard, E. (1958). Influence of linoleic and linolenic acids on symptoms of vitamin E deficiency in chicks. *Nature* **182,** 802.

Dayton, S., Haskimoto, S., Rosenblum, D. and Pearse, M. L. (1965). Vitamin E status of humans during prolonged feeding of unsaturated fats. *J. Lab. Clin. Med.* **65,** 739.

Desai, I. D. and Scott, M. L. (1965). Mode of action of selenium in relation to biological activity of tocopherols. *Arch. Biochem. Biophys.* **110,** 309.

Dinning, S. (1952). Leucocytosis in vitamin E deficient rabbits. *Proc. Soc. Exp. Biol. Med.* **79,** 231.

Dinning, J. and Day, P. L. (1957). Vitamin E deficiency in the monkey. I Muscular dystrophy, haematologic changes and the excretion of urinary nitrogenous constituents. *J. Exp. Med.* **105,** 395.

Diplock, A. T., Cawthorne, M. A., Murrell, E. A., Green, J. and Bunyan, J. (1968). Measurements of lipid peroxidation and α-tocopherol destruction *in vitro* and *in vivo* and their significance in connection with the biological function of vitamin E. *Br. J. Nutr.* **22,** 465.

Diplock, A. T., Baum, H. and Lucy, J. A. (1971). The effect of vitamin E on the oxidation state of selenium in rat liver. *Biochem. J.* **123,** 721.

Draper, H. H. (1959). Biopotency of non-tocopherol compounds in vitamin E deficiency disease. *Proc. Soc. Exp. Biol. Med.* **102,** 737.

Draper, H. H. and Saari Csallany (1969). A simplified hemolysis test for vitamin E deficiency. *J. Nutr.* **98,** 390.

Evans, H. M. (1962). The pioneer history of vitamin E. *Vit. Horm.* **20,** 379.

Evans, H. M. and Bishop, K. S. (1922). On the relation between fertility and nutrition I and II. *J. Metabol. Res.* **1,** 319 and 335.

Evans, H. M., Emerson, G. A. and Telford, I. R. (1938). Degeneration of cross striated musculature in vitamin E-low rats. *Proc. Soc. Exp. Biol. Med.* **38,** 625.
Fitch, C. D., Porter, F. S. and Ebert, R. V. (1964). Studies of the anemia of vitamin E deficiency. *J. Lab. Clin. Med.* **64,** 856.
Forbes, R. M. and Draper, H. M. (1958). Production and study of vitamin E deficiency in the baby pig. *J. Nutr.* **65,** 535.
Friedman, L., Weiss, W., Wherry, F. and Kline, O. L. (1958). Bioassay of vitamin E by the dialuric acid method. *J. Nutr.* **65,** 143.
Gerber, G. B., Gerber, G., Koszalka, T. R. and Emmel, V. M. (1952). Creatine metabolism in vitamin E deficiency in the rat. *Am. J. Physiol.* **202,** 453.
Giese, E., Erzoy, E. and Hill, H. (1965). Der Einfluss von Selen und Vitamin E auf dem Hämoglobin- und Myoglobingehalt sowie auf am Muskelstoffwechsel beteiligte Fermente bei Küken. *Deut. Tierärztl. Wschr.* **72,** 464.
Gilbert, J. J. and Birky, C. W. (1971). Sensitivity and specificity of the Asplanchna response to dietary α-tocopherol. *J. Nutr.* **101,** 113.
Gitler, C., Sunde, M. L. and Baumann, C. A. (1958). Effect of certain necrosis-preventing factors on haemolysis in vitamin E deficient rats and chicks. *J. Nutr.* **65,** 397.
Glavind, J., Christensen, F. and Sylvén, C. (1971). Intestinal absorption and *in vivo* formation of lipoperoxides in vitamin E deficient rats. *Acta Chem. Scand.* **25,** 3220.
Goettsch, M. and Pappenheimer, A. M. (1931). Nutritional muscular dystrophy in the guinea-pig and rabbit. *J. Exp. Med.* **54,** 145.
Goldstein, J. and Scott, M. L. (1956). An electrophoretic study of exudative diathesis in chicks. *J. Nutr.* **60,** 349.
Gordon, H. H. and Nitowsky, H. M. (1956). Some studies of tocopherol in infants and children. *Am. J. Clin. Nutr.* **4,** 391.
Green, J. (1972). Vitamin E and the biological antioxidant theory. *Ann. N.Y. Acad. Sci.* **203,** 29.
Green, J., Diplock, A. T., Bunyan, J., McHale, D. and Muthy, I. R. (1967). Vitamin E and stress: I. Dietary unsaturated fatty acid stress and the metabolism of α-tocopherol in the rat. *Brit. J. Nutr.* **21,** 69.
Gross, R. T., Bracci, R., Rudolph, N., Schroeder, E. and Kochen, J. A. (1967). Hydrogen peroxide toxicity and detoxification in the erythrocytes of newborn infants. *Blood* **29,** 481.
György, P., Cogan, G. and Rose, C. S. (1952). Availability of vitamin E in the newborn infant. *Proc. Soc. Exp. Biol. Med.* **81,** 536.
Hanna, F. M., Jackson, R. L. and Chinn, R. (1965). Vitamin E in the nutrition of the premature newborn infant. *Am. J. Clin. Nutr.* **16,** 384.
Harris, R. S. (1962). Influences of storage and processing on vitamin E. *Vit. Horm.* **20,** 603.
Harris, P. L. and Embree, N. D. (1963). Quantitative consideration of the effect of polyunsaturated fatty acid content of the diet upon the requirements for vitamin E. *Am. J. Clin. Nutr.* **13,** 385.
Hayes, K. C. and Rousseau, J. E. (1970). Dialuric acid haemolysis as an index of plasma tocopherol concentrations in the dog. *Lab. Animal Care* **20,** 48.
Herting, D. C. and Drury, E. J. E. (1963). Vitamin E content of vegetable oils and fats. *J. Nutr.* **81,** 335.
Hill, E. G. (1963). Dietary antioxidants in young swine. *J. Am. Oil Chem. Soc.* **40,** 360.
Holman, R. T. (1954). Autoxidation of fats and related substances. *In* "Progress in the Chemistry of Fats and other Lipids". Vol. 2 (R. T. Holman, W. O. Lundberg and T. Malkin, eds), p. 73. Pergamon Press, Oxford.

Holman, R. T. (1960). The ratio of trienoic: tetraenoic acids in tissue lipids as a measure of essential fatty acid requirement. *J. Nutr.* **70**, 405.

Horwitt, M. K. (1960). Vitamin E and lipid metabolism in Man. *Am. J. Clin. Nutr.* **8**, 451.

Horwitt, M. K. (1965). Role of vitamin E, selenium and polyunsaturated fatty acids in clinical and experimental muscle disease. *Fedn Proc. Fedn Am. Socs. Exp. Biol.* **24**, 68.

Horwitt, M. K., Harvey, C. C., Duncan, G. D. and Wilson, W. C. (1956). Effects of limited tocopherol intake in man with relationship to erythrocyte haemolysis and lipid oxidations. *Am. J. Clin. Nutr.* **4**, 408.

Horwitt, M. K., Century, B. and Zeman, A. A. (1963). Erythrocyte survival time and reticulocyte levels after tocopherol depletion in man. *Am. J. Clin. Nutr.* **12**, 99.

Houchin, O. B. and Mattill, H. A. (1942). *In vitro* effect of α-tocopherol phosphate on oxygen consumption of muscle from vitamin E-deficient animal. *Proc. Soc. Exp. Biol. Med.* **50**, 216.

Hove, E. L., Fry, G. S. and Schwarz, K. (1958). Ineffectiveness of factor 3-active selenium compounds in muscular dystrophy of rabbits on vitamin E-free diets. *Proc. Soc. Exp. Biol. Med.* **98**, 27.

Howes, E. L., Price, H. M. and Blomberg, J. M. (1964). The effects of a diet producing lipochrome pigment (ceroid) on the ultrastructure of skeletal muscle in the rat. *Am. J. Path.* **45**, 599.

Hutcheson, L. M., Hill, D. C. and Jenkins, K. I. (1963). Influence of dietary fat on the efficacy of agents protecting against muscular dystrophy in the chick. *Poultry Sci.* **42**, 846.

Jacob, H. S. and Jandl, J. H. (1966). Effect of sulfhydryl inhibition on red blood cells. Glutathione in the regulation of the hexose monophosphate pathway. *J. Biol. Chem.* **241**, 4243.

Jacob, H. S. and Lux, S. E. (1968). Degradation of membrane phospholipids and thiols in peroxide haemolysis; Studies in vitamin E deficiency. *Blood* **32**, 549.

Jager, F. C. (1968). Determination of vitamin E requirement in rats by means of spontaneous haemolysis *in vitro*. *Nutr. Dieta* **10**, 215.

Jager, F. C. (1969a). Vitamin E deficiency and polyunsaturated fatty acids. *Lancet* **ii**, 380.

Jager, F. C. (1969b). Vitamin E and polyunsaturated fatty acids. *Acta Physiol. Pharmacol. Neerl.* **15**, 47.

Jager, F. C. (1969c). High linoleic acid intake and vitamin E requirement in rats. *Nutr. Dieta* **11**, 270.

Jager, F. C. (1972a). Long-term dose-response effects of vitamin E in rats. Significance of the *in vitro* haemolysis test. *Nutr. Metabol.* **14**, 1.

Jager, F. C. (1972b). Effect of dietary linoleic acid and selenium on the requirement of vitamin E in ducklings. *Nutr. Metabol.* **14**, 210.

Jager, F. C. (1972c). Linoleic acid intakes and vitamin E requirement in rats and ducklings. *Ann. N.Y. Acad. Sci.* **203**, 199.

Jager, F. C. and Houtsmuller, U. M. T. (1970). Effect of dietary linoleic acid on vitamin E requirement and fatty acid composition of erythrocyte lipids in rats. *Nutr. Metabol.* **12**, 3.

Jager, F. C. and Verbeek-Raad, J. A. (1970). Methods for determining vitamin E requirement in ducklings. II. Myopathy, serum enzymes and serum proteins. *Int. J. Vit. Res.* **40**, 597.

Jager, F. C. and Vles, R. O. (1970). Methods for determining vitamin E requirement

in ducklings. I. Myopathy, *in vitro* haemolysis and leucocyte count. *Int. J. Vit. Res.* **40,** 592.
Jager, F. C., Njio, K. D., Verbeek, J. A. and Vles, R. O. (1969). Dose response effects of vitamin E in ducklings. *Acta Physiol. Pharm. Neerl.* **15,** 406.
Jenkins, K. J., Hill, D. C., Hutcheson, L. M. and Branion, H. (1962). Relation of arginine and sulphur amino acids to the development of muscular dystrophy in the chick. *Poultry Sci.* **41,** 61.
Jones, T. C. and Reed, W. O. (1948). Muscular dystrophy in a foal. *J. Am. Vet. Med. Ass.* **113,** 170.
Jungherr, E. and Pappenheimer, A. M. (1937). Nutritional myopathy of the gizzard in turkeys. *Proc. Soc. Exp. Biol. Med.* **37,** 520.
Krishnamurty, S. and Bieri, J. G. (1961). An effect of dietary selenium on haemolysis and lipid autoxidation of erythrocytes from vitamin E deficient rats. *Biochem. Biophys. Res. Commun.* **4,** 384.
Leonard, P. J. and Losowsky, M. S. (1967). Relationship between plasma vitamin E level and peroxide haemolysis test in human subjects. *Am. J. Clin. Nutr.* **20,** 795.
Losowsky, M. S. and Kelleher, J. (1970). Vitamin E research in man in the U.K. *Brit. J. Nutr.* **24,** 1033.
Lucy, J. A. (1972). Functional and structural aspects of biological membranes: A suggested structural role for vitamin E in the control of membrane permeability and stability. *Ann. N.Y. Acad. Sci.* **203,** 4.
Machlin, L. J. and Shalkop, W. T. (1956). Muscular degeneration in chickens fed diets low in vitamin E and sulphur. *J. Nutr.* **60,** 87.
Madsen, L. L., McCay, C. M. and Maynard, L. A. (1933). Possible relationship between cod liver oil and muscular degeneration of herbivora fed synthetic diets. *Proc. Soc. Exp. Biol. Med.* **30,** 1434.
Majaj, A. S., Dinning, J. S., Azzam, S. A. and Darby, W. J. (1963). Vitamin E responsive megaloblastic anemia in infants with protein-calorie malnutrition. *Am. J. Clin. Nutr.* **12,** 374.
Marvin, H. N. (1963). Erythrocyte survival of rats deficient in vitamin E or vitamin B6. *J. Nutr.* **80,** 185.
Mason, K. E. and Hartsough, F. R. (1951). "Steatitis" or "Yellow fat" in mink and its relation to dietary fats and inadequacy of vitamin E. *J. Am. Vet. Med. Ass.* **119,** 72.
Menge, H. (1970). Comparative requirements of linoleic acid for male and female chicks. *Poultry Sci.* **49,** 178.
Metzger, H. J. and Hagan, W. A. (1927). The so-called stiff lambs. *Cornell Vet.* **17,** 35.
Mils, G. C. (1957). Hemoglobin catabolism: I. Glutathione peroxidase, an erythrocyte enzyme which protects hemoglobin from oxidative breakdown. *J. Biol. Chem.* **229,** 189.
Molenaar, I., Hommes, F. A., Braams, W. G. and Polman, H. A. (1968). Effect of vitamin E on membranes of the intestinal cell. *Proc. Natn Acad. Sci. U.S.* **61,** 982.
Molenaar, I., Vos, J., Jager, F. C. and Hommes, F. A. (1970). The influence of vitamin E deficiency on biological membranes. An ultrastructural study on the intestinal epithelial cells of ducklings. *Nutr. Metabol.* **12,** 358.
Molenaar, I., Vos. J. and Hommes, F. A. (1972). Effect of vitamin E deficiency on cellular membranes. *Vit. Horm.* **30,** 45.
Moore, T. and Sharman, I. M. (1964). The mode of action of vitamin E and its substitutes. *Int. J. Vit. Res.* **34,** 317.

Moore, T., Sharman, I. M. and Ward, R. J. (1957). The destruction of vitamin E in flour by chlorine dioxide. *J. Sci. Food Agric.* **8,** 97.

Nafstad, J. (1965). Studies of haematology and bone marrow morphology in vitamin E deficient pigs. *Path. Vet.* **2,** 277.

Naito, H., Johnson, B. and Johnson, B. C. (1966). Some effects of methyl linoleate hydroperoxide on oxidative phosphorylation in rat liver mitochondria. *Proc. Soc. Exp. Biol. Med.* **122,** 545.

Nitowski, H. M. and Tildon, J. T. (1956). Some studies of tocopherol deficiency in infants and children: III. Relation of blood catalase activity and other factors to hemolysis of erythrocytes in hydrogen peroxide. *Am. J. Clin. Nutr.* **4,** 397.

Olcott, H. S. (1938). The paralysis in the young of vitamin E deficient female rats. *J. Nutr.* **15,** 221.

Oliveira, M. M. and Vaughan, M. (1964). Incorporation of fatty acids into phospholipids of erythrocyte membranes. *J. Lipid Res.* **5,** 156.

Oski, F. A. and Barness, L. A. (1967). Vitamin E deficiency; A previously unrecognized cause of haemolytic anemia in the premature infant. *J. Pediat.* **70,** 211.

Pappenheimer, A. M. (1939). The pathology of nutritional muscular dystrophy in young rats. *Am. J. Pathol.* **15,** 179.

Pappenheimer, A. M. (1940). Prevention of nutritional myopathy of ducklings by α-tocopherol. *Proc. Exp. Biol. Med.* **45,** 457.

Pappenheimer, A. M. and Goettsch, M. (1934). Nutritional myopathy in ducklings. *J. Exp. Med.* **59,** 35.

Porter, F. S., Fitch, C. D. and Dinning, J. S. (1962). Vitamin E deficiency in the monkey: IV. Further studies of the anemia with emphasis on bone marrow morphology. *Blood* **20,** 471.

Poukka, R. K. H. and Bieri, J. G. (1970). Blood α-tocopherol: Erythrocyte and plasma relationships *in vitro* and *in vivo*. *Lipids* **5,** 757.

Proctor, J. F., Maplesden, D. C., Hogue, D. E. and Loosli, J. K. (1961). Relation of vitamin E, selenium and other factors to muscular dystrophy in the rabbit. *Proc. Soc. Exp. Biol. Med.* **108,** 77.

Pudelkiewicz, W. J. and Nakiya, M. (1969). Some relationships between plasma, liver and excreta tocopherol in chicks fed graded levels of alpha-tocopherylacetate. *J. Nutr.* **97,** 303.

Ringler, D. H. and Abrams, G. D. (1971). Laboratory diagnosis of vitamin E deficiency in rabbits fed a faulty commercial ration. *Lab. Animal Sci.* **21,** 383.

Rose, C. S. and György, P. (1950a) Haemolysis with alloxan and alloxan-like compounds and the protective action of tocopherol. *Blood* **5,** 1062.

Rose, C. S. and György, P. (1950b). Tocopherol requirement of rats by means of the haemolysis test. *Proc. Soc. Exp. Biol. Med.* **74,** 411.

Rose, C. S. and György, P. (1952). Specificity of haemolytic reaction in vitamin E deficient erythrocytes. *Am. J. Physiol.* **168,** 414.

Schwarz, K. and Foltz, C. M. (1957). Selenium as an integral part of factor 3 against dietary necrotic liver degeneration. *J. Am. Chem. Soc.* **79,** 3292.

Scott, M. L. (1962). Vitamin E in health and disease of poultry. *Vit. Horm.* **20,** 621.

Scott, M. L. (1970). Nutritional and metabolic interrelationships involving vitamin E, selenium and cystine in the chicken. *Int. J. Vit. Res.* **40,** 334.

Scott, M. L. and Calvert, C. C. (1962). Evidence of a specific effect of cystine in the prevention of nutritional muscular dystrophy in vitamin E deficient chicks. *J. Nutr.* **77,** 105.

Scott, M. L., Olson, G., Krook, L. and Brown, W. R. (1967). Selenium-responsive myopathies of myocardium and of smooth muscle in the young poult. *J. Nutr.* **91,** 573.

Silber, R., Winter, R. and Kayden, H. J. (1969). Tocopherol transport in the rat erythrocyte. *J. Clin. Invest.* **48,** 2089.

Slover, H. T. (1971). Tocopherols in foods and fats. *Lipids* **6,** 291.

Smith, C. L., Kelleher, J., Losowsky, M. S. and Morrish, N. (1971). The content of vitamin E in British diets. *Brit. J. Nutr.* **26,** 89.

Søndergaard, E. and Dam, H. (1966). Influence of the level of dietary linoelic acid on the amount of D-α-tocopheryl acetate required for protection against encephalomalacia. *Z. Ernaehrungswiss.* **6,** 253.

Søndergaard, E. and Dam, H. (1970). The vitamin E activity of 5 different tocopheramines on muscular dystrophy in chicks. *Z. Ernaehrungswiss.* **10,** 71.

Swern, D. (1969). Structure and composition of fats and oils. *In* "Bailey's Industrial Oil and Fat Products" (D. Swern, ed.), p. 40. Interscience Publ. London.

Tappel, A. L. (1962). Vitamin E as the biological lipid antioxidant. *Vit. Horm.* **20,** 493.

Tappel, A. L. (1965). Free-radical lipid peroxidation damage and its inhibition by vitamin E and selenium. *Fedn Proc. Fedn Am. Socs. Exp. Biol.* **24,** 73.

Tappel, A. L. (1970). Biological antioxidant protection against lipid peroxidation damage. *Am. J. Clin. Nutr.* **23,** 1137.

Theorell, H. and Ehrenberg, A. (1952). The reaction between catalase, azide and hydrogen peroxide. *Arch. Biochem.* **41,** 462.

Tsen, C. C. and Collier, H. B. (1960). The protective action of tocopherol against hemolysis of rat erythrocytes by dialuric acid. *Can. J. Biochem. Physiol.* **38,** 957.

Van Vleet, J. F., Hall, B. V. and Simon, J. (1968). Vitamin E deficiency. A sequential light and electron microscopic study of skeletal muscle degeneration in weaning rabbits. *Am. J. Path.* **52,** 1067.

Vawter, L. R. and Records, E. (1947). Muscular dystrophy (white muscle disease) in young calves. *J. Am. Vet. Med. Ass.* **110,** 152.

Vles, R. O. and Jager, F. C. (1970). Etude expérimentale des besoins en vitamin E lors d'ingestion élevée d'acide linoléique. *Int. J. Vit. Res.* **40,** 138.

Vogtmann, H. and Prabucki, A. L. (1971). Über den Einfluss der Art des Futterfettes auf das Fettsäuremuster der Leberlipide sowie auf den Vitamin-A- und -E-Gehalt der Leber von Legehennen. *Int. J. Vit. Nutr. Res.* **41,** 33.

Vos, J. (1972). Cellulaire membranen bij vitamine E gebrek. Thesis. University of Groningen. The Netherlands.

Vos, J., Molenaar, I., Searle-van Leeuwen, M. and Hommes, F. A. (1972). Mitochondrial and microsomal membranes from livers of vitamin E-deficient ducklings. *Ann. N.Y. Acad. Sci.* **203,** 74.

Waku, K. and Lands, W. E. M. (1968). Control of lecithin biosynthesis in erythrocyte membranes. *J. Lipid. Res.* **9,** 12.

Walker, B. L. (1972). Deposition of erucic acid in rat tissue lipids. *Nutr. metabol.* **14,** 8.

Walker, B. L. and Kummerow, F. A. (1964). Dietary fat and the structure and properties of rat erythrocytes. *J. Nutr.* **82,** 323.

Walter, E. D. and Jensen, L. S. (1964). Serum glutamic-oxaloacetic transaminase levels, muscular dystrophy and certain haematological measurements in chicks and poults as influenced by vitamin E, selenium and methionine. *Poultry Sci.* **43,** 919.

Ward, R. J. (1963). Sex differences in the α-tocopherol requirement of rats as shown by the haemolysis test. *Brit. J. Nutr.* **17,** 135.

Ways, P. and Hanahan, D. (1964). Characterization and quantification of red cell lipids in normal man. *J. Lipid Res.* **5,** 318.

Weber, F., Gloor, U. and Wiss, O. (1962). Vitamin E und essentielle Fettsäuren. *Fette Seifen Anstrichmittel* **64,** 1149.

Weber, F. and Weiser, H. (1967). Vitamin E bedarf. *Wissen. Veröffent. Deut. Ges. Ern.* **16,** 139. Steinkopff Verlag, Darmstadt.

Weber, F., Weiser, H. and Wiss, O. (1964). Bedarf an Vitamin E in Abhängigkeit von der Zufuhr an Linolsäure. *Z. Ernaehrungswiss.* **4,** 245.

Whitaker, J. A., Fort, E. G., Vimokesant, S. and Dinning, J. S. (1967). Haematologic response to vitamin E in the anemia associated with protein-caloric malnutrition. *Am. J. Clin. Nutr.* **20,** 783.

Wittels, B. and Hochstein, P. (1966). The effect of primaquine on lecithin metabolism in human erythrocytes. *Biochem. Biophys. Acta* **125,** 594.

Witting, L. A. (1965). Biological availability of tocopherol and other antioxidants at the cellular level. *Fedn Proc. Fedn Am. Socs. Exp. Biol.* **24,** 912.

Witting, L. A. (1970). The interrelationship of polyunsaturated fatty acids and anti-oxidants *in vivo*. *In* "Progress in the Chemistry of Fats and Other Lipids", Vol IX. (R. T. Holman, ed.), p. 519. Pergamon Press, Oxford.

Witting, L. A. (1972). Recommended dietary allowance for vitamin E. *Am. J. Clin. Nutr.* **25.** 257.

Witting, L. A., Century, B. and Horwitt, M. K. (1967). *In* "Nutrition and Health", Vol. 1. (Kuhnau, J., ed.), pp. 199–202. Pergamon Press, Oxford.

Witting, L. A. and Horwitt, M. K. (1964a). Effect of degree of fatty acid unsaturation in tocopherol deficiency-induced creatinuria. *J. Nutr.* **82,** 19.

Witting, L. A. and Horwitt, M. K. (1964b). Effects of dietary selenium, methionine, fat level and tocopherol on rat growth. *J. Nutr.* **84,** 351.

Witting, L. A., Likhite, V. N. and Horwitt, M. K. (1967). The effect of antioxidant-deficiency on tissue lipid composition in the rat: III. Testes. *Lipids* **2,** 103.

Wolf, E., Kollonitsch, V. and Kline, C. H. (1963). A survey of selenium treatment in livestock production. *J. Agr. Food Chem.* **11,** 355.

Zalkin, H., Tappel, A. L., Caldwell, K. A., Shibko. S. and Holliday, T. A. (1962). Increased lysozomal enzymes in muscular dystrophy of vitamin E-deficient rabbits. *J. Biol. Chem.* **237,** 2678.

# 10 Nutritional Aspects of Rapeseed Oil

R. O. VLES

*Unilever Research, Vlaardingen, The Netherlands*

# I. INTRODUCTION

## A. Rapeseed Market

Cruciferous oilseed crops play an important role in the international market of vegetable oils, meals and seeds. They are grown successfully in an area extending from the northernmost farming areas of Canada and Europe to the subtropics (Downey, 1971). Oils extracted from these seeds, particularly from current varieties of the genus *Brassica*, have a long history of consumption by man. Rape (*Brassica napus*) and turnip rape (*Brassica campestris*) are commercially the most important species. Furthermore both have winter and spring varieties. India, China, Canada, France, Pakistan, Germany, Poland and Sweden are the major producers of rapeseed. The world production of rapeseed oil places its tonnage in fifth place as an edible oil after soyabean, sunflowerseed, groundnut and cottonseed oil (Lesieur, 1971). It accounts for about 4% of the total fat production. In the past ten years, the world production of rapeseed increased from 3·6 to 5·6 million metric tons. There has been a steep rise of rapeseed production in the last two decades. The rise is likely to continue in future as the plant is well adapted to a wide range of climatic conditions. Another factor of agricultural importance is the insertion of the rapeseed crop in cereal-grass rotation, which arrests the build-up of cereal diseases (Downey, 1971).

Most of the oil extracted from rapeseed is used in the food market for products such as salad oils, cooking oils, margarine and shortenings, but there seem to exist substantial opportunities for industrial purposes, especially for the oils with a high erucic acid content like crambe oil which is extracted from the seed of *Crambe abyssinica* (Craig, 1971; Tallent, 1972). These oils are used as lubricants and lubricant additives. Moreover, derivatives and products from cleavage of erucic acid can be obtained, giving many useful chemicals (Nieschlag and Wolff, 1971).

## B. Rapeseed Composition

The seeds of the Cruciferae have a characteristic chemical composition due to the presence of large amounts of erucic acid in their triglycerides and to their content of thioglucosides, precursors of goitrogenic compounds and other toxins which restrict the use of rapeseed meal as a protein source.

*1. Seed Lipids*

*a. Fatty acid composition of the oils.* Erucic acid (*cis*-13-docosenoic acid)—a fatty acid with 22 carbon atoms and one double bond at the ninth carbon atom relative to the methyl end of the molecule (22:1 *n*–9)—usually constitutes more than 40% of the total fatty acid content in a large number of wild species and current varieties of the genus *Brassica* (Uzzan and Arondel, 1965; Appelqvist, 1972). Other long-chain fatty acids with 20, 22 and 24 carbon atoms and 0, 1 or 2 double bonds have been detected in rapeseed oil (Ackman, 1966; Haeffner, 1970; Conacher and Page, 1972); the level of saturated fatty acids, particularly palmitic acid (16:0), is low.

Variety and environment can influence the fatty acid composition of the oil and the fat content of the seed. However, the fatty acid composition of the seed is mainly controlled by the genetic constitution of the developing embryo. This has been demonstrated for erucic (22:1 *n*–9) and eicosenoic (20:1 *n*–9) acids in the seed oil of *B. campestris*. The two steps of the elongating system that convert oleic acid via eicosenoic acid into erucic acid have been found to be controlled by a single gene with a series of multiple alleles which act in an additive manner. One recessive allele blocks the chain lengthening. This allele, when present in a homozygous form, consequently causes the absence of erucic acid (Dorrel and Downey, 1964; Downey and Craig, 1964; Rollier, 1973). Similarly, elongation of palmitic acid is most probably involved in the synthesis of saturated and monounsaturated fatty acids of the *n*–7 series. In the maturing seeds the conversion of oleic via linoleic into linolenic acid (Dutton and Mounts, 1966) makes it possible to increase the level of linoleic acid and to lower the linolenic acid content. The fact that only half a rapeseed provides sufficient fatty material to be analysed in detail by gas liquid chromatography greatly facilitates selection for improved fatty acid composition. It is possible to analyse one of the cotyledons and to raise a plant from the other seed half. In 1961, the first report of rapeseed plants producing "zero" erucic oil appeared. This oil, practically free of erucic acid, has been named Canbra oil, a contraction of the words Canada and Brassica (Downey *et al.*, 1969). However, the term "Lear" is rapidly replacing the word Canbra when describing *l*ow *e*rucic *a*cid *r*apeseed.

*b. Glyceride structure.* Oils with a high erucic acid content have a unique glyceride structure. Long-chain monounsaturated acids (erucic and eicosenoic) of rapeseed oil are almost exclusively esterified to the 1- and 3-positions of glycerol (Mattson and Volpenhein, 1961). Plants yielding oils with a high erucic acid content seem to lack the proper biosynthetic pathways for attaching erucic acid at position 2, which suggests an upper limit of about 67 mole per cent of acids with more than 18 carbon atoms in the triglycerides of Cruciferae seeds (Appelqvist, 1968). The glyceride structure of Canbra oil, however, is more closely related to that of peanut oil and olive oil since oleic acid, which replaces erucic and eicosenoic acids in this oil, does not follow such a distribution (Rocquelin *et al.*, 1971; Sergiel, 1973).

*2. Seed Meal*

After extraction of the oil, the Cruciferae seed meal constitutes a good-quality protein for livestock and poultry. Rapeseed meal contains about 40% protein. Unfortunately, the thioglucoside content and the high fibre content due to the thickness of the seed coats severely restrict the use of the meal as a high-protein feed supplement.

*a. Thioglucosides.* Contents and types of thioglucoside (glucosinolate) differ with the various rape species. Environmental conditions similarly influence the thioglucoside content. Goitrogenic and other toxic compounds are formed by enzymatic hydrolysis of these glucosinolates. The hydrolysis is catalysed by thioglucoside hydrolases (myrosinase) which give rise to thiocyanates, isothiocyanates and nitriles (Van Etten *et al.*, 1969; Tallent, 1972). These derivatives cause considerable changes in the thyroids, the lesions being especially evident in growing chickens. Rapeseed meal has no marked goitrogenic influence in cattle, but it is less palatable and less readily digested than other high-protein oilseed meals. Sheep and pigs tolerate rapeseed meal less well than cows (Rutkowski, 1971). Various industrial methods are available to detoxify either the seed, before processing, or the meal, after processing, but these treatments substantially decrease the biological value of the protein or remove only part of the toxic substances. Almost complete removal of thioglucosides is possible by plant breeding and one may expect varieties with greatly improved quality of the meal to become available in the near future. Contrary to the inheritance pattern of erucic acid, the thioglucoside content in rapeseed is largely determined by the genotype of the maternal plant (Krzymanski, 1970). The Polish Bronowski variety is serving as a source for genotypes which are extremely low in thioglucosides. Low thioglucoside content can be combined with low erucic acid content, yielding the "double-zero varieties" (Rutkowski, 1970; Downey, 1971).

*b. Crude fibre.* Crude fibre, due to the thick coat of the seed, constitutes a balast component which is digested with difficulty; it contributes to the low metabolizable energy content of rapeseed meal for chickens (Lodhi *et al.*, 1970; Bell, 1970). Lower percentage and less pigmentation of the seed coats are the next objectives of rapeseed breeding (Lööf and Appelqvist, 1972).

### C. Scope of This Review

Although rapeseed oil has a weak reputation, at least in Europe, as a source of edible fat, its production and use in human nutrition is still increasing. The possible consequences of this increase have lately been questioned since it has been found that this oil not only causes poor growth but also produces pathological effects, especially in the hearts of various laboratory animal species. Comprehensive reviews have been published on the rather extensive literature dealing with the chemical and biological characteristics of rapeseed oil. (Beare, 1957; Rocquelin and Potteau, 1968; Jacquot *et al.*, 1969; Rocquelin *et al.*, 1971; Aaes-Jørgensen, 1972). Rocquelin and Cluzan (1971), Abdellatif (1972) and Rocquelin *et al.* (1973a, b) more specifically surveyed the effects of rapeseed oil on heart muscle. This chapter does not pretend to be a complete bibliographical review; it will attempt to explain and correlate present knowledge on the nutritional, physiopathological and biochemical properties of (very) long-chain fatty acids, particularly of those present in rapeseed oil.

## II. NUTRITIVE VALUE

### A. Effects on Growth

There is general agreement in the literature that rapeseed oil and erucic acid retard the growth of young rats in proportion to the amount in the diet (Jacquot *et al.*, 1969); this depression of growth becomes important at levels of rapeseed oil equal to or exceeding 15% by weight in the diet. The poor growth performances have been mainly related in the past to decreased feed consumption (Thomasson, 1955a). However, it has now become clear that the low appetite is only partly responsible for the retarded growth; recent data indicate that poor digestibility and low caloric efficiency also contribute to the low nutritive value of rapeseed oil with a high erucic acid content. The preference of the rat for oils and fats other than rapeseed oil becomes only of any importance at dietary levels of 20% by weight or more (Rocquelin and Potteau, 1968). Depressed growth corresponding to lower feed efficiency (weight gain in g per g ingested feed multiplied by 100) has been found in rat experiments in which no influence of rapeseed oil on feed consumption was noted (Cheniti *et al.*, 1967a; Rocquelin and Cluzan, 1968; Pipy *et al.*, 1972). Recently, Hornstra (1972) found that rats fed diets containing 31·5% by weight of rapeseed oil *ad libitum* for 64 weeks, required more feed to achieve lower growth than rats on a similar sunflowerseed oil diet.

The growth-depressing effects of dietary rapeseed oil have also been observed in other animal species. In three-month-old pigs, a diet in which 28% of the calories (28 cal%) were supplied by rapeseed oil, induced poorer growth and lower feed efficiency than a diet containing isocaloric amounts of soyabean oil (Roine *et al.*, 1960). Thoron (1969) found no growth depression in pigs fed 15% by weight of rapeseed oil for eight months; the feed intake of the animals was, however, somewhat higher and consequently the feed efficiency lower. A long-term experiment with rabbits similarly pointed to poor growth as a result of lower feed efficiency of a diet containing rapeseed oil (Abdellatif and Vles, 1971b).

Differences in growth between mice and hamsters fed butterfat and rapeseed oil were significant at a 40 cal% rapeseed oil level; 50 cal% rapeseed oil caused important growth retardation in ten-week-old guinea-pigs in comparison with butterfat or rapeseed oil (Thomasson *et al.*, 1970). Abdellatif and Vles (unpublished data) found that mice fed rapeseed oil needed more feed per unit of weight gain than mice fed sunflowerseed oil.

In one-day-old Pekin ducklings, diets with 20, 40 and 60 cal% butterfat, or rapeseed oil containing 40% erucic acid, induced mortality and growth depression in the groups fed 40 and 60 cal% rapeseed oil (Abdellatif and Vles, 1970b). In one-week-old Pekin ducklings fed 10, 20, 25, 30, 35 and 40 cal% rapeseed oil containing 50% erucic acid, Abdellatif and Vles (1970b) similarly observed a high rate of mortality and significant growth depression in the group fed 40 cal% rapeseed oil.

At 20% by weight of rapeseed oil in the diet, depression of growth and lower feed consumption were noticed in turkey poults and chicks as compared with birds fed rapeseed oil with a low erucic acid content (Canbra oil) (Walker *et al.*, 1970). Salmon (1969a, b) similarly observed depressed growth in turkey poults and chicks fed diets containing 9 and 10% by weight of rapeseed oil respectively; the turkey poults fed the 9% rapeseed oil diet consumed more feed in the first 14 days than those receiving the 9% soyabean oil diet. Salmon and O'Neil (1971) later confirmed the growth-depressing effect in these birds fed 11·4% dietary rapeseed oil in comparison with palm oil. Older birds are less susceptible to the growth-depressing effect of rapeseed oil, as is shown by Blakely *et al.* (1965) in 20 to 24-week-old finishing turkeys. Sheppard *et al.* (1971), studying the nutritive value of crambe oil (54% erucic acid) in comparison with rapeseed oil (32% erucic acid) and corn oil, found that diets containing 16% by weight of the crambe and rapeseed oils produced poorer growth and lower feed efficiency than a 16% corn oil diet in one-day-old White Plymouth Rock and White Leghorn chicks.

Vogtmann *et al.* (1973a), investigating in chicks the utilization of lard, soyabean oil and rapeseed oils of high and low erucic acid content at 5, 10 and 15% levels in isocaloric and isonitrogenous starter rations, found that feeding 15% regular rapeseed oil containing 21·4% erucic acid depressed growth. This growth depression was not associated with a decreased feed efficiency but due to lower feed consumption.

## B. Digestibility

As early as 1948, Deuel *et al.* related the poor growth performance of rats fed 10% rapeseed oil to poor digestibility, which was in turn thought to be due to the characteristically high content of erucic acid in this oil. There is now well documented evidence that the low digestibility of rapeseed oil in rats is mainly the result of the poor digestibility of the erucic acid fraction (Caroll, 1958; Savary and Constantin, 1966; Rocquelin and Leclerc, 1969; Demarne *et al.*, 1971). Rocquelin and Leclerc (1969) showed that 75% of the recovered faecal fatty acids is erucic acid which was preferentially excreted as free fatty acid or mono- and diglycerides.

The position of the long-chain monoenoic fatty acids in the rapeseed oil triglycerides is of importance in this context of digestibility. Interesterification of rapeseed triglycerides, which may shift 31·7% of erucic acid chains from the original 1–3 esterification positions to the 2-position, improves the digestibility significantly, suggesting a fairly good absorption of 2-monoerucin (Rocquelin *et al.*, 1971; Rocquelin, 1973).

The poorer digestion of rapeseed oil is not compensated for by a better digestion of other non-fatty dietary components (Hornstra, 1972). The low digestibility of rapeseed oil in the rat appears to be insufficient to explain the differences in growth in paired feeding experiments.

McDonald (1972) found that in the pig rapeseed oil was digested more slowly than coconut oil and lard, confirming the slower rate of absorption observed by Deuel *et al.* (1940), Thomasson (1956) and Ziemlanski *et al.* (1972a, b) in the rat. McDonald (1972) found erucic and behenic acids to make up 50% of the faecal fatty acids of pigs rapeseed oil.

Walker and Stokes (1970) showed that in the milk-fed lamb also other fatty acids in rapeseed oil had reduced digestibilities. The same conclusion can be drawn from the data of Vogtmann *et al.* (1973a) for poultry. In turkeys, Salmon (1970) observed a better absorption of the saturated fatty acids when the fat mixture contained 75% rapeseed oil than when rapeseed oil was fed alone.

## C. Caloric Efficiency and Metabolizable Energy

Hornstra (1972) found that in rats the digested calories of a 60 cal% rapeseed oil diet were less efficiently used than those of a 60 cal% sunflowerseed diet. This difference was manifest only in experiments lasting less than seven weeks. After this period the developing difference in body weight between the groups probably masked the differences in caloric efficiency, animals of divergent body weights having different requirements of calories for maintenance. The observed increased relative feed intake coincides with the concept of improper utilization of absorbed calories. Njaa *et al.* (1971), feeding rats 50 cal% hydrogenated rapeseed oil and hydrogenated marine oils containing 38 and 20% C22-acids respectively, found a less efficient utilization of absorbed calories in comparison with lard, mixtures of coconut oil and tallow or hydrogenated soyabean oil. Supplementation with sunflowerseed oil improved the caloric efficiency but did not result in caloric efficiencies equal to those found for the control fats. Monoenoic fatty acids with 20 and 22 carbon atoms appeared to be responsible for this residual difference. Crampton *et al.* (1960) showed that guinea-pigs and swine behaved similar to rats in their inability to efficiently utilize dietary rapeseed oil.

Salmon (1969a, b, 1970), Walker *et al.* (1970) and Sheppard *et al.* (1971) studied the metabolizable energy of diets containing rapeseed oil in turkeys and chicks. In fat nutrition, this metabolizable energy is related to the digestible energy owing to the fact that breakdown products of fat metabolism are not excreted to any extent via the urine. Diets containing 3–9% rapeseed oil (23·7% erucic acid) depressed the dietary metabolizable energy in turkeys during the second week but not during the sixth week of the experiment (Salmon, 1969a). In chicks (Salmon, 1969b), diets containing 5 and 10% rapeseed oil at two different protein levels, did not depress the dietary metabolizable energy in comparison with soyabean oil; the low-protein diets were significantly higher in metabolizable energy than the high-protein diets. Substitution of 10% rapeseed oil for 10% soyabean oil reduced the body weight. So, equal metabolizable energy and depressed growth in chickens and turkeys support the concept of improper utiiization of absorbed energy when rapeseed-oil-containing diets are fed. Walker *et al.* (1970) showed that rapeseed oil which contains no erucic acid is higher in energy value than oils containing erucic acid. Sheppard *et al.* (1971) similarly concluded from experiments with 16% oil in the diet, that crambe and rapeseed oils are inferior to corn oil as energy sources for the chick. Vogtmann *et al.* (1973a) did not notice real differences in the efficiency of energy utilization between chicken fed rapeseed oil (21·4% erucic acid), soyabean oil or lard.

## D. Effects of Saturated Fatty Acids

Thomasson and Boldingh (1955) showed erucic acid to be responsible for the growth-retarding action of rapeseed oil. Thomasson (1955a) did not exclude the possibility that eicosenoic acid (20:1), also present in rapeseed oil, and other long-chain fatty acids as present in owalanut oil, whale oil and herring oil, would also be partly responsible for the lower growth action. The possibility that this growth retardation would further be due to the unbalanced ratio of unsaturated to saturated fatty acids (Hopkins *et al.*, 1955) and/or the low level of palmitic acid, which characterizes rapeseed oil (Beare *et al.*, 1963b), stimulated a series of experiments. Thomasson *et al.* (1970) showed that the addition of palmitic and myristic acids to rapeseed oil induced a better growth than the addition of butterfat. However, no improvement in weight gain was attained when Canbra oil, which contains hardly any erucic acid and has a palmitic acid content similar to that of rapeseed oil, was blended with tripalmitin, tristearin, palm oil or lard (Craig and Beare, 1968). Rocquelin *et al.* (1970, 1971) and Abdellatif and Vles (1970c) showed that Canbra oil of low palmitic and erucic acid content promotes body weight gains in rats similar to those in animals fed peanut oil or sunflowerseed oil. Unbalanced ratio of saturated to monounsaturated fatty acids only influenced the growth of rats when the dietary linoleic acid supply was equal to or lower than 10% of the total fatty acid content (Rocquelin *et al.*, 1970, 1971).

It can be concluded that the observed growth depression in rats fed rapeseed oil is mainly due to the presence of erucic acid in the diet; lower digestibility, prolonged absorption time (Deuel *et al.*, 1940; Thomasson, 1956) and inefficient energetic utilization of the monoenoic long-chain fatty acids appear to determine the lower growth performances. Growth can be improved by the addition of palmitic acid, especially when the linoleic acid level in the fat mixture is low.

Salmon (1969a) reported that turkeys given diets containing 1 or 2% tallow and equal levels of erucic acid overcame the growth-depressing effect of rapeseed oil much more effectively than did turkeys given 1 or 2% soyabean oil and equal levels of erucic acid; this confirms the finding of Beare *et al.* (1963b) that erucic acid is not the sole factor involved in the low growth performance of rats fed rapeseed oil. Abdellatif and Vles (1971a) did not observe appreciable differences in growth among groups of ducklings given 40 cal% rapeseed oil either alone or in combination with olive oil or sunflowerseed oil, whereas the groups fed a mixture of rapeseed oil and tallow grew significantly better. Supplementing diets containing erucic acid with increasing levels of hardened palm oil or glyceryl trilaurate showed that hardened palm oil improved growth response in proportion to its level in the diet whereas glyceryl trilaurate aggravated the growth depression. Supplementation of rapeseed oil with hardened palm oil overcame the growth depression of ducklings more effectively than supplementation with isocaloric amounts of soyabean oil (Abdellatif *et al.*, 1972). However, a low level of palmitic acid in a rapeseed oil low in erucic acid (Abdellatif and Vles, 1973b) did not impair the growth of ducklings compared with groups fed sunflowerseed oil; this confirms similar observations in rats (Craig and Beare, 1968; Rocquelin *et al.*, 1970; Abdellatif and Vles, 1970c), chicks and turkey poults (Walker *et al.*, 1970). Walker *et al.* (1970) and Lall and Slinger (1973a) also observed that chicks, turkey poults and rats utilize mixtures of rapeseed oil and tallow more effectively than could be anticipated from the fats fed singly, which points to a synergistic effect in energy utilization. A similar synergism in fat utilization was found in chicks fed mixtures of palmitic and stearic acids with rapeseed oil. Identical results have been obtained in laying hens (Lall and Slinger, 1973b). This synergistic effect seems to be due to the improved digestibility of the mixture in comparison with the palmitic- and erucic-acid-containing oils fed singly. As a matter of fact, Salmon (1970) showed that the absorption of palmitic and stearic acid was significantly greater when the fat mixture contained 75% rapeseed oil than when rapeseed oil or beef tallow was fed alone.

## E. Longevity

Undernutrition or restriction of feed intake may lengthen the life-span of experimental animals. At dietary levels of 50 cal% rapeseed oil, the feed intake of rats distinctly decreases, so the life-span may be expected to be prolonged. In accordance with this working hypothesis, Thomasson (1955b), using Wistar rats fed 50 cal% fat, observed a longer life-span in the animals on rapeseed oil than in those on a butterfat diet. However, in experiments in which 10, 20, 30, 40, 50, 60 and 72 cal% butterfat or rapeseed oil was administered, no relationship between fat content or type of fat on the one hand and the life-span of the animals on the other hand, could be found (Thomasson *et al.*, 1970). Vles and Abdellatif (1970a), using specific pathogen-free rats from the same Wistar strain, did not find significant differences either in the mortality during the experiment or in the average life-span between groups of 24 animals fed 60 cal% coconut oil, butterfat, corn oil, soyabean oil, rapeseed oil or whale oil. The mean life-span for the different dietary fats was 830, 747, 827, 787, 769 and 814 days respectively. However, in an 89-week experiment with male Swiss mice fed 10, 20, 30, 40, 50, 60 and 70 cal% rapeseed oil or butterfat, the diets containing 40 cal% rapeseed oil or more both retarded the growth and prolonged the life-span (Thomasson *et al.*, 1970). No differences in calorie intake were found between the groups; unfortunately, the gross energy digestion coefficient or the absorption of total calories was not determined. It is conceivable that, similar to the rat, the lower digestibility and lower caloric efficiency of diets containing rapeseed oil are responsible for the longer life-span of mice on a rapeseed oil diet compared with animals on a butterfat diet.

Abdellatif and Vles (1973b) recently found in a three-month experiment with Pekin ducklings that a group fed 35 cal% rapeseed oil (50% erucic acid) grew significantly less than a control group fed 35 cal% sunflowerseed oil; 90% of the animals fed rapeseed oil died in the course of the experiment. No mortality was observed in a third group fed 50 cal% of a rapeseed oil low in erucic acid (8·5% erucic acid) and in the group on a sunflowerseed oil diet.

The data collected for rats and mice support the statement that high levels of rapeseed oil do not seem to shorten the life-span of rats and mice under *ad libitum* feeding conditions.

## III. METABOLISM OF ERUCIC ACID

In order to place precisely the status of rapeseed oil as a food, data on the metabolism of erucic acid in mammalian tissue were considered to be indispensable. The lack of this type of information greatly stimulated further research. Unfortunately, as it will become clear when in this chapter the histopathological effects are described, the majority of biochemical studies prior to 1970 did not include cardiac and muscle tissue, for which organs fatty acids constitute an important source of energy. Mainly two approaches have been followed to clarify the metabolic pathway of erucic acid: first, the group of experiments which studied the incorporation of erucic acid into different tissue lipids and depot fat, and secondly, those which traced the *in vivo* transformation and distribution of labelled erucic acid and measured its oxidation rate.

## A. Incorporation in Tissue Lipids

*1. Rats*

Rats fed rapeseed oil incorporate only a small proportion of dietary erucic acid into their tissue lipids. Wagner *et al.* (1958) found no true accumulation of erucic acid in adult rats maintained for six months on a diet containing rapeseed oil and they concluded that erucic acid behaved as a fatty acid normally metabolized. In rats fed diets containing 20% rapeseed oil or corn oil for 21 weeks, the fatty acid composition of depot fat reflected that of administered dietary oil except for palmitic, palmitoleic, oleic and erucic acids (Craig *et al.*, 1963). The fatty acid analysis of abdominal, cutaneous and carcass fat indicated a physiological tendency to maintain an amount of palmitic acid in the body fat which is not related to the amount in the dietary fat. Less erucic and more oleic acid was found in the tissue lipids than in the diet, which suggests a conversion of erucic acid into oleic acid. Craig and Beare (1968) later showed in a 24-day experiment that 10% eicosenoic acid and 11·4% erucic acid were recovered in total body fat of rats fed 20% rapeseed oil. Rocquelin *et al.* (1970) found that dietary oils of different fatty acid composition hardly changed the level of total saturated and monounsaturated fatty acids of depot fats and other tissue lipids except for cardiac fatty acids. The heart of animals fed rapeseed oil contained more unsaturated fatty acids and less saturated ones. Appreciable amounts of erucic (and eicosenoic) acids were found in abdominal fat (7·4% erucic acid), heart (7·6%) and muscle (5·7%) of young male Wistar rats fed 15% rapeseed oil (44·7% erucic acid) for two months. In male weanling Wistar rats fed 12% rapeseed oil (24·6% erucic acid) for 18 weeks, the greatest deposition of erucic acid occurred in the adrenals (11·7%), decreasing amounts being found in spleen (4·6%), heart (3·1%), plasma (2·9%), kidney (2·3%), erythrocyte (2·2%), testis (2·1%), liver (1·3%) and brain (0·7%) (Walker *et al.*, 1970; Walker, 1972a).

Hornstra (1972), determining the fatty acid spectrum of subcutaneous fat in rats fed 60 cal% rapeseed oil (51·5% erucic acid) for 64 weeks, found that even on prolonged feeding of high levels of rapeseed oil, no considerable amounts of erucic acid are stored (4·2% erucic acid). Studying in great detail the influence of rapeseed, peanut or Canbra oils and mixtures of simple synthetic triglycerides on the composition of liver lipids, Martin (1972) concluded that feeding these fats for periods of two months had practically no quantitative or qualitative effects on the composition of total liver lipids or that of the different lipid classes, the phospholipids in particular. These observations have been largely confirmed by Struijk (1972), Rocquelin (1972, 1973), Quan and Le Breton (1973a, b), Beare *et al.* (1972a) and Kramer *et al.* (1973). Prolonged administration of rapeseed oil similarly led to low incorporation of erucic acid into liver lipids (Hornstra, 1972; Collomb *et al.*, 1973). Data referring to cardiac lipids will be discussed extensively in Section V.

In conclusion, the deposition of erucic acid in rat tissue is, in general, limited. In depot fat of older animals it seldom exceeds 7% of total fatty acids even when a diet high in erucic acid is fed. In young animals, the energetic expense related to body weight is higher than in adults and leads to a faster mobilization and renewal of depot fats. This makes depot fat of a young animal more diet-dependent than that of adults, which explains the somewhat higher incorporation of erucic and eicosenoic acids.

*2. Pigs and Dogs*

Similar low deposition of erucic acid has been found in the pig by Jacquot *et al.* (1967). Young male pigs, fed 15% refined rapeseed oil (45% erucic acid) for six months, showed a very low incorporation of erucic acid into depot triglycerides (2–3%). Linolenic acid from rapeseed oil was incorporated at a relatively higher level (7%). No eicosatrienoic acid (20:3 *n*–9) was found in the male pig genital organs, which suggests a normal utilization of essential fatty acids. Walker (1972b) investigated tissue fatty acids of Yorkshire-type swine, five weeks old, fed 10% rapeseed oil or 10% corn oil for six weeks. The erucic and eicosenoic acid contents of tissue lipids in pigs receiving rapeseed oil were fairly comparable with those reported for rat tissue (Walker, 1972a). The level of erucic acid was highest in the plasma and adipose tissue, where it accounted for over 7% of total fatty acids. In the spleen, adrenal, erythrocyte and heart, erucic acid comprised 3–5% of total fatty acids. In the ovary, liver, kidney and testis 1–3% erucic acid was found. A similar study in the growing pig has been performed by Molnar *et al.* (1972). In dogs fed 60–100 g rapeseed oil/day for 50–76 days, subcutaneous fat contained 6–14% erucic acid, perirenal fat 10–15%, mesenterial fat 7–18% and in one animal an amount of 20% erucic acid was found in the pericardial fat. Practically no erucic acid was found in the phospholipid fraction of kidneys and liver (Bernhard *et al.*, 1960).

*3. Birds*

Chomyszyn (1954) found subcutaneous and peritoneal fat resembling rapeseed oil in consistency, odour, iodine number and melting point in geese that had been fed rapeseed oil. Appreciable quantities of eicosenoic acid (5–8%) and erucic acid (5–6%) were found in adipose tissue of 8-week-old chickens fed the low levels of 4 and 8% rapeseed oil (31·5% erucic acid) in the diet (Sell and Hodgson, 1962), while in chickens fed 6% and 12% rapeseed oil for only 16 days, the content of erucic acid in the depot fat was 14·7 and 16% respectively (Chudy and Batura, 1966). Salmon (1969b) showed that the erucic acid level in depot fat of chickens fed 2·5, 5·0, 7·5 or 10% rapeseed oil (22% erucic acid) for six weeks, was about 50% of that in the dietary fat. There was no major change in the eicosenoic acid content but oleic acid increased in proportion to the disappearance of dietary erucic acid. This is possibly due to the partial degradation of erucic acid through eicosenoic acid to oleic acid, as suggested by Craig and Beare (1967) for the rat.

The data on the fatty acid deposition in chickens differ from those reported for turkeys of the same age by Salmon (1969a; 1970). In the carcass fat of turkeys, 80% of the dietary level of erucic acid was deposited and the remaining 20% was matched by an increase in eicosenoic acid. Turkeys deposit long-chain dietary fatty acids to a larger extent than do chickens. This difference might be due to the more advanced physiological development of chickens in comparison with turkeys at the age of six weeks.

Vogtmann *et al.* (1974) investigated the effects of feeding different levels of rapeseed oils of high and low erucic acid content on the fatty acid composition of various tissues in 4-week-old chickens. The level of eicosenoic and erucic acid in the diet particularly influenced the content of these fatty acids in the spleen lipids. In heart and breast muscle lipids the influence was less marked and in liver lipids it was smallest.

In the laying hen fed erucic acid, Leclercq (1971) noticed a reduction of egg production and egg weight, while no incorporation of erucic acid could be demonstrated in egg lipids. These findings were extended by Vogtmann *et al.* (1973b) who determined the effects of different types of rapeseed oil on egg weight. Regardless of the level of erucic acid in the diet, only traces of erucic acid were found in the egg. Lall and Slinger (1973b) showed a depressing effect of rapeseed oils not only on egg production and egg weight but also on hatchability. Rapeseed oil low in erucic acid exerted no detrimental effects. Leclercq (1972) observed a decrease in egg and yolk weight at an erucic acid level as low as 2% in the diet. It is worthwhile to note in this context that rats fed rapeseed oil, although they continued to reproduce, had fewer and smaller offspring than rats fed control diets, and that eicosenoic and erucic acids were present in the milk of rats receiving rapeseed oil (Beare *et al.*, 1961). Foetuses obtained by cesarian section from mother rats fed rapeseed oil for several days did not contain appreciable amounts of erucic acid, indicating that this fatty acid does not pass through the placental barrier (Houtsmuller, personal communication).

*4. Preruminant Lambs and Veal Calves*

Studying the nutritive value of rapeseed oil in the diet of milk-fed lamb, Stokes and Walker (1970) found more than 17, 21 and 24% very long-chain unsaturated fatty acids in skin, subcutaneous and perirenal lipids respectively. Very long-chain unsaturated fatty acids from sources other than rapeseed oil, like hydrogenated fish oil, which is used in milk replacers for veal calves, were deposited in the adipose tissues of veal calves without significant modifications (Veen, 1972).

It can be concluded that, in comparison with the rat, the meat-producing animal species show a somewhat larger incorporation of erucic acid into their body fat. On the other hand, when comparing the experimental results in a given species, the age of the animal has to be considered. In rats and mice, the highest incorporation of erucic acid seems to take place into the adrenal cholesterol esters (Caroll, 1962a; Walker, 1972a). The subsequent elevation of esterified cholesterol does not take place in the rabbit, guinea-pig, dog or chicken (Carroll, 1957). However, in the rabbit fed 40 cal% rapeseed oil for longer periods, Abdellatif and Vles (1971b) found a fast and persistent rise of total serum cholesterol.

## B. *In Vivo* Oxidation

The work of Hopkins *et al.* (1957), Craig *et al.* (1963) and Craig and Beare (1967) strongly suggested that in animals oleic acid would be the main metabolic product of erucic acid, while Downey and Craig (1964) demonstrated that in the developing rapeseeds eicosenoic and erucic acids were formed by elongation of oleic acid. Carreau *et al.* (1968) proved the *in vivo* conversion of erucic acid into oleic acid by injecting 14-$^{14}$C-erucic acid; in the liver oleic acid appeared to be a metabolic product of erucic acid. So erucic acid was considered to be "neutralized" after conversion into oleic acid, an endogenous fatty acid normally metabolized in the body. The existence of this conversion, however, did not give any idea about the rate of oxidation of erucic acid in comparison with other exogenous fatty acids. Caroll (1962b) investigated the radioactivity in respiratory carbon dioxide at various intervals, after oral administration of 1-$^{14}$C-palmitic acid, 2-$^{14}$C-erucic acid or 2-$^{14}$C-nervonic acid to rats. Radioactive palmitic acid appeared to be catabolized to respiratory carbon dioxide more rapidly than radioactive erucic or nervonic acid. When given either by mouth or by tail vein injection, highest activities were generally observed in tissue lipids of rats given palmitic acid. Carroll (1966) later showed that 2-$^{14}$C-erucic acid and 2-$^{14}$C-nervonic acid, when administered by tail vein, were deposited in the liver as free fatty acids and were metabolized more slowly than 1-$^{14}$C-oleic acid. Bach *et al.* (1969) measured the specific activity of the carbon dioxide expired by the rat following ingestion of 14-$^{14}$C-erucic acid and 10-$^{14}$C-oleic acids labelled at the double bond instead of at the carboxyl group or at the second carbon atom as did Carroll (1962b). Both acids were oxidized at the same rate but the overall yield from erucic acid oxidation was lower than that from oleic acid oxidation. The rate of oxidation of erucic acid appeared to be influenced by the diet previously fed to the animals. A lipid-free diet yielded a lower percentage of radioactivity recovered as carbon dioxide in comparison with a diet containing high amounts of rapeseed oil (Bach *et al.*, 1969). Lapous *et al.* (1970) studied the incorporation of labelled erucic acid into liver, spleen, kidneys, brain, testicles and seminal vesicles of the rat. Erucic acid rapidly disappeared from all the tissues except from the spleen. The heart and adrenals were not investigated. No interference was found between erucic acid and essential fatty acid metabolism.

Recently, more attention has been given to the myocardium. Using macroscopical autoradiography, Martinelli *et al.* (1973) investigated the distribution of 14-$^{14}$C-erucic acid and 10-$^{14}$C-oleic acid administered orally or intravenously to normal and pregnant mice. Radioactivity was mainly found in liver, brown adipose tissue, myocardium, kidney, spleen, bone marrow and placenta. Measurements of specific activity revealed for erucic acid 100 times more radioactivity in the heart of the mother than in that of the 18-day-old foetus. The radioactivity of erucic origin found in the myocardium of the foetus was half as intense as that of oleic origin. Ketevi *et al.* (1973) administered orally to rats 14-$^{14}$C-erucic acid or 10-$^{14}$C-oleic acid and found by radioscanning of the myocardial lipid homogenates a slower metabolism of 14-$^{14}$C-erucic acid in the rat heart. Boucrot and Bézard (1973) compared the metabolic conversion of injected 10-$^{3}$H-oleic and 14-$^{14}$C-erucic acids in various organs of rats fed rapeseed, Canbra or groundnut oil. Two to nineteen hours after injection of tracer molecules, the remaining $^{14}$C-radioactivity was more intense than the $^{3}$H-radioactivity in liver, heart, spleen, lungs, muscle, adipose tissue, kidneys, brain and testicles. The recovered $^{3}$H-radioactivity was carried on by oleic acid whereas the $^{14}$C-radioactivity was distributed among several fatty acids; C 16:1,

C 18:1, C 20:1, C 22:1 and C 24:1, in varying proportions depending on the organ studied. Erucic acid is not only converted into oleic acid but also into shorter or longer monounsaturates.

### C. Conclusion

Except for its tendency to form cholesterol esters, especially in the adrenal cortex of the rat, erucic acid shows in general a relatively low rate of deposition in tissue triglycerides and a weak incorporation into structural phospholipids. After non-quantitative intestinal absorption, erucic acid rapidly disappears from liver and kidneys but not from spleen and adrenals. Its fate in the myocardium will be fully discussed in the following sections of this chapter.

## IV. HISTOPATHOLOGICAL EFFECTS

Numerous experiments on the nutritive value of rapeseed oil have been performed in the past 30 years. In some of these studies, selected organs have been examined microscopically. More systematic histopathological studies were started when it became apparent that rapeseed oil produces cardiopathogenic effects in various animal species.

### A. Studies on Selected Organs

#### *1. Adrenals*

Carroll (1951) noted pale and enlarged adrenals in rats fed rapeseed oil, which was later confirmed by Alexander and Mattson (1966). The increase in adrenal weight was associated with an increase in the cholesterol content of this organ. Carroll (1953) showed that erucic acid was the cause of the cholesterol accumulation; erucic acid was deposited in the adrenals primarily as cholesteryl erucate (Carroll, 1962a). In a recent study of the adrenal function, Walker and Carney (1971) found that the increase in plasma corticosterone in response to cold stress was smaller in animals fed ethyl erucate than in those receiving olive oil. Cholesteryl erucate, which was the major adrenal ester in the animals fed ethyl erucate, was poorly utilized in response to stress. This could well account for the low growth performances and high mortality of rats fed rapeseed oil and maintained at 4°C (Beare *et al.*, 1963a; Beare-Rogers, 1972). Carney *et al.* (1972) determined the effect of dietary rapeseed oil on the *in vitro* production of prostaglandins by rat adrenal tissue. Stimulation of prostaglandin production by adrenocorticotrophin was considerably lower in adrenals from rats receiving rapeseed oil than in those receiving corn oil. As expected, the inclusion of rapeseed oil in the diet increased the deposition of cholesteryl erucate in the adrenal but this compound was not deposited at the expense of cholesteryl arachidonate (20:4 *n*–6) and adrenate (22:4 *n*–6). Consequently, the lower production of prostaglandin cannot be attributed to a lack of the major prostaglandin precursor, arachidonic acid.

*2. Reproductive Organs*

Carroll and Noble (1957) reported testicular degeneration in Sprague Dawley rats fed 10% erucic acid for five months. No degeneration was observed in the same rats fed 25% rapeseed oil (Carroll and Noble, 1957) nor in Wistar rats given 20% rapeseed oil for 5 weeks (Beare *et al.*, 1959). The testicular lesions observed after feeding 10% erucic acid appeared to be caused by a lack of essential fatty acids, although an increased need for essential fatty acids after feeding very long-chain monoenoic fatty acids should not be excluded (Martin, 1972). The effects of rapeseed oil on the reproductive organs have later been re-examined in the rat and in the pig. Cheniti *et al.* (1967b) did not find any specific effect of rapeseed oil on testicular development and spermatogenesis in the rat. Thoron (1969) observed an important decrease in weight of the Cowper glands in the pig and, to a lesser extent, of the testicles plus epididymides, suggesting an interference of erucic acid with the androsteroid synthesis.

## B. Systematic Histopathological Studies

*1. Rats*

Besides the above-mentioned isolated findings, the only systematic study before 1968 of the histopathological effects of feeding rapeseed oil is that of Roine *et al.* (1960). These authors described the presence of inflammatory changes in the hearts of rats fed various amounts of rapeseed oil. In 1968, Rocquelin and Cluzan confirmed the presence of myocardial changes in 7-month-old male and female rats fed 15% rapeseed oil for six months. Abdellatif and Vles (1970a) demonstrated that these lesions are preceded by severe intracellular lipid deposition, which explains the creamed colour of the heart as noticed on autopsy (Figs 1 and 2). This lipid deposition reaches its maximum intensity after three to six days and decreases afterwards but then necrotic foci and histiocytic infiltrations develop. If the dietary supply of rapeseed oil is maintained for longer periods, fibroblastic proliferation and fibrosis ensue. The skeletal muscles are lighter in colour and show fatty deposition which, however, disappears after four weeks of feeding rapeseed oil. As was also observed by Carroll (1951), the adrenals have a pale appearance showing microscopically enlarged cortical cells with increased fat content. Fine droplet vacuolation is seen in the pancreatic acinar cells

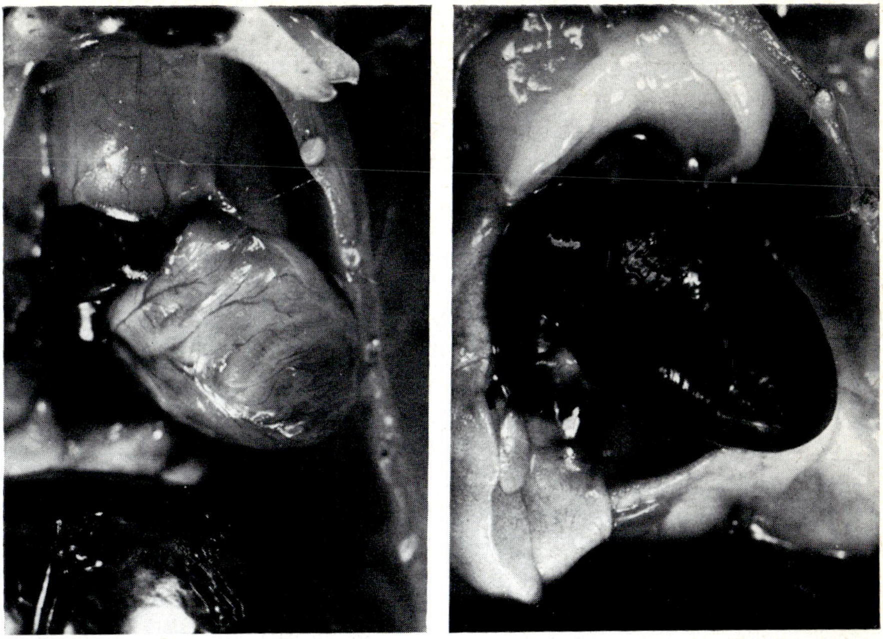

Fig. 1. Macroscopical appearance of heart of a rat fed 50 cal% rapeseed oil for three days (left) and of a control rat 50 cal% sunflowerseed oil (right).

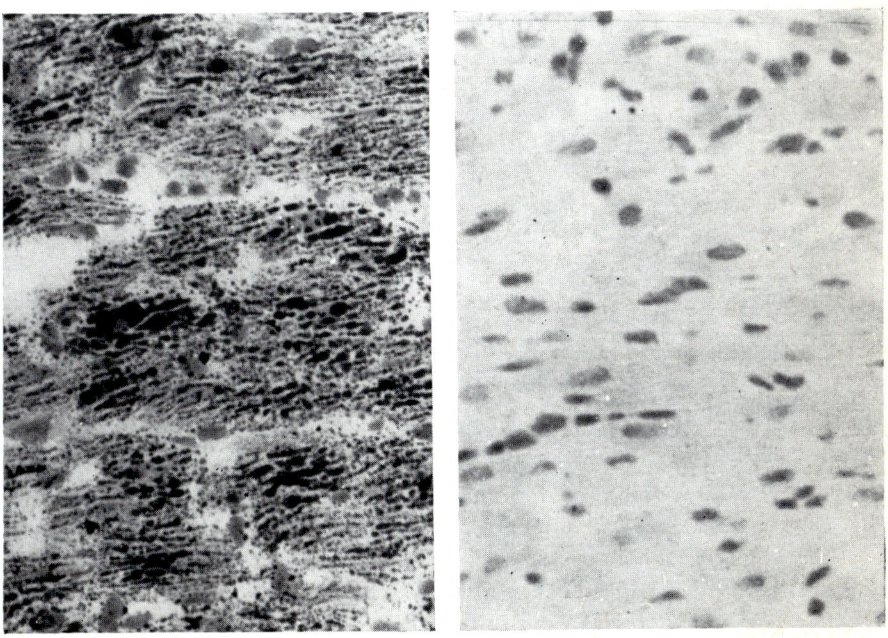

Fig. 2. Massive fatty deposition in heart of a rat fed rapeseed oil (left). Absence of fat droplets in control (right). Sudan red (40×).

and renal changes comprising the presence of proteinaceous material in the lumen of renal tubules, droplet vacuolation of the tubular epithelium, tubular dilatation and increased interstitial collagen deposition are found, the two latter features becoming prominent when the period of feeding rapeseed oil was prolonged to 64 weeks (Abdellatif and Vles, 1970c, 1971b). After long-term feeding of 60 cal% rapeseed oil, the thyroids, adrenals, heart and kidneys are heavier in the animals fed rapeseed oil than in control animals fed sunflowerseed oil. Histologically, the enlarged thyroids show somewhat distended follicles with a flattened epithelium suggesting hypothyroidism. This finding is in agreement with the observation of Niemi and Roine (1960) who suggested that the insaponifiable fraction of rapeseed oil contains a factor which interferes with the ability of the thyroid gland to accumulate iodine from plasma, leading to a reduction of thyroxine synthesis and an increase of thyrotrophic hormone, the result being hypothyroidism. The fatty droplets infiltration of liver, observed particularly after 64 experimental weeks, is more severe in the rapeseed oil group than in the animals fed sunflowerseed oil.

The present histopathological observations especially those involving the myocardium, which are potentially of great concern for human nutrition, prompted further experimentation in various animal species and with other dietary sources of docosenoic (and eicosenoic) fatty acids (Beare-Rogers, 1970; Rocquelin *et al.*, 1970; Rocquelin and Cluzan, 1970, 1971; Beare-Rogers *et al.*, 1971; Nera *et al.*, 1971; Booth *et al.*, 1972; Beare-Rogers and Nera, 1972; Beare-Rogers *et al.*, 1972a, b; Ziemlanski *et al.*, 1972c, d; Lall *et al.*, 1972; Bodak, 1972; Levillain *et al.*, 1972; Vodovar *et al.*, 1972b, 1973; Kramer *et al.*, 1973; and Dallochio *et al.*, 1973). From experiments with rats, it became evident that oils, fats or fat mixtures rich in monoenoic fatty acids with 20 and more carbon atoms like rapeseed or crambe oil, partially hydrogenated rapeseed oil, partially hydrogenated herring oil or mixture of glyceryl trierucate with glyceryl tripalmitate and/or glyceryl trioleate, glyceryl trierucate with sunflowerseed oil and synthesized oils containing a high proportion of eicosenoic or docosenoic acid, induce early fatty deposition which may progress to foci of myocytolysis, necrosis and fibrosis, the latter being a predominant feature of a prolonged and high intake of docosenoic fatty acids (Fig. 3).

Besides the level and duration of feeding rapeseed oil, the age of the animals is of some importance when evaluating the pathological response. The myocardial fatty deposition in 3-week-old male Wistar rats is almost equal in intensity to that found in 11-week-old (mature) animals fed rapeseed oil for three days. After six days, however, fatty

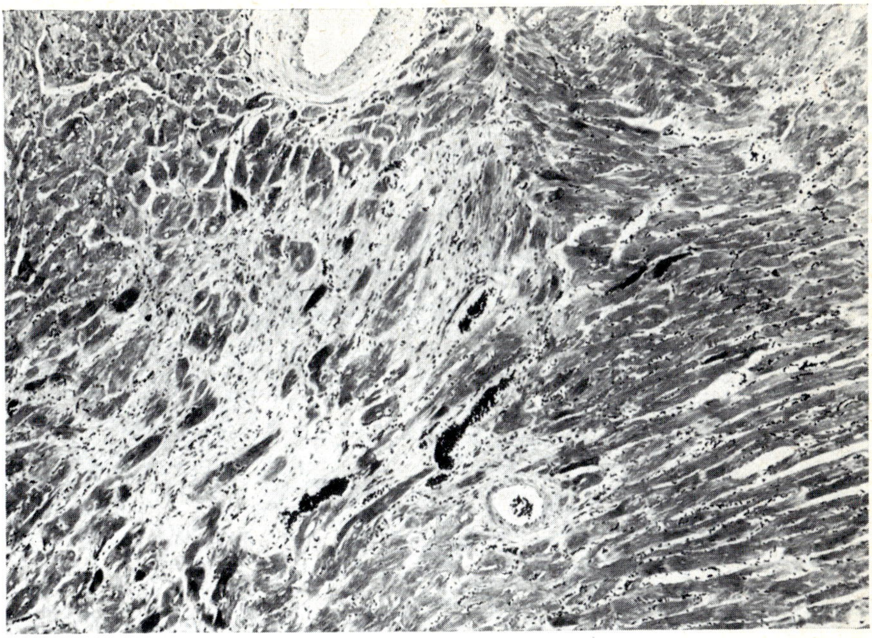

Fig. 3. Fibrosis in heart of a rat fed 50 cal% rapeseed oil for 64 weeks (4×).

deposition is more severe in the young than in the mature rat. This faster decrease in the mature rat is associated with higher scores for myolysis and cell proliferation (Abdellatif and Vles, 1970c). In 18-month-old Wistar rats fed 40 cal% rapeseed oil for six days, fatty deposition and some cell infiltration are still found (Abdellatif and Vles, unpublished data). Consequently, the pathological picture resulting from short-term feeding of rapeseed oil definitely cannot be regarded as a "neonatal disease", as has been suggested by Staron (1972).

*2. Poultry*

Ducklings were found to be highly susceptible to the effects of dietary rapeseed oil which produced high mortality and in addition to lipid accumulation in myocardium and skeletal muscles, severe hydropericardium, cirrhotic changes of the liver associated with hypoalbuminaemia and an increase of the reticulocyte count of the blood (Vles, 1969; Vles and Abdellatif, 1970; Abdellatif and Vles, 1970b, 1971b; Abdellatif *et al.*, 1972). A positive relationship was found between heart weight and caloric percentage rapeseed oil in the diet. The liver weights also increased with increasing levels of dietary rapeseed oil up to 30 cal% (Hypertrophic cirrhosis) but decreased as the rapeseed oil was further increased, corresponding to an atrophic cirrhosis of the liver. Similarly, measurement of the weights of heart and liver in turkeys fed 10 or 7·5% rapeseed oil for six weeks revealed enlargement of these organs. No histological study of these animals has been reported yet (Salmon, 1970). In chicks, Sheppard *et al.* (1971) reported heavier hearts and livers after feeding 16% crambe or rapeseed oil in comparison with corn oil; no histology was reported.

In experiments involving 4-week-old chickens fed 5, 10 or 15% rapeseed oil of high (regular) or low erucic acid content for 28 days, Vogtmann *et al.* (1974) showed that regular rapeseed oil did not influence heart-to-body weight ratio but increased liver-to-body weight ratio by more than 10%. Lall *et al.* (1972) reported fatty accumulation of myocardial fibres in one-day-old chicks fed 20% rapeseed oil for three days, six days and two weeks. No abnormalities were found at eight weeks of age. Similarly, histopathological examination of heart, liver, adrenals, pancreas, spleen, kidney and ovaries of laying hens fed 10 and 20% regular rapeseed oil or 10% rapeseed oil of low erucic acid content for 12 weeks showed no abnormalities which could be related to the diet (Lall and Slinger, 1973b).

*3. Other Species*

Hamsters and guinea-pigs fed rapeseed oil displayed similar fatty changes in the myocardium (Vles, 1969; Thomasson *et al.*, 1970). Moreover, rapeseed oil caused haemolytic anaemia in guinea-pigs, the severity of which was closely related to the amount of rapeseed oil in the diet (Vles and Abdellatif, 1970b). Short-term feeding of rapeseed oil or glyceryl trierucate to adult rabbits and of rapeseed oil or fats containing high amounts of docosenoic acid to young mice induced fatty deposition in the myocardium (Abdellatif and Vles, unpublished data). Long-term feeding of 40 cal% rapeseed oil caused diffuse fibrosis of the myocardium and liver cirrhosis in rabbits. The serum lipid pattern in this animal species revealed an increase in the total lipids which was mainly due to the increase in the free and esterified cholesterol and phospholipid fractions (Abdellatif and Vles, 1971b).

Rabbits fed 6% rapeseed oil (40% erucic acid) or corn oil in diets containing 2% cholesterol for two months did not show differences in average cholesterol level and cholesterol-induced atherosclerosis; no histopathology was performed and the conclusion was drawn that at the level and time period of feeding, rapeseed oil did not exert a deleterious effect on the rabbits (Kritchevsky *et al.*, 1972).

Diffuse fibrosis was also noticed in adult mice from different strains after feeding 50 cal% rapeseed oil for three months (Vles, unpublished data). Similar myocardial lipid droplet deposition has been described in miniature pigs and commercial piglets (*Sus scrofa*), squirrel monkeys (*Saimiri sciureus*) and gerbils (*Meriones unguiculatus*) after feeding rapeseed oil (Beare-Rogers, 1970; Beare-Rogers and Nera, 1972). Gerbils receiving a diet containing 6% erucic acid showed a peak in lipid deposition after four days (Beare-Rogers *et al.*, 1972b) while a diet with 20% Canbra oil from Oro seed, a variety of Brassica napus containing 1·9% eicosenoic acid and 2·3% erucic acid, did not induce stainable fat droplets in the gerbils' myocardia (Beare-Rogers and Nera, 1972). Although some differences were observed in the extent and pattern of response between all species investigated, Beare-Rogers and Nera (1972) concluded that none has been found so far to be free from cardiac alteration.

## C. Ultrastructural Studies

### *1. Intestine*

Various studies have revealed the lower digestibility of rapeseed oil and of its main fatty acid, erucic acid, in the rat (Deuel *et al.*, 1948; Savary and Constantin, 1966; Rocquelin and Leclerc, 1969; Demarne *et al.*, 1971; Hornstra, 1972). Other experiments have shown the lower rate of intestinal absorption of rapeseed oil not only in the rat (Deuel *et al.*, 1940; Thomasson, 1956; Ziemlanski *et al.*, 1972a) but also in the pig (McDonald, 1972). These results incited Vodovar *et al.* (1972a) to investigate the ultrastructural aspect of the intestine during rapeseed oil absorption; 45 and 60 min after ingestion of rapeseed oil, numerous large lipid droplets were found in the supranuclear region of the jejunal cell while in the animal given corn oil a picture of normal lipid transit was observed. This supranuclear accumulation of large lipid droplets, as found in various cases of lipid malabsorption, is accompanied by infranuclear clusters of mitochondria. Moreover, a large number of desquamated absorbing cells containing important amounts of lipids is seen in the intestinal lumen. The presence of these dequamated cells can be due to a retarded transport of rapeseed fatty acids through the intestinal cell, while the passage from lumen to absorbing cell seems to be normal. The cause of this impaired transfer resulting in lipid accumulation, desquamation, lower absorption rate and lower digestibility remains unexplained.

### *2. Myocardium*

Electron-microscope studies of the myocardium of rats fed diets containing rapeseed oil for three and seven days confirmed the changes observed by light microscopy. Excessive amounts of lipid droplets characterize the ultrastructure of rat heart after short-term feeding of rapeseed oil (Figs 4 and 5). These fatty droplets are disseminated between the mitochondria, in the intermyofibrillar spaces. The diameter of the inclusions varies between 0·3 and 2·5 $\mu$m. Mitochondria, myofibrils and nuclei are often distorted by large droplets. A membrane-like structure limits the fatty droplet. Slight alterations of the myofibrillar structure and lipid-loaded macrophages are observed particularly on the seventh day of feeding rapeseed oil (Vodovar *et al.*, 1972b).

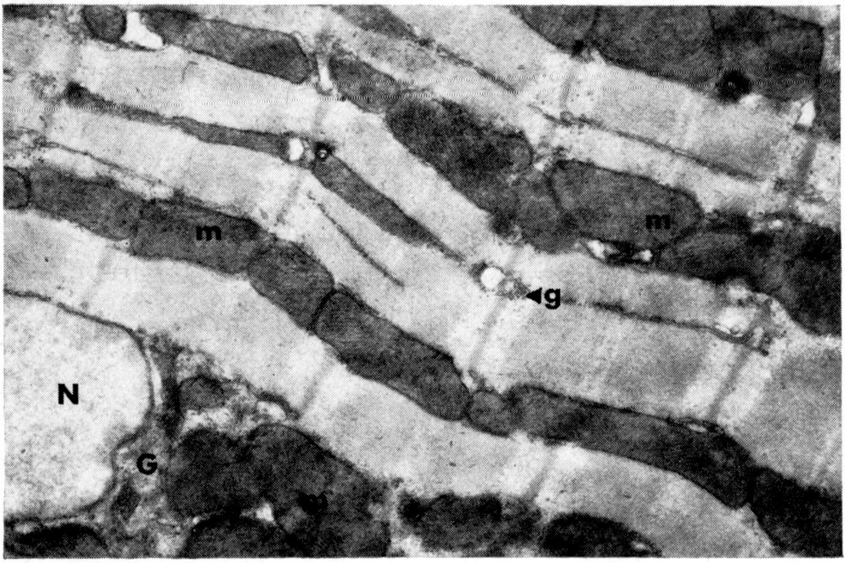


Fig. 4. Rat heart muscle (15,000×). The rat had been fed 50 cal% sunflowerseed oil for 3 days. N: nucleus; G: Golgi apparatus; m: mitochondria; g: glycogen granules.

Similarly, ultrastructural studies of Jager and Boom (unpublished observations from our laboratory) revealed that feeding 50 cal% rapeseed oil for three days induced fat deposition which occupied about 25% of the surface of myocardial section. The counting of mitochondria and evaluation of their size distribution indicated a marked increase in the percentage of small mitochondria, the structure of which displayed no abnormalities.

Ziemlanski *et al.* (1973) noted lipid droplets in the myocardial cells as early as three hours after rapeseed oil administration. The number and size of lipid droplets increased with time. After 48 hours, the droplets often fused, compressing and deforming the contractile elements and the mitochondria. No further damage was noted at this stage of feeding. The ultrastructural aspects of the myocardial changes in rats and pigs fed rapeseed oil for longer periods of time have been further documented by Bodak (1972), Levillain *et al.* (1972) and Vodovar *et al.* (1973). These authors confirmed the sequence of rapid and intense fat deposition, subsequent degenerative changes of the myocardial fibres, proliferation of connective tissue elements followed by mutilating areas of fibrosis. Finally, Bodak and Hatt (1973) have emphasized the sub-epicardial localization of the degenerative foci, the presence of fat droplets in histiocytes and macrophages, the increase of volume occupied by the mitochondria and the occurrence of megamitochondria.

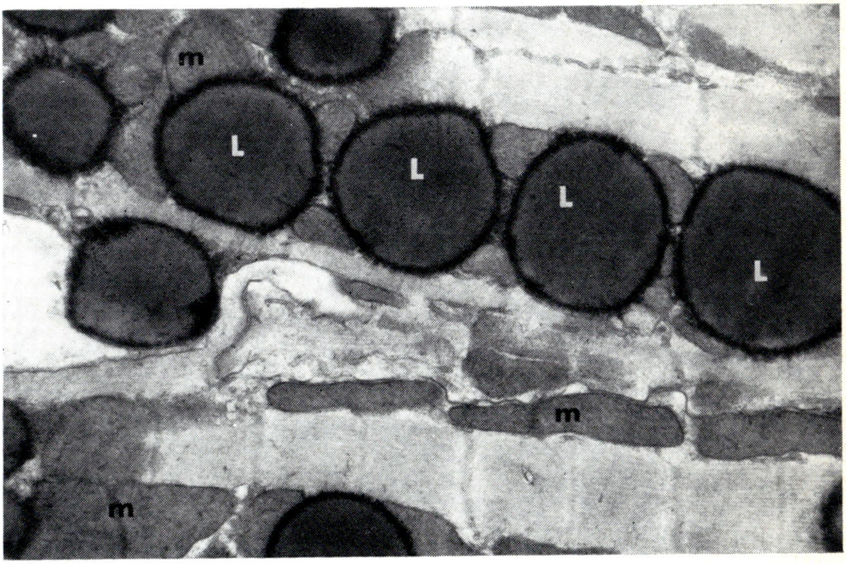


Fig. 5. Rat heart muscle (15,000×). The rat had been fed 50 cal% rapeseed oil for 3 days. L: lipid droplet; m: mitochondria.

## V. PATHOGENESIS OF MYOCARDIAL CHANGES

### A. Nature and Cause of Lipid Deposition

*1. Cardiac Lipids*

Biochemical studies of myocardial tissue lipids in rats fed various sources of very long-chain fatty acids confirmed the histologically observed sequence of early fatty deposition followed by a decrease of the lipid content to the development of degenerative lesions in the heart (Houtsmuller *et al.*, 1970; Beare-Rogers, 1970; Rocquelin *et al.*, 1970; Beare-Rogers *et al.*, 1971; Beare-Rogers and Nera, 1972; Beare-Rogers *et al.*, 1972a, b; Rocquelin, 1972, 1973; Rocquelin *et al.*, 1973c; Jaillard *et al.*, 1973). In eight-week-old male Wistar rats fed 50 cal% rapeseed oil (48% erucic acid) for different periods, the fat content of the heart reached its maximum after three experimental days; the total lipid content increasing from an initial 3% to 8% of the wet tissue weight. This increase was mainly due to a tenfold rise of the triglyceride content; the free fatty acid content also increased, but to a lesser extent. Gas–liquid chromatography showed that erucic acid constituted 27% of the fatty acids of total lipids after three days' feeding; this level gradually fell to about 15% in the following 39 days (Houtsmuller *et al.*, 1970). A fatty acid analysis of the triglycerides and the free fatty acid fraction showed a high percentage of erucic acid, namely, 40 and 25% respectively. No important shifts were observed in the amounts of phospholipids, cholesterol and cholesterol esters. The analysis of liver fat revealed no changes in the total lipid content nor in lipid classes. The decrease of fat content in the heart became important after six days of feeding (Houtsmuller *et al.*, 1972; Struijk, 1972).

Beare-Rogers *et al.* (1971) similarly determined the composition of the cardiac fatty acids in rats receiving docosenoic acid provided by 40 cal% liquid or partially hydrogenated rapeseed oil or partially hydrogenated herring oil. The lipid deposited in the heart within the first week contained high levels of monoenoic acid. Beare-Rogers *et al.* (1972a) later evaluated the relative effects of oleic (18:1 *n*–9), eicosenoic (20:1 *n*–9), erucic (22:1 *n*–9) and cetoleic (22:1 *n*–11) acids by feeding random triglycerides of tailored fatty acid composition to rats. The dietary docosenoic acids (erucic and cetoleic) caused a pronounced accumulation of cardiac lipid after one week of experimental feeding. A positive relationship was found between total fatty acids and erucic acid in the heart; all dietary fatty acids present with erucic acid accumulated in the heart and no interference was noted with arachidonic acid synthesis. The fatty acids of the accumulated triglycerides in the heart reflected the dietary fatty acids, suggesting an inhibited oxidation of all the dietary fatty acids coming to the heart. Changing the level of saturated fatty acids did not modify the accumulation of cardiac lipids produced by the dietary intake of erucic acid. These results are in agreement with those of histological studies in ducklings and guinea-pigs fed erucic acid sources combined with variable amounts of palmitic acid (Vles and Abdellatif, 1970b; Abdellatif *et al.*, 1972). A high intake of eicosenoic acid also induced some fat deposition. Feeding whale or seal oils low in C22 fatty acids, had hardly any effect on the amounts of lipids in the hearts of rats or gerbils (Beare-Rogers *et al.*, 1972a, b). The most important factor in the accumulation of cardiac lipids appeared to be the dietary intake of docosenoic acids (Teige and Beare-Rogers, 1973).

Short-term experiments with synthetic fatty acids (Houtsmuller *et al.*, 1972) and with fatty acid fractions obtained from fish oils before and after partial hydrogenation (unpublished data from our laboratory) led to the same conclusion: early cardiac fatty acid deposition is mainly due to dietary docosenoic acids. The role of eicosenoic and C22-polyenoic acids other than the *cis-cis* methyl-interrupted polyunsaturated fatty acids which are still present after partial hydrogenation, should however, not be neglected. No lipid deposition was observed after the administration of unhardened fish oil fractions containing very long all *cis*-polyenoic fatty acids.

In similar short-term feeding experiments, Rocquelin (1972, 1973) investigated the effects of 30 cal% refined and unrefined rapeseed oil (48% erucic acid) or refined Canbra oil (3% erucic acid). He noticed a rapid and important accumulation of triglycerides rich in erucic acid in the myocardium of newly weaned Wistar rats after feeding both the refined and the unrefined rapeseed oil. Canbra oil did not produce this short-term effect, which confirms the previous observations by Abdellatif and Vles (1970c), Beare-Rogers (1970) and Beare-Rogers *et al.* (1971).

Quan and Le Breton (1972a, b) investigated in detail the myocardial lipids of rats fed rapeseed oil for three days, paying special attention to the effects of fasting and of lipotropic factors. The preferential deposition of erucic acid in the neutral lipids and its low incorporation in the phospholipids was confirmed. Fasting hardly influenced the neutral fatty acid and erucic acid contents as a percentage of total fatty acids. Erucic acid deposition did increase after extra addition of lipotropic factors. Rocquelin (1973), studying the effects of interesterification, showed that interesterified rapeseed oil increased the magnitude of the fat accumulation; 27% more lipids were found in the myocardium in comparison with refined rapeseed oil. After interesterification, a shift of erucic acid from external positions, in the triglyceride molecule to the internal position may lead, during digestion to a higher yield of 2-monoerucin which is better absorbed than the free erucic acid. Consequently, an increased availability of erucic acid seems to be responsible for the more severe lipid accumulation. Slinger *et al.* (1973) observed that the deposition of fat in the myocardium of rats fed erucic acid is accompanied by a decrease in cardiac glycogen which appears to substitute for fat as a source of cardiac energy. The concentration of cardiac glycogen remains low as long as high erucic acid rapeseed oil is fed.

Beare-Rogers (1972) also investigated the changes in cardiac phospholipids in rats fed 20 % rapeseed oil or olive oil for 20 weeks. Although no changes were observed in lipid phosphorus, the amount of sphingomyelin in the hearts of the rats fed rapeseed oil was increased. These biochemical changes which point to alterations of the membrane lipids, correspond fairly well with the degenerative lesions observed histologically at that stage of long-term feeding of rapeseed oil.

*2. Causes of Deposition*

Triglycerides accumulate in the heart muscle when this organ takes up more fatty acids than it can oxidize. Factors that may influence the equilibrium between influx and utilization are the concentrations and/or composition of plasmatic free fatty acids, the binding of these fatty acids to plasma albumin, the rate of oxidation by the myocardial mitochondria and the carnitine content of the heart (Opie, 1968).

*a. Plasmatic free fatty acids.* Muscle tissue takes up fatty acids in proportion to their concentration in the plasma. Analysis of the blood lipids received therefore much attention (Houtsmuller *et al.*, 1972; Struijk, 1972; Rocquelin *et al.*, 1974). The plasma content of total lipid, triglycerides, phospholipids, non-esterified fatty acids and cholesterol esters appeared not to be influenced by feeding rapeseed oil for various periods of time. On the other hand, an important shift in fatty acid composition was noticed; particularly, the incorporation of erucic and eicosenoic acids in the triglyceride and free fatty acid fractions was fairly high and constant. Normally, most of the free fatty acids in the plasma are complexed to albumin. The affinity of this protein for erucic acid is looser than that for other fatty acids. A shift in free fatty acid composition in favour of erucic acid and the relatively low binding capacity of albumin for erucic acid may contribute to an increased uptake by and accumulation in the heart muscle (Houtsmuller *et al.*, 1972; Gumpen and Norum, 1973; Swarttouw, 1974).

*b. Rate of oxidation by mitochondria.* From the work of Houtsmuller *et al.* (1970, 1972), Christophersen and Bremer (1972), Lemarchal *et al.* (1972), Pinson and Padieu (1973) and Swarttouw (1974) it is evident that erucic acid is metabolized by heart mitochondria at a distinctly slower rate than are palmitic and oleic acid. Very long-chain monoenoic fatty acids are apparently poor substrates for mitochondria. Three major enzymatic steps are involved in the metabolism of fatty acids by mitochondria: acyl-CoA synthetase, carnitine acyl transferase and the enzyme complex of the $\beta$-oxidation. *In vitro*, these three steps display a lower activity towards erucic acid than towards palmitic acid (Swarttouw, 1974). *In vivo*, however, the erucic acid accumulates in the heart muscle as triglycerides, indicating that the formation of erucyl-CoA cannot be greatly hampered. To determine which of the two remaining enzymatic steps would be rate limiting, studies on the carnitine content of hearts of rats fed rapeseed oil were performed.

*c. Carnitine content.* Carnitine (3-trimethylammonium-2-hydroxy-butyrate stimulates the oxidation of long-chain fatty acids through formation of long-chain acyl carnitine esters which facilitates the transport of the acyl moiety across the inner mitochondrial membrane. Variations in the acyl carnitine levels are likely to reflect alterations in the rate of fatty acid oxidation. Struijk (1972) determined the carnitine content of heart and liver in rats fed rapeseed oil or sunflowerseed oil for various days. In both groups the carnitine content of the heart fell during the first day, the decrease in the rapeseed oil group being largest. The differences were mainly due to changes in the free carnitine fractions. The amount of short-chain and long-chain acyl carnitine esters were hardly affected. This is in full agreement with findings by Gumpen and Norum (1973), who found no differences in the amount of long-chain acyl carnitines relative to the total carnitine content (fractional amount) in the hearts of rats fed rapeseed oil or corn oil for four days or four weeks. These findings indicate that the triglyceride accumulation in the myocardium is not likely to be due to inhibition of the $\beta$-oxidation.

Struijk (1972) and Houtsmuller *et al.* (1972, 1974) found a relatively low long-chain acyl carnitine free carnitine ratio in the hearts of rats fed erucic acid. They concluded that the low affinity of carnitine acyl transferase for erucic acid, which decreases the transport of activated fatty acids into the mitochondria, underlies the process of lipid accumulation.

### 3. *Mechanism of Removal*

Equally intriguing as the cause of muscular fatty deposition is the mechanism by which the accumulated fat slopes down on continuous feeding of erucic acid. The decrease in triglyceride content in the heart during the experimental time is not due to an improved capacity of the cardiac mitochondria to oxidize erucic acid (Swarttouw, personal communication), neither can it be explained by modifications of the plasma triglycerides or non esterified fatty acid concentrations and/or their fatty acid composition (Rocquelin *et al.*, 1974). It has been investigated whether a lipolytic enzyme, present in different organs and which appears in the blood after intravenous heparin injection, plays a role in the removal of accumulated fat in heart muscle. Struijk *et al.* (1973) showed that 50 cal% rapeseed oil fed to rats for periods of one to fourteen days, increased the postheparin lipoprotein lipase activity in the plasma by about 45% after three to six days. This rise in enzyme activity, which coincides with the rapid decrease in triglyceride content of the myocardium, strongly suggests a causative relationship with respect to the removal of fat from the myocardium.

## B. Degenerative Changes

Dietary fat mixtures rich in docosenoic acid promote early fatty deposition of triglycerides in the rat. In a later stage of feeding, this fatty accumulation decreases but never disappears completely. Multiple foci of myocytolysis and/or necrosis with various degrees of myoblastic and histiocytic proliferation develop. When feeding rapeseed oil is maintained for still longer periods, collagen is deposited in the lesion area. The pathogenesis of the later degenerative lesions is far from clear. It is still unknown whether any of the stages—fatty deposition, cellular infiltration, fibrosis—necessarily incites the next one. It is true that severe fibrosis has never been observed without preceding steatosis. However, while the severity of the fat deposition is remarkably uniform, the fibrotic response greatly varies from one animal to another (Abdellatif, 1972). When maximum fat deposition is reached and the feeding of rapeseed oil to growing rats is discontinued, neither fatty deposition, nor myocardial necrosis, nor fibrosis will be observed later. This indicates that degenerative lesions are not due to early fat deposition but are rather the result of continuous exposure to dietary docosenoic acids (Beare-Rogers, 1970; Abdellatif and Vles, 1970a). As mentioned earlier in this chapter, mature rats develop a severer mononuclear cell response to short-term feeding of rapeseed oil than do newly weaned rats, and the accumulated fat seems to decrease more rapidly in older rats (Abdellatif and Vles, 1970c). Recent studies in our laboratory on the fate of the heart changes induced by rapeseed oil strongly support the pathogenetic concept suggested by Abdellatif (1972): erucic acid and similar very long-chain monoenoic fatty acids are rapidly taken up by heart muscle after intestinal absorption. The inability of cardiac tissue to readily metabolize these fatty acids leads to their incorporation into triglycerides which are deposited *in situ*. Some myocardial cells undergo degenerative changes (cytomyolosis, necrosis) and repair, the repair being easier when the animal is younger. In the course of this regenerative process, myogenic cells (myocytes) as well as Anitschkow cells which are commonly observed in heart injury, represent an attempt to cardiac tissue repair. Meanwhile, the heart acquires a mechanism to dispose of the accumulated fat (Struijk *et al.*, 1973); histiocytes with their macrophagic function may help in decreasing the fat deposition. In course of time, the arising collagen deposition or fibrosis should be considered as the balance between repair and the failure to accomplish repair. Continuous supply by plasma of uncomplexed free erucic acid to—and its removal from—heart cell through interstitial tissue by lymphatic drainage seems to cause permanent irritation and continuous induction of mesenchymal response, which can be particularly important at the points of confluence of larger lymphatics (subepicardial localizations).

There is much evidence that erucic acid and other very long-chain monoenoic fatty acids are responsible for fat deposition after short-term feeding. Doubts on the causative role of erucic acid as being the sole factor responsible for the long-term effects have been expressed by Rocquelin and Cluzan (1968) who found myocardial degenerative changes in rats fed Canbra oil low in erucic acid, while no heart lipid accumulation had been found at an early stage of feeding this oil (Rocquelin, 1972). Recent work has confirmed residual long-term effects of rapeseed oils low in erucic acid (Rocquelin *et al.*, 1973c; Levillain *et al.*, 1972; Pipy *et al.*, 1972). However, the fact that these lesions were delayed, and were less frequent and less severe than those observed in animals fed rapeseed oils as well as results from experiments with mixtures of triglycerides (Rocquelin *et al.*, 1970, 1971) and with other sources of docosenoic acids (Beare-Rogers *et al.*, 1972a, b) and studies on the long-term effects of glyceryl trierucate and of increasing levels of rapeseed oil (Abdellatif and Vles, 1973a) strongly point an accusing finger toward the docosenoic fatty acids as far as the fibrotic response to their prolonged administration is concerned. One can only speculate on the possible fibrogenic role of eicosenoic acid and of the very long-chain polyenoic fatty acids which do not have the all-*cis* configuration.

## C. Functional Disorders

### *1. Isolated Heart Mitochondria*

The oxidation rate of various substrates by mitochondria isolated from hearts of rats fed erucic acid, is depressed (Houtsmuller *et al.*, 1970). This depression, expressed as a decrease in the rate of ATP synthesis, is proportional to the amount of erucic acid absorbed by the rat but is not specific for this fatty acid. Qualitatively, the same effect was obtained by homologues of erucic acid, namely, eicosenoic acid (20:1 *n*–9), nervonic acid (24:1 *n*–9) and the positional isomers of erucic acid (22:1 *n*–7) and cetoleic acid (22:1 *n*–11) (Houtsmuller *et al.*, 1972). A relationship was found between the magnitude of the decrease in ATP synthesis and the chain length on the one hand, and the position of the double bond on the other. In the *n*–9 series of fatty acids (20:1, 22:1,

24:1), the quality of mitochondria decreased with increasing chain length. For identical chain length, a similar decrease in the rate of ATP synthesis was observed when shifting the double bond from the position *n*–11 to *n*–7.

### 2. *Isolated Heart*

Besides the decreased capacity of isolated mitochondria to oxidize substrate, the myocardial function of rats fed rapeseed oil for a short term was studied using isolated left ventricular papillary muscle and heart-lung preparation (Ten Hoor *et al.*, 1973). It was found that dietary rapeseed oil considerably reduced the contractile force of isolated rat myocardium in comparison with sunflowerseed oil.

In the heart-lung preparation, the left ventricular stroke work of rats fed rapeseed oil was lower than that of controls. Long-term feeding of diets rich in erucic acid recently appeared to have similar effects on papillary muscle function (Quadt *et al.*, 1974), which indicates that it is not the fatty deposition that is responsible for the dysfunction.

### 3. *Myocardial Enzymes*

In rats fed 15% rapeseed oil, Canbra oil or peanut oil for periods of two to fifteen days, Dallochio *et al.* (1973) studied the activities of the myocardial enzymes lactate dehydrogenase, malate dehydrogenase, hydroxybutyrate dehydrogenase, glucose-6-phosphate dehydrogenase, ATP-ases and creatine phosphatase finding no differences in enzymatic activites between the experimental groups.

Using newly weaned Wistar rats, Cresteil *et al.* (1972) administered per stomach tube 0·5 or 1·0 ml rapeseed or olive oil per day, for three days. After sacrifice, a significantly weaker adenylcyclase activity of cardiac tissue was noticed in the rats fed rapeseed oil than in the control animals. This lower activity was shown to be related to a decrease in catalytic units rather than to an inhibition of their activity. Considering the role of cyclic AMP in the regulation of cardiac lipid metabolism, the possibility that rapeseed oil promotes lipid accumulation by decreasing the lipid "clearance" capacity of the myocardium should not be discarded.

# VI. IMPLICATIONS FOR HUMAN NUTRITION

## A. Extrapolation to Man

Fatty accumulation has been found to follow the ingestion of various sources of docosenoic acid in rats, rabbits, ducklings, guinea-pigs, hamsters, mice, gerbils, miniature pigs, piglets and squirrel monkeys.

Sometimes the extent and pattern of response varies, but none of these species was resistant to the effects of feeding rapeseed oil or erucic acid. The involvement of ten species undoubtedly increases the likelihood that the response in man will be similar. Although there is no, and probably never will be any evidence that rapeseed oil causes harm to humans, it is difficult to prove that such an effect does not occur. From epidemiological studies and retrospective enquiries on mortality cases carried out by the French National Institute for Health and Medical Research (Anonymus, 1972), it appeared impossible to link the consumption of rapeseed oil with a certain type of non-obstructive idiopathic cardiomyopathy which might have certain similarities with lesions found in laboratory animals. The absence of correlation between the consumption of rapeseed oil and any human heart illness as seems to have been stated in French cardiological centres, does not exclude a potential hazard and therefore the French Higher Council of Public Health requested complementary research in order to estimate the nutritive value of rapeseed oil in comparison with other edible oils. Similarly, in Canada and Sweden, where increasing amounts of rapeseed oil were intended to be used as cooking oils and/or processed fats, it was considered prudent to limit the erucic acid intake (to 5 and 7% of total fatty acids, respectively) by lowering the incorporation of regular rapeseed oil in edible oils and fats and by stimulating the breeding and culture of Brassica seed strains low in erucic acid (Weinberg, 1972). Moreover, considering the particular susceptibility of young animals to the effects of very long-chain fatty acids, it was recommended to withdraw rapeseed oil from infant formula.

## B. Experiments in Man

Available evidence from experimental animals as well as a forecasted steep increase in the production and consumption of rapeseed made better knowledge of the metabolism of erucic acid in man a matter of urgency. Data in this field are still scarce and mainly refer to the digestibility of rapeseed oil or erucic acid and to the effects of a single dose of rapeseed oil on the respiratory function and on the uptake of free erucic acid by the myocardium.

### *1. Digestibility*

McDonald (1972) determined the digestibility of erucic acid in adult experimental subjects fed 20–22% of total calories from rapeseed oil and rapeseed-oil margarine and shortening. The apparent digestibility of erucic acid ranged from 98 to 100%. Vaisey *et al.* (1973), investigating the digestibility of high and low erucic-acid rapeseed oils in a mixed

Canadian diet, found that while erucic acid accounted for 20% of the fat, 99 to 100% appeared to be absorbed. This high utilization of erucic acid agrees well with older data from Deuel *et al.* (1949) who found the digestibility of rapeseed oil to be 99%. However, Gompertz and Sammons (1961), feeding to four subjects dietary fat randomly esterified with erucic acid, found a somewhat lower absorption of erucic acid (92–96%) although the faecal fat was not raised above normal level.

*2. Respiratory Quotient*

In normal resting human adults, a single dose of 0·5 g/kg body weight of rapeseed oil—covering 13% of daily total calories—after 150 minutes induced an increased oxidation of fatty acids, probably taking place in the liver, in comparison with groundnut oil (Trémolières *et al.*, 1971). The ratio of plasmatic hydroxybutyrate/acetoacetate and lactate/pyruvate indicates that the mitochondrial capacity to oxidize fatty acids at rest and carbohydrates during exercise remains sufficient under the experimental conditions used. Maximal plasmatic concentrations of erucic acid and eicosenoic acids were found between 150 and 210 minutes after rapeseed oil intake. No accumulation of erucic acid was noticed in red blood cells after a single administration (Trémolières *et al.*, 1972). Trémolières and Carré (1972) later confirmed the increased oxidation of rapeseed oil fatty acids in comparison with those of groundnut oil. Four hours after rapeseed oil ingestion, oxygen consumption showed a 24% increase in the resting state. These authors believe that prior to the mitochondrial oxidation, erucic acid has to be submitted to a microsomal oxidation which takes place in the liver and not in myocardial or in muscular tissue, these tissues being devoid of adequate microsomal systems. However, the possibility should not be overlooked that the increased oxygen consumption is due to partial uncoupling of mitochondria by free fatty acids. Moreover, it has been proved that heart mitochondria as well as isolated heart are able to carry out the $\beta$-oxidation of erucic acid, be it at a lower rate than oleic acid or palmitic acid (Houtsmuller *et al.*, 1972). Trémolières *et al.* (1971) noticed a laxative effect in five out of the eight experimental subjects after administration of a single rapeseed oil dose. This effect was absent from the groundnut oil group, neither were electrocardiographic abnormalities observed after exercise in any participant.

*3. Myocardial Uptake*

In seven human patients, Jaillard *et al.* (1973) studied the extraction of free erucic acid compared with other common fatty acids from plasma by the myocardium, three hours after the patients had consumed a rapeseed oil meal. No preferential uptake of free erucic acid by the human myocardium could be demonstrated, and the authors argued that the accumulation of erucic acid observed in the myocardium of various animals is not due to an increased rate of erucic acid uptake compared with that of ordinary fatty acids.

#### *4. Acceptable Dietary Level*

There are no reported cases of toxicity nor indications in the literature that erucic acid causes changes in man similar to those observed in experimental animals. The interpretation of autopsy findings in exposed populations requires some caution, since the expected changes are not very specific, but are rather common for a series of diseases, intoxications and nutritional conditions. It will remain difficult to prove or disprove that they have been induced by erucic acid intake.

Moreover, data on the average intake by populations should not be overemphasized since there always will be important groups of individuals with higher or lower intake than the average, while also special risk groups regarding age, sex and disease have to be considered. For instance in a dietary study performed by Vaisey *et al.* (1973), fostering maximum use of rapeseed oil available in market forms, the average daily consumption of rapeseed oil was 72 g, which is considerably more than the estimated average Canadian rapeseed oil intake of 7 g. On the other hand, accurate determination of a no-effect level is complicated by the fact that the available biochemical and histopathological techniques when applied to laboratory animals already reveal some effect even at the lowest given dose. Also the possibility of a cumulative effect after long-term administration of low doses should not be overlooked. The total exclusion of erucic acid from human food seems unnecessary and probably too unrealistic, since docosenoic acids are transferred into the food chain by valuable protein sources like fish and by meat-producing animals that have in turn been fed these fatty acids. Chicken, turkeys, lambs and calves, for example, show appreciable amounts of incorporated erucic acid after feeding rapeseed oil or marine fat.

## C. Conclusion

The presented experimental evidence strongly suggests that erucic acid is not the proper substrate for energy production by muscle tissue, its oxidation rate at the mitochondrial site being rather limited. In man, high and/or prolonged intake of docosenoic acids, in analogy with alcohol, should be avoided in order to limit their potential toxicity.

## REFERENCES

Aaes-Jørgensen, E. (1972). Nutritional value of rapeseed oil. *In* "Rapeseed. Cultivation, Composition, Processing and Utilization" (L. A. Appelqvist and R. Ohlson, eds), pp. 301–353. Elsevier Publishing Company, Amsterdam.

Abdellatif, A. M. M. (1972). Cardiopathogenic effects of dietary rapeseed oil. *Nutr. Rev.* **30,** 2–6.

Abdellatif, A. M. M. and Vles, R. O. (1970a). Pathological effects of dietary rapeseed oil in rats. *Nutr. Metabol.* **12,** 285–295.

Abdellatif, A. M. M. and Vles, R. O. (1970b). Pathological effects of dietary rapeseed oil in ducklings. *Nutr. Metabol.* **12,** 296–305.

Abdellatif, A. M. M. and Vles, R. O. (1970c). Physiopathological effects of rapeseed oil and canbra oil in rats. *In* "Proceedings Int. Conf. Sci. Technol. Marketing Rapeseed and Rapeseed Products. Ste Adèle, Québec, Canada, September 1970", pp. 423–434. Rapeseed Association of Canada and Department of Industry, Trade and Commerce, Ottawa.

Abdellatif, A. M. M. and Vles, R. O. (1971a). The effects of various fat supplements on the nutritional and pathogenic characteristics of diets containing erucic acid in ducklings. *Nutr. Metabol.* **13,** 65–74.

Abdellatif, A. M. M. and Vles, R. O. (1971b). Long-term pathological effects of dietary rapeseed oil in rats and rabbits. *Voeding* **32,** 602–611.

Abdellatif, A. M. M. and Vles, R. O. (1973a). Short- and long-term pathological effects of glyceryl trierucate and of increasing levels of dietary rapeseed oil in rats. *Nutr. Metabol.* **15,** 219–231.

Abdellatif, A. M. M. and Vles, R. O. (1973b). Pathological effects of dietary rapeseed oils with high or low erucic acid content in ducklings. *Poultry Sci.* **52,** 1932–1936.

Abdellatif, A. M. M., Starrenburg, A. and Vles, R. O. (1972). Effects of hardened palm oil and protein on the pathological and hematological characteristics of ducklings fed rapeseed oil. *Nutr. Metabol.* **14,** 17–27.

Ackman, R. G. (1966). Analysis of the monoethylenic fatty acids of rapeseed oil by open tubular gas chromatography. *J. Am. Oil Chem Soc.* **43,** 483–486.

Alexander, J. C. and Mattson, F. H. (1966). A nutritional comparison of rapeseed oil and soybean oil. *Can. J. Biochem.* **44,** 35–43.

Anonymus (1972). Valeur nutritionnelle de l'huile de Colza. *Rev. Franç Corps Gras* **19,** 70.

Appelqvist, L.-A. (1968). Lipid patterns in Cruciferae. *Acta Univ. Lund.* **11,** 1–25.

Appelqvist, L.-A. (1972). Chemical constituents of rapeseed. *In* "Rapeseed. Cultivation, Composition, Processing and Utilization" (L.-A. Appelqvist and R. Ohlson, eds), pp. 123–173. Elsevier Publishing Company, Amsterdam.

Bach, A., Métais, P., Raulin, J. and Jacquot, R. (1969). Métabolisme de l'acide érucique. II. Vitesse d'oxydation. *Bull. Soc. Chim. Biol.* **51,** 167–175.

Beare, J. L. (1957). Rapeseed oil as a food. *Food Manuf.* **32,** 378–384.

Beare, J. L., Murray, T. K., Grice, H. C. and Campbell, J. A. (1959). A comparison of the utilization of rapeseed oil and corn oil by the rat. *Can. J. Biochem. Physiol.* **37,** 613–621.

Beare, J. L., Gregory, E. R. W., Smith, D. M. and Campbell, J. A. (1961). The effect of rapeseed oil on reproduction and on the composition of rat milk fat. *Can. J. Biochem. Physiol.* **39,** 195–201.

Beare, J. L., Murray, T. K., McLaughlan, J. M. and Campbell, J. A. (1963a). Relative effects of rapeseed oil and corn oil on rats subjected to adrenalectomy, cold, or pyridoxine deprivation. *J. Nutr.* **80,** 157–161.

Beare, J. L., Campbell, J. A., Youngs, C. G. and Craig, B. M. (1963b). Effects of saturated fat in rats fed rapeseed oil. *Can. J. Biochem. Physiol.* **41,** 605–612.

Beare-Rogers, J. L. (1970). Nutritional aspects of long-chain fatty acids. *In* "Proceedings Int. Conf. Sci. Technol. Marketing Rapeseed and Rapeseed Products. Ste Adèle, Québec, Canada, September 1970", pp. 450–465. Rapeseed Association of Canada and Department of Industry, Trade and Commerce, Ottawa.

Beare-Rogers, J. L. (1972). Nutritional effects of docosenoic acid. Abstract no. 61, *In* Abstracts of papers. The 11th World Congress of the International Society for Fat Research. Göteborg, Sweden; 18–22 June, 1972.

Beare-Rogers, J. L. and Nera, E. A. (1972). Cardiac fatty acids and histopathology of rats, pigs, monkeys and gerbils fed rapeseed oil. *Comp. Biochem. Physiol.* **41** B, 793–800.

Beare-Rogers, J. L., Nera, E. A. and Heggtveit, H. A. (1971). Cardiac lipid changes in rats fed oils containing long-chain fatty acids. *Can. Inst. Food Sci. Technol. J.* **4,** 120–124.

Beare-Rogers, J. L., Nera, E. A. and Craig, B. M. (1972a). Accumulation of cardiac fatty acids in rats fed synthesized oils containing $C_{22}$ fatty acids. *Lipids*, **7,** 46–50.

Beare-Rogers, J. L., Nera, E. A. and Craig, B. M. (1972b). Cardiac lipids in rats and gerbils fed oils containing $C_{22}$ fatty acids. *Lipids*, **7,** 548–552.

Bell, J. M. (1970) New developments concerning nutritional characteristics of rapeseed meal. *In* "Proceedings Int. Conf. Sci. Technol. Marketing Rapeseed and Rapeseed Products. Ste Adèle, Québec, Canada, September 1970", pp. 516–524. Rapeseed Association of Canada and Department of Industry, Trade and Commerce, Ottawa.

Bernhard, K., Lindlar, F. and Wagner, H. (1960). Zur Verteilung Körperfremder Fettsäuren in Tierkörper: Die Beteiligung der Erucasäure am Aufbau der Organ- und Depotfette nach längeren Gaben von Rapsöl. *Z. Ernaehrungswiss.* **1,** 48–53.

Blakely, R. M., MacGregor, H. I. and Hanel, D. (1965). Performance of turkeys on finishing diets containing different fats. *Can. J. Anim. Sci.* **45,** 59–61.

Bodak, A. (1972). M.D. Thesis. Etude au microscope électronique des lésions cellulaires myocardiques induites par une surcharge en huile de colza chez le rat. Académie de Paris.

Bodak, A. and Hatt, P. Y. (1973). Myocardial lesions induced by dietary rapeseed oil in the rats. Ultrastructural aspects. Abstracts of Papers, 6th Annual Meeting of the International Study Group for Research in Cardiac Metabolism. Sept. 25–28 1973, Freiburg i. Br. Germany. Paper No 90.

Booth, A. N., Robbins, D. J., Gumbmann, M. R., Gould, D. H., Tallent, W. H. and Wolff, T. A. (1972). Crambe and rapeseed oil chronic toxicity study in rats. *J. Am. Oil Chem. Soc.* **49,** 304A.

Boucrot, P. and Bezard, J. (1973). Incorporation et transformations métaboliques de l'acide érucique —$^{14}$C, *in vivo*, dans les lipides de plusieurs organes et tissus de rats soumis à un régime à base d'huile de colza, ou de canbra ou d'arachide. *Arch. Sci. Physiol* **27,** 1–24.

Carney, J. A., Lewis, A., Walker, B. L. and Slinger, S. J. (1972). Effect of dietary rapeseed oil on the adrenocorticotrophin-induced production of prostaglandins in the rat adrenal. *Biochim. Biophys. Acta* **280,** 211–214.

Carreau, J. P., Thoron, A., Lapous, D. and Raulin, J. (1968). Métabolisme de l'acide érucique. I. Conversion en acide oléique. *Bull. Soc. Chim. Biol.* **50,** 1973–1981.

Carroll, K. K. (1951). Effect of dietary fats and oils on adrenal cholesterol. *Endocrinology* **48,** 101–110.

Carroll, K. K. (1953). Erucic acid as the factor in rape oil affecting adrenal cholesterol in the rat. *J. Biol. Chem.* **200,** 287–292.

Carroll, K. K. (1957). Rape oil and cholesterol metabolism in different species with reference to experimental atherosclerosis. *Proc. Soc. Exp. Biol. Med.* **94,** 202–205.

Carroll, K. K. (1958). Digestibility of individual fatty acids in the rat. *J. Nutr.* **64,** 399–410.

Carroll, K. K. (1962a). Studies on the mechanisms by which erucic acid affects cholesterol metabolism. Distribution of erucic acid in adrenal and plasma lipids. *Can. J. Biochem. Physiol.* **40,** 1115–1122.

Carroll, K. K. (1962b). Levels of radioactivity in tissues and in expired carbon dioxide after administration of 1-$C^{14}$-labelled palmitic acid, 2-$C^{14}$-labelled erucic acid, or 2-$C^{14}$-labelled nervonic acid to rats, *Can. J. Biochem. Physiol.* **40,** 1229–1238.

Carroll, K. K. (1966). Metabolism of $^{14}C$-labelled oleic acid, erucic acid, and nervonic acid in rats. *Lipids* **1,** 171–175.

Carroll, K. K. and Noble, R. L. (1957). Influencc of a dietary supplement of erucic acid and other fatty acids on fertility in the rat. *Can J. Biochem. Physiol.* **35,** 1093–1105.

Cheniti, T., Bourdel, G. and Jacquot, R. (1967a). Valeur alimentaire des huiles de colza raffinées ou hydrogénées et de leurs composants principaux. Etude chez le rat mâle en croissance. *Rev. Franç. Corps Gras.* **14,** 151–166.

Cheniti, T., Bourdel, G. and Jacquot, R. (1967b). Effets de l'huile de colza sur la fonction sexuelle chez le Rat mâle. *Rev. Franç. Corps Gras* **14,** 401–402.

Chomyszyn, M. (1954). The influence of Feed on the Quality of Fat in Geese. Cited in Nutrition Abstr. Rev. **25,** 855.

Christophersen, B. O. and Bremer, J. (1972). Erucic acid—an inhibitor of fatty acid oxidation in the heart. *Biochim. Biophys Acta,* **280,** 506–514.

Chudy, J. and Batura, J. (1966). Nutrition Studies on Rapeseed Oil. I. Storage of Erucic Acid in the Depot Fat in Chickens Fed Rapeseed Oil. Cited in *Chem. Abs.* **65,** 20588 h.

Collomb, M. H., Trémolières, A. and Manchon, Ph. (1973). Etude biochimique du foie chez le rat ingérant de l'huile de colza. II. Les acides gras du foie. *Cah. Nut. Diét.* **8,** 75–76.

Conacher, H. B. S. and Page, B. D. (1972). Studies on the isomers of major monoenoic acids in rapeseed and partially hydrogenated rapeseed oil. *J. Am. Oil Chem. Soc.* **49,** 283–286.

Craig, B. M. (1971). Production and utilization of rapeseed in Canada. *J. Am. Oil Chem. Soc.* **48,** 737–739.

Craig, B. M. and Beare, J. L. (1967). The $\beta$-oxidative degradation of docosenoic acids to eicosenoic and octadecenoic acids in the rat. *Can. J. Biochem. Physiol.* **45,** 1075–1079.

Craig, B. M. and Beare, J. L. (1968). Nutritional properties of Canadian canbra oil. *Can. Inst. Food Sci. Technol. J.* **1,** 64–67.

Craig, B. M., Youngs, C. G., Beare, J. L. and Campbell, J. A. (1963). Fatty acid composition and glyceride structure in rats fed rapeseed oil or corn oil. *Can. J. Biochem. Physiol.* **41,** 43–49.

Crampton, E. N., Shaw, R. K., Mackay, V. G. and Schad, D. C. (1960). Comparative feeding value of common edible fats as measured by the growth of prematurely weaned pups, guinea-pigs and swine *J. Nutr.* **70,** 81–90.

Cresteil, T., Ketevi, P. and Lapous, D. (1972). Modulation de l'activité adenylcyclase du coeur de rat par ingestion d'huile de colza. *C.R. Acad. Sci. Paris* **275,** 1443–1445. Série D.

Dallochio, M., Larrue, J., Rabaud, M., Razaka, G., Crockett, R. and Bricaud, H.

(1973). Modifications du myocarde de Rat sous l'effet de régimes contenant différentes huiles (arachide, canbra, colza). *C.R. Soc. Biol. (Paris)* **167,** 257–262.

Demarne, Y., Sacquet, E., Flanzy, J., Garnier, H. and Francois, A.-C. (1971). Type de matière grasse et stéatorrhée. II. Effet de l'ingestion d'huile de colza. *Ann. Biol. Anim. Bioch. Biophys.* **11,** 729–731.

Deuel, H. J., Jr., Hallman, L. and Leonard, A. (1940). The comparative rate of absorption of some natural fats. *J. Nutr.* **20,** 215–226.

Deuel, H. J., Jr., Cheng, A. L. S., Morehouse, M. G. (1948). The digestibility of rapeseed oil in the rat. *J. Nutr.* **35,** 295–300.

Deuel, H. J., Jr., Johnson, R. M., Calbert, C. E., Gardner, J., Thomas, B. (1949). Studies on the comparative nutritive value of fats: XII. The digestibility of rapeseed and cottonseed oils in human subjects. *J. Nutr.* **38,** 369–379.

Dorrel, D. G. and Downey, R. K. (1964). The inheritance of erucic acid content in rapeseed (*Brassica campestris*). *Can. J. Plant. Sci.* **44,** 499–504.

Downey, R. K. (1971). Agricultural and genetic potentials of cruciferous oilseed crops. *J. Am. Oil Chem. Soc.* **48,** 718–722.

Downey, R. K. and Craig, B. M. (1964). Genetic control of fatty acid biosynthesis in rapeseed (*Brassica napus L.*). *J. Am. Oil Chem. Soc.* **41,** 475–478.

Downey, R. K., Craig, B. M. and Youngs, C. G. (1969). Breeding rapeseed for oil and meal quality, *J. Am. Oil Chem. Soc.* **46,** 121–123.

Dutton, H. J. and Mounts, T. L. (1966). Desaturation of fatty acids in seeds of higher plants. *J. Lipid Res.* **7,** 221–225.

Gompertz, S. M. and Sammons, H. G. (1961). Relation between the composition of the fatty acids in the diet and in the faeces. *Biochem. J.* **80,** 30 p.

Gumpen, S. A. and Norum, K. R. (1973). The relative amounts of long-chain acylcarnitines, short-chain acylcarnitines and carnitine in heart, liver and brown adipose tissue from rats fed on rapeseed oil. *Biochim. Biophys. Acta* **316,** 48–55.

Haeffner, E. W. (1970). Isolation and structural determination of the $C_{20}$ and $C_{22}$ unsaturated fatty acids of rapeseed oil. *Lipids* **5,** 430–433.

Hopkins, C. Y., Murray, T. K. and Campbell, J. A. (1955). Optimum ratio of saturated to monounsaturated fatty acids in rat diets. *Can. J. Biochem. Physiol.* **33,** 1047–1054.

Hopkins, C. Y., Chisholm, M. J., Murray, T. K. and Campbell, J. A. (1957). Assimilation of dietary eicosenoic and erucic acid esters. *J. Am. Oil Chem. Soc.* **34,**505–508.

Hornstra, G. (1972). Digestibility, efficiency and other metabolic effects of dietary rapeseed oil in rats. *Nutr. Metabol.* **14,** 282–297.

Houtsmuller, U. M. T. (1974). Biological effects of erucic acid. Lecture Meeting Soc. Chem. Ind. London, 23 January 1974.

Houtsmuller, U. M. T., Struijk, C. B. and van der Beek, A. (1970). Decrease in rate of ATP synthesis of isolated rat heart mitochondria induced by dietary erucic acid. *Biochim. Biophys. Acta* **218,** 564–566.

Houtsmuller, U. M. T., Struijk, C. B. and van der Beek, A. (1972). Biochemical effects of dietary very long chain fatty acids on rat heart and liver *J. Am. Oil Chem. Soc.* **49,** 304 A.

Jacquot, R., Raulin, J. and Thoron, A. (1967). Effets physiopathologiques des constituants inhabituels des graisses. Problème relatif à l'huile de colza. *Rev. Franç. Corps Gras* **14,** 441–443.

Jacquot, R., Rocquelin, G. and Potteau, B. (1969). L'huile de colza et son usage alimentaire. *Cah. Nutr. Diet.* **4,** 51–78. suppl. fasc. 2.

Jaillard, J., Sezille, G., Dewailly, P., Fruchart, J. C. and Bertrand, M. (1973).Etude expérimentale chez l'homme et chez l'animal du métabolisme de l'acide érucique:

extraction myocardique chez l'homme, après surcharge en huile de colza et lipides tissulaires chez le rat, après surcharge en triérucine. *Nutr. Metabol.* **15,** 336–347.

Ketevi, P., Lapous, D. and Loriette, C. (1973). Huile de colza marquée et radioactivité des éléments subcellulaires du myocarde. *J. Physiol. Paris* **67,** 200A–201A.

Kramer, J. K. G., Mahadevan, S., Hunt, J. R., Sauer, F. D., Corner, A. H. and Charlton, K. M. (1973). Growth rate, lipid composition, metabolism and myocardial lesions of rats fed rapeseed oils (*Brassica campestris* var. Arlo, Echo and Span, and *B. napus* var. Oro). *J. Nutr.* **103,** 1696–1708.

Kritchevsky, D., Kim, H. K. and Tepper, S. A. (1972). Cholesterol vehicle in experimental atherosclerosis part 12. Rapeseed oil. *Atherosclerosis* **15,** 101–105.

Krzymanski, J. (1970). Inheritance of thioglucoside content by rapeseed (Brassica napus) *In* "Journées Internationals sur le Colza, Paris 26–30 mai 1970—Exposés et Discussions", pp. 212–225. C.E.T.I.O.M., Paris.

Lall, S. P. and Slinger, S. J. (1973a). The metabolizable energy content of rapeseed oils and rapeseed oil foots and the effect of blending with other fats. *Poultry Sci.* **52,** 143–151.

Lall, S. P. and Slinger, S. J. (1973b). Nutritional evaluation of rapeseed oils and rapeseed soapstocks for laying hens. *Poultry Sci.* **52,** 1729–1740.

Lall, S. P., Pass, D. and Slinger, S. J. (1972). Effect of high and low erucic acid rapeseed oil on biochemical and histopathological changes in heart muscle of chickens. *Poultry Sci.* **51,** 1828.

Lapous, D., Carreau, J.-P. and Raulin, J. (1970). Métabolisme de l'acide érucique. Sort de l'acide érucique 14–$^{14}$C dans différents organes et fractions subcellulaires du rat. *Arch. Sci. Physiol.* **24,** 125–131.

Leclercq, B. (1971). Les corps gras dans les aliments composés pour la volaille. *Rev. Franç. Corps Gras* **18,** 753–768.

Leclercq, B. (1972). Influence de l'acide érucique alimentaire chez la poule pondeuse. Diminution du poids de l'oeuf. *Ann. Biol. Anim. Bioch. Biophys.* **12,** 505–508.

Lemarchal, Ph., Clouet, P. and Blond, J.-P. (1972). $\beta$-oxydations comparées des acides érucique et oléique par les mitochondries de coeur de Rat in vitro. *C.R. Acad. Sci. Paris* **274,** 1961–1963. Série D.

Lesieur, B. (1971). Production and use of rapeseed in Europe. *J. Am. Oil Chem. Soc.* **48,** 869–871.

Levillain, R., Vodovar, N., Flanzy, J. and Cluzan, R. (1972). Altérations cardiaques observées chez des porcs ayant absorbé de l'huile de Colza ou de l'huile de Canbra. *C.R. Soc. Biol.* (*Paris*) **166,** 1633–1635.

Lodhi, G. N., Renner, R. and Clandinin, D. R. (1970). Factors affecting the metabolizable energy content of rapeseed meal. *In* "Journées Internationales sur le Colza, Paris 26–30 mai 1970. Exposés et Discussions", pp. 440–445. C.E.T.I.O.M., Paris.

Lööf, B and Appelqvist, L.-A. (1972). Plant breeding for improved yield and quality. *In* "Rapeseed. Cultivation, Composition, Processing and Utilization" (L.-A. Appelqvist and R. Ohlson, eds), pp. 101–122. Elsevier Publishing Company, Amsterdam.

Martin, B. (1972). Ph.D. Thesis. Influence des Huiles de Colza et de Canbra et de mélanges de triglycerides homogènes reproduisant certaines caractéristiques de ces huiles sur les lipides hépatiques du rat. Université de Dijon. E.U.E.R. de Nutrition.

Martinelli, M., Merlin, L. and Cohen, Y. (1973). Distribution de l'acide érucique $^{14}$C chez la Souris normale ou gestante. *C.R. Acad. Sci. Paris* **276,** 853–856. Série D.

Mattson, E. H. and Volpenhein, R. A. (1961). The specific distribution of fatty acids in the glycerides of vegetable fats. *J. Biol. Chem.* **236,** 1891–1894.

McDonald, B. E. (1972). Digestion and metabolism of rapeseed oil by the human and other species. *J. Am. Oil Chem Soc.* **49,** 304A.

Molnar, S., Ter Meulen, U. and Rosenow, H. (1972). Untersuchungen über die Beeinflussung der Fettsäuremuster der Organlipide des wachsenden Schweines nach 5 wöchiger Zufütterung von Kokos-Palmkern, Sojaöl und Rapsöl. *Z. Tierphysiol. Tier. Futt.* **29,** 196–204.

Nera, E. A., Beare-Rogers, J. L. and Heggtveit, H. A. (1971). Cardio-toxicity of rapeseed oil. *Am. J. Path.* **62,** 34a.

Niemi, U. M. and Roine, P. (1960). The effect of rapeseed oil on the thyroid function of rats. *Z. Ernaehrungswiss.* **1,** 164–170.

Nieschlag, H. J. and Wolff, I. A. (1971). Industrial uses of high erucic oils. *J. Am. Oil Chem. Soc.* **48,** 723–727.

Njaa, L. R., Braekkan, O. R., Lambertsen, G. and Utne, F. (1971). Hydrogenated marine fat, effect on growth and liver weight in young rats given a high fat, low protein ration. *Nutr. Metabol.* **13,** 207–221.

Opie, L. H. (1968). Metabolism of the heart in health and disease. Part I. *Am. Heart J.* **76,** 685–698.

Pipy, B., Gaillard, D. and Derache, R. (1972). Influence de régimes contenant des huiles de colza et de canbra sur le système réticuloendothelial du Rat. *J. Physiol. Paris* **64,** 439–456.

Pinson, A. and Padieu, P. (1973). Erucic acid metabolism by cultured beating heart cell of the postnatal rat. Abstracts of Papers, 6th Annual Meeting of the International Study Group for Research in Cardiac Metabolism. Sept. 25–28 1973, Freiburg i. Br. Germany. Paper No 91.

Quadt, J. F. A., van de Graaf, H. M. and Ten Hoor, F. (1974). Short- and long-term effects of dietary erucic acid on the isometric contractile force of the isolated papillary muscle of the rat. Lecture, 15de Federatieve Vergadering Medisch-Biologische Verenigingen, Nijmegen 17–20 April 1974.

Quan, P.-C. and Le Breton, E. (1972a). Composition des acides gras totaux (AGT) et des acides gras neutres (AGN) du myocarde du Rat ayant ingéré, dès le sevrage, un temps court, diverses huiles alimentaires. Effets du jeûne et des lipotropes. *C.R. Acad. Sci. Paris* **275,** 1183–1186. Série D.

Quan, P.-C. and Le Breton, E. (1972b). Répartition et composition en AG des classes de phospholipides (PL), dans le myocarde du Rat ayant ingéré, durant 3 jours, un régime contenant de l'huile d'arachide, de canbra ou de colza. Influence du jeûne et des lipotropes. *C.R. Acad. Sci. Paris* **275,** 1271–1274. Série D.

Quan, P.-C and Le Breton, E. (1973a). Etude des acides gras totaux et des acides gras non phosphorés du foie de rats soumis, après le sevrage, durant 3 jours, à des régimes contenant diverses huiles alimentaires. Effets du jeûne et des lipotropes. Comparaison entre le myocarde et le foi. *C.R. Acad. Sci. Paris* **276,** 61–64. Série D.

Quan, P.-C. and Le Breton, E. (1973b). Etude de la composition en AG des trois classes principales de PL du foie, chez le Rat ayant ingéré, après le sevrage, durant 3 ou 45 jours, des régimes contenant diverses huiles. Effets du jeûne et des lipotropes. Comparaison avec les phospholipides cardiaques. *C.R. Acad. Sci. Paris* **276,** 1585–1588. Série D.

Rocquelin, G. (1972). L'huile de colza et l'huile de canbra: effets à très court terme sur les lipides cardiaques et hépatiques du rat sevré. *C.R. Acad. Sci. Paris* **274,** 592–595. Série D.

Rocquelin, G. (1973). Effets à très court terme de l'huile de colza sur les lipides cardiaques et hépatiques du rat sevré: influence du raffinage et de l'interesterification. *Ann. Biol. Anim. Bioch. Biophys.* **13,** 151–154.

Rocquelin, G. and Cluzan, R. (1968). L'huile de colza riche en acide érucique et l'huile de colza sans acide érucique: valeur nutritionnelle et effets physiologiques chez le rat. I. Effets sur la croissance, l'éfficacité alimentaire et l'état de différents organes. *Ann. Biol. Anim. Bioch. Biophys.* **8,** 395–406.

Rocquelin, G. and Cluzan, R. (1970). Compared nutritional and physiopathological effects of rapeseed oil (having a high content of erucic acid) and "zero erucic acid" rapeseed oil in the rat. *In* "Proceedings of the International Symposium for the Chemistry and Technology of Rapeseed Oil and Other Cruciferae Oils. Gdansk, September 19th-23rd, 1967, Warszawa 1970", pp. 405–411.

Rocquelin, G. and Cluzan, R. (1971). L'huile de colza: ses effets particuliers au niveau du myocarde. *Cah. Nutr. Diét.* **6,** 85–95.

Rocquelin, G. and Leclerc, J. (1969). L'huile de colza riche en acide érucique et l'huile de colza sans acide érucique. II. Utilisation digestive comparée chez le rat. *Ann. Biol. Anim. Bioch. Biophys.* **9,** 413–426.

Rocquelin, G. and Potteau, B. (1968). La valeur nutritionnelle et les effets physiopathologiques de l'huile de colza. Influence de sa teneur en acide érucique. *Ann. Nutr. Aliment.* **22,** 191–244.

Rocquelin, G., Martin, B. and Cluzan, R. (1970). Comparative physiological effects of rapeseed and canbra oils in the rat: influence of the ratio of saturated to monounsaturated fatty acids. *In* "Proceedings Int. Conf. Sci. Technol. Marketing Rapeseed and Rapeseed Products. Ste Adèle, Québec, Canada, September 1970", pp. 405–422. Rapeseed Association of Canada and Department of Industry, Trade and Commerce, Ottawa.

Rocquelin, G., Sergiel, J. P., Martin, B., Leclerc, J. and Cluzan, R. (1971). The nutritive value of refined rapeseed oils: a review. *J. Am. Oil Chem. Soc.* **48,** 728–732.

Rocquelin, G., Cluzan, R., Vodovar, N. and Levillain, R. (1973a). Recherches récentes sur les effets physiopathologiques des huiles de colza et de canbra au niveau du myocarde et d'autres organes. *Cah. Nut. Diét.* **8,** 103–116.

Rocquelin, G., Cluzan, R., Levillain, R., Vodovar, N. and Causeret, J. (1973b). Aspects biochimiques et anatomo-pathologiques du myocarde chez différentes espèces animales ingérant de l'huile de colza. *Arch. Mal. Coeur* **66,** 1085–1100.

Rocquelin, G., Sergiel, J. P., Astorg, P. O. and Cluzan, R. (1973c). Effets des huiles de colza et de canbra sur les lipides et l'anatomie du myocarde du rat: étude à court terme (de 0 à 60 jours). *Ann. Biol. Anim. Bioch. Biophys.* **13,** 587–609.

Rocquelin, G., Astorg, P. O., Peleran, J. C. and Juaneda, P. (1974). Influence des huiles de colza et de canbra sur les lipides plasmatiques du rat. *Nutr. Metabol.* **16,** 305–316.

Roine, P., Uksila, E., Teir, H. and Rapola, J. (1960). Histopathological changes in rats and pigs fed rapeseed oil. *Z. Ernaehrungswiss.* **1,** 118–124.

Rollier, M. (1973). La sélection du colza. *Oléagineux* **28,** 405–408 and 461–466.

Rutkowski, A. (1970). Effect of processing on the chemical composition of rapeseed meal. *In* "Proceedings Int. Conf. Sci. Technol. Marketing Rapeseed and Rapeseed Products. Ste Adèle, Québec, Canada, September 1970", pp. 496–515. Rapeseed Association of Canada and Department of Industry, Trade and Commerce, Ottawa.

Rutkowski, A. (1971). The feed value of rapeseed meal. *J. Am. Oil Chem. Soc.* **48,** 863–868.

Salmon, R. E. (1969a). Soybean versus rapeseed oil in turkey starter diets. *Poultry Sci.* **48,** 87–93.

Salmon, R. E. (1969b). The relative value of rapeseed and soybean oils in chick starter diets. *Poultry Sci.* **48,** 1045–1050.

Salmon, R. E. (1970). Rapeseed oil in poultry diets. *In* "Proceedings Int. Conf. Sci. Technol. Marketing Rapeseed and Rapeseed Products. Ste Adèle, Québec, Canada, September 1970", pp. 369–376. Rapeseed Association of Canada and Department of Industry, Trade and Commerce, Ottawa.

Salmon, R. E. and O'Neil, J. B. (1971). The effect of the level and source of dietary fat on the growth, feed efficiency, grade and carcass composition of turkeys. *Poultry Sci.* **50,** 1456–1467.

Savary, P. and Constantin, M. J. (1966). Sur la résorption intestinale des chaînes eruciques et leur incorporation dans les chylomicrons lymphatiques du rat. *Biochim. Biophys. Acta,* **125,** 118–128.

Sell, J. L. and Hodgson, G. C. (1962). Comparative value of dietary rapeseed oil, sunflowerseed oil, soybean oil and animal tallow for chickens. *J. Nutr.* **76,** 113–118.

Sergiel, J. P. (1973). Structure glycéridique de l'huile de canbra. *Rev. Franç. Corps Gras* **20,** 137–141.

Sheppard, A. J., Fritz, J. C., Hooper, W. H., Roberts, T., Hubbard, W. D., Prossei, A. R., and Boehne, J. W. (1971). Crambe and rapeseed oils as energy sources for rats and chicks and some ancillary data on organ weights and body cavity fat composition. *Poultry Sci.* **50,** 79–84.

Slinger, S. J., Coates, B. J., Carney, J. A. and Walker, B. J. (1973). Effect of dietary rapeseed oil on cardiac glycogen in the growing rat. *Nutr. Rep. Int.* **8,** 245–250.

Staron, T. (1972). *In* "Table ronde sur le rôle de la recherche". *Cah. Nutr. Diét.* **7,** 235.

Stokes, G. B. and Walker, D. M. (1970). The nutritive value of fat in the diet of the milk-fed lamb: 2. The effect of different dietary fats on the composition of the body fats. *Brit. J. Nutr.* **24,** 435–440.

Struijk, C. B. (1972). The effect of dietary erucic acid on rat heart and liver. Abstracts of Papers, 15th International Conference on the Biochemistry of Lipids. ICBL The Hague (Netherlands) Aug. 28–Sept. 1, 1972, A 31.

Struijk, C. B., Houtsmuller, U. M. T., Jansen, H. and Hülsmann, W. C. (1973). Increase in post-heparin lipoprotein-lipase activity in rat plasma by dietary erucic acid. *Biochim. Biophys. Acta* **296,** 253–256.

Swarttouw, M. A. (1974). The oxidation of erucic acid by rat heart mitochondria. *Biochim. Biophys. Acta* **337,** 13–21.

Tallent, W. H. (1972). Improving high-erucic oilseeds: chemically or genetically. *J. Am. Oil Chem. Soc.* **49,** 15–19.

Teige, B. and Beare-Rogers, J. L. (1973). Cardiac fatty acids in rats fed marine oils. *Lipids* **8,** 584–587.

Ten Hoor, F., van de Graaf, H. M. and Vergroesen, A. J. (1973). Effects of dietary erucic and linoleic acid on myocardial function in rats. *In* "Myocardial Metabolism, Recent Advances in Studies on Cardiac Structure and Metabolism" (N. S. Dhalla, ed.), pp. 59–72. University Park Press Baltimore, London, Tokyo.

Thomasson, H. J. (1955a). The biological value of oils and fats: I. Growth and food intake on feeding with natural oils and fats. *J. Nutr.* **56,** 455–468.

Thomasson, H. J. (1955b). The biological value of oils and fats: III. The longevity of rats fed rapeseed oil or butterfat-containing diets. *J. Nutr.* **57,** 17–27.

Thomasson, H. J. (1956). The biological value of oils and fats: IV. The rate of intestinal absorption. *J. Nutr.* **59,** 343–352.

Thomasson, H. J. and Boldingh, J. (1955). The biological value of oils and fats: II. The growth-retarding substance in rapeseed oil. *J. Nutr.* **56,** 469–475.

Thomasson, H. J., Gottenbos, J. J., van Pijpen, P. L. and Vles, R. O. (1970). Nutritive value of rapeseed oil. *In* "Proceedings of the International Symposium for the Chemistry and Technology of Rapeseed Oil and Other Cruciferae Oils. Gdansk, September 19th–23rd, 1967, Warszawa 1970", pp. 381–402.

Thoron, A. (1969). Interpretation du caractère nutritionnel particulier de l'huile de colza. Essais sur le porc et le rat. *Ann. Nutr. Aliment.* **23,** 103–116.

Trémolières, J., Lowy R., Griffaton, G. and Carré, L. (1971). Effets métaboliques de deux huiles alimentaires chez l'homme. Part des glucides et des lipides dans la dépense d'énergie. *Cah. Nutr. Diét.* **6,** 70–74.

Trémolières, A., Collomb, M. H. and Trémolières, J. (1972). Effets métaboliques de l'huile de colza chez l'homme II. Evolution des concentrations d'acides gras sanguins. *Cah. Nutr. Diét.* **7,** 67–71.

Trémolières, J. and Carré, L. (1972). Effets de l'huile de colza riche en acide érucique sur les échanges respiratoires de l'homme. *Cah. Nutr. Diét.* **7,** 156–157.

Uzzan, A. and Arondel, M. T. (1965). Influence de la variété, due lieu et des conditions culturales de certaines graines oléagineuses sur la composition en acides gras de leur huile. *Rev. Franç. Corps Gras* **12,** 323–332.

Vaisey, M., Latta, M., Bruce, V. M. and McDonald, B. E. (1973). Assessment of the intake and digestibility of high and low erucic acid rapeseed oils in a mixed Canadian diet. *Can. Inst. Food Sci. Technol. J.* **6,** 142–147.

VanEtten, C. H., Daxenbichler, M. E. and Wolff, I. A. (1969). Natural glucosinolates (thioglucosides) in foods and feeds. *J. Ag. Food. Chem.* **17,** 483–491.

Veen, W. A. G. (1972). Animal and vegetable fats in milk replacers for veal calves: 5. Fatty acid patterns in various adipose tissues. *Z. Tierphysiol. Tier. Futt.* **30,** 1–19.

Vles, R. O. (1969). Pathology of ducklings and guinea-pigs fed rapeseed oil. Abstracts of Papers, V-13. 8th International Congress of Nutrition, Prague, 1969.

Vles, R. O. and Abdellatif, A. M. M. (1970a). Long-term effects of rapeseed oil in rats and rabbits. *J. Am. Oil Chem. Soc.* **47,** 338A.

Vles, R. O. and Abdellatif, A. M. M. (1970b). Effects of hardened palm oil on rapeseed oil-induced changes in ducklings and guinea-pigs. *In* "Proceedings Int. Conf. Sci. Technol. Marketing Rapeseed and Rapeseed Products. Ste Adèle, Québec, Canada, September 1970", pp. 435–449. Rapeseed Association of Canada and Department of Industry, Trade and Commerce, Ottawa.

Vodovar, N., Desnoyers, F. and Flanzy, J. (1972a). Absorption intestinale de l'huile de colza. Aspect ultrastructural. *C.R. Acad. Sci. Paris* **274,** 1743–1745. Série. D.

Vodovar, N., Desnoyers, F., Cluzan, R., Marson, A.-M. and Levillain, R. (1972b). Accumulation de lipides dans le myocarde des rats ayant reçu de l'huile de colza dans leur régime. Aspect ultrastructural. *C.R. Acad. Sci. Paris* **274,** 3109–3112. Série D.

Vodovar, N., Desnoyers, F., Levillain, R. and Cluzan, R. (1973). Accumulation lipidique et altérations cellulaires du myocarde des porcs ayant reçu de l'huile de colza dans leur régime. Etude ultrastructurale. *C.R. Acad. Sci. Paris* **276,** 1597–1600. Série D.

Vogtmann, H., Clandinin, D. R. and Hardin, R. T. (1973a). Utilization of rapeseed oils of high and low erucic acid contents: 1. Digestibility and energy utilization. *Nutr. Metabol.* **15,** 252–266.

Vogtmann, H., Clandinin, D. R. and Robblee, A. R. (1973b). Low and high erucic acid rapeseed oils in rations for laying hens. *Poultry Sci.* **52,** 955–962.

Vogtmann, H., Clandinin, D. R. and Hardin, R. T. (1974). Utilization of rapeseed oils of high and low erucic acid contents: 2. Influence on tissues. *Nutr. Metabol.* **17,** 136–147.

Wagner, H., Seelig, E. und Bernhard, K. (1958). Verteilung und Halbwertzeit der Erucasäure nach Rapsölgaben an Ratten. *Z. Physiol. Chem.* **312,** 104–110.

Walker, B. L. (1972a). Deposition of erucic acid in rat tissue lipids. *Nutr. Metabol.* **14,** 8–16.

Walker, B. L. (1972b). Deposition of erucic acid in swine tissue lipids. *Can. J. Anim. Sci.* **52,** 713–719.

Walker, B. L. and Carney, J. A. (1971). Response of rat adrenal cholesteryl esters to cold stress. *Lipids* **6,** 797–804.

Walker, B. L., Lall, S. P., Slinger, S. J. and Bayley, H. S. (1970). Nutritional aspects of rapeseed oil: digestibility, processing and influence of erucic acid on tissue lipids. *In* "Proceedings Int. Conf. Sci. Technol. Marketing Rapeseed and Rapeseed Products. Ste Adèle, Québec, Canada, September 1970", pp. 377–404. Rapeseed Association of Canada and Department of Industry, Trade and Commerce, Ottawa.

Walker, D. M. and Stokes, G. B. (1970). The nutritive value of fat in the diet of the milk fed lamb: 1. The apparent and corrected digestibilities of different dietary fats and of their constituent fatty acids. *Brit. J. Nutr.* **24,** 425–433.

Weinberg, B. (1972). Processing of low-erucic acid rapeseed and of canbra oil. *Can. Inst. Food Sci. Technol. J.* **5,** A57–A60.

Ziemlanski, S., Cieslakowa, D. and Palaszewska, M. (1972a). Effect of certain fats on protein digestion and absorption of amino acids in the digestive tract. *Polish Med. J.* **11,** 881–889.

Ziemlanski, S., Opuszynska, T., Bulhak-Jachymczyk, B., Okolska, G., Bartlet, H., Olszewska, I., and Budzynska-Topolowska, J. (1972b). Biological evaluation of the nutritive value of edible fats: I. Effect of selected fats on the consumption, fat digestibility coefficients, gain of body weight and some enzymatic tests in the serum and liver of experimental animals. *Polish Med. J.* **11,** 1602–1611.

Ziemlanski, S., Bulhak-Jachymczyk, B., Kucharczyk, B., Rusiecka M., Opuszynska, T., Budzynska-Topolowska, J., Piekarzewska, A., Jakubowski, A., Krasnodebski, P. (1972c). Biological evaluation of the nutritive value of edible fats: II. Effect of certain fats on serum lipid fractions, composition of fatty acids and the level of trans isomers in lipids of some organs. *Polish Med. J.* **11,** 1612–1624.

Ziemlanski, S., Opuszynska, T., and Krus, S. (1972). Biological evaluation of the nutritive value of edible fats. III. Effects of selected fats on the morphology of certain organs. *Polish Med. J.* **11,** 1625–1633.

Ziemlanski, S., Rosnowski, A. and Opuszynska-Freyer, T. (1973). Ultrastructure of early fatty infiltration in the myocardium after administration of rapeseed oil in the diet. *Acta Med. Pol.* **14,** 279–290.

# Subject Index

F

## I

## N